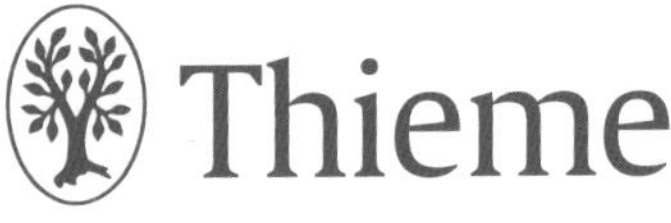

Comprehensive Board Review in Orthopaedic Surgery

Robin N. Kamal, MD
Assistant Professor
Chase Hand and Upper Limb Center
Department of Orthopaedic Surgery
Stanford University
Palo Alto, California

Arnold-Peter Weiss, MD
R. Scot Sellers Scholar of Hand Surgery
Vice Chairman and Professor of Orthopaedics
Warren Alpert Medical School of Brown University
Rhode Island Hospital
Providence, Rhode Island

With 433 Figures

Thieme
New York • Stuttgart • Delhi • Rio de Janeiro

Executive Editor: William Lamsback
Managing Editor: Elizabeth Palumbo
Editorial Assistant: Haley Paskalides
Director, Editorial Services: Mary Jo Casey
Production Editor: Barbara Chernow
International Production Director: Andreas Schabert
Vice President, Editorial and E-Product Development: Vera Spillner
International Marketing Director: Fiona Henderson
International Sales Director: Louisa Turrell
Director of Sales, North America: Mike Roseman
Senior Vice President and Chief Operating Officer: Sarah Vanderbilt
President: Brian D. Scanlan
Illustrations: Markus Voll and Karl Wesker
Compositor: Carol Pierson, Chernow Editorial Services, Inc.

Library of Congress Cataloging-in-Publication Data

Names: Kamal, Robin N., editor. | Weiss, Arnold-Peter C., editor.
Title: Comprehensive board review in orthopaedic surgery / [edited by] Robin N. Kamal, Arnold-Peter Weiss.
Description: New York : Thieme, [2016] | Includes index.
Identifiers: LCCN 2016000132| ISBN 9781604069044 (alk. paper) | ISBN 9781604069051 (e-book)
Subjects: | MESH: Orthopedic Procedures | Outlines
Classification: LCC RD731 | NLM WE 18.2 | DDC 617.5–dc23
LC record available at http://lccn.loc.gov/2016000132

Important note: Medicine is an ever-changing science undergoing continual development. Research and clinical experience are continually expanding our knowledge, in particular our knowledge of proper treatment and drug therapy. Insofar as this book mentions any dosage or application, readers may rest assured that the authors, editors, and publishers have made every effort to ensure that such references are in accordance with **the state of knowledge at the time of production of the book.**

Nevertheless, this does not involve, imply, or express any guarantee or responsibility on the part of the publishers in respect to any dosage instructions and forms of applications stated in the book. **Every user is requested to examine carefully** the manufacturers' leaflets accompanying each drug and to check, if necessary in consultation with a physician or specialist, whether the dosage schedules mentioned therein or the contraindications stated by the manufacturers differ from the statements made in the present book. Such examination is particularly important with drugs that are either rarely used or have been newly released on the market. Every dosage schedule or every form of application used is entirely at the user's own risk and responsibility. The authors and publishers request every user to report to the publishers any discrepancies or inaccuracies noticed. If errors in this work are found after publication, errata will be posted at www.thieme.com on the product description page.

Some of the product names, patents, and registered designs referred to in this book are in fact registered trademarks or proprietary names even though specific reference to this fact is not always made in the text. Therefore, the appearance of a name without designation as proprietary is not to be construed as a representation by the publisher that it is in the public domain.

Thieme Publishers New York
333 Seventh Avenue, New York, NY 10001 USA
+1 800 782 3488, customerservice@thieme.com

Thieme Publishers Stuttgart
Rüdigerstrasse 14, 70469 Stuttgart, Germany
+49 [0]711 8931 421, customerservice@thieme.de

Thieme Publishers Delhi
A-12, Second Floor, Sector-2, Noida-201301
Uttar Pradesh, India
+91 120 45 566 00, customerservice@thieme.in

Thieme Publishers Rio de Janeiro, Thieme Publicações Ltda.
Edifício Rodolpho de Paoli, 25º andar
Av. Nilo Peçanha, 50 – Sala 2508
Rio de Janeiro 20020-906 Brasil
+55 21 3172 2297

Printed in China by Asia Pacific Offset 5 4 3 2 1

ISBN 978-1-60406-904-4

Also available as an e-book:
eISBN 978-1-60406-905-1

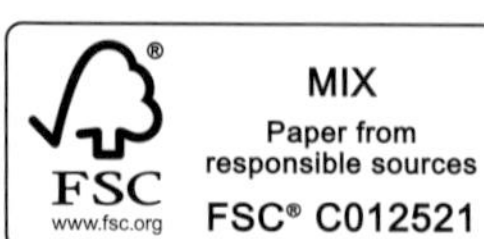

Contents

Preface

Preparing for the Orthopaedics In-Training Exam (OITE) and passing Part 1 of the American Board of Orthopaedic Surgery (ABOS) continues to be challenging, with the boards having a failure rate upward of 20%. Likewise, orthopaedic surgery continues to be one of the most competitive specialties for a medical student to enter. Although the scope of orthopaedic surgery continues to expand on a daily basis, the fundamental information required to pass orthopaedic electives or orthopaedic exams such as the OITE or ABOS Maintenance of Certification remains largely unchanged. We created this book for the medical student, orthopaedic resident, or practicing surgeon to serve as a comprehensive yet succinctly written review of the fundamentals of orthopaedic surgery. The content of the book is based on information that has previously appeared on orthopaedic exams, has been asked in the operating room, or is thought to be highly testable information. We have weighted the content of the book to emphasize those subjects that are frequently tested or asked in the operating room. Half of the material and concepts found in the book were seen on a previous orthopaedic exam, and half is composed of information that is fundamental to the field of orthopaedic surgery.

Chapters are separated by subspecialty, and information is supplied in an easy-to-read bullet format that allows you to organize, synthesize, and memorize the information with ease. Shading is used to highlight test-taking and clinical pearls, and figures are specifically used to help you understand and memorize difficult concepts. Pertinent anatomy has uniquely been illustrated and described in each subspecialty chapter to enable you to better memorize the structure and function of the normal and pathological musculoskeletal system. There is enough background information so that the book can be used by the medical student preparing for an orthopaedic elective, while also including the high-yield details needed to answer specific exam questions for the orthopaedic resident or surgeon preparing to take the OITE, Part 1 of the ABOS, or the Maintenance of Certification exams.

We wish to thank the contributors. All of them have been very close to the experience of knowledge preparation and are very familiar with classic content pearls and essentials.

Robin N. Kamal, MD
Arnold-Peter Weiss, MD

Acknowledgments

This review book demonstrates the dedication and commitment of the Brown University Department of Orthopaedics toward education. It would not have been possible without the support of my mentor and friend, Peter Weiss. Thank you to my parents and my siblings Arif, Afrin, Jennifer, Sana, Nimah, and Daanish for your encouragement and guidance. Lastly, to my wife Fahmeedah, I am forever grateful for your steadfast and unconditional support, day in and day out.

Robin N. Kamal, MD

Writing or editing a book is filled with hard work. Fortunately, for me, Rob Kamal was my partner in this project. He really did the heavy lifting and gave the vast majority of the timeless hours required to provide a useful and efficient book. While he is younger than I am by a couple of decades, his ability to synthesize and execute are mature. Thanks, Rob.

The editorial team at Thieme worked tirelessly to get to the vision needed for an effective product. It is not always an easy task. Without them, the result would not have been the same.

Lastly, to my wife and five children. They have suffered through countless publication projects for no easy to grasp reward. They just know it makes me happy to teach. I am grateful.

Arnold-Peter Weiss, MD

Contributors

Jason T. Bariteau, MD
Assistant Professor
Department of Orthopedics
Emory University School of Medicine
Atlanta, Georgia

Todd Borenstein, MD
Department of Orthopaedics
Warren Alpert Medical School of Brown University
Providence, Rhode Island

Melissa A. Christino, MD
Children's Orthopedics of Atlanta
Atlanta, Georgia

Eric Cohen, MD
Department of Orthopaedics
Warren Alpert Medical School of Brown University
Providence, Rhode Island

Alan H. Daniels, MD
Assistant Professor
Department of Orthopaedics
Warren Alpert Medical School of Brown University
Providence, Rhode Island

Matthew E. Deren, MD
Department of Orthopaedics
Warren Alpert Medical School of Brown University
Providence, Rhode Island

Christopher W. DiGiovanni, MD
Visiting Professor of Orthopaedics
Harvard Medical School
Massachusetts General Hospital
Boston, Massachusetts

Craig Eberson, MD
Associate Professor and Division Chief
Pediatric Orthopedics and Scoliosis
Hasbro Children's Hospital
Program Director, Orthopedic Residency
Warren Alpert Medical School of Brown University
Providence, Rhode Island

Paul Fadale, MD
Professor and Chief of Sports Medicine
Department of Orthopaedic Surgery
Warren Alpert Medical School of Brown University
Rhode Island Hospital
Providence, Rhode Island

Amanda Fantry, MD
Department of Orthopaedics
Warren Alpert Medical School of Brown University
Providence, Rhode Island

John Froehlich, MD, MBA
Associate Clinical Professor
Director
Joint Replacement Center
Miriam Hospital
Warren Alpert Medical School of Brown University
Providence, Rhode Island

Stacey Elisa Gallacher, MD
St. Luke's University Health Network
East Stroudsburg, Pennsylvania

Andrew Green, MD
Associate Professor
Chief
Division of Shoulder and Elbow Surgery
Warren Alpert Medical School of Brown University
Providence, Rhode Island

Roman Hayda, MD
Co-Director, Division of Orthopedic Trauma
Associate Professor
Warren Alpert Medical School of Brown University
Providence, Rhode Island

Raymond Hsu, MD
Department of Orthopaedics
Warren Alpert Medical School of Brown University
Providence, Rhode Island

Robin N. Kamal, MD
Assistant Professor
Chase Hand and Upper Limb Center
Department of Orthopaedic Surgery
Stanford University
Palo Alto, California

Stephen Klinge, MD
Orthopedic Surgery
Farmington, Connecticut

Craig R. Lareau, MD
New England Orthopedic Surgeons
Springfield, Massachusetts

Byung J. Lee, MD
Irving Orthopedics and Sports Medicine
Irving, Texas

Peter Kaveh Mansuripur, MD
Department of Orthopaedics
Warren Alpert Medical School of Brown University
Providence, Rhode Island

Philip McClure, MD
Texas Scottish Rite Hospital for Children
Department of Orthopedic Surgery
Dallas, Texas

Matthew McDonnell, MD
Clinical Assistant Professor
Department of Orthopaedic Surgery
Rutgers University-Robert Wood Johnson Medical School
Somerset, New Jersey

Matthew Miller, MD
Clinical Assistant Professor
Orthopaedic Surgery
Stanford School of Medicine
Los Gatos, California

Mark A. Palumbo, MD
Associate Professor
Department of Orthopaedic Surgery
Chief, Division of Spine Surgery
Warren Alpert Medical School of Brown University
Providence, Rhode Island

Michael J. Rainbow, PhD
Assistant Professor
Mechanical & Materials Engineering
Queen's University
Kingston, Ontario
Canada

Scott Ritterman, MD
Department of Orthopaedics
Warren Alpert Medical School of Brown University
Providence, Rhode Island

Gregory A. Sawyer, MD
Orthopedic Surgery
Falmouth, Maine

Alan Schiller, MD
Chairman and Professor, Department of Pathology
John A. Burns School of Medicine
University of Hawaii
Honolulu, Hawaii

Richard M. Terek, MD
Associate Professor
Department of Orthopaedics
Warren Alpert Medical School of Brown University
Rhode Island Hospital
Providence, Rhode Island

Josh Vaughn, MD
Department of Orthopedic Surgery
Brown University/Rhode Island Hospital
Providence, Rhode Island

Gregory R. Waryasz, MD
Department of Orthopaedics
Warren Alpert Medical School of Brown University
Providence, Rhode Island

Arnold-Peter Weiss, MD
R. Scot Sellers Scholar of Hand Surgery
Vice Chairman and Professor of Orthopaedics
Warren Alpert Medical School of Brown University
Rhode Island Hospital
Providence, Rhode Island

1

Basic Science

Raymond Hsu, Matthew E. Deren, and Richard M. Terek

I. Bone and Joint Physiology

1. Cell types **(Table 1.1, Fig. 1.1)**
   - Osteoblasts
     a. Originate from mesenchymal lineage; produce type I collagen; produce alkaline phosphatase
     b. Wnt/β-catenin pathway: Wnt protein binds and activates lipoprotein receptor-related protein (LRP) 5/6 at the cell surface and activates an intracellular cascade involving translocation of β-catenin into the nucleus to activate transcription of genes that control osteoblast differentiation.
     c. Runx2 (Cbfa1) and Osx: transcription factors required for differentiation of mesenchymal stem cells into osteoblasts
     d. Secrete receptor activator of nuclear factor kappa B ligand (RANKL) and macrophage colony-stimulating factor (MCSF) to activate osteoclasts.
     e. Stimulated by estrogens and 1,25-(OH)2-vitamin D; produce osteocalcin
     f. Downregulated by glucocorticoids, prostaglandins, leptin, parathyroid hormone (PTH)
   - Osteoclasts
     a. Originate from monocyte/macrophage lineage
     b. Use lysosomal enzymes including cathepsin K, matrix metalloproteinase, and carbonic anhydrase to resorb bone
        - Carbonic anhydrase produces hydrogen ions that are pumped into the ruffled border.
     c. Directly inhibited by calcitonin
     d. Responsible for pathological absorption of bone in multiple myeloma and metastatic disease
     e. Stimulated by interleukin-1 (IL-1) and RANKL
   - Osteocytes
     a. Originate as osteoblasts that become trapped in matrix
     b. 90% of cells in mature skeleton
     c. Canaliculi have gap junctions for communication between osteocytes.
     d. Stimulated by calcitonin, inhibited by PTH
2. Bone matrix
   - 60–70% inorganic: compressive strength; 25–30% organic: tensile strength (90% collagen); 5–8% water
   - Osteocalcin: expressed by mature osteoblasts, specific marker of osteoblast phenotype and differentiation, involved in calcium homeostasis. Levels increase with increasing bone mineral density when treating osteoporosis.

Table 1.1 Cell Types of Bone

Cell Type	Origin	Role	Important Hormones
Osteoprogenitor	Mesenchymal stem cells	– ↓Strain/↑O_2 → osteoblasts – Intermediate strain/↓O_2 → cartilage – ↑Strain → fibrous tissue	
Osteoblasts	Mesenchymal stem cells	– Form bone: synthesize bone matrix – Synthesize RANKL	– Runx2 directs MSC to become osteoblasts (Cbfa1/Runx2 is key transcription factor) – PTH: stimulate osteoclast by second messenger through activation of adenylyl cyclase – Estrogen: ↑bone production, ↓resorption – Prostaglandins: activate adenylyl cyclase – Glucocorticoids: inhibit protein, DNA and collagen synthesis – 1,25$(OH)_2$ Vit D_3: matrix, alkaline phosphatase, bone protein production – Osteocalcin expressed by mature osteoblasts
Osteoclasts	Hematopoietic cells in macrophage lineage	Ruffled border: resorption of bone (cathepsin K, carbonic anhydrase)	– RANKL: stimulates mature osteoclasts to ↑bone resorption – Calcitonin: inhibits bone resorption – Osteoprotegerin (OPG): binds RANKL to inhibit resorption IL-1: ↑bone resorption IL-10: ↓bone resorption Vitronectin: receptor aids in osteoclast attachment to bone
Osteocytes	Mesenchymal stem cells (former osteoblasts)	– Maintain bone – Majority of cells – Control extracellular calcium and phosphate homeostasis	Calcitonin: stimulate PTH: inhibit

Abbreviations: IL, interleukin; MSC, mesenchymal stem cells; PTH, parathyroid hormone; RANKL, receptor activator of nuclear factor kappa B ligand.

- Osteonectin: calcium-binding glycoprotein secreted by platelets and osteoblasts
- Mineralization occurs as crystals form a lattice in the hole zones between collagen fibrils. The formation of the critical nucleus requires the most energy in this process.

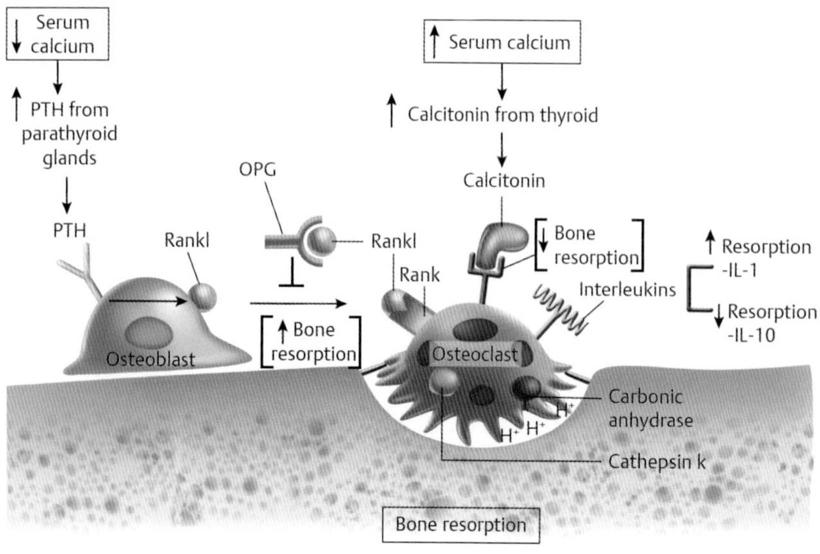

Fig. 1.1 Activators and inhibitors of osteoblasts and osteoclasts. IL, interleukin; OPG, osteoprotegerin; PTH, parathyroid hormone; RANK, receptor activator of nuclear factor kappa B; RANKL, receptor activator of nuclear factor kappa B ligand.

3. Types of bone **(Fig. 1.2)**
   - Lamellar: normal, mature, cortical, or cancellous
     a. Cortical
        - Majority of skeleton
        - Higher Young's modulus
        - Connection of haversian canals

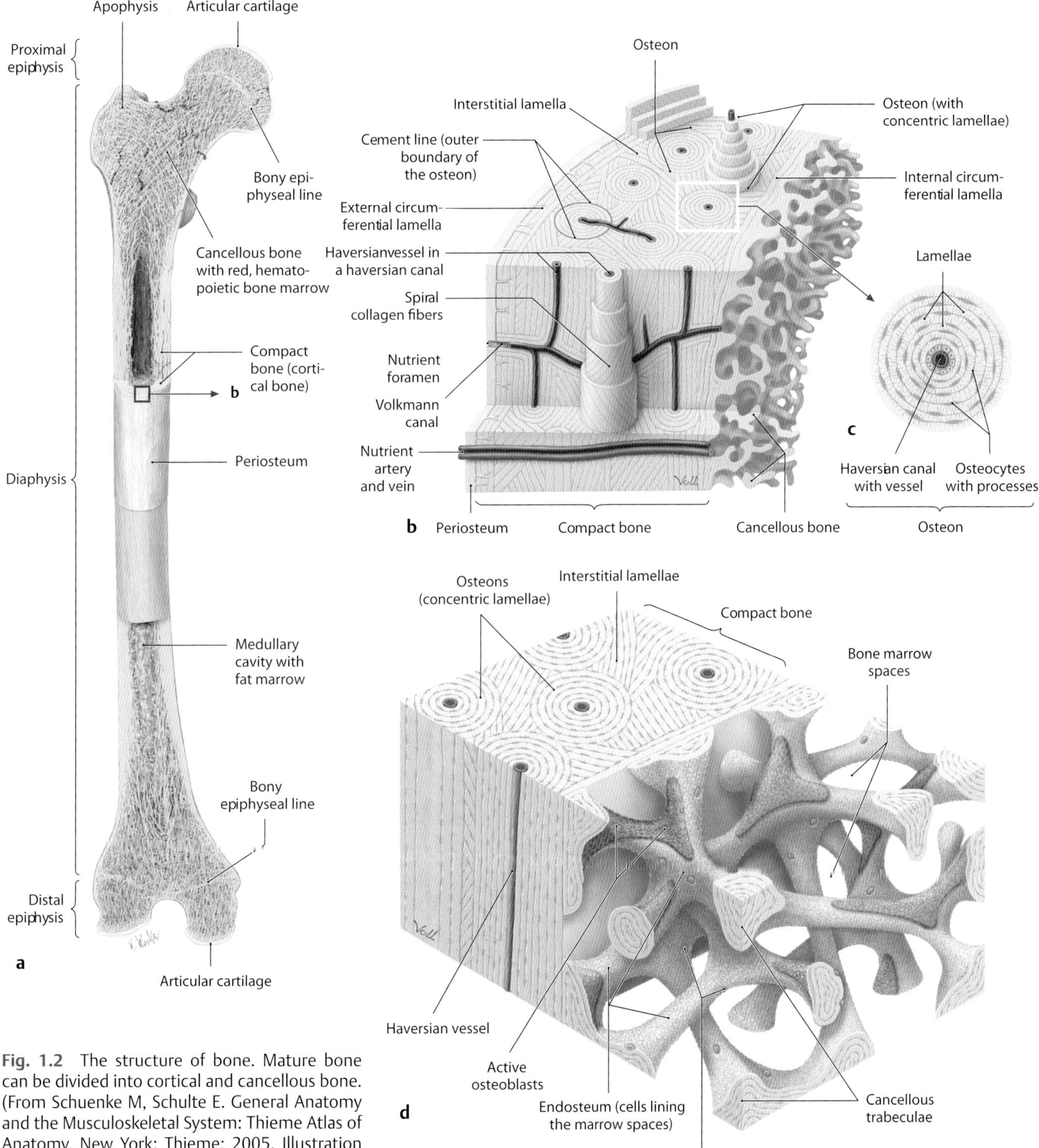

Fig. 1.2 The structure of bone. Mature bone can be divided into cortical and cancellous bone. (From Schuenke M, Schulte E. General Anatomy and the Musculoskeletal System: Thieme Atlas of Anatomy. New York: Thieme; 2005. Illustration by Karl Wesker.)

- Cement lines = outer border of osteon
  - ♦ Interstitial lamellae connect osteons

b. Cancellous
   - Higher turnover
   - Less dense
   - Modeled along stress lines
     - ♦ **Wolff's law: form follows function, bone responds to stress by increasing formation**

- Woven: random; pathological or immature
- **Biopsy of fracture callus can be confused with osteosarcoma because they both have woven bone.**

4. Blood supply of bone (two supplies)
   - Nutrient artery: traverse cortices through nutrient foramen, arise from major arteries, supply inner two thirds of cortex; high-pressure system
   - Periosteum: capillaries supplying outer one third of cortex; low-pressure system
   - Metaphyseal-epiphyseal blood supply

     a. Growth plate supplied by perichondral artery (nutrients) and epiphyseal artery (supplying proliferative zone of physis)

5. Bone formation (three types)
   - **Endochondral: cartilage model replaced by bone**

     a. Occurs in nonrigid fracture callus, physis, and formation of long bones
        - Associated with type X collagen
        - Sox-9: key gene for regulation of chondrogenesis, expressed earliest in endochondral ossification
   - **Intramembranous: mesenchymal stem cells differentiate into osteoblasts to form bone**

     a. Occurs in formation of flat bones (skull, clavicle), healing of fractures repaired with semirigid stability (plating), and distraction osteogenesis
   - **Appositional: Laying new bone on preexisting bone by osteoblasts occurs in bone remodeling and periosteal enlargement of bone (creating increased thickness).**

6. Physis **(Fig. 1.3)**
   - Zones of physis:

     a. Reserve/resting: coordinates organization and development of chondrocytes, marked by abundant matrix and cell inactivity

     b. Proliferative: longitudinal growth of cells, high oxygen tension and ionized calcium, significant endoplasmic reticulum from aerobic metabolism

     c. Hypertrophic: enlarged cells, calcification of the matrix, alkaline phosphatase, and type X collagen abundant

     d. Maturation: removal of mineralized cartilage and formation of primary spongiosa
   - **Groove/zone of Ranvier: periphery of physis responsible for appositional bone growth of the physis and provides structural stability in first 2 years of life**
   - Perichondral ring of La Croix: thick fibrous band surrounding and providing stability to physis
   - **Achondroplasia: affects the proliferative zone**
   - **Gigantism: affects the proliferative zone by action of growth hormone**

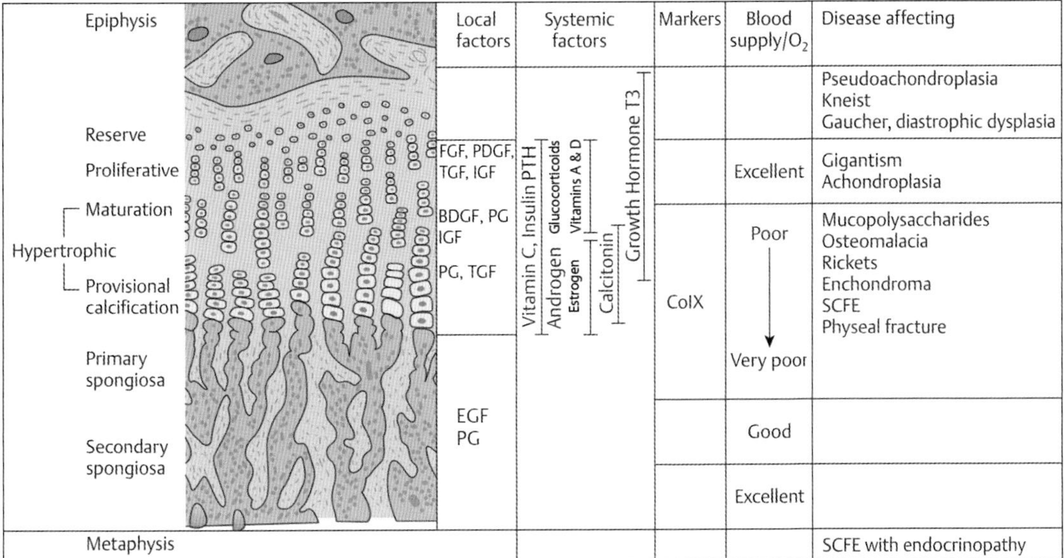

Fig. 1.3 Zones of the physis. BDGF, bone-derived growth factor; Col X, collagen X; EGF, epidermal growth factor; FGF, fibroblast growth factor; IGF, insulin-like growth factor; PDGF, platelet-derived growth factor; PG, prostaglandin; SCFE, slipped capital femoral epiphysis; TGF, transforming growth factor. (From Schuenke M, Schulte E. General Anatomy and the Musculoskeletal System: Thieme Atlas of Anatomy. New York: Thieme; 2005. Illustration by Marcus Voll.)

- **Physeal fractures occur through the zone of provisional calcification in the hypertrophic zone.**

7. Fracture repair
   - Types of healing (dependent on rigidity/strain)
     a. Primary ("cutting cones," haversian remodeling)
        - Requires contact and absolute stability (compression plates)
     b. Intramembranous healing (direct bone formation, no intermediate)
        - Semirigid fixation (locked plating, intramedullary nails)
     c. Endochondral healing (cartilage intermediate and then bone formation)
        - Nonrigid fixation (casts, external fixation)
        - Intramedullary nails: combination of endochondral and intramembranous based on stability and bony contact
     d. In general, less rigid fixation is associated with more callous (endochondral).
   - Stages of fracture healing
     a. Reactive/inflammation (24–72 hours)
        - Hematoma provides source of growth factors and fibroblasts and mesenchymal precursors of osteoblasts.
        - **Inhibition of cyclooxygenase-2 (COX 2) in mice and rabbits increases time to healing.**
     b. Repair (2 weeks)
        - Callous formation, type and amount depend on extent of immobilization
        - Nonrigid fixation: initial soft callous formation from fibroblasts followed by chondroblasts (type II collagen and then type I collagen). Type X collagen expressed by hypertrophic chondrocytes as matrix undergoes endochondral calcification.
        - Rigid fixation: minimal callous, primarily haversian remodeling
        - Protein deprivation in rats limits callous formation.
     c. Remodeling (7 years)
        - Wolff's law: remodeling in response to mechanical stress

- **Piezoelectric mechanism**
  - **Compression side is negatively charged, stimulating osteoblast activity.**
  - **Tension side is positively charged, stimulating osteoclast activity (upper part of "t" = +).**

8. Biological fracture treatments
   - Bone morphogenic proteins (BMPs)
     a. Extracellular proteins that belong to the transforming growth factor-β (TGF-β) family act by binding serine-threonine kinase surface receptors that activate intracellular signaling molecules called SMADs.
        - **BMP-2: used to treat acute open tibial fractures**
        - **BMP-7: used to treat tibial nonunions**
   - Smoking/nicotine decreases blood flow and callous strength while increasing time to union and risk of nonunion.
   - Low-intensity pulsed ultrasound stimulation (LIPUS) produces nanomotion to stimulate bone formation.
     a. 30 mW/cm^2 pulsed-wave at 1.0 kHz
     b. Increases intracellular calcium, increasing proteoglycan synthesis
     c. Decreases time to union in nonoperatively treated radial shaft, distal radius, scaphoid, and tibial fractures
     d. No demonstrated benefit for intramedullary fixed tibia shafts
   - Capacitative coupling (CC) stimulation uses electrodes with an alternating current to create an electric field to stimulate bone formation.
     a. Stimulates transmembrane calcium translocation through voltage-gated calcium channels
     b. Calcium activates calmodulin and upregulates cytokines for bone formation.
   - Direct current stimulation reduces local oxygen concentration and increases local tissue pH, decreasing osteoclast and increasing osteoblast activity.
   - Nonunion treatment
     a. Hypertrophic: adequate biology, inadequate immobilization
        - Treatment: increase mechanical stability (e.g., compression plating of previously nailed fracture)

     b. Atrophic: inadequate biology
        - Treatment: take down of nonunion, restabilize, and bone graft/BMP
9. Bone grafts
   - Properties:
     a. Osteoconductive: provides structural framework for bone growth
     b. Osteoinductive: contains growth factors that stimulate bone growth
     c. Osteogenic: contains cells that produce bone (osteoblasts or mesenchymal stem cells)
   - Autograft: osteoconductive, osteoinductive, and osteogenic
     a. Gold standard
     b. Cancellous: less structural integrity, more osteoconductive, rapid incorporation by creeping substitution
     c. Cortical: more structural support, incorporates slowly by remodeling of haversian system (cutting cones)
        - Includes vascularized bone grafts
     d. Iliac crest bone graft: anterior harvest has higher complication rate than posterior harvest (can be cancellous or cortical).

e. Femoral intramedullary reaming contents equivalent to iliac crest cancellous autograft
f. Bone marrow aspirate: only other osteogenic source

- Allografts: osteoconductive (osteoinductive depends on processing)
  a. Antigenicity dependent on cell-surface glycoproteins and matrix macromolecules.
  b. Fresh used for osteochondral defects
  c. Frozen bulk allograft used in tumor reconstruction and revision arthroplasty.
    - Some osteoinduction
    - Higher immunogenicity and risk of disease transmission
  d. Freeze dried much more common
    - Osteoconductive, no osteoinduction but decreased immunogenicity/disease
    - Fewer impactions to maximal stiffness compared with fresh-frozen, therefore possibly more mechanically efficient
  e. Routinely screened for HIV, hepatitis B, hepatitis C, and syphilis
  f. Risk of transmission (estimated from blood transmission)
    - HIV: 1:1,000,000–1,500,000
    - **Hepatitis C: 1:100,000**
    - Hepatitis B: 1:50,000–60,000
  g. Massive cortical structural allograft
    - Only the ends are incorporated by creeping substitution ("cutting cones")
    - May eventually be encapsulated by callous but the bulk of the graft remains avascular
    - Stress fractures occur in ~ 25% (no remodeling)
  h. Cartilage allograft
    - Cartilage architecture maintained for first 2–3 years
    - Cartilage graft remains completely acellular
    - Pannus of host fibrocartilage can form over the graft
  i. Demineralized bone matrix: produced by acid extraction
    - Removal of inorganic component exposes more osteoinductive proteins, but efficacy of proteins is also partially lost in processing.
- Synthetics: osteoconductive only
  a. Calcium phosphate and calcium sulfate
    - High compressive strength
    - Low tensile/sheer/torsional properties
    - Ca phosphate: very slow resorption (1 year), cement form available, popular for subchondral support of fractures
    - Ca sulfate: fast resorption (4–12 weeks), essentially plaster of Paris, can cause increased serous drainage from surgical incisions
  b. Subsets of calcium phosphate
    - Tricalcium phosphate
      - Resorbs more rapidly, less compressive strength, and weaker than hydroxyapatite
      - Partially converted to hydroxyapatite
    - **Hydroxyapatite: $Ca_{10}(PO_4)_6(OH)_2$**
      - Ceramic preparation very resistant to resorption
      - Can be converted from calcium carbonate (marine coral)

◆ Porous preparation enables neovascularization and appositional new bone growth.

◆ Resorbed by foreign body giant cell

10. Bone metabolism
  - Calcium homeostasis **(Fig. 1.4)**
    a. Requirements for Ca intake **(Table 1.2)**
    b. Calcitonin: directly inhibits osteoclasts, decreases serum calcium
  - Hormone effects and interactions
    a. Estrogen
      - **Most important hormone for peak bone mass in females**
      - Inhibits bone absorption and increases bone formation

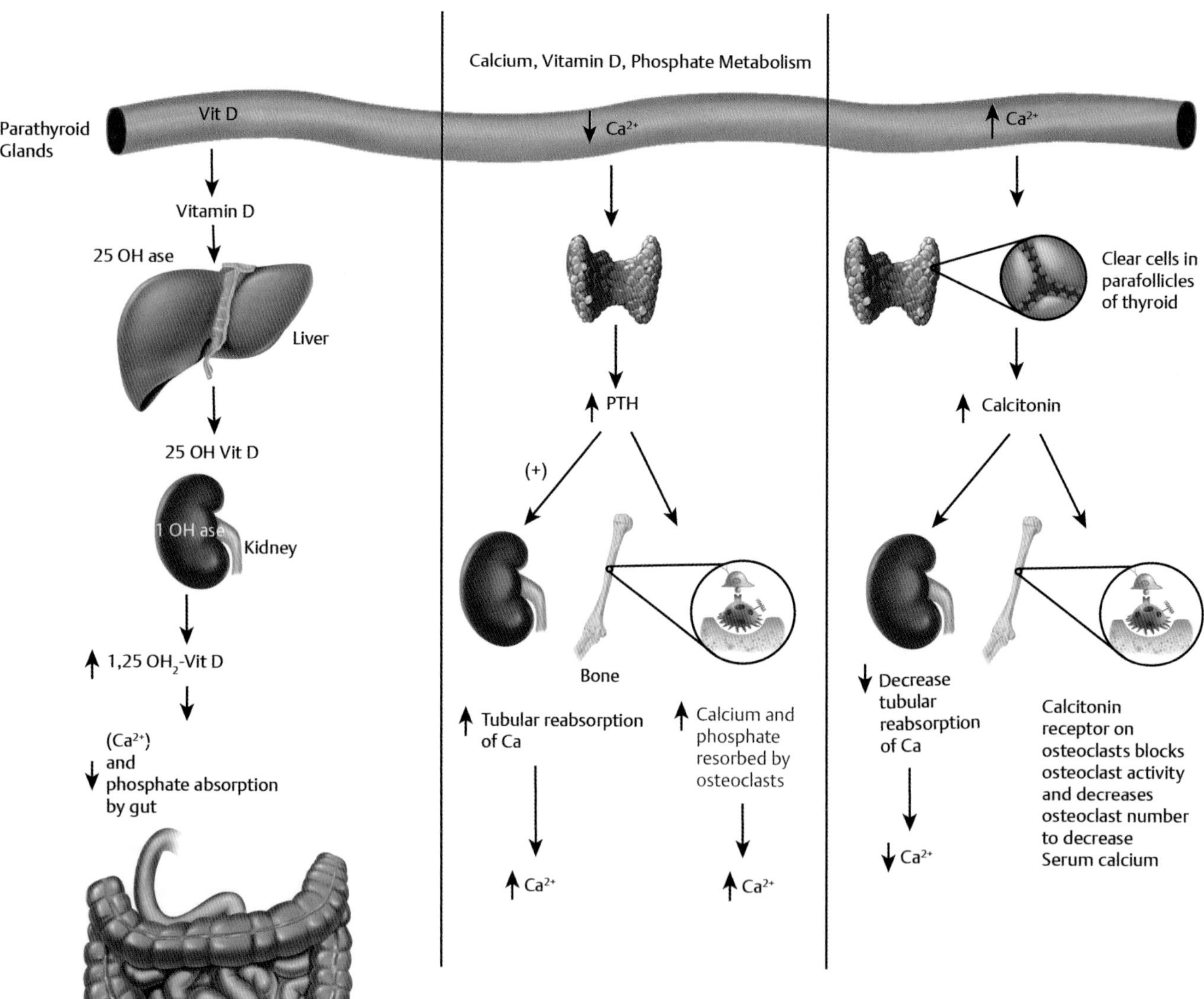

Fig. 1.4 Calcium, phosphate, and vitamin D metabolism and homeostasis are a complex interaction of parathyroid hormone (PTH), calcitonin, vitamin D, and calcium (Ca^{2+}). Low serum calcium stimulates the parathyroid gland to release PTH, which increases renal reabsorption of calcium, causes osteoblasts to activate osteoclasts through the receptor activator of nuclear factor kappa B ligand (RANKL), and increases renal production of 1,25-(OH)2-vitamin D, with resultant increased intestinal absorption of calcium. Vitamin D is metabolized by hepatocyte enzyme 25-hydroxylase to 25-(OH)-vitamin D, which in the kidney is metabolized by 1α-hydroxylase to active 1,25(OH)2-vitamin D.

Table 1.2 Recommended Daily Calcium Intake Requirements

Age	Male	Female	Pregnant
0–6 months	200 mg	200 mg	
7–12 months	260 mg	260 mg	
1–3 years	700 mg	700 mg	
4–8 years	1,000 mg	1,000 mg	
9–13 years	1,300 mg	1,300 mg	
14–18 years	1,300 mg	1,300 mg	1,300 mg
19–50 years	1,000 mg	1,000 mg	1,000 mg
51–70 years	1,000 mg	1,200 mg	
71+ years	1,200 mg	1,200 mg	

Source: Reproduced from the National Institutes of Health (NIH) Dietary Fact Sheets (nih.gov).

   - Associated decreased risk of heart disease and increased risk of endometrial and breast cancer

  b. Corticosteroids
   - Decreases gut absorption of calcium, increases bone loss (decreases bone formation from inhibition of osteoblast collagen synthesis)

  c. Thyroid hormones
   - Thyroxine: high doses can result in osteoporosis
   - Affect physeal growth by increasing chondrocyte growth, collagen X synthesis, and alkaline phosphatase; increases both proliferation and hypertrophy of the growth plate

  d. Growth hormone
   - Insulin-like growth factor-I (IGF-I) induces linear growth by engendering proliferation in physis.

- Growth factor signaling types
  a. Autocrine: affects the same cell that secreted the growth factor
  b. Paracrine: affects adjacent cells
  c. Endocrine: affects cells at distant site

11. Metabolic bone disease **(Table 1.3)**
- Malignancy/metastasis
   - Tumor cells secrete parathyroid hormone–related protein (PTHrP), interleukins, macrophage inflammatory protein (MIP), tumor necrosis factor-α (TNF-α), prostaglandin E_2 (PGE_2) to activate osteoblastic production of RANKL, or directly secrete RANKL. Increased ratio of RANKL/osteoprotegerin (OPG) activates osteoclasts.
   - Bone resorption by osteoclasts releases TGF-β from bone matrix, feeding back to tumor cells to release more PTHrP (leading to increased lysis).
- Hyperthyroidism
  a. Causes hypercalcemia by increased production of calcitonin from thyroid parafollicular clear cells that binds to osteoclasts to decrease activity and number, resulting in increased serum calcium
- Vitamin D toxicity
  a. Excessive vitamin D intake leads to increased 25(OH)-vitamin D, with subsequent increased intestinal absorption of calcium and resultant hypercalcemia.
  b. Treatment: correct intake of vitamin D
- Hypoparathyroidism
  a. Decreased PTH production by parathyroid chief cells leads to decreased serum calcium, increased phosphate, decreased 1,25-(OH)2-vitamin D levels

Table 1.3 Metabolic Bone Diseases

Disease	Serum Ca	Serum Phos	25(OH) Vit D	1,25(OH)2 Vit D	Urine Ca	PTH	Alk Phos
Primary hyperparathyroidism	↑	= or ↓	=	= or ↑	↑	↑	= or ↑
Malignancy/metastasis	↑	= or ↑	=	= or ↓	↑	= or ↓	= or ↑
Rickets/osteomalacia							
– Vitamin D deficiency	↓ or =	↓	↓	↓	↓	↑	↑
– Calcium deficiency	↓ or =	↓	=	= or ↑	↓	↑	↑
– Phosphate deficiency	=	↓	=	↑↑	=	=	↑
Hereditary Vit-D–dependent rickets	↓	↓	= or ↑	↓↓ (type 1) ↑↑(type 2)	↓	↑	↑
Hypophosphatasia	↑	↑↑	=	=		=	↓↓
Renal osteodystrophy							
– High bone turnover	= or ↓	↑↑	=	↓		↑↑	↑
– Low bone turnover	= or ↑	= or ↑	=	↓		= or ↑	↑
Osteopenia/osteoporosis	=	=	= or ↓	= or ↓	= or ↑		
Hyperthyroidism	↑						
Vitamin D toxicity	↑	= or ↑	↑↑	=	↑	= or ↓	= or ↑
Hypoparathyroidism	↓	↑	=	↓	↓	↓	=
Pseudohypoparathyroidism	↓	↑	=	↓	↓	= or ↑	=
Albright hereditary osteodystrophy	=	↓↓	=	=	= or ↑	=	↑
Hyperthyroidism	↑	=	=	=	↑	= or ↓	=

Abbreviations: Alk, alkaline; Ca, calcium; Phos, phosphatase; PTH, parathyroid hormone; Vit, vitamin.

b. Treatment: calcium and vitamin D supplementation

- Pseudohypoparathyroidism
  a. Genetic disorder of ineffective PTH receptor causing normal to elevated PTH levels
- Albright hereditary osteodystrophy
  a. A form of pseudohypoparathyroidism due to a defective maternal *GNAS1* gene with resultant exostoses, short fourth and fifth metacarpals and metatarsals, brachydactyly, obesity, low intelligence, short stature
- Vitamin D deficiency rickets/osteomalacia
  a. Rickets: children with open growth plates
    - Widened growth plates from accumulation of nonmineralized osteoid and cartilage
    - **Causes widening of the anterior ribs (rachitic rosary)**

  b. Osteomalacia: adults with closed growth plates
  c. Mechanism: dietary deficiency of vitamin D leads to decreased intestinal calcium absorption.
  d. Results in increased PTH, increased bone resorption (alkaline phosphatase)
  e. Low to normal serum calcium, low phosphate, low Vitamin D
  f. Treatment: 5,000 IU vitamin D daily
- Primary hyperparathyroidism
  a. Primary pathology is increased PTH, such as from a parathyroid adenoma
  b. Accumulation of fibrous tissue in metaphysis can mimic widened growth plates of rickets.
  c. Erosions around growth plate
  d. Brown tumor of hyperparathyroidism

- Secondary hyperparathyroidism (renal osteodystrophy)
  a. Primary pathology is renal failure
     - Inability to convert vitamin D_3 to active calcitriol leads to hypocalcemia and osteomalacia
     - Failure to adequately excrete phosphate leading to uremia-related phosphate retention
  b. Insoluble calcium phosphate forms, removing calcium from the circulation.
  c. Low serum calcium/high serum phosphate causes secondary hyperparathyroidism.
  d. Two types:
     - High bone turnover: increased PTH, parathyroid hyperplasia leading to osteitis cystica; continues after correction of kidney disease
     - Low bone turnover: common in dialysis, low PTH, and low bone formation (frontal bossing, genu varum, metaphyseal enlargement)
  e. "Rugger jersey" spine: sclerosis of end plates of the vertebrae seen on X-ray
- Osteogenesis imperfecta
  a. Mutation in collagen type 1 (*COL1A1* or *COL1A2* genes)
  b. Hearing defects, blue sclera, fractures, scoliosis, poor dentition
  c. Olecranon apophysis fractures relatively common
  d. Bisphosphonates reduce bone pain and fracture incidence, increase bone density and overall function
- Hereditary vitamin D–dependent rickets
  a. Genetics: autosomal recessive
  b. Type I: loss of function mutation in 25-hydroxyvitamin D hydroxylase gene [decreased levels of 1,25-(OH)2-vitamin D]
  c. Type II: defective intracellular receptor for 1,25-(OH)2-vitamin D_3 [increased levels of 1,25-(OH)2-vitamin D_3]
  d. Decreased serum calcium and phosphorus, increased PTH, increased alkaline phosphatase
- X-linked hypophosphatemic (vitamin D–resistant) rickets
  a. Genetics: X-linked dominant
  b. Mechanism: mutated *PHEX* gene (X-chromosome) causing inability of renal proximal tubules to reabsorb phosphate (phosphate diabetes)
  c. Low serum phosphorus, elevated alkaline phosphatase, normal PTH levels, low or normal calcium levels
  d. Treatment: High-dose vitamin D_3
- Oncogenic osteomalacia
  a. Mesenchymal tumors secrete fibroblast growth factor-23 (FGF-23) or phosphatonin, which inhibits phosphate reabsorption and increases excretion at the proximal renal tubules.
- Hypophosphatasia
  a. Genetics: autosomal recessive
  b. Mechanism: Defect in tissue-nonspecific isoenzyme of alkaline phosphatase leading to decreased levels of alkaline phosphatase and hypomineralization
  c. Diagnosis by elevated urinary phosphoethanolamine
- Osteoporosis
  a. Chronic progressive disease associated with low bone mass and decreased bone strength
  b. Genetics: multiple associated polymorphisms in genes, including calcitonin receptor, estrogen receptor-1, vitamin D receptor, type 1 collagen α-chain, IL-1, IL-10, IGF-II, TGF-β, TNF-α, TNF receptor 2

c. Bone structure with age:
  - Loss of density in both cortical and cancellous bone but more in cancellous (thinned trabeculae, decreased interconnections)
  - Decreasing cortical thickness and enlarging medullary canal diameter in long bones
  - Estrogen most important hormone for peak bone mass, which usually occurs at between 16 and 25 years of age

d. Bone mineral density (BMD):
  - Dual-energy X-ray absorptiometry (DEXA) testing: determines bone density (defined as standard deviations) in hip and lumbar spine
  - Recommended for all women of ages 65 and older and all men of ages 70 and older
  - T-score is in comparison to a healthy 25-year-old of same sex and ethnicity (peak bone age)
    - Osteopenia: T-score between –1 and –2.5
    - Osteoporosis: T-score ≤ –2.5
  - Z-score is in comparison to same age, sex, and ethnicity.
    - For diagnosis of metabolic bone diseases
  - Osteoarthritis can falsely elevate spinal BMD values.

e. Workup after a fragility fracture:
  - DEXA, 25-OH vitamin D levels, calcium levels
  - Metabolic workup and arrange follow-up with osteoporosis clinic

f. History of any fragility fracture (spine, hip, or wrist)
  - Most predictive of future fractures (more so than vitamin D level, T-score, family history, or other risk factors)
  - Vertebral body fractures
    - Most predictive of future vertebral body fractures (as compared with hip and wrist fractures)
    - Higher overall mortality than previously recognized
    - Overall mortality twice that of controls
    - Greater increase in mortality risk in men than women and with younger age

g. FRAX (fracture risk assessment tool) score
  - Developed by World Health Organization (WHO)
  - Calculates clinical risk of fracture using BMD at femoral neck, body mass index (BMI), current smoking activity, history of parental hip fracture, and prior personal history of fracture before age 50
  - Does not use BMD of spine

h. Medications that increase risk of osteoporosis:
  - Oral corticosteroids
  - Androgen-deprivation therapy, aromatase inhibitors
  - Protease inhibitors
  - Selective serotonin reuptake inhibitors, prolactin-raising antiepileptics (carbamazepine, phenytoin, valproic acid)

i. Dietary treatments:
  - Daily calcium intake for osteoporosis treatment/prevention: 1,000–1,500 mg (starting from age 9) (only lactating women require more: 2,000 mg/day)
  - Daily vitamin D intake for adults > 50 years: 1,000 units
    - With age, decreased dietary intake, decreased conversion via the skin, and decreased conversion in the kidney
  - Protein-enriched diet

j. Pharmacological treatments
    - Bisphosphonates (see dedicated section below)
    - Teriparatide (Forteo) (recombinant 1–34 amino acid sequence at the N-terminus of parathyroid hormone)
        - ♦ Activates osteoblasts, which release RANKL and IL-6 to activate osteoclasts
        - ♦ Intermittent dosing: increased coupling of osteoblast activity to osteoclast resorption, net bone formation (maximum treatment 2 years)
        - ♦ Continuous dosing: net bone resorption
    - Calcitonin: directly inhibits osteoclasts
    - Denosumab: anti-RANKL monoclonal antibody

- Lead toxicity
  a. Stored in bone and released slowly over decades
  b. Inhibits parathyroid hormone–related peptide (PTHrP) causing decreased bone mineral density
- Osteopetrosis: abnormal osteoclast number and function
  a. decreased bone turnover and remodeling (fractures, Erlenmeyer flask deformity)
  b. *CLCN7* and *TC1RG1* genes
- Scurvy: deficiency of vitamin C, which is required for cross-linking during collagen synthesis
  a. Bleeding from fragile capillaries
  b. Growth plate affected primarily at primary spongiosa
  c. Radiographs show dense band at metaphyseal/growth plate junction: white line of Frankel.
- Fibrodysplasia ossificans progressiva (FOP): characterized by massive spontaneous heterotopic bone formation
  a. Altered BMP-4 signal transduction
  b. Diagnosis is clinical; biopsy worsens process

12. Heterotopic ossification
    - Bone formation in extraskeletal tissue
    - Risk factors: prolonged ventilator time, brain injury, spinal cord injury, neurologic compromise, burns, blast injury, and amputation through zone of injury
    - **Prophylaxis: irradiation with 700 cG or indomethacin 25 mg oral t.i.d. for 6 weeks**
13. Bisphosphonates
    - Pyrophosphate analogues that inhibit osteoclast resorption of bone
    - Accumulate in high concentrations in bone due to affinity for hydroxyapatite crystals, then taken up by osteoclasts
    - Nitrogen-containing
      a. Alendronate/Fosamax, pamidronate/Aredia, risedronate/Actonel, zoledronate/Zometa
      b. Inhibit farnesyl diphosphate synthase (FPPS), preventing protein prenylation of small guanosine triphosphatases (GTPases) in the cholesterol synthetic pathway
        - Also inhibits geranylgeranyl diphosphate synthase (GGPPS) and undecaprenol diphosphate synthase (UPPS)
    - Non-nitrogen containing
      a. Etidronate/Didronel, clodronate, tiludronate
      b. Metabolized form replaces terminal pyrophosphate of adenosine triphosphate (ATP), which forms an analogue that competes with ATP and causes osteoclast apoptosis

- Indications: osteoporosis, history of fragility fractures, osteogenesis imperfecta, Paget's disease, metastatic bone disease, idiopathic hyperphosphatasia, avascular necrosis
- Results for osteoporosis:
  a. Vertebral fractures: 65% reduction after 1 year and 40% reduction after 3 years
  b. Nonvertebral fractures: 40% reduction after 3 years
- Metabolism:
  a. Minimal gastrointestinal (GI) absorption (recommendation: take 1 hour prior to meal)
  b. Excreted by kidneys
- Complications:
  a. Subtrochanteric stress reaction and fractures:
     - Symptoms: lateral thigh pain
     - Imaging: lateral cortical thickening, beaking, "dreaded black line" (stress fracture)
     - Treatment: discontinuation of bisphosphonate, contralateral imaging, consider prophylactic intramedullary fixation for impending fracture
  b. Osteonecrosis of the jaw
  c. Reduced fusion rates in spine fusion surgery
  d. Osteopetrosis-like bone when used in children

14. The joint
- Articular cartilage **(Fig. 1.5)**
  a. Deep zone: highest concentration of proteoglycans and lowest concentration of water
  b. Overall concentrations: water > collagen > proteoglycan > noncollagenous proteins > chondrocytes.
  c. Collagen oriented parallel in superficial zone and perpendicular in the calcified zone
  d. 65–80% water
     - **Water effectively stress shields matrix from compression.**
  e. Osteoarthritis changes in cartilage versus changes in aging **(Table 1.4)**
  f. Proteoglycans: 10–15% of wet weight, viscoelastic with molecular two-tiered brush-like structure **(Fig. 1.6)**
     - Hyaluronate: a complex sugar, composes the core
     - Aggrecan: major proteoglycan in cartilage, aggregates onto hyaluronic acid with link proteins
     - Glycosaminoglycan chains: attached to the core aggrecan
       - ♦ Chondroitin sulfate and keratin sulfate
       - ♦ Glucosamine serves as substrate for formation of chondroitin sulfate.
       - ♦ Increase in the knee with moderate exercise
- Effect of aging:
  a. Decreased proteoglycan synthesis and water
  b. Decreased chondrocyte number
  c. Keratin sulfate increases until age 30, then levels off.
  d. Chondroitin sulfate decreases.
- Collagen types throughout the body:
  a. Type I: major form in tendon, bone, and meniscus
  b. Type II: major collagen of articular cartilage
     - Very stable, half-life > 25 years
     - Adults have only a 5% rate of synthesis in articular cartilage as compared with teenagers.

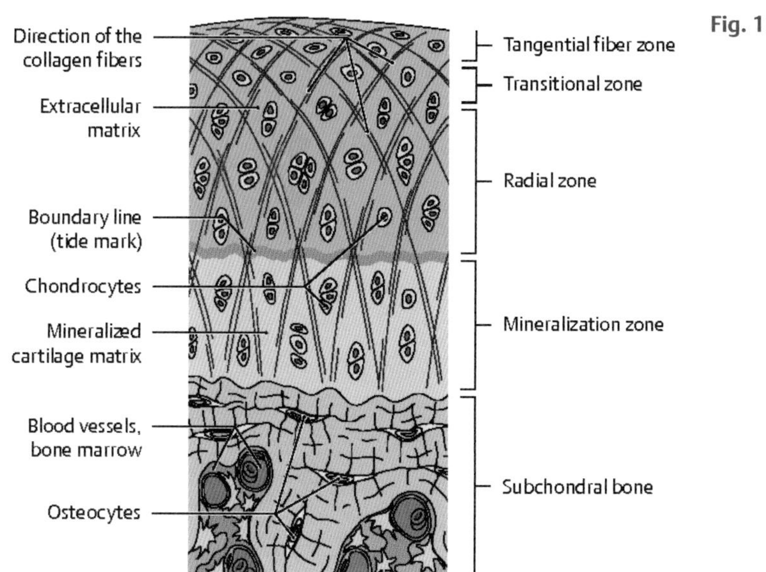

a

Layers of articular cartilage

	Zone	Direction	Concentrated	Special characteristics	Healing
	Gliding	Tangential	- Col II - Collagen Fibers	Highest conversion of collagen fibers Articular cartilage progenitor cells	Limited because articular
	Transitional	Oblique		Compression	
	Radial	Vertical		Compression	
	Tidemark	Tangential		Division of nutritional source for chondrocytes	
	Mineralisation (calcified)		Hypertrophic chondrocytes + Col X	Anchor	Fibrocartilage from modification MSCs (Mesenchymal stem cells)
	Subchondral bone				

b

Fig. 1.5 Layers of articular cartilage.

Table 1.4 Changes in Concentrations of Articular Cartilage

	Aging	Osteoarthritis (OA)
Water content	↓	↑
Proteoglycan content	↓	↓
Collagen content	=	Relative concentration due to loss of proteoglycans ↓ in severe OA
Proteoglycan synthesis	=	↑
Proteoglycan degradation	↓	↑↑
Chondroitin sulfate	↓	↑
Keratin sulfate	↑	↓
Chondrocyte density	↓	Transiently increased than decreased

c. Type III: early tendon healing (also in skin and vessels)

d. Type IV: basement membranes

e. Type X: hypertrophic chondrocytes: enchondral ossification, heterotopic ossification, early osteoarthritis, and calcified cartilaginous tumors

f. Articular cartilage also contains types V, VI, IX

- Chondrocytes

a. Sit in lacunae in cartilage matrix

b. 2% of total volume of adult articular cartilage

c. SOX-9: key transcription factor in differentiation of chondrocytes

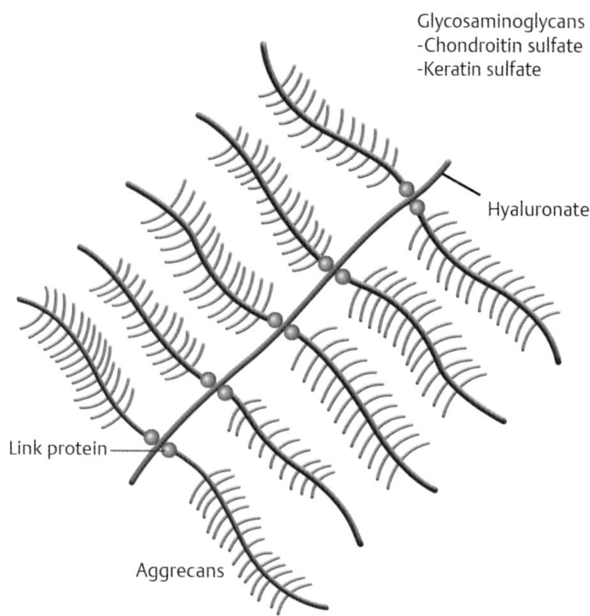

Fig. 1.6 The structure of proteoglycans including hyaluronate, aggrecans, and glycosaminoglycans.

- Types of lubrication

a. Elastohydrodynamic lubrication: function of fluid as well as surface under compressive load

  - Elastic deformation of articular surface combined with a thin film of fluid separating surfaces during motion
  - Predominant mechanism during dynamic joint function

b. Boundary lubrication: primarily a function of the surfaces

  - Bearing surface is largely nondeformable without a continuous fluid film (part of surfaces are in direct contact)
  - Mechanism when starting from rest or with slow motion
  - Lubricin, found in superficial zone of cartilage, believed to play a large role
  - Superficial zone protein: similar primary structure to lubricin but different posttranslational modifications

c. Others:

  - Hydrodynamic: thin film of fluid completely separates surfaces during motion, but (unlike elastohydrodynamic lubrication) there is no elastic deformation of the surfaces
  - Weeping: similar to elastohydrodynamic lubrication but fluid weeps out of the surface (cartilage) with loading and separates the surfaces by hydrostatic pressure
  - Squeeze film: layer of fluid is slowly squeezed from between surfaces

- Cartilage healing

a. Above tidemark: limited due to avascular cartilage

b. Below tidemark: fibrocartilage produced by marrow mesenchymal stem cells as the laceration involves subchondral bone—the theory behind microfracture and abrasion chondroplasty

- Synovium

a. Vascularized connective tissue with no basement membrane, functions to allow nutrient exchange of the joint

b. Synovial fluid

  - Combination of ultrafiltrate of blood plasma and fluid secreted by synovial cells
  - Contains hyaluronic acid, lubricin, proteinases, and collagenases
  - Provides nourishment by diffusion
  - Non-newtonian fluid: viscosity is not constant, it increases as shear rate decreases

c. Type A synovial cell: phagocytic role

d. Type B synovial cell: fibroblast-like cell that secretes synovial fluid

Table 1.5 Inflammatory and Noninflammatory Arthritides

	WBC Count	Glucose	Color	Viscosity	Gram Stain
Noninflammatory	$200/mm^3$, 25% PMNs	Equal to serum	Clear, straw	High	Negative
Inflammatory	$2{,}000–75{,}000/mm^3$, 50% PMNs	Decreased compared with serum	Yellow-green, cloudy	Low	Negative
Septic	$>80{,}000/mm^3$, 75% PMNs	Low	Opaque	Low	Positive

Abbreviations: PMN, polymorphonuclear cells; WBC, white blood cell.

15. Inflammatory versus noninflammatory arthritides **(Table 1.5)**
   - Noninflammatory
     a. Osteoarthritis (OA)
        - Decreased proteoglycan content, higher water content, lower compressive modulus, and higher permeability
        - In early OA, collagen type X is increased in the deep zone.
        - Genetic linkage has been found to certain molecules, including collagen type IX and aggrecanase ADAMTS-5 (a disintegrin and metalloproteinase with thrombospondin motifs).
        - Passive glycation of articular cartilage stiffens and degrades collagen over time, playing a role in OA.

     b. Neuropathic (Charcot)
        - Causes: diabetes mellitus, syringomyelia, leprosy, neurosyphilis, myelomeningocele
        - Recurrent trauma from loss of proprioception and sensation
        - **Diabetes: most common cause overall**
        - **Syringomyelia: most common cause in upper extremity**

     c. Hemophilia
        - Hemophilia A (factor VIII deficiency) and B (factor IX deficiency)
        - X-linked recessive
        - Repeated hemarthrosis causes synovitis, cartilage destruction, and dense synovial scar
        - Treatment: factor treatment, synovectomy, total joint replacement
   - Inflammatory
     a. Rheumatoid arthritis
        - Rheumatoid factor: autoimmune immunoglobulin M (IgM) antibody against IgG, which forms complexes that deposit in tissues; nonspecific, may be elevated in other autoimmune conditions
        - Associated with human leukocyte antigen (HLA)-DR4 and HLA-DW4
        - May have increased viral load of Epstein-Barr virus due to impaired ability to control infection
        - Radiography characterized by periarticular erosions and osteopenia
        - Pathology shows synovial hyperplasia, increased vascularity, and abundant lymphocytes with rare neutrophils. Pannus, itself, has no lymphocytes.
        - Treatment:
          - First-line: low-dose corticosteroids
          - Second-line: disease modifying antirheumatic drugs (DMARDs) **(Table 1.6)**
          - Anti-TNF medications (etanercept, adalimumab) should be discontinued 4 weeks before planned surgery because of the risk of infection.
          - Methotrexate combined with tetracycline is more effective than methotrexate alone.

Table 1.6 Disease Modifying Antirheumatic Drugs (DMARDs)

Methotrexate	Folate analogue	Anti-inflammatory, anti-neovascularization combined with tetracyclines (anti-collagenase activity)
Sulfasalazine		Mechanism unknown
Hydroxychloroquine		Blocks Toll-like receptor activity
Leflunomide		Inhibits pyrimidine synthesis
Etanercept	TNF antagonist (decoy receptor)	
Adalimumab	TNF antagonist (antibody to receptor)	
Infliximab	TNF antagonist (antibody to receptor)	
Golimumab	TNF antagonist (antibody to receptor)	
Certolizumab	TNF antagonist (antibody to receptor)	
Rituximab	CD20 antibody	Inhibits B cells
Abatacept	Binds CD80 and CD86	Inhibits B cells
Tocilizumab	IL-6 receptor inhibitor (antibody to receptor)	
Anakinra	IL-1 receptor antagonist	

Abbreviations: IL, interleukin; TNF, tumor necrosis factor.

b. Systemic lupus erythematosus
   - Chronic inflammatory disease, frequently HLA-DR3 and antinuclear antibody (ANA) positive
   - Most common in African-American women
   - Symptoms: butterfly malar rash, polyarthritis, nephritis, pancytopenia
   - Treatment: corticosteroids, possibly DMARDs

c. Polymyalgia rheumatica
   - Inflammatory condition causing stiffness and pain of shoulder and pelvic girdle
   - Elevated erythrocyte sedimentation rate (ESR), anemia
   - Associated with temporal arteritis, which may cause blindness if untreated; requires biopsy
   - Treatment: corticosteroids

d. Seronegative spondyloarthropathies
   - Negative rheumatoid factor titer and positive HLA-B27
   - Includes ankylosing spondylitis, psoriatic arthritis, and Reiter's syndrome (reactive arthritis), enteropathic arthritis (Crohn's and ulcerative colitis)

e. Ankylosing spondylitis
   - Positive for HLA-B27
   - Bilateral sacroiliitis, hip pain, rigid kyphotic spine deformity, and uveitis
   - Radiographic findings: sclerosis of sacroiliac joints, squaring of vertebrae, and vertebral syndesmophytes
   - Treatment: nonsteroidal anti-inflammatory drugs (NSAIDs), physical therapy, total hip arthroplasty (THA), and spine deformity correction

f. Psoriatic
   - HLA-B27 positive in about half of patients
   - Psoriatic plaques, entheses, dactylitis (sausage digits), tendonitis, plantar fasciitis, nail pitting
   - Treatment: DMARDs, possible operative intervention if failure including fusion, arthroplasty, or osteotomy.

g. Reiter's syndrome (reactive arthritis)
   - Oligoarticular arthritis, conjunctivitis, urethritis

- HLA-B27 in 80–90%
- Treatment: NSAIDs, physical therapy

h. Crystal deposition
- Gout
  - Monosodium urate crystals: negatively birefringent, needle-shaped crystals
  - Deposition in joints causing inflammation and pain, most common in first metatarsophalangeal joint
  - Radiographic findings: asymmetric polyarthropathy, well-defined erosions with sclerotic margins, overhanging bony edges, tophi
  - Treatment: oral NSAIDs (indomethacin), allopurinol or colchicine for chronic treatment
  - Surgical debridement indications: failure of nonoperative treatment
- Pseudogout
  - Calcium pyrophosphate deposition (CPPD): positively birefringent, rhomboid crystals
  - Associated with chondrocalcinosis
  - Calcified menisci and triangular fibrocartilage complex (TFCC)
- Ochronosis: caused by alkaptonuria, disorder of phenylalanine and tyrosine metabolism, causing build up of homogentisic acid
  - Deposition of homogentisic acid in joints and spine causes black coating on cartilage and arthritis
  - Black urine from excretion of homogentisic acid

II. Soft Tissue Physiology

1. Skeletal muscle
   - Muscle body architecture
     a. Epimysium surrounds muscles bundles.
     b. Perimysium surrounds muscle fascicles.
     c. Endomysium surrounds individual fibers.
   - Muscle body > fascicles > fibers (myoblast cell) > myofibrils > sarcomere
   - Sarcomere: basic contractile unit, bordered by Z lines **(Fig. 1.7)**
     a. Myosin, thick filament that contracts
     b. Actin, thin filament with docking points for myosin
     c. H band: only thick filaments (myosin)
     d. M line: attachment of thick filaments
     e. I band: only thin filaments (actin)
     f. Z line: attachment of thin filaments
     g. A band: entire length of thick filament, overlaps with ends of thin filament
   - Contraction sequence from motor neuron to muscle tension
     a. Action potential travels down axon and depolarizes motor end plate of motor neuron.
     b. Depolarization causes acetylcholine release from presynaptic vesicles into synaptic cleft.
        - **Botulinum A injections block presynaptic acetylcholine release.**
     c. Acetylcholine binds to receptor on muscle membrane, causing depolarization of muscle cell including sarcoplasmic reticulum.
        - Myasthenia gravis is caused by antibodies that block acetylcholine receptors.

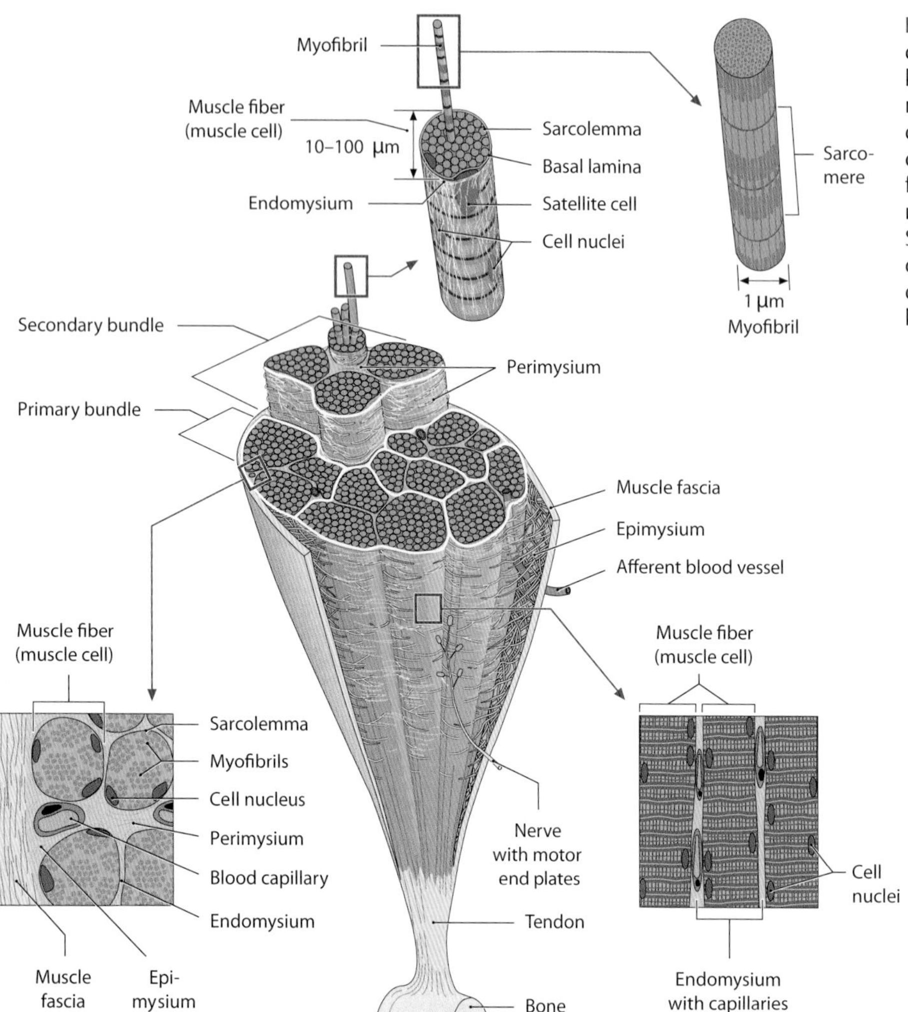

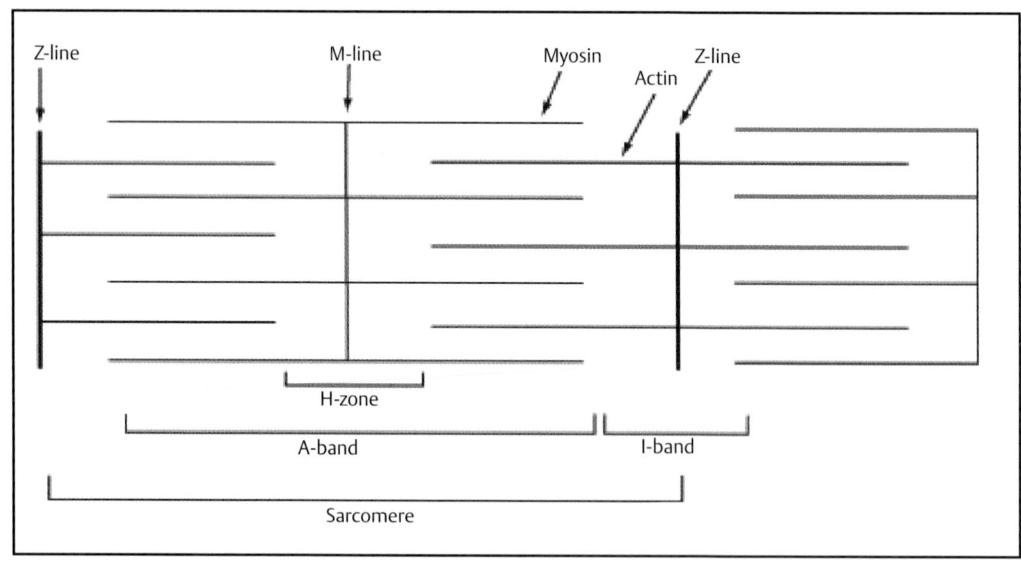

Fig. 1.7 Muscle structure. The muscle consists of basic subunits combined to form larger units, beginning with sarcomere to myofibril, fibers, fascicles, and finally muscles body. The endomysium surrounds individual fibers, the perimysium surrounds fascicles, and the epimysium surrounds muscle bundles. (**a:** From Schuenke M, Schulte E. General Anatomy and the Musculoskeletal System: Thieme Atlas of Anatomy. New York: Thieme; 2005. Illustration by Marcus Voll.)

- Depolarizing paralytics (e.g., succinylcholine) bind acetylcholine receptors, causing temporary depolarization.
- Nondepolarizing paralytics (e.g., curare) competitively inhibit acetylcholine receptor.

d. Depolarization causes release of calcium from sarcoplasmic reticulum, including transverse or t-tubules, into cytoplasm.

e. Calcium binds to troponin on actin filaments, which causes structure change in tropomyosin, exposing myosin binding site on actin.

f. Myosin binds to binding sites on actin in repetitive manner, causing contraction.

- Rigor mortis is caused by lack of ATP, which is required for release at each site.
- **Muscle that is overstretched is unable to generate maximal tension due to decreased overlap of actin and myosin.**

- Types of muscle contraction

a. Isotonic: constant muscle tension

b. Isometric: constant muscle length

c. Isokinetic: constant velocity

d. Concentric: muscle shortening

e. Eccentric: muscle lengthening

- Most efficient way to strengthen muscle; highest risk for tear/injury

f. Plyometric: rapid rate of contractions

- Muscle fiber types

a. Type 1 (red, slow-twitch, slow oxidative)

- Slow contraction, low strength, fatigue resistant, aerobic
- Small motor unit, high capillary density
- Perform endurance activities, posture/balance: first to be lost without rehabilitation

b. Type 2A (white, fast-twitch, fast oxidative glycolytic)

- Fast contraction, high strength, fatigable, anaerobic/aerobic mix
- Medium-size motor unit, high capillary density

c. Type 2B (fast glycolytic)

- Fast contraction, high strength, most fatigable, anaerobic
- Large motor unit, low capillary density

d. Type 2 (in general): high-intensity, short-duration activities, sprinting

- Energy chemical systems

a. Aerobic: Krebs cycle and oxidative phosphorylation

- Activity of longer duration

b. Anaerobic: lactic acid system

- Activity of 20–120 seconds

c. ATP: creatine phosphate system (phosphagen system)

- Activity of less than 20 seconds
- Basis for creatine phosphate supplementation

- Endocrine

a. Insulin: anabolic

b. Glucagon: catabolic

- Force of muscle contraction

a. Primarily dictated by cross-sectional area of muscle

b. Muscle length (amount stretched) affects contraction force through Blix curve

   c. Muscle fiber type primarily affects duration and speed of contraction, not force
- Types of exercise/training
   a. Sprint/strength training: motor unit recruitment, hyperplasia, and hypertrophy of type 2B fibers
   b. Endurance training: increase in muscle capillary density and hypertrophy of type 1 fibers
- Muscle injuries
   a. Contusion and soreness: resident mononucleated cells release signals to cause massive influx of neutrophils that in turn release inflammatory cytokines and free radicals. Macrophages follow to phagocytose debris.
   b. Strains: occur most often at myotendinous junction and with eccentric load

2. Nervous system (also see Chapter 9)
- Nerve architecture **(Fig. 1.8)**
   a. Epineurium: surrounds nerve
   b. Perineurium: covers nerve fascicle, provides tensile strength and prevents injury from edema by limiting diffusion
   c. Endoneurium: covers each fiber (nerve axon, Schwann cell, and myelin sheath)
- Charcot-Marie-Tooth (CMT) disease: progressive motor and sensory neuropathy
   a. Notable for cavo varus feet from anterior tibialis and peroneus brevis weakness
   b. Type I: demyelination, detectable by nerve conduction velocities
   c. Type II: axonopathy, minimal change to nerve conduction velocities
- Sensory receptors types
   a. Merkel's disks: cutaneous slowly adapting skin receptors that detect steady pressure, texture, and low frequency vibration, best evaluated by static two-point discrimination
   b. Meissner's corpuscles: cutaneous rapidly adapting skin receptors that are highly sensitive to touch

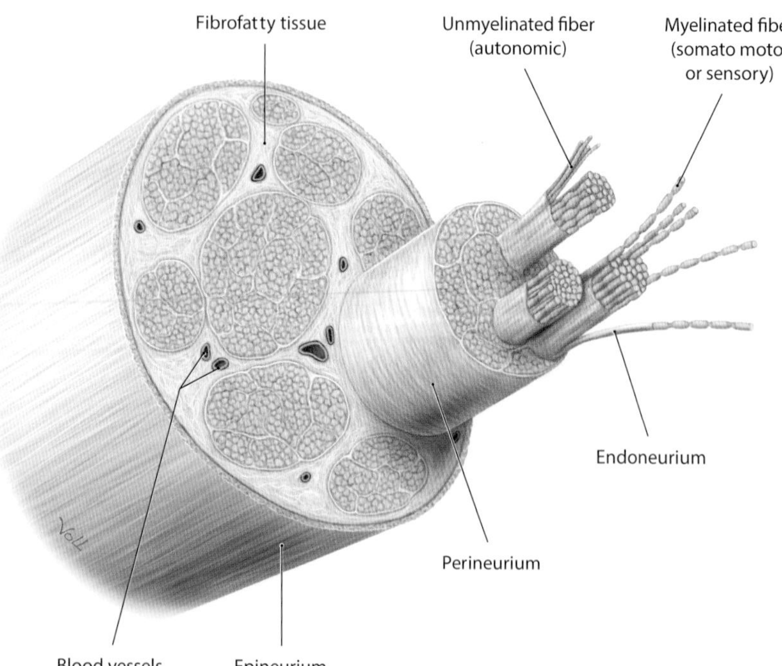

Fig. 1.8 Nerve structure. (From Schuenke M, Schulte E. General Anatomy and the Musculoskeletal System: Thieme Atlas of Anatomy. New York: Thieme; 2005. Illustration by Marcus Voll.)

c. Ruffini terminals: subcutaneous slowly adapting receptors that detect skin stretch
d. Pacinian corpuscles: subcutaneous large ovoid receptors that detect high-frequency vibrations and rapid indentations
e. Free nerve endings: pain

- Nerve injury (Seddon classification)
  a. Neurapraxia (first degree): reversible conduction block with no axonal disruption, good prognosis
  b. Axonotmesis (second degree): disruption of axon and myelin sheath but epineurium remains intact, fair prognosis
  c. Neurotmesis (third degree): complete disruption including epineurium, poor prognosis, may benefit from surgical repair
- Wallerian degeneration: distal axon and myelin sheath degeneration after second- or third-degree injuries
- Chronic compression syndromes
  a. Characterized by Schwann cell proliferation and apoptosis
  b. Not primary axonal pathology, not wallerian degeneration
- Nerve repair and regeneration
  a. Regenerative potential in restoring motor function after graft repair dependent on length of nerve
     - Radial, musculocutaneous, and femoral more favorable
     - Median, ulnar, and tibial moderate
     - Peroneal least favorable
- Vitamin B12 deficiency causes peripheral sensory neuropathy.
- Nerve conduction velocity (NCV): detect speed of impulse along axon
  a. Measures distal motor latency, distal sensor latency, and conduction velocity
- Electromyography (EMG): detect electrical potential in activated muscle cells
  a. Measures fibrillations, sharp waves, motor recruitment, and insertional activity of muscle

3. Tendons/ligaments
   - Primarily type I collagen
   - Type III collagen found in early healing
   - Direct insertion—four zones:
     a. Zone 1: ligament/tendon (type I collagen)
     b. Zone 2: fibrocartilage (mostly type II and III collagen)
     c. Zone 3: calcified fibrocartilage (type II and X collagen)
     d. Zone 4: bone (type I collagen)
   - Indirect insertion (more common): superficial fibers insert into periosteum and deep fibers insert directly into bone via Sharpey fibers.
   - Anisotropic as mechanical properties vary with the direction of loading
   - Immobilization results in decreased tendon weight, stiffness, and strength
   - Platelet-rich plasma: no consensus on efficacy
     a. Calcium chloride is used to activate platelets and release growth factors.

III. Basic Biology

1. Cells
   - DNA: bases are ATGC, always double-stranded, found in nucleus
   - RNA: bases are AUGC, may be single- or double-stranded, found in nucleus or cytoplasm

- Four phases of cell cycle
  a. G1: initial growth/gap phase, diploid cells
  b. S: DNA replication and synthesis, tetraploid cells
  c. G2: second gap phase, tetraploid cells
  d. M: mitosis

2. Molecular biology tools
   - Cytogenetic analysis: detect chromosomal number, translocations, and rearrangements
   - Southern blot: detect presence and number of a specific DNA gene
   - Northern blot: detects presence and number of messenger RNAs (mRNAs)
   - **Western blot: detects protein and phosphorylation states**
   - Enzyme-linked immunosorbent assay (ELISA): detects the presence of a protein using antibodies, more sensitive than Western blot
   - Flow cytometry: sorts cells based on cell surface markers or cell cycle phase
   - Polymerase chain reaction (PCR): used to detect presence of a DNA sequence by amplifying a sequence using specific primers and DNA polymerase
   - Reverse transcription (RT)-PCR: mRNA reverse-transcribed to complementary DNA (cDNA), which can then be amplified with PCR to determine gene expression
     a. Real-time RT-PCR: more sensitive, can be done quantitatively to measure gene expression (mRNA) relative to a housekeeping gene
   - Plasmids: circular, extrachromosomal DNA that replicate independently and may be used to introduce genes into a cell

3. Cancer
   - Oncogenes
     a. Gene for proteins that stimulate growth
     b. Proto-oncogenes are the wild-type normal version of an oncogene that does not cause cancer unless mutated or overexpressed.
   - Tumor suppressor genes
     a. Restrain growth by regulating the cell cycle (e.g., p53, Rb)
   - Important tumor molecules
     a. E-cadherin, a cell adhesion molecule (CAM): decreased in tumor cells to allow release into bloodstream
     b. Integrin, also a CAM: on tumor cells, allows attachment to matrix
     c. Matrix metalloproteinases (MMPs): allow invasion of basement membrane
     d. CD44 glycoprotein: cell surface cytokine that allows binding to subendothelial basement membranes
     e. Vascular endothelial growth factor (VEGF): induces angiogenesis
     f. Chemokine ligand 12 (CXCL12): secreted by stromal cells of bone marrow, acts as a target for certain tumor cells that preferentially metastasize to bone
     g. Multidrug resistance gene 1 (*MDR1*): codes for membrane p-glycoprotein, an efflux pump that is associated with resistance to hydrophobic chemotherapy agents
     h. TNF-α: secreted by tumor cells to induce osteoblasts to secrete RANKL
     i. RANKL: secreted by tumor cells directly or by osteoblasts to activate osteoclasts
     j. TGF-β: when released from bone matrix by osteoclasts, acts as positive feedback to further activate tumor cells

4. Immunology
   - Innate immune response

   a. Complement system
   b. Involved in fracture, injury, and foreign body reaction; targeted by anti-inflammatory medication
   c. Initial defense against infections
- Cell-mediated immune response
   a. Antigen-presenting cells present antigen to the T cell through the major histocompatibility complex receptors, which activate the T cell.
- Humoral antibody-mediated immune response
   a. IgG most abundant (most commonly produced in multiple myeloma as well)
   b. IgM first to appear in serum after antigen exposure
   c. IgA found in secretions such as mucus, tears, saliva
   d. IgE prominent in allergic reactions and antiparasitic functions
   e. IgD role is unclear
- Hypersensitivity reactions
   a. Type I (immediate anaphylactic) mediated by IgE
   b. Type II (antibody dependent, cytotoxic) mediated by IgM and IgG
   c. Type III (immune complex) mediated by IgG and IgM antibodies bound to antigen and deposited in host tissues
   d. Type IV (delayed) occurs after 2–3 days and can be in response to orthopaedic metal implants

5. Genetics
   - Mendelian inheritance **(Fig. 1.9)**
   - Autosomal dominant (AD): one allele is mutated or absent to express phenotype, affects both sexes equally, does not skip generations
   - Autosomal recessive (AR): need both alleles mutated or absent to express phenotype, affect both sexes equally, may skip generations as unaffected parents may produce affected offspring
   - X-linked: affect males born to mothers whom are carriers of the disease, does not skip generations (unless no males)

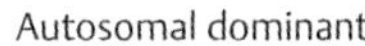

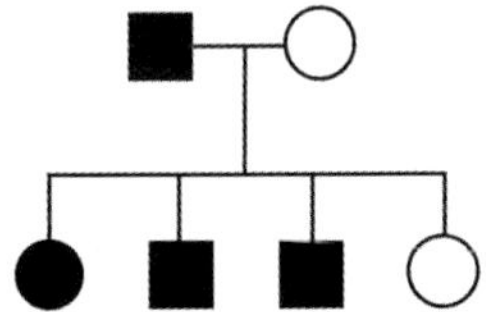

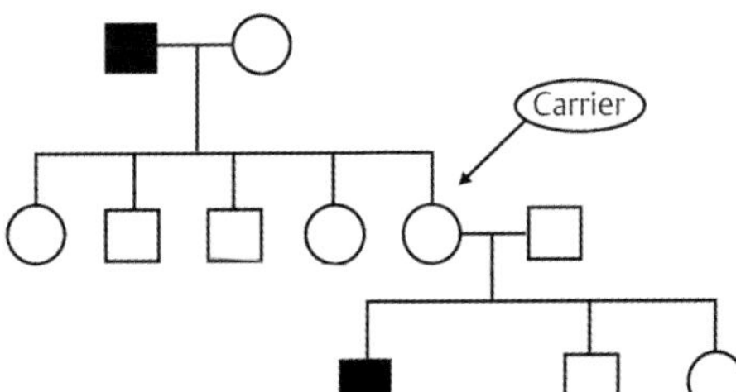

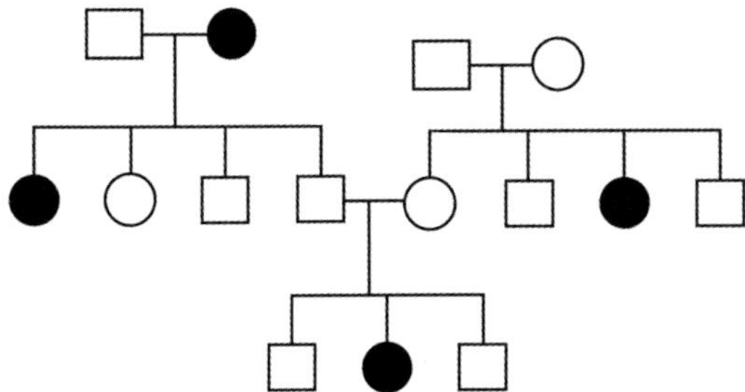

Fig. 1.9 Examples of pedigrees demonstrating different inheritance patterns.

- **Anticipation: occurs in hereditary diseases in which the disease presents earlier and more severely in affected offspring than in their parents**
  a. Example: Huntington's disease: CAG repeat on chromosome 4
- **Genomic imprinting: disease dependent on which parent contributes gene**
  a. Angelman: maternal defective gene (smiling facies, tremor, epilepsy)
  b. Prader-Willi: paternal defective gene (hypotonia, obesity, hyperphagism, hypogonadism)
- Prenatal testing performed by cytogenetic analysis of chromosomes to evaluate for number and quality.
- Commonly tested genetic diseases **(Table 1.7)**
  a. Achondroplasia [AD, FGF receptor 3 (FGFR-3), chondrocyte inhibition]
     - Gain of function increase in tyrosine kinase activity inhibiting chondrocyte differentiation in zone of proliferation
     - Rhizomelic (proximal) dwarfism, genu varum, foramen magnum stenosis, kyphosis, and spinal stenosis
  b. Diastrophic dysplasia [AR, *SLC26A2* gene, diastrophic dysplasia sulfate transporter (DTDST)]
     - Decreased sulfate groups on proteoglycans in cartilage causing defects
     - Cauliflower ear, tracheomalacia, abducted hitchhiker thumb, symphalangism (finger stiffness), C-spine kyphosis
  c. Cleidocranial dysplasia (AD, *CBFA1/Runx2*, osteoblast differentiation)
     - Dysplasia of midline bones formed by intramembranous ossification: skull, clavicles
  d. Schmid metaphyseal chondrodysplasia (type X collagen, enchondral ossification)
     - Short limbs and bowing of legs aggravated by walking
  e. Apert's syndrome (AD, FGFR-2, increased osteoblast activity)
     - Craniosynostosis and syndactyly
  f. Multiple epiphyseal dysplasia [AD, cartilage oligometric matrix protein (COMP)]
     - Short stature, irregular epiphyseal ossification, early-onset osteoarthritis
  g. Pseudoachondroplasia (AD, COMP)
     - Short stature, fragmented epiphyses, early arthritis

Table 1.7 Inheritance of Commonly Tested Orthopaedic Diseases

Autosomal Recessive	Autosomal Dominant	X-Linked Dominant	X-Linked Recessive
Osteogenesis imperfecta (types II and III)	Syndactyly/polydactyly	Hypophosphatemic rickets	Duchenne's muscular dystrophy
Sickle cell	Marfan's syndrome	Leri-Weill dyschondrosteosis	Becker's muscular dystrophy
Gaucher's	Achondroplasia		Hunter's syndrome
Friedreich's ataxia	Ehlers Danlos syndrome		Hemophilia
Diastrophic dysplasia	Osteogenesis imperfecta (types I and IV)		Spondyloepiphyseal dysplasia (SED)
Spinal muscular atrophy	Cleidocranial dysostosis		
Hypophosphatasia	Hereditary multiple exostosis		
Malignant, infantile osteopetrosis	Multiple epiphyseal dysplasia		
	Schmid and Jansen metaphyseal chondrodysplasia		
	Kniest dysplasia		
	Malignant hyperthermia		
	Osteochondromatosis		
	Mild, tarda osteopetrosis		

h. Mucopolysaccharidosis (lysosomal storage)
   - Hunter's syndrome (X-linked R, dermatan/heparan sulfate urinary excretion)
   - Hurler's syndrome (AR, α-L-iduronidase, dermatan/heparan sulfate urinary excretion)
   - Morquio syndrome (AR, lysosomal storage, keratan sulfate urinary excretion)

i. Gaucher's disease (AR, β-glucocerebrosidase, lysosomal storage, lipid storage)
   - Accumulation of cerebrosidase in cells
   - Bone pain, hepatosplenomegaly
   - Osteopenia, "moth-eaten" trabeculae
   - Avascular necrosis of the femoral head
   - Erlenmeyer flask deformity of the distal femur

j. Neurofibromatosis [NF; AD, NF1 (chromosome 17) codes neurofibromin, a tumor suppressor gene; NF2 (chromosome 22)]
   - Café-au-lait macules, neurofibromas, axillary or inguinal freckling, optic glioma, Lisch nodules (iris hamartomas)
   - Scoliosis, anterolateral tibial bowing and pseudarthrosis, and bone tumors
   - 5–13% lifetime risk of malignant peripheral nerve sheath tumor for NF1

k. Multiple hereditary exostoses [AD, exostosis 1 (EXT1) and EXT2/EXT3]
   - **Greater burden of disease and risk of malignancy with EXT1**

l. Charcot-Marie-Tooth type 1 (CMT 1) (AD, chromosome 1 or 17, demyelination)
   - Progressive motor and sensory neuropathy
   - Weakness of muscles innervated by peroneal nerve: anterior tibialis and peroneus brevis: causes cavo varus feet

6. Embryology
   - Limb development
     a. Apical ectodermal ridge (AER)
        - Directs proximal/distal growth of underlying mesoderm
        - Directs interdigital apoptosis
        - Congenital vascular injury causes a complete transverse absence of the limb.
     b. Zone of polarizing activity (ZPA): part of mesoderm
        - Sonic hedgehog *(Shh)* gene directs both anterior-posterior and radio-ulnar patterning (higher activity radial)
     c. Other genes
        - Homeobox *(Hox)* genes in mesoderm direct anterior-posterior
        - *Wnt* genes in non–apical ectodermal ridge (AER) direct dorsal-ventral (higher activity dorsal)
   - Spine development
     a. Somites: 52 paired mesodermal structures that develop cranial to caudal around the notochord and neural tube
     b. Somite layers
        - Sclerotome: forms vertebral bodies and annulus fibrosis (nucleus pulposus forms from notochord)
        - Myotome: forms muscle
        - Dermatome: forms skin
     c. Gene activity
        - *Hox* genes direct somatization

- *Shh* secreted by notochord in inducing development of surrounding tissue and more active ventral
- *Wnt* more active dorsal (same as in limbs)

IV. Infectious Disease

1. Septic arthritis
   - Pediatric
     a. Higher risk due to seeding in metaphysis from sluggish blood flow that then can erupt into joint
     b. *Staphylococcus aureus* most common across all age groups
     c. Newborn to 3 months
        - *S. aureus*, group B streptococcus, *Neisseria gonorrhoeae*, and Enterobacteriaceae
        - Treatment: nafcillin, oxacillin, or vancomycin [if concerned about methicillin-resistant *S. aureus* (MRSA)] with a third-generation cephalosporin
        - Blood cultures often positive
     d. Children
        - *S. aureus*, *Streptococcus pneumoniae*, group A streptococci, and *Haemophilus influenzae*
        - Treatment: vancomycin and a third-generation cephalosporin
   - Adolescent/adult
     a. Higher risk with rheumatoid arthritis, intravenous drug use
     b. *S. aureus*, *N. gonorrhoeae* (if sexually active), streptococci, gram-negative bacilli
     c. Treatment: vancomycin with a third-generation cephalosporin
        - If Gram stain shows only gram-positive cocci, replace cephalosporin with fluoroquinolone.
   - Treatment:
     a. Narrow antibiotics from culture (blood or synovial)
     b. Surgical (open or arthroscopic) debridement or daily aspiration
2. Acute hematogenous osteomyelitis: from vascular seeding
   - Pediatric
     a. Newborn to 3 months
        - Same bacteria as for septic joint but no *N. gonorrhoeae*
        - Treatment: same coverage as for septic joint, and blood cultures often positive
     b. Children
        - *S. aureus* and group A streptococci
        - Treatment: nafcillin, oxacillin, or vancomycin (third-generation cephalosporin only necessary if suspicion for gram-negative bacilli)
   - Adult
     a. Most common *S. aureus*
     b. Treatment: nafcillin, oxacillin, or vancomycin
   - **Sequestrum: avascular necrotic bone**
   - **Involucrum: healthy bone from the periosteum that walls off sequestrum**
   - Treatment
     a. Narrow the antibiotic options based on blood culture or deep culture (aspiration or drainage).
     b. Debridement if abscess or no improvement with antibiotics

3. Acute direct osteomyelitis: from direct open wound/fracture/surgical site
   - *S. aureus, Pseudomonas aeruginosa,* gram-negative bacilli, but often polymicrobial in immunocompromised patient
   - Treatment: empiric vancomycin and third-generation cephalosporin until cultures return
4. Subacute osteomyelitis
   - Unlike acute osteomyelitis, no systemic signs, minimal local signs, and white blood cell count (WBC) and blood cultures often normal
   - Brodie's abscess: most often in metaphysis of femur or tibia
   - Treatment: surgical drainage and antibiotics (usually for *S. aureus*)
5. Chronic osteomyelitis
   - Often characterized by occult infection with acute flares, resulting from missed or inappropriately treated acute osteomyelitis
   - Cierny classification
     a. Anatomic type
        - Stage 1: medullary
        - Stage 2: superficial
        - Stage 3: localized
        - Stage 4: diffuse
     b. Physiological type
        - A: Normal host
        - B: Systemically compromised (Bs), locally compromised host (Bl)
        - C: Treatment is worse than the infection for the host.
   - *S. aureus, P. aeruginosa,* Enterobacteriaceae
   - Treatment: requires deep debridement and intravenous antibiotics directed by results of culture (does not require empiric coverage prior to culture)
6. Specific tested infections **(Table 1.8)**
   - **Sickle cell osteomyelitis and septic arthritis**
     a. *Salmonella* most characteristic
     b. *Staphylococcus* most common
   - Necrotizing fasciitis
     a. Swelling, pain out of proportion to exam, crepitus, bullae, "dishwater pus," sepsis

Table 1.8 Culture Medium Requirements for Different Bacteria

Organism	Culture Medium
Staphylococcus aureus	Blood
Streptococcus	Blood
Kingella kingae	Blood
Mycobacterium tuberculosis	Lowenstein Jensen
Mycobacterium avium	Lowenstein Jensen or Middlebrook
Neisseria	Thayer-Martin
Escherichia coli	Luria Bertani
Haemophilus	Blood
Actinobacillus	Blood
Cardiobacterium	Blood
Eikenella	Blood
Propionibacterium acnes	Blood (extended, 14–21 days)

b. Diabetes is the most common risk factor, but half of cases occur in healthy patients.

c. Most commonly polymicrobial

d. Group A β-hemolytic streptococci most common in otherwise healthy patients

e. Treatment: debridement back to healthy tissue, antibiotics, resuscitation

- Bites
  a. Human bite associated with *Eikenella corrodens*
  b. Cat bite associated with *Pasteurella multocida*
    - Cat scratch is from *Bartonella henselae*, associated with epitrochlear adenopathy
  c. Tick (*Ixodes dammini* or *Ixodes pacificus*) bite associated with *Borrelia burgdorferi* in lime disease
- Rabies: from saliva of rabid animals
  a. Treatment: infiltrate immunoglobulin around bite with remainder injected intramuscularly (IM) and vaccine IM (five doses over 4 weeks)
  b. Healthy dog or cat bite: observe animal for 10 days and if begins to have symptoms, initiate treatment
  c. Suspected rabid dog or cat bite: initiate treatment
  d. Bites from wild animal associated with rabies (bats, raccoons, foxes): initiate treatment
- Foot puncture wounds (through glue in shoe): *P. aeruginosa*
- Intravenous drug use: MRSA, *P. aeruginosa*
- Renal dialysis: *S. aureus*
- Marine exposure: brackish water and shellfish associated with *Vibrio vulnificus*, treat with third-generation cephalosporin; also *Mycobacterium marinum*
- Intestinal and hematologic malignancy: associated with *Clostridium septicum* infection
- Health care related exposure from contaminated needle
  a. HIV: 0.3% risk
  b. Hepatitis C: 3% risk
  c. Hepatitis B: 30% risk

7. Antibiotic prophylaxis
- Perioperative prophylaxis (controversial)
  a. General practice to give 24 hours coverage in patients having implants, bone graft, or large dissection
  b. No evidence to support use beyond first preoperative dose
- Dental prophylaxis after total joint arthroplasty (also controversial)
  a. Previous recommendations:
    - 2 g amoxicillin or cephalexin 1 hour prior to procedure
    - If penicillin allergic, 600 mg of clindamycin
    - First 2 years after surgery for all patients
    - Lifetime if immunocompromised or susceptible, including inflammatory arthropathy, diabetes, and previous joint infection
  b. Current American Academy of Orthopaedic Surgeons/American Dental Association (AAOS/ADA) recommendations
    - Consider changing from dental prophylaxis (strength: limited)
    - Maintain good oral hygiene (strength: consensus)
- Open fractures

a. Indicated treatments: immediate antibiotic prophylaxis and early adequate surgical debridement (no defined time frame)

b. Gustilo and Anderson classification

- **Grade I and II: first-generation cephalosporin**
- **Grade III: add aminoglycoside (although no literature)**
- **Farm or fecal contamination: add penicillin**

c. Tetanus vaccine if three or more vaccines in the past (completed series) but the last one over 3 years ago. Tetanus vaccine and immunoglobulin if less than three vaccines in the past (incomplete series).

d. No evidence to support: antibiotics in irrigation solution or high-pressure pulsatile lavage

- Postsplenectomy

a. Vaccines: pneumococcal, meningococcal group C, and *H. influenzae* type B

b. Lifelong antibiotic prophylaxis (controversial)

8. Specific antibiotic (mechanism of action, coverage, complications)

- Penicillins (penicillin, ampicillin, nafcillin, piperacillin)

a. Bactericidal, inhibits transpeptidate involved in cell wall synthesis/cross-linking

b. Treatment: gram-positive coverage (piperacillin for gram negative)

c. Complications: hypersensitivity reaction, hemolytic anemia

d. Resistance: *mecA* gene, found in MRSA, provides resistance to β-lactam antibiotics

- Cephalosporins

a. Same mechanism and allergic reaction as penicillins

b. First generation (cefazolin, cephalexin): gram positive

c. Second generation (cefoxitin): more gram negative

d. Third generation (ceftriaxone, cefepime): gram negative, less gram positive

- Vancomycin

a. Bactericidal/bacteriostatic, inhibits cell wall synthesis (cross-linking)

b. Treatment: gram positive, MRSA, *Clostridium difficile*

c. Complications: red man syndrome, ototoxic, nephrotoxic

d. When mixed with polymethylmethacrylate, maximum amount is 5% by weight or 2 g in 40 g of cement before affecting mechanical strength

- Aminoglycosides (gentamicin, tobramycin)

a. Bactericidal, irreversibly binds ribosome (30s subunit)

b. Treatment: gram negative and polymicrobial

c. Complications: ototoxic (auditory and vestibular), nephrotoxic

- Tetracyclines (tetracycline, doxycycline, minocycline)

a. Bacteriostatic, blocks transfer RNA (tRNA) from ribosome (30s subunit)

b. Treatment: *Rickettsia*, *Mycoplasma*, Lyme

c. Complications: hepatotoxicity, impairs growth, tooth discoloration

- Macrolides (erythromycin, azithromycin, clarithromycin)

a. Bacteriostatic, reversibly binds ribosome (50s subunit)

b. Treatment: gram positive

c. Complications: ototoxic

- Clindamycin

a. Bacteriostatic, binds ribosome (50s subunit)

b. Treatment: gram positive

c. Separate class from macrolides but some cross-resistance, determined by D-zone test (positive test denotes resistance to erythromycin and inducible resistance to clindamycin)

- Linezolid
  a. Bactericidal/bacteriostatic, binds ribosome [23S ribosomal RNA (rRNA) of 50s subunit]
  b. Treatment: resistant gram positive
  c. Complications: is a monoamine oxidase inhibitor (MAOI) and can induce serotonin syndrome: treated with benzodiazepines
- Fluoroquinolones (ciprofloxacin, levofloxacin)
  a. Bactericidal, inhibits DNA gyrase, inhibiting DNA unwinding to allow replication
  b. Treatment: gram negative, some gram positive
  c. Equivalent in intravenous and oral formulations
  d. Complications: risk of tendon rupture, concern for cartilage erosion in pediatrics, toxic to chondrocytes in animal model
- Rifampin
  a. Bactericidal, inhibits RNA polymerase, RNA transcription
  b. Treatment: for *Staphylococcus* and tuberculosis
  c. Complications: hepatotoxic
  d. Lipophilic structure allows high cellular penetration, effective in conjunction with other antibiotics
  e. Rapid resistance development when used alone
  f. Often used for *S. aureus* in conjunction with another antibiotic when hardware is present
- Trimethoprim/sulfamethoxazole
  a. Bacteriostatic, inhibits folate metabolism
  b. Treatment: urinary flora, gram negative, MRSA
  c. Complications: anemia, thrombocytopenia
- Bacitracin
  a. Bactericidal
  b. Treatment: gram-positive bacteria, particularly *S. aureus*
  c. Topical use only, systemically toxic

9. Mechanisms of antibiotic resistance
   - Beta-lactamase hydrolyzes β-lactams (resistance to penicillin, ampicillin)
   - *mecA* mutation alters the target penicillin binding protein (PBPa) to have a low affinity to penicillins (MRSA resistance to all penicillins)
   - Altered cell wall permeability (tetracyclines, quinolones, trimethoprim, penicillins)
   - Efflux pumps (erythromycin and tetracycline)
   - Altered peptidoglycan subunits (vancomycin)

V. Perioperative Complications

1. Deep venous thrombosis (DVT)/pulmonary embolism (PE)
   - Mechanism
     a. Virchow's triad—hypercoagulable state, venous stasis, endothelial injury—increases the risk of thromboembolic events.
     b. Thromboplastin released after damage to endothelial vessel walls: activates extrinsic clotting pathway, factor VII, ultimately leading to conversion of fibrinogen to fibrin and clot formation

c. Risk factors: previous DVT/PE, hypercoagulable states (factor V Leiden, prothrombin gene mutation, protein C/S deficiency, antithrombin III (ATIII) deficiency, phospholipid antibodies: lupus anticoagulant, cancer, elevated homocysteine levels)

- Prophylaxis

a. AAOS 2013 recommendations for total joint arthroplasty
   - Postoperative DVT screening ultrasound not recommended
   - Discontinue antiplatelet medications preoperatively
   - Pharmacological agents or mechanical compressive devices should be used routinely
   - No specific recommendation against or in favor of specific pharmacological agents
   - Patients with prior thromboembolic event should receive both pharmacological and mechanical prophylaxis
   - Patients with bleeding disorder or active liver disease should receive mechanical prophylaxis
   - Early mobilization
   - No clear evidence for inferior vena cava (IVC) filters in patients with contraindication to pharmacological prophylaxis

b. American College of Chest Physicians 2012 recommendations
   - For total joint arthroplasty, heparin, low-molecular-weight heparin (LMWH), fondaparinux, apixaban, dabigatran, rivaroxaban, Coumadin, aspirin, or mechanical compression device
   - For hip fracture surgery, heparin, LMWH, fondaparinux, Coumadin, aspirin, or mechanical compression device
   - LMWH should be stopped before 12 hours preoperatively and started after 12 hours postoperatively
   - LMWH is pharmacological agent that is preferred [THA and total knee arthroplasty (TKA)]
   - Prophylaxis should be for 35 days postoperatively
   - For inpatient setting, recommend pharmacological agent and mechanical device
   - For high bleeding risk patients, recommend mechanical device alone or no prophylaxis
   - For injuries distal to knee and knee arthroscopy, recommend no pharmacological prophylaxis
   - Similar to AAOS, no role for IVC filter even if contraindications exist for pharmacological prophylaxis and no role for routine DVT screening

c. All pharmacological prophylaxis: risk of major bleeding if recent GI bleed, recent hemorrhagic stroke, or bleeding disorder

- Specific anticoagulants **(Fig. 1.10)**

a. Coumadin (warfarin)
   - Does not directly inhibit vitamin K, which acts as a cofactor in the carboxylation of clotting factors
   - Acts by inhibiting vitamin K 2,3-epoxide reductase, enzyme that reduces the oxidized "used" vitamin K epoxide into active vitamin K hydroquinone
   - Affects vitamin K–dependent clotting factors (II, VII, IX, X, protein C and S). Mnemonic: 2 (II) + 7 (VII) = 9 (IX) plus one more = 10 (X).
   - If protein C or S deficient, will have transient hypercoagulability with initiation of treatment
   - **Warfarin-induced skin necrosis: rapid reduction in protein C causes hypercoagulable state with fibrin thrombi forming in cutaneous vessels.**
   - Vitamin K given to reverse action of Coumadin

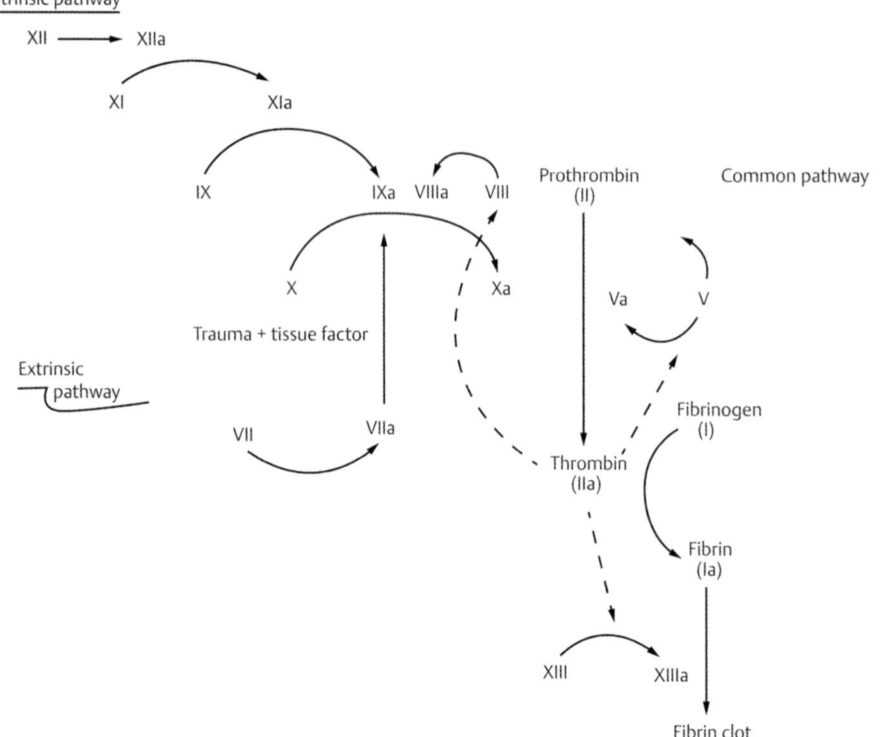

Fig. 1.10 The normal clotting cascade with intrinsic and extrinsic pathways.

b. Heparin
   - Increases activity of antithrombin III, which then inhibits factor Xa (primarily) and IIa
   - LMWH (enoxaparin): increased risk (similar to Coumadin) of postoperative hematoma, retroperitoneal hematoma, and wound complications as compared with aspirin, clopidogrel, or mechanical compressive devices.
   - **Protamine: neutralizes heparin/LMWH by forming stable compound**

c. Fondaparinux (Arixtra): similar mechanism as heparin but complex with antithrombin III specifically targets Xa

d. Rivaroxaban (Xarelto): direct factor Xa inhibitor, no antidote

e. Aspirin
   - Irreversible inhibition of thromboxane A_2 formation leading to diminished platelet aggregation

f. Gingko and ginseng inhibit platelets, increasing bleeding and postoperative hematoma

g. Hirudin: inhibits thrombin

- Workup of pulmonary embolism
  a. Symptoms: calf pain, fever, tachypnea, tachycardia (most common symptom)
  b. Signs: Hypoxia ($Pao_2 < 80$ mm Hg), hypocapnic ($Paco_2 < 35$ mm Hg), high A-a gradient (> 20 mm Hg). Pulse oximetry is not reliable compared with arterial blood gas values, as hyperventilation can maintain normal pulse oximetry values.
  c. Duplex venous ultrasound: most sensitive and specific test for DVT

d. Helical chest computed tomography (CT): first-line imaging study for identifying PE

- Pneumatic compression devices

  a. Increase venous blood flow, decrease venous compliance

  b. Enhance endothelial derived fibrinolysis

2. Fat embolism
   - Embolic marrow fat damages endothelium of pulmonary capillary beds
   - Risk factors: long bone fracture, intramedullary nailing, hip and knee arthroplasty, intramedullary cutting alignment guides for arthroplasty, cement pressurization of femoral canal
   - Signs: tachycardia, tachypnea, hypoxemia, altered mental status, axillary and subconjunctival petechiae, respiratory failure, acute respiratory distress syndrome (ARDS)
   - Imaging: CT angiography normal
   - Treatment: supportive
   - Prevention: early fracture stabilization
3. Wound healing (also see Chapter 10)
   - Wagner grading system for diabetic foot ulcers
     a. Grade 0: intact skin
     b. Grade 1: superficial ulcer
     c. Grade 2: deep ulcer with exposed ligaments, tendon, capsule, or deep fascia without abscess or osteomyelitis
     d. Grade 3: deep ulcer with abscess or osteomyelitis
     e. Grade 4: localized gangrene
     f. Grade 5: extensive gangrene
   - Negative predictors of healing:
     a. Transcutaneous oxygen < 30–40 mm Hg
     b. Ankle brachial index < 0.5
     c. Albumin < 3.0 g/dL
     d. Total lymphocyte count < 1,500/mm^3
   - Hyperbaric oxygen therapy
     a. Increased oxygen gradient for greater diffusion
     b. For adjunctive treatment of gas gangrene, crush injury, compartment syndrome, necrotizing fasciitis, chronic osteomyelitis, burns, and flaps
     c. Contraindications: pneumothorax, ongoing chemotherapy or radiation therapy, bleomycin, chronic obstructive pulmonary disease, and pressure-sensitive implanted medical devices (e.g., insulin pump, pacemaker)

VI. Anesthesia/Pain Control

1. Anesthesia issues/complications
   - Nitrous oxide, used as induction agent, crosses from blood into the bowel and causes gaseous abdominal distention.
     a. Should be avoided in cases that require fluoroscopy of the lower spine or pelvis
2. Local anesthetics: blocks depolarization phase of neuron action potential
   a. Amides (lidocaine/Xylocaine, bupivacaine/Marcaine)
   b. Esters (procaine/Novocain, ethyl aminobenzoate/Benzocaine)
   - Intra-articular infusions of lidocaine have been documented to cause chondrolysis, particularly in the shoulder.

- Interscalene block: targets brachial plexus between anterior and middle scalene muscles
  a. Most common complication is sensory neuropathy
- Supraclavicular block: targets brachial plexus superior to clavicle
  a. Complications include pneumothorax

3. Narcotics
   - In obese patients, intravenous narcotics should be dosed by ideal body weight and not actual body weight for safe and appropriate dosing
4. Nonsteroidal anti-inflammatory drugs (NSAIDs) **(Fig. 1.11)**
   - Inhibits constitutively expressed cyclooxygenase-1 (COX-1) and inducible COX-2
     a. Both COX-1 and -2 convert arachidonic acid into prostaglandins.
     b. COX-1 expressed as "housekeeping" gene throughout body:
        - Protection of gastric mucosa
        - Vasodilation of renal afferent arterioles
        - Platelet aggregation
     c. COX-2 unexpressed in most cells but elevated in inflammation
   - Indications: pain, fever, heterotopic ossification
   - Contraindications: renal disease, gastric ulcers, congestive heart failure
   - Types:
     a. COX inhibitors (ibuprofen, naproxen)
        - Reversible inhibition of COX-1 and -2
     b. Aspirin
        - Irreversible inhibition of COX (upstream of thromboxane A_2)
     c. COX-2 selective inhibitors (celecoxib/Celebrex)
        - Spares COX-1 activity in stomach, kidneys, and platelets
        - Specific concern for cardiac toxicity
   - Complications:
     a. Renal failure, gastric ulcers, platelet inhibition, congestive heart failure exacerbation
     b. Gastric bleeding is a particular issue due to the combination of both increasing gastric ulcers and decreasing platelet activity.
     c. COX-2 downregulation in mice shown to delay endochondral ossification of fracture healing, but no conformational human studies
     d. Increases risk of nonunion in posterior spinal fusion

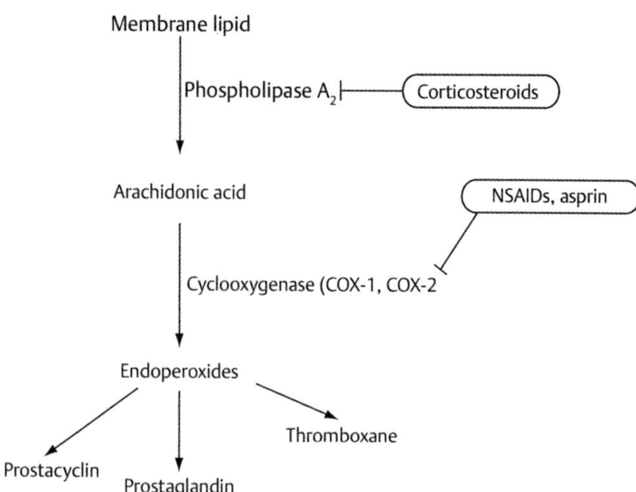

Fig. 1.11 The arachidonic acid pathway with the site of corticosteroid and nonsteroidal anti-inflammatory medication effects. NSAID, nonsteroidal anti-inflammatory drug.

5. Acetaminophen **(Fig. 1.10)**
   - Inhibits prostaglandin E_2 production through IL-1β, no effect on cyclooxygenase
6. **Corticosteroids (Fig. 1.10)**
   - Inhibit phospholipase A_2 to inhibit arachidonic acid formation (works upstream of NSAIDs)
   - Induces osteoporosis by inhibiting osteoblast, activating osteoclasts, and causing secondary hyperparathyroidism
   - **Complications of injections: pain, bleeding, local flare, skin pigmentation changes, fat atrophy, facial flushing, elevated blood sugars**
7. Iontophoresis: direct current drives ions and medications into deep tissue

VII. Imaging Studies

1. Nuclear medicine
   - Technetium-99m phosphate bone scan: initially in blood and then deposited in bone
     a. First phase: immediate, blood flow in arterial system
     b. Second phase: 30 minutes, blood pool, distribution in vasculature
     c. Third phase: 4 hours, accumulation in bone
     d. Detects infection, occult fractures, tumor, arthroplasty loosening, avascular necrosis
   - WBC labeled bone scan (indium-111 or technetium-99m)
     a. Detects infections
2. Magnetic resonance imaging (MRI)
   - **T1-weighted**
     a. Fat is bright
     b. High signal-to-noise ratio, good for anatomic definition
   - **T2-weighted**
     a. Water is bright (cerebrospinal fluid, blood, soft tissue tumor)
     b. Contrasts pathology best (edema)
   - Gadolinium contrast
     a. Enhances edema in T1-weighted images
   - Field strength
     a. 3.0 tesla (T) has nine times the field strength of 1.5-T machine
     b. Higher field strength leads to higher signal-to-noise ratio
     c. 3.0 T no difference in sensitivity or specificity for meniscal or anterior cruciate ligament (ACL) tears compared with 1.5 T

VIII. Clinical Trials

1. Types of trials
   - Randomized controlled trial (RCT): subjects are divided randomly into controls and experimental groups; reduces selection bias, reduces confounders, and allows for blinding
     a. Double-blinded RCT: patient and physician/evaluator blinded to treatment group; for surgical trial would require sham surgery
   - Case-control study: subjects and controls selected based on having or not having a disease and risk factors are examined retrospectively; produces odds ratio (OR) statistics
   - Cohort study: follows subjects (prospectively or retrospectively) after a particular event; produces relative risk (RR) statistics
   - Case series: retrospective review of outcomes of a series of patients with a particular disease or condition
2. Types of bias
   - Crossover: patients from one treatment arm change to the other treatment being tested
   - Washout period: time between two therapies in a crossover study allows for the first therapy to "wear off"
   - Recall: different likelihood of test subjects in recalling exposures
   - Detection: more careful attention to outcomes in one group compared with other treatment groups
   - Selection: due to inappropriate selection of subjects in treatment groups, avoided by RCT

3. Levels of evidence

- **Level 1: high-quality RCT; meta-analysis**
- **Level 2: lesser quality RCTs: RCTs that are unblinded, improperly randomized, have less than 80% follow-up; prospective cohort studies (with exposure or treatment beginning after the onset of the study)**
- **Level 3: retrospective cohort and case-control studies**
- **Level 4: case series**
- **Level 5: case reports, expert opinion, anecdotal evidence**

4. Other factors
   - Power: important for ensuring that a study has enough patients to be clinically relevant and to detect statistically significant differences in results
   - Intention to treat: analysis of results based on original randomization or assignment, eliminates crossover bias but more difficult to demonstrate a difference between groups
   - Inclusion/exclusion criteria
     a. Stricter criteria: more homogeneous but less generalizable
     b. Less stringent criteria: less homogeneous but more generalizable

2

Musculoskeletal Oncology and Pathology

Amanda Fantry, Alan Schiller, Robin N. Kamal, and Richard M. Terek

I. Workup and Staging

A. Workup for Bone Lesion (Fig. 2.1)

1. Biopsy should be performed by treating surgeon at a sarcoma center.
2. Common reason for referral to orthopaedic oncologist is incomplete excision of an unknown sarcoma. Always refer suspicious lesions to surgeon at a sarcoma center.
3. Regardless of a known primary, a new lesion without a previous diagnosis of metastatic bone disease should be biopsied.

B. Workup for Soft Tissue Sarcoma

See Soft Tissue Tumors section, below.

C. Staging

Stage is the most important prognostic factor for survival.

1. Enneking staging for malignant bone tumors **(Table 2.1)**
2. Enneking staging for benign bone tumors
   - Stage 1: latent [nonossifying fibroma (NOF), enchondroma]
   - Stage 2: active [aneurysmal bone cyst (ABC)/unicameral bone cyst (UBC), chondroblastoma]
   - Stage 3: aggressive (giant cell tumor of bone)
3. American Joint Committee on Cancer (AJCC) staging for malignant bone tumors **(Table 2.2)**
   - Stage is most important prognostic factor for survival.
   - Presence or absence of metastatic disease has most significant impact on long-term survival of a primary bone sarcoma.
4. AJCC staging for soft tissue sarcomas **(Table 2.3)**

D. Treatment

1. Goal is to remove lesion with minimal risk of recurrence.

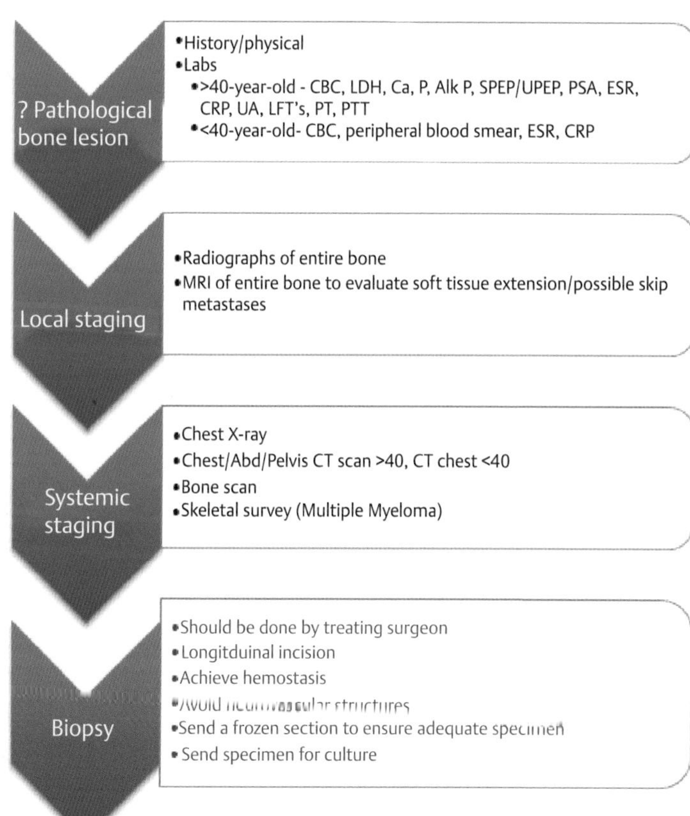

Fig. 2.1 Workup of bone lesion. Abd, abdomen; Alk P, alkaline phosphatase; Ca, calcium; CBC, complete blood count; CRP, C-reactive protein; CT, computed tomography; ESR, erythrocyte sedimentation rate; LDH, lactate dehydrogenase; LFT, liver function test; MRI, magnetic resonance imaging; P, phosphorus; PSA, prostate-specific antigen; PT, prothrombin time; PTT, partial thromboplastin time; SPEP, serum protein electrophoresis; UA, uranalysis; UPEP, urine protein electrophoresis.

Table 2.1 Enneking System for Staging Malignant Bone Tumors

Stage	Description
IA	Low grade, intracompartmental (no soft tissue involvement)
IB	Low grade, extracompartmental (penetration of cortex)
IIA	High grade, intracompartmental
IIB	High grade, extracompartmental
IIIA	Metastasis, intracompartmental
III B	Metastasis, extracompartmental

Note: Low grade: well or moderately differentiated. High grade: poorly differentiated.

- Local control versus amputation: must be equal in outcomes and remaining limb must be functional
- Criteria for amputation:
    a. Cannot obtain adequate surgical margin
    b. Unacceptably high morbidity
    c. Nonfunctional resulting limb
    d. Continued tumor growth
    e. Tumor encases major neurovascular bundles (relative)
        - Sciatic nerve involvement does not necessitate amputation, as balanced palsy can be managed with orthoses.

2. Surgical margins **(Fig. 2.2)**
    - Intralesional: within tumor
    - Marginal: through reactive zone around tumor
    - Wide: cuff of normal tissue surrounding
    - Radical: removal of entire compartment
3. Adjuvant therapy
    - Chemotherapy: multiagent chemotherapy for osteogenic sarcoma and Ewing's sarcoma with improved survival and limb salvage
        a. Mechanism of chemotherapy: induction of apoptosis
        b. For both osteogenic sarcoma and Ewing's sarcoma, preoperative chemotherapy followed by restaging, surgery, and then additional chemotherapy
        c. Chemotherapy controversial for soft tissue sarcomas
        d. Common chemotherapy agents **(Table 2.4)**
    - Radiation: used for Ewing's sarcoma, lymphoma, myeloma, metastatic bone disease, soft tissue sarcoma
        a. Preoperative versus postoperative radiation risks and benefits for sarcoma

Table 2.2 American Joint Committee on Cancer (AJCC) System for Staging Malignant Bone Tumors

Stage	Description
IA	Low grade, < 8 cm
IB	Low grade, > 8 cm
IIA	High grade, < 8 cm
IIB	High grade, > 8 cm
III	Discontinuous tumor; skip lesions (any grade)
IVA	Metastasis to lungs (any grade)
IVB	Metastasis to regional lymph nodes, or another distant site (any grade)

Note: Low grade: well or moderately differentiated. High grade: poorly differentiated.

Table 2.3 American Joint Committee on Cancer (AJCC) System for Staging Soft Tissue Sarcomas

Stage	Description
IA	Low grade, < 5 cm
IB	Low grade, > 5 cm
IIA	High grade, < 5 cm
IIB	High grade, > 5 cm
III	Metastasis to regional lymph nodes (any grade)
IV	Distant metastasis (any grade)

Note: Tumors are staged as T1 (< 5 cm in greatest dimension) or T2 (> 5 cm in greatest dimension). Tumor further qualified as T1a/T2a (superficial tumor) or T1b/T2b (subfascial tumor).

- Preoperative radiation
  - Benefits: requires lower dose than postoperative (50 Gy), decreased surrounding edema, capsule formation around tumor
  - Risks: delayed wound healing, wound complication (30%), infection
- Postoperative radiation
  - Risks: fibrosis, fractures, joint stiffness, wound healing complications, higher dose of radiation required (66 Gy) to larger treatment field

b. Risk factors for pathologic fracture postradiotherapy: female, higher dose of radiation (> 60 Gy), age > 60 years, periosteal stripping during tumor excision

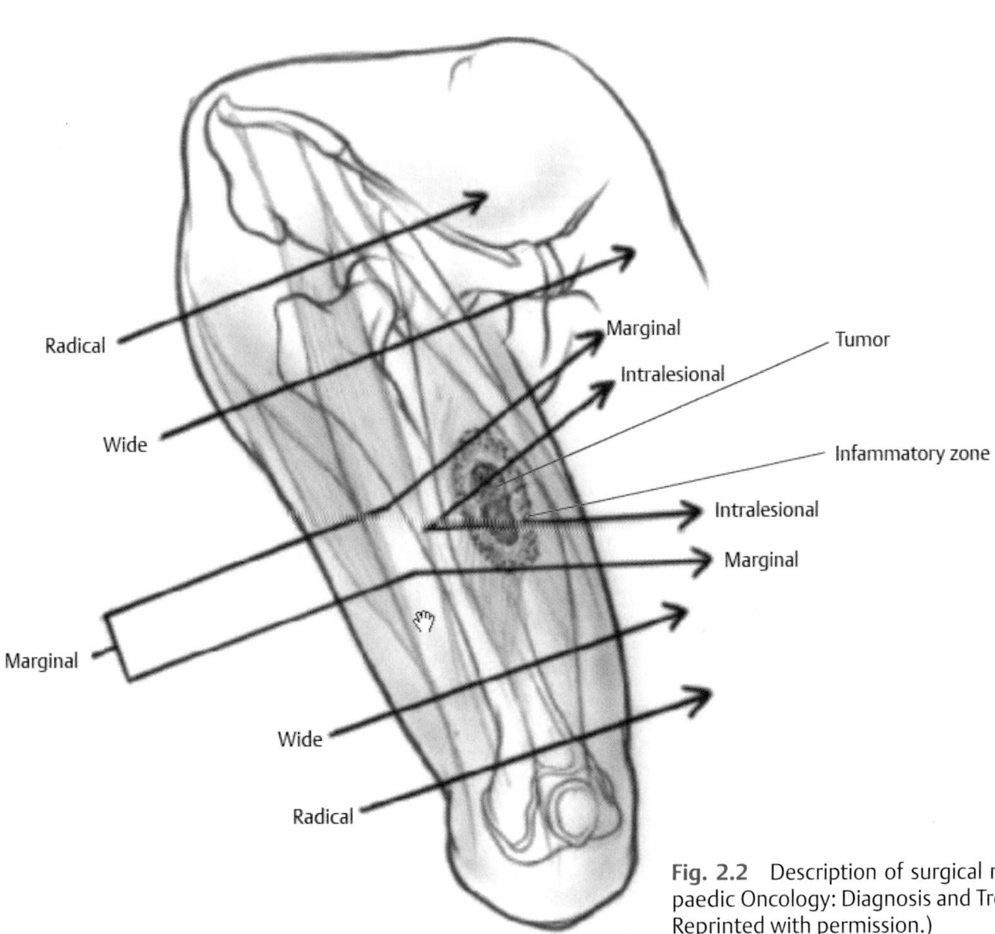

Fig. 2.2 Description of surgical margins. (From Conrad EU. Orthopaedic Oncology: Diagnosis and Treatment. New York: Thieme; 2008. Reprinted with permission.)

Table 2.4 Common Chemotherapy Agents

Drug	Mechanism of Action	Toxicity	Tumor
Adriamycin/doxorubicin	Blocks DNA/RNA synthesis by inhibiting topoisomerase II	Cardiotoxicity	Osteogenic sarcoma
Cis-platinum	DNA cross-linking, interrupts covalent bonding	Nephrotoxicity, ototoxicity, neurotoxicity	Osteogenic sarcoma
Methotrexate	Inhibits dihydrofolate reductase	Ulcerative stomatitis, leukopenia, cystitis	Osteogenic sarcoma
Ifosfamide	DNA alkylating agent	Nephrotoxicity, encephalopathy	Osteogenic sarcoma and Ewing's sarcoma
Vincristine	Vinca alkyloid, disrupts microtubule assembly	Peripheral neuropathy	Ewing's sarcoma
Etoposide	Topoisomerase II inhibitor	Bone marrow suppression	Ewing's sarcoma
Cyclophosphamide	DNA alkylating agent	Myelosuppression, hemorrhagic cystitis	Ewing's sarcoma
Actinomycin	Transcription inhibitor	Bone marrow suppression	Ewing's sarcoma

c. Radiation-associated sarcoma usually occurs > 5 years after therapy in the field of radiation treatment, with different histology than the initial lesion.

E. Chromosomal Translocations (Table 2.5)

Table 2.5 Common Tumor Chromosomal Translocations

Tumor	Translocation/gene
Ewing's sarcoma	t(11;22). *EWS, FLI1*
Clear cell sarcoma	t(12;22). *EWS, ATF1.*
Myxoid liposarcoma	t(12;16). *CHOP, TLS*
Alveolar rhabdomyosarcoma	t(2;13). *PAX3*
Synovial sarcoma	t(X;18). *SYT, SSX*
Aneurysmal bone cyst	*USP6*

II. Bone

A. Benign Bone Producing Tumors

1. Osteoid osteoma (**Figs. 2.3, 2.4, 2.5**)

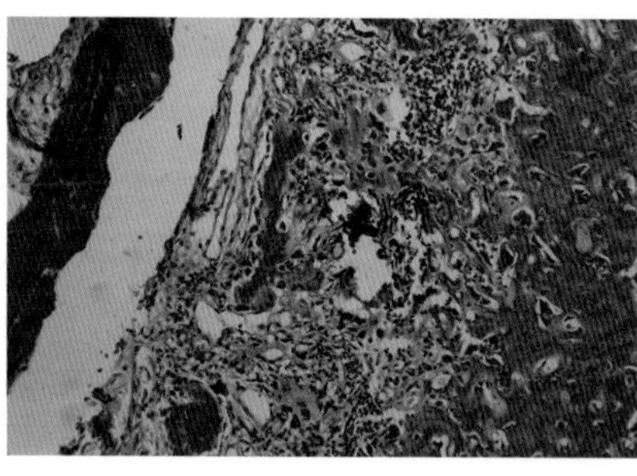

Fig. 2.3 High-power view of nidus showing osteoblastic activity with occasional blood vessel and giant cells. (From Conrad EU. Orthopaedic Oncology: Diagnosis and Treatment. New York: Thieme; 2008. Reprinted with permission.)

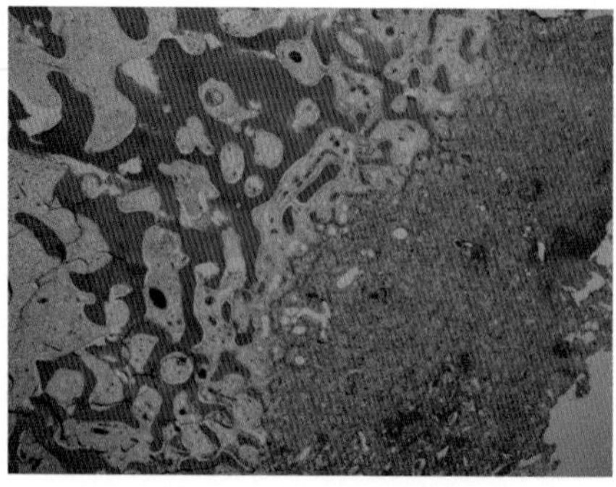

Fig. 2.4 Osteoid-osteoma. Low-power view with the nidus *(right)* and the reactive bone and remnants of the cortex *(left)*.

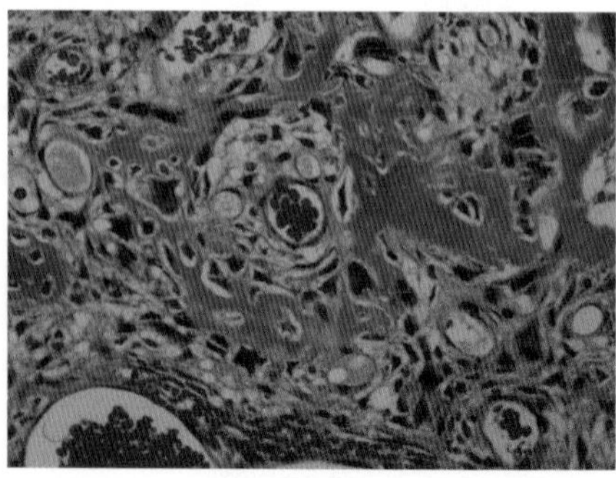

Fig. 2.5 The nidus under high power has a disorganized pattern of woven bone with prominent osteoblastic rimming or palisading and benign fibrovascular stroma. Several large osteoclasts are present.

- Demographic: young patients (ages 5–30 years), male-to-female ratio = 2:1
- Presentation: increasing pain, worse at night
- Relieved by nonsteroidal anti-inflammatory drugs (NSAIDs)/aspirin
- **Tumor releases prostaglandins, so NSAIDs uniquely relieve pain in this tumor.**
- Locations: proximal femur, tibial diaphysis, posterior elements of spine
  a. Can cause scoliosis: lesion at center of concavity of curve
- Imaging: computed tomography (CT) superior to magnetic resonance imaging (MRI); nidus of bone surrounded by reactive bone
  a. Hot on bone scan
  b. Nidus always < 1–1.5 cm
- Histology: thin osteoid seams, immature trabeculae; fibrovascular rim surrounding nidus
- Treatment: radiofrequency ablation (RFA), observation/NSAIDs, or open excision
  a. RFA contraindicated for lesions in digits secondary to risk of thermal necrosis and damage to neurovascular bundles.
- Prognosis: usually self limited to 3–5 years

2. Osteoblastoma **(Figs. 2.6, 2.7, 2.8, 2.9)**
   - Demographic: young (ages 10–30 years), male-to-female ratio = 2:1
   - > 2 cm
   - **"Big brother" lesion to osteoid osteoma**
   - Presentation: dull, aching pain not relieved by NSAIDs
   - Locations: posterior elements of spine, proximal humerus, femur, tibia, hip, mandible
     a. May be blastic or lytic

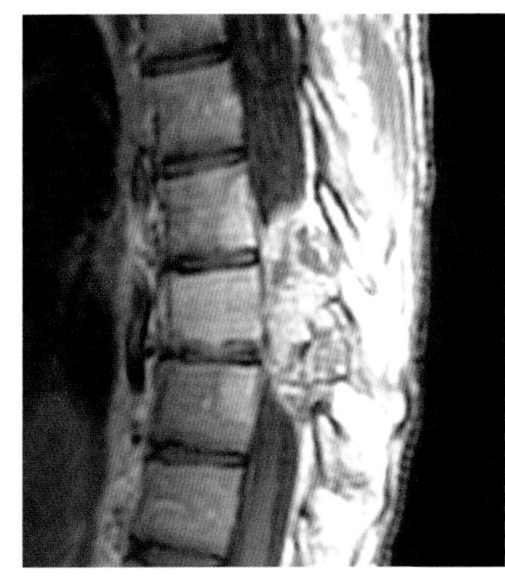

Fig. 2.6 Sagittal magnetic resonance imaging (MRI) of a T10 pedicle lesion. (From Conrad EU. Orthopaedic Oncology: Diagnosis and Treatment. New York: Thieme; 2008. Reprinted with permission.)

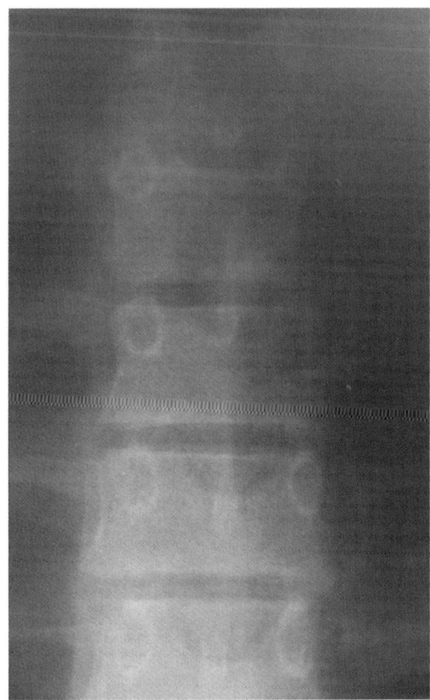

Fig. 2.7 The pedicle is missing in a 12-year-old girl. (From Conrad EU. Orthopaedic Oncology: Diagnosis and Treatment. New York: Thieme; 2008. Reprinted with permission.)

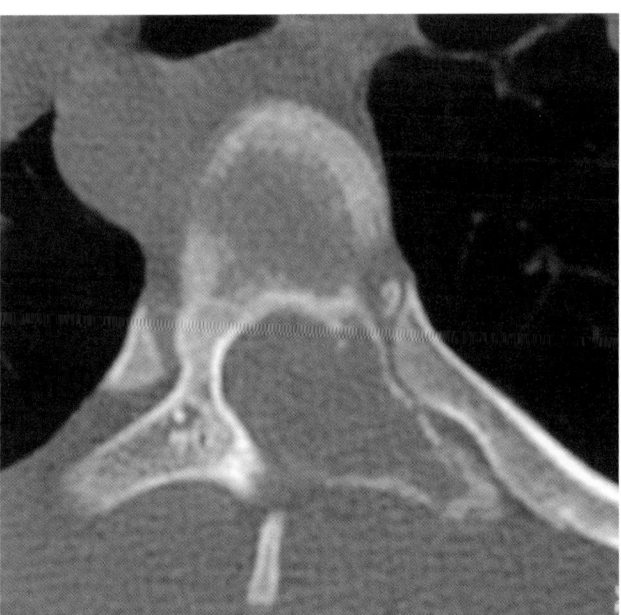

Fig. 2.8 A cystic pedicle lesion at T10 in a 12-year-old. (From Conrad EU. Orthopaedic Oncology: Diagnosis and Treatment. New York: Thieme; 2008. Reprinted with permission.)

- **Tumors of vertebral body: multiple myeloma, chordoma, osteosarcoma, giant cell tumor of bone (sacrum), eosinophilic granuloma, hemangioma, Ewing's sarcoma**
- **Tumors of posterior elements of spine: osteoid osteoma, osteoblastoma, ABC**

- Imaging: radiolucent lesion, > 2 cm in size, typically two thirds are cortically based, well marginated; hot on bone scan
- Differential: osteosarcoma, ABC, osteoid osteoma, osteomyelitis
- Histology: similar to osteoid osteoma but less organized: irregular osteoid with fibrovascular stroma and giant cells

- **Presence of normal osteoblasts producing osteoid differentiates osteoblastoma from osteosarcoma where malignant cells produce osteoid.**

- Treatment: curettage and bone grafting

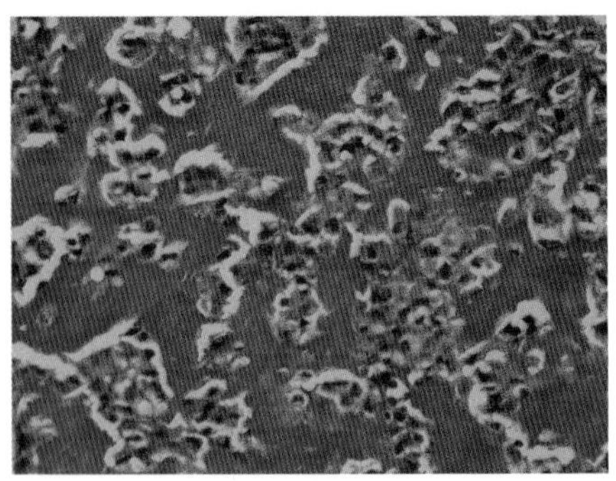

Fig. 2.9 Osteoblastoma with a chaotic arrangement of woven bone, prominent osteoblasts, and bland cells without mitoses.

3. Myositis ossificans **(Figs. 2.10, 2.11, 2.12)**
   - Reactive process typically caused by trauma, characterized by proliferation of fibroblasts, cartilage, bone within muscle.
   - Demographic: ages 15–35 years, males > females
   - Presentation: pain, swelling, decreased range of motion, increasing in size over several months
   - Locations: muscles surrounding diaphysis of long bones (quadriceps, brachialis, gluteal muscles)
   - Imaging: peripheral mineralization with central lucent area, not attached to bone; may initially be only periosteal reaction
     a. Differential diagnosis: extraskeletal or parosteal osteosarcoma

- **Myositis ossificans: mineralizes from outside in with mature bone initially at periphery of lesion; opposite of osteosarcoma, which mineralizes from inside out**
- **Myositis ossificans (MO): mature from outside inwards**

   - Histology: woven bone in zonal pattern with mature bone at periphery and immature fibrous tissue at center; may be confused with osteosarcoma

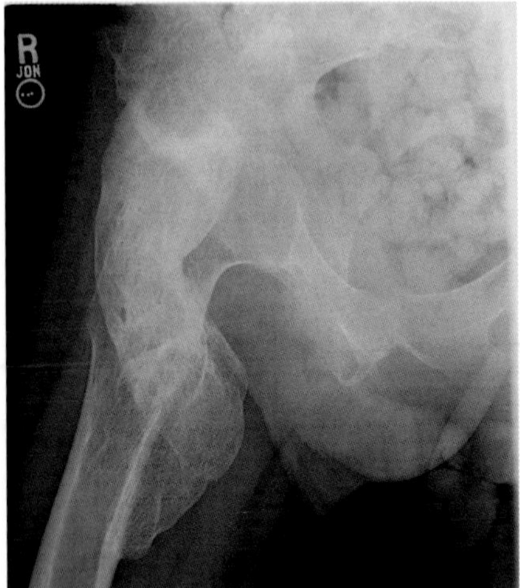

Fig. 2.10 Dense myositis ossificans in 22-year-old head-injured patient. (From Conrad EU. Orthopaedic Oncology: Diagnosis and Treatment. New York: Thieme; 2008. Reprinted with permission.)

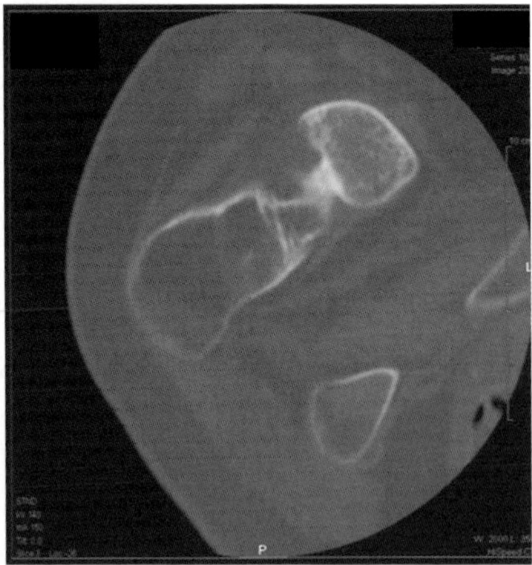

Fig. 2.11 Computed tomography (CT) of the proximal thigh in a 22-year-old man. (From Conrad EU. Orthopaedic Oncology: Diagnosis and Treatment. New York: Thieme; 2008. Reprinted with permission.)

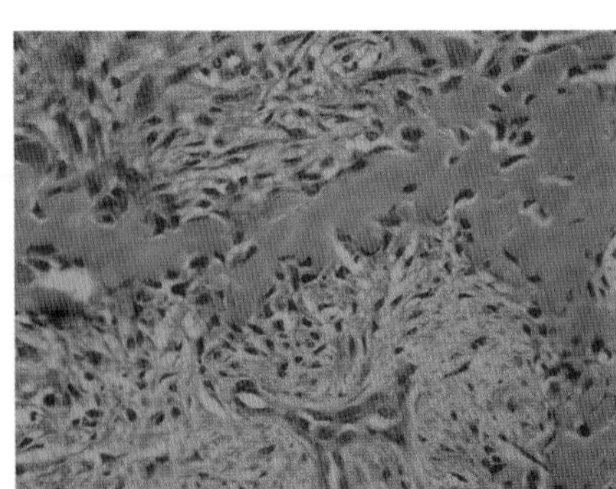

Fig. 2.12 In myositis ossificans, centrally, woven bone and abundant fibrovascular tissue is found. This zonation (peripheral well-defined bone and central poorly defined woven bone) is characteristic of myositis ossificans.

- Treatment: observation, repeat radiographs; may excise when lesion is mature (typically 6–12 months)

4. Melorheostosis **(Fig. 2.13)**
   - Rare disorder of new periosteal bone formation on surface of multiple bones
   - Demographic: discovered at age < 40 years
   - Presentation: significant pain, decreased range of motion (ROM)
   - Location: long bones, feet
   - Imaging: "dripping candle wax" with wavy appearance, can involve joint
   - Treatment: can excise hyperostotic areas to improve ROM or observe if asymptomatic

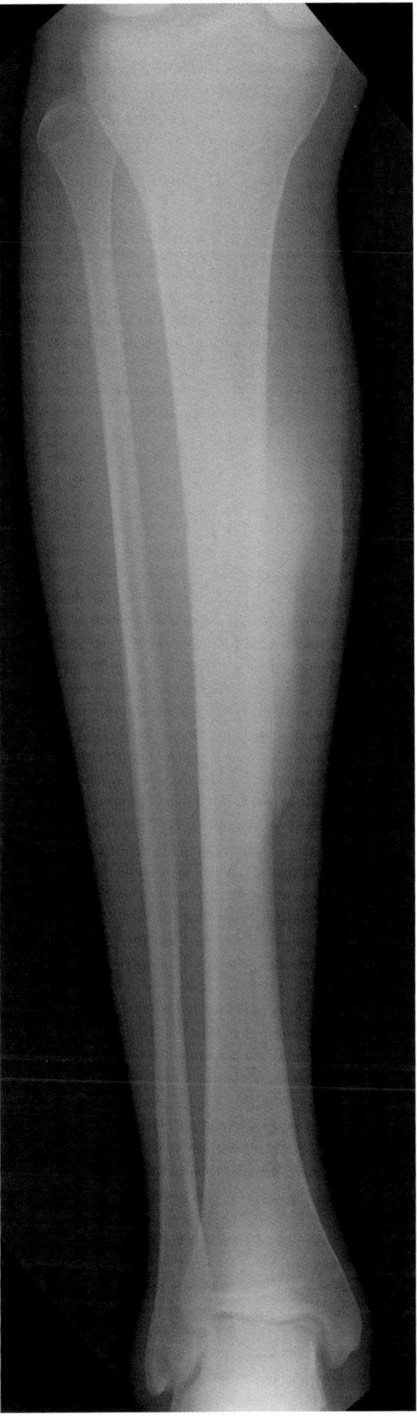

Fig. 2.13 Melorheostosis. X-ray showing thick and wavy bone consistent with melorheostosis.

B. Benign Reactive Lesions of Bone

1. Aneurysmal bone cyst **(Table 2.6, Figs. 2.14, 2.15, 2.16)**
   - Benign, locally aggressive lesion of bone
   - May be primary or in association with other tumors [giant cell tumor (GCT), chondroblastoma, chondromyxoid fibroma, fibrous dysplasia (FD)]
   - Genetics: upregulation of ubiquitin-specific protease (USP)-6
   - Demographic: age < 20 years
   - Presentation: pain, swelling
   - Location: distal femur, proximal tibia, pelvis, posterior elements of spine (25%)
   - Imaging: eccentric, lytic, expansile area of destruction in metaphysis, typically with rim of new bone surrounding lesion
     a. Expands wider than physis
     b. MRI: fluid–fluid levels
     c. Differential: UBC, telangiectatic osteosarcoma
   - Histology: cavernous blood-filled spaces, no endothelial lining, + giant cells, septations
   - **Must evaluate histology to differentiate from telangiectatic osteosarcoma**
   - Treatment: curettage, bone grafting
   - Risk of recurrence
   - Factors leading to increased risk of recurrence: young age, open physes, high stage, positive margin at time of excision
2. Unicameral bone cyst **(Table 2.6, Figs. 2.17** and **2.18)**
   - Demographic: age < 20 years
   - Presentation: pain, usually after fracture from minor trauma

Table 2.6 Aneurysmal Bone Cyst Versus Unicameral Bone Cyst

	Aneurysmal Bone Cyst	Unicameral Bone Cyst
Presentation	Pain, swelling	Pathologic fracture
Location	Distal femur, proximal tibia, pelvis, posterior elements of spine	Proximal humerus, proximal femur
Imaging	Metaphyseal lytic lesion, wider than physis MRI: fluid–fluid levels	Metaphyseal, lytic lesion, less than width of physis Falling leaf sign
Treatment	Curettage, bone graft	Methylprednisolone Curettage/bone graft (proximal femur)

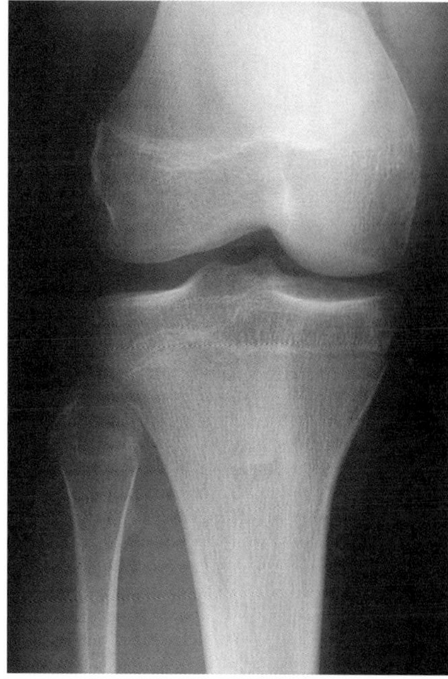

Fig. 2.14 Subtle tibial cortical lesion in a 16-year-old boy. (From Conrad EU. Orthopaedic Oncology: Diagnosis and Treatment. New York: Thieme; 2008. Reprinted with permission.)

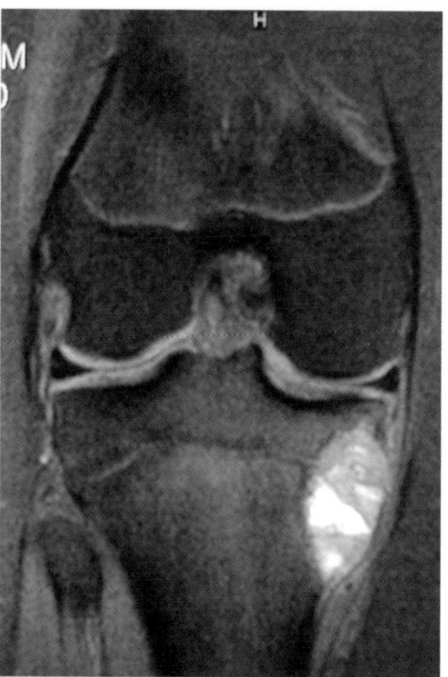

Fig. 2.15 Coronal MRI showing septations and fluid–fluid levels. (From Conrad EU. Orthopaedic Oncology: Diagnosis and Treatment. New York: Thieme; 2008. Reprinted with permission.)

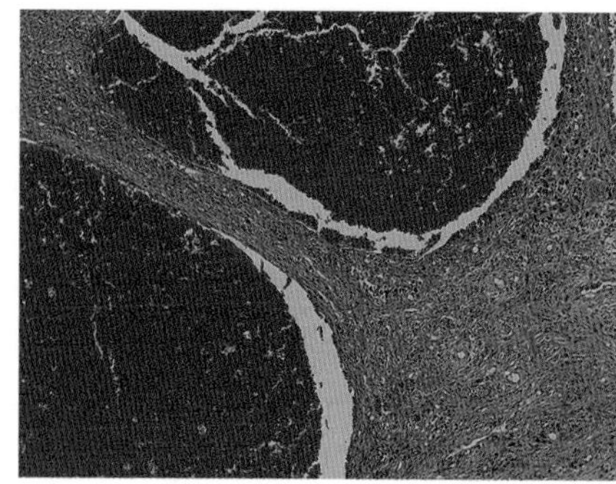

Fig. 2.16 Aneurysmal bone cyst (ABC) is composed of large blood-filled spaces surrounded by fibrous tissue, often with bony spicules. The spaces are not lined by endothelial cells, which are seen in vascular structures.

- **UBC commonly discovered after proximal humerus fracture with throwing injury.**
- Location: proximal humerus most common, then proximal femur, distal tibia, tarsal bones of feet
- Imaging: lytic lesion with symmetric cystic expansion, thinning of cortices, bone no wider than physis
  a. Falling leaf sign: pathognomonic for UBC (scattered, horizontal bone wisps in cystic cavity)
  b. Active (cyst abuts physeal plate) versus latent (normal bone intervenes)
- Histology: thin, fibrous lining (fibrous tissue, giants cells, hemosiderin)
- Treatment: observation, curettage/bone graft, aspiration and injection: methylprednisolone acetate, bone marrow, synthetic bone graft. Only aspirate and inject after pathologic fracture has healed. There is a risk of recurrence with any treatment.

C. Malignant Bone Producing Tumors

1. High-grade intramedullary osteosarcoma **(Figs. 2.19, 2.20, 2.21, 2.22, 2.23, 2.24, 2.25)**
   - High-grade, intermediate-grade, low-grade variants
     a. High-grade variants: osteoblastic, fibroblastic [differentiate from malignant fibrous histiocytoma (MFH)], chondroblastic (differentiate from chondrosarcoma), telangiectatic (differentiate from ABC), small cell (differentiate from Ewing's sarcoma), giant cell rich (differentiate from giant cell tumor of bone)
     b. No difference in prognosis between high-grade variants
     c. All grades may be intramedullary or surface lesions.

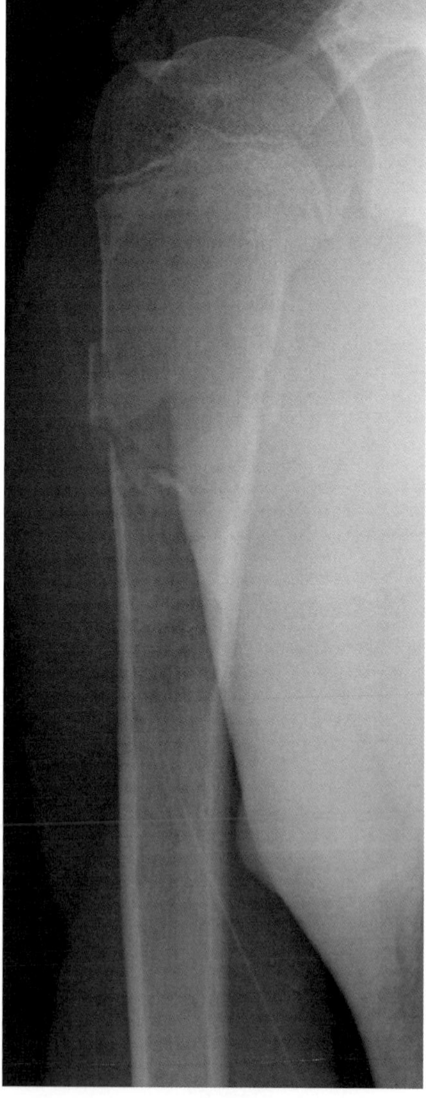

Fig. 2.17 Proximal humerus demonstrating a fracture through a well-marginated, lucent cyst in the metaphysis.

- **Most common primary sarcoma of bone**

- Demographic: bimodal; affects young patients (10–20 years) and older patients (Paget's osteosarcoma); male-to-female ratio = 1.5:1
- Genetics: associated with retinoblastoma (Rb) and p53 mutations (Li-Fraumeni syndrome)
- Risks: prior radiation, Paget's disease
- Presentation: pain, mass
- Location: distal femur > proximal tibia > proximal humerus
- Staging: most common stage: IIB (75%): high grade, extracompartmental
  a. 10–20% with metastases (stage III)
- Imaging: mixed appearance (both lytic and blastic) originating in medullary canal or classic "sunburst" appearance, Codman triangle
  a. MRI: extension into soft tissue, skip metastases (2–3%)
  b. Differential: osteomyelitis, Ewing's sarcoma
- Histology: malignant spindle cells forming osteoid in existing trabeculae with mitotic figures, pleomorphism; may have giant cells or cartilage
- Workup: plain films (lytic or blastic), CT chest, MRI of entire bone (skip metastases), laboratories
- Treatment: Neoadjuvant chemotherapy (Adriamycin/doxorubicin, methotrexate, cis-platinum, Ifofsamide), wide surgical resection, adjuvant chemo

- **Chemotherapy drugs induce apoptosis between G1 and S phases of cell cycle.**

- Survival: 60–70%
  a. Poor prognostic factors: age < 14 years, high alkaline phosphatase, tumor volume > 200 mL, two-drug chemotherapy, inadequate margins, poor histological response to radiation, +p-glycoprotein
  b. Metastasis: lungs most commonly, then bone
  c. Presence of distant bone metastasis has poor prognosis, equivalent to lung metastasis

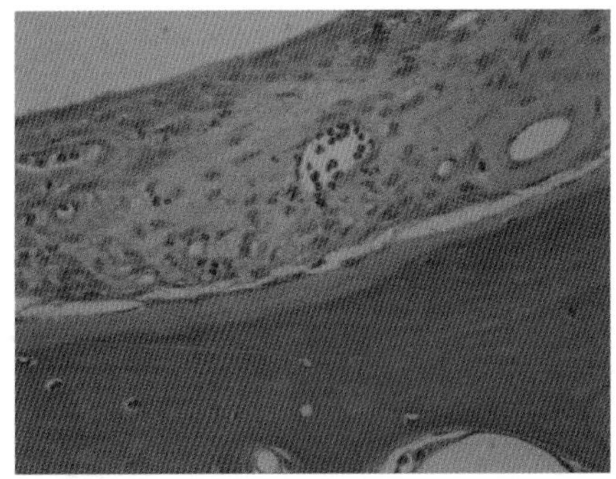

Fig. 2.18 Unicameral bone cyst (UBC) with a thin lining of fibrous tissue and some vessels. There is usually no reactive bone production as seen in an ABC.

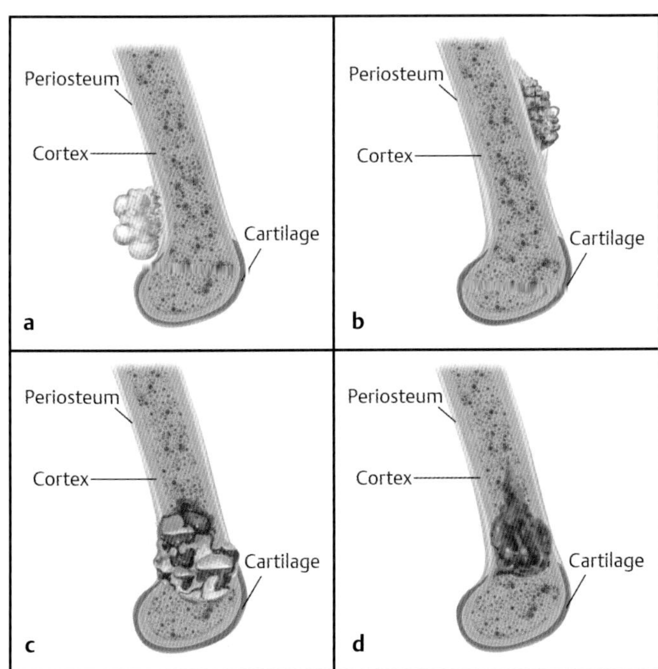

Fig. 2.19 **(a)** Parosteal osteosarcoma arises from the surface of the bone (usually the posterior femur). **(b)** Periosteal osteosarcoma arises from the surface with mineralization and a sunburst pattern. **(c)** Telangiectatic osteosarcoma arises from the metaphysis as a lytic mass, with areas of hemorrhage that create fluid–fluid levels on imaging. **(d)** High-grade intramedullary osteosarcoma is the most common primary sarcoma of bone and arises from the intramedullary canal as a lytic and blastic lesion with cortical destruction and soft tissue mass.

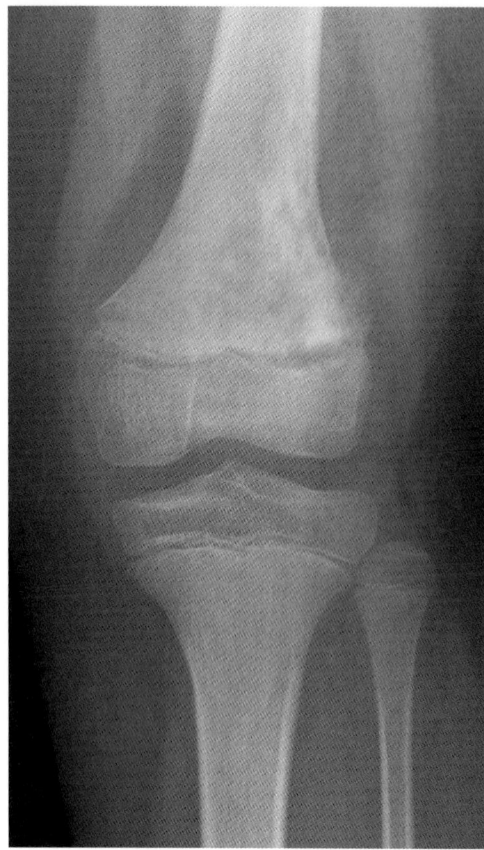

Fig. 2.20 Intramedullary osteosarcoma. Anteroposterior (AP) X-ray demonstrating a lytic and blastic lesion of the distal femur with the suggestion of a soft tissue mass.

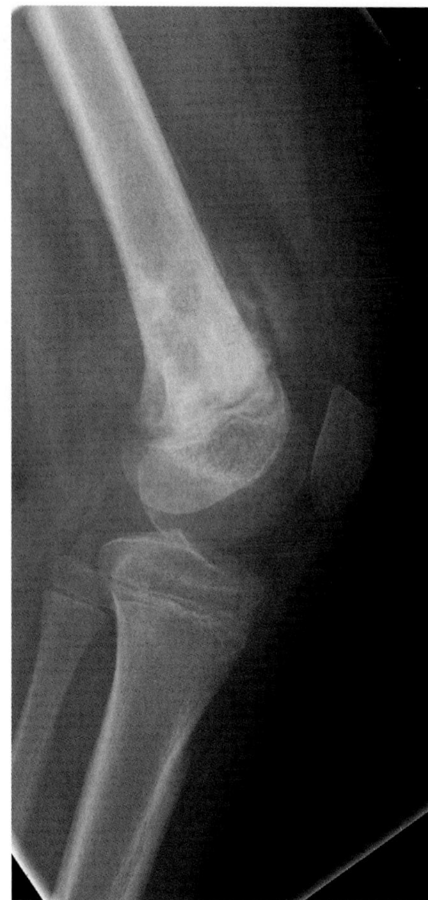

Fig. 2.21 Lateral X-ray of the lesion in Fig. 2.20.

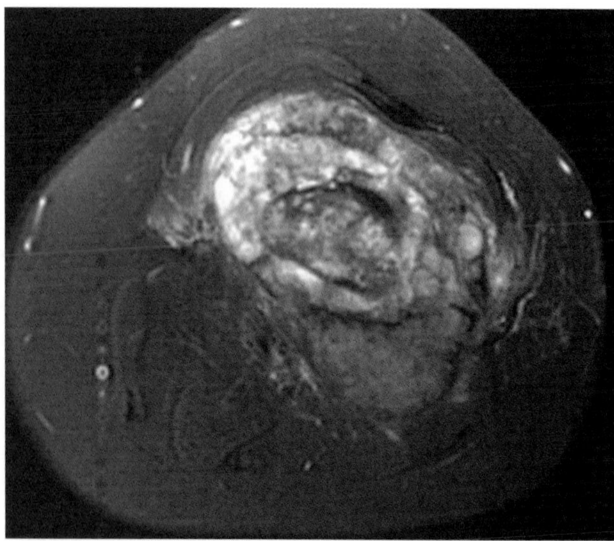

Fig. 2.22 Axial T2 MRI showing soft tissue extension of the intramedullary in Fig. 2.20.

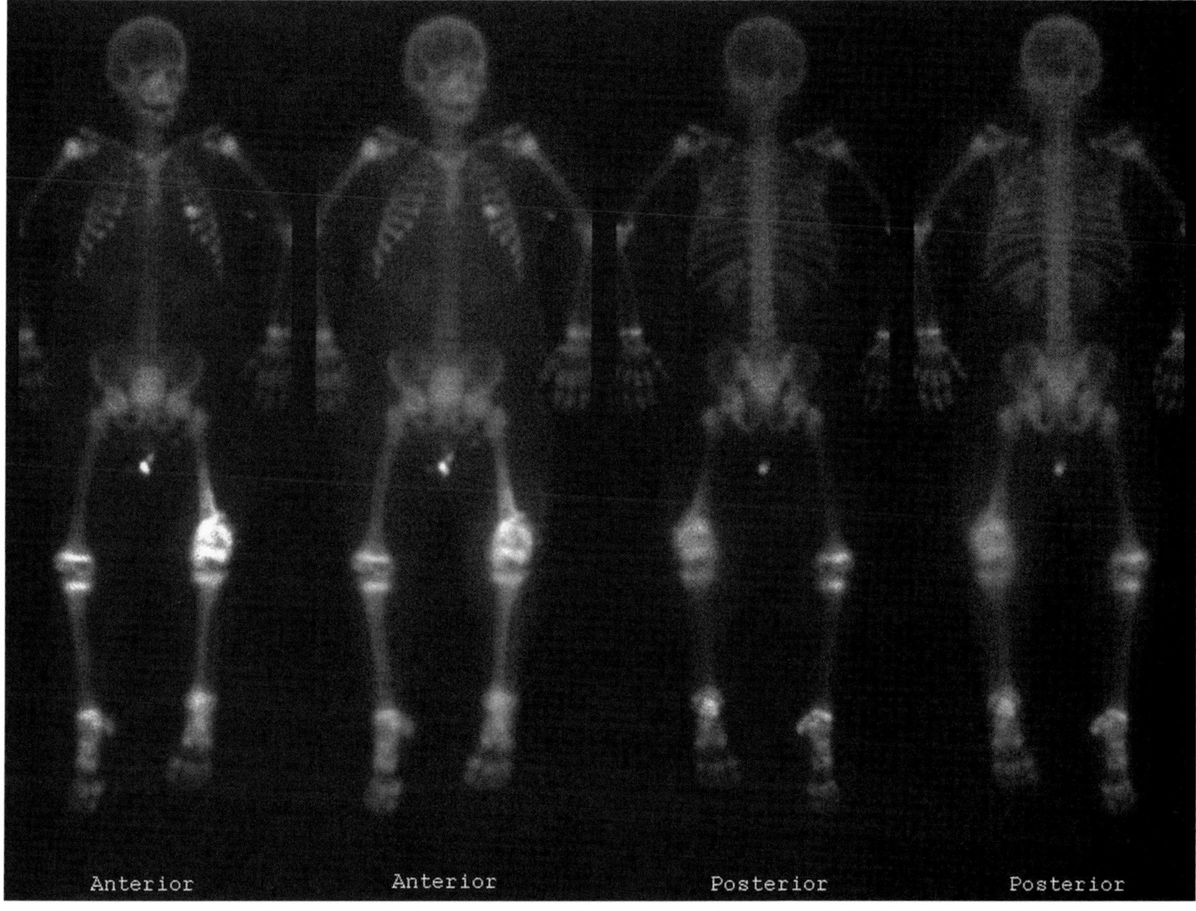

Fig. 2.23 Bone scan showing increased signal in the distal femur of the lesion in Fig. 2.20; used to evaluate for skip lesions or metastatic disease.

2. Telangiectatic osteosarcoma (**Figs. 2.26** and **2.27**)
   - Rare variant of osteosarcoma containing cavernous blood-filled spaces
   - Demographics: ages 10–30 years
   - Location: knee, proximal femur, proximal humerus—same as ABC
   - Imaging: destructive, lytic lesion; MRI demonstrates fluid–fluid lesions
     a. Differential: ABC

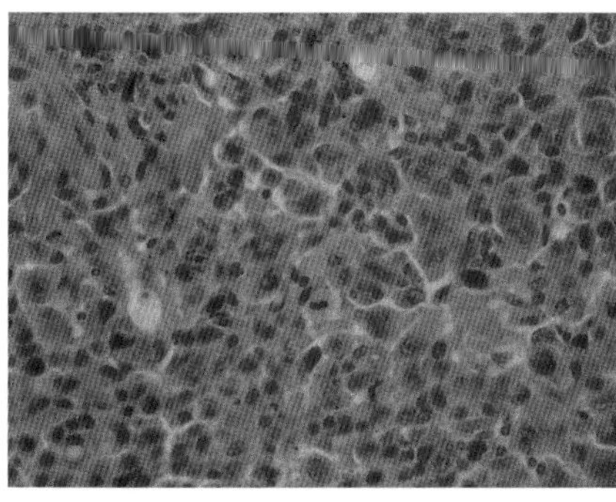

Fig. 2.24 Osteosarcoma, high grade, is composed of pleomorphic cells with hyperchromatic nuclei producing scattered woven bone trabeculae.

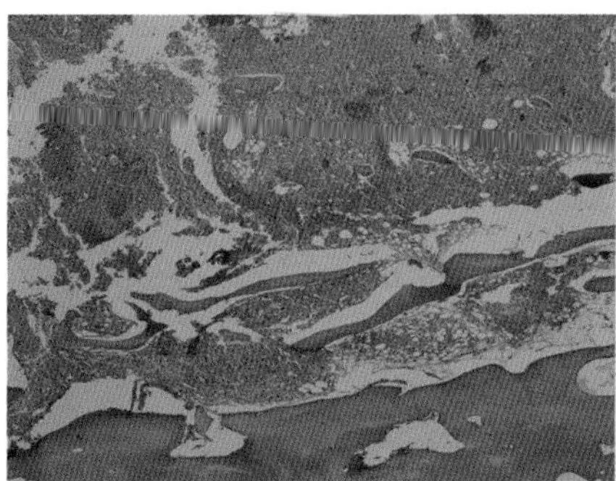

Fig. 2.25 Osteosarcoma, low power, replacing the marrow cavity and extending into the cortical vascular spaces. Remnants of marrow lamellar bone trabeculae are seen within the tumor.

Differentiate from ABC

- Histology: few cellular elements, blood filled ("bag of blood"); septa with high-grade sarcoma, pleomorphic cells, and multiple mitoses
- Treatment: neoadjuvant chemotherapy, wide resection, adjuvant chemotherapy

3. Parosteal osteosarcoma
   - Low-grade surface osteosarcoma; can rarely transform to dedifferentiated high-grade lesion
   - Genetics: may have supernumerary ring chromosomes
   - Demographic: ages 20–30 years, more common in females
   - Presentation: painless or dull, chronic pain and swelling
   - Location: metaphysis of posterior distal femur (80%), proximal tibia, proximal humerus
   - Imaging: ossified, lobulated mass arising from cortex with no cortical or medullary invasion (75%) and central density, "stuck-on appearance"; 25% with intramedullary invasion
   - **On imaging, parosteal osteosarcoma appears to be a bony mass stuck on the femur.**
     a. "String sign": cleavage plane between portions tumor and cortex of bone
     b. Hot on bone scan
     c. Differential: myositis ossificans, osteochondroma
   - Histology: regularly arranged trabeculae with atypical spindle cells and bland stroma invading skeletal muscle at periphery of tumor
     a. Dedifferentiated high-grade parosteal osteosarcoma seen with area of highly cellular spindle cells
   - **Treatment: wide resection, no chemotherapy if low grade (low-grade parosteal osteosarcoma does not require chemotherapy)**
     a. If high grade, neoadjuvant chemotherapy, wide surgical excision, adjuvant chemotherapy

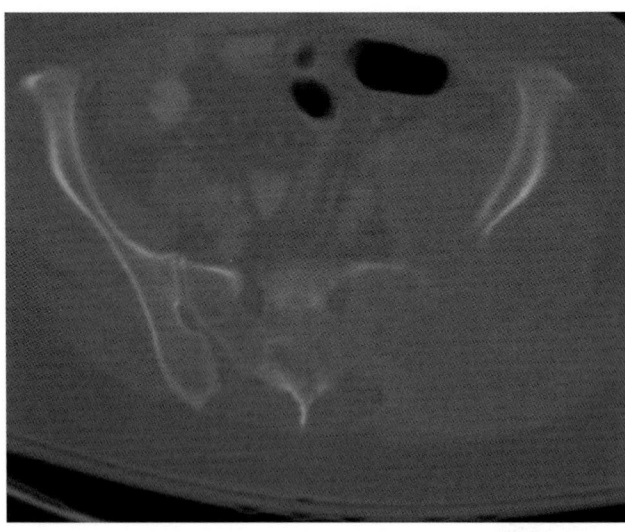

Fig. 2.26 Axial CT showing a lytic, destructive lesion, found in telangiectatic osteosarcoma.

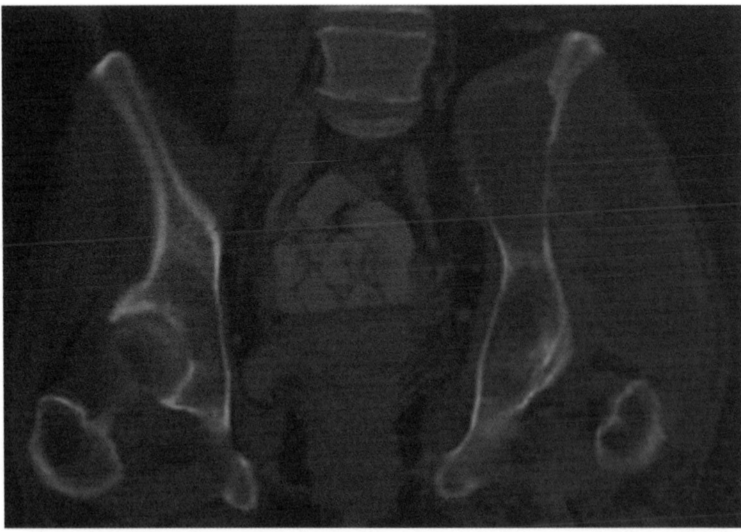

Fig. 2.27 Coronal CT of the lesion in Fig. 2.26.

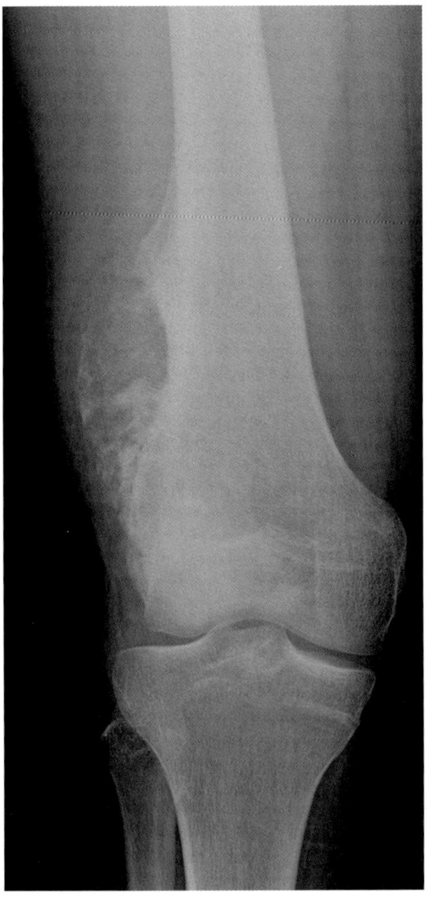

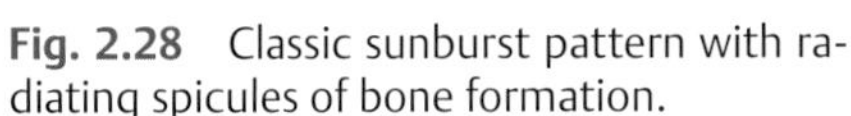

Fig. 2.28 Classic sunburst pattern with radiating spicules of bone formation.

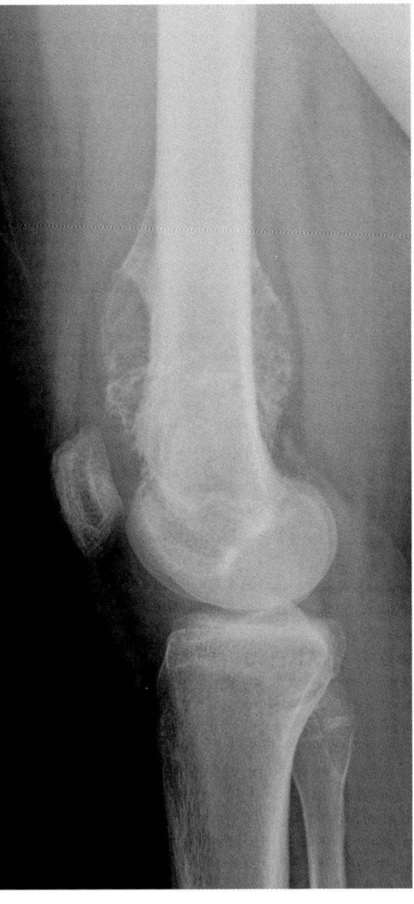

Fig. 2.29 Classic sunburst pattern with radiating spicules of bone formation.

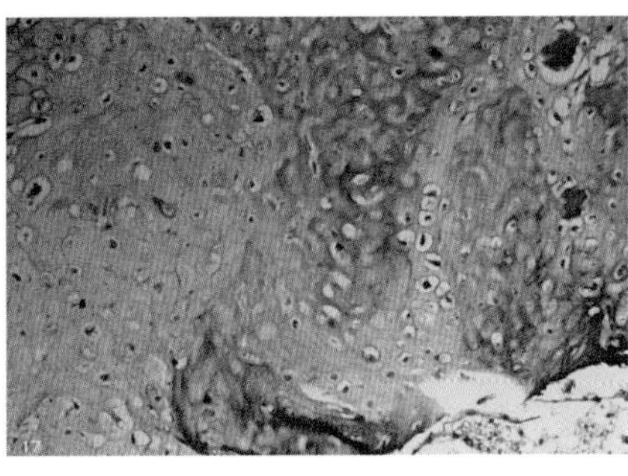

Fig. 2.30 Osteosarcoma photomicrograph demonstrating chondroid matrix. (From Conrad EU. Orthopaedic Oncology: Diagnosis and Treatment. New York: Thieme; 2008. Reprinted with permission.)

4. Periosteal osteosarcoma **(Figs. 2.28, 2.29, 2.30)**
   - Demographic: ages 10–20 years
   - Presentation: pain
   - Location: diaphysis of long bones (femur/tibia)
   - Imaging: sunburst lesion overlying cortical depression
   - Histology: typically high grade, chondroblastic matrix, osteoid
   - Treatment: neoadjuvant chemotherapy, wide resection, adjuvant chemotherapy

D. Benign Cartilage Producing Lesions

1. Periosteal chondroma
   - Benign cartilage tumor on surface of bone
   - Location: 50% proximal humerus, femur
   - Imaging: eccentric, cortically based lesion eroding the underlying cortex, producing a saucer-like defect
     a. Differential diagnosis: osteochondroma (but without stalk) or myositis ossificans
   - Histology: chondroid matrix and lacunae with multiple chondrocytes
   - Treatment: marginal excision including underlying cortex
2. Enchondroma **(Figs. 2.31, 2.32, 2.33, 2.34)**
   - Benign cartilage lesion in medullary cavity

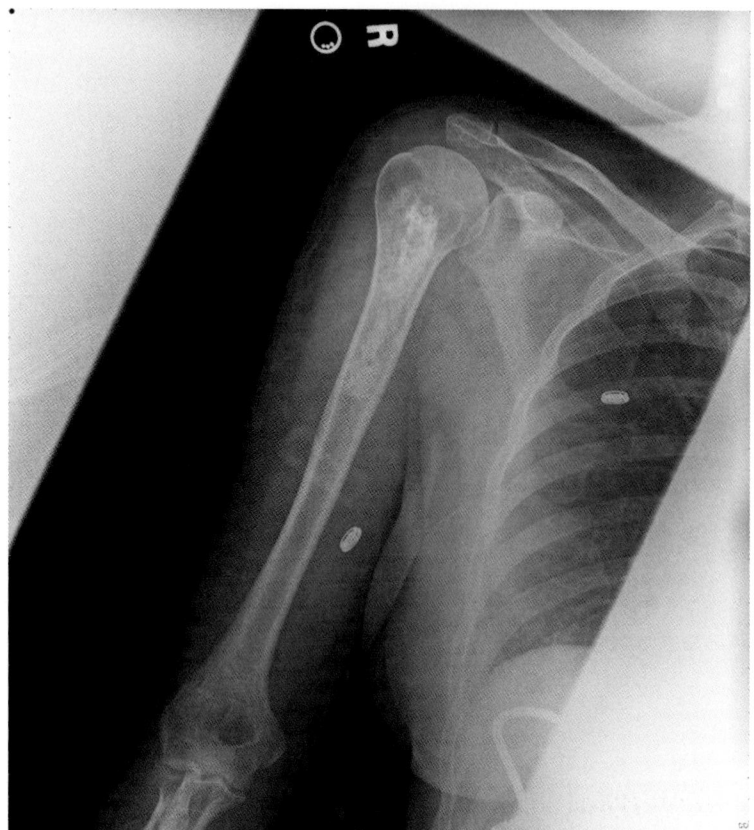

Fig. 2.31 Dense calcified lesion of proximal humerus (enchondroma). (From Conrad EU. Orthopaedic Oncology: Diagnosis and Treatment. New York: Thieme; 2008. Reprinted with permission.)

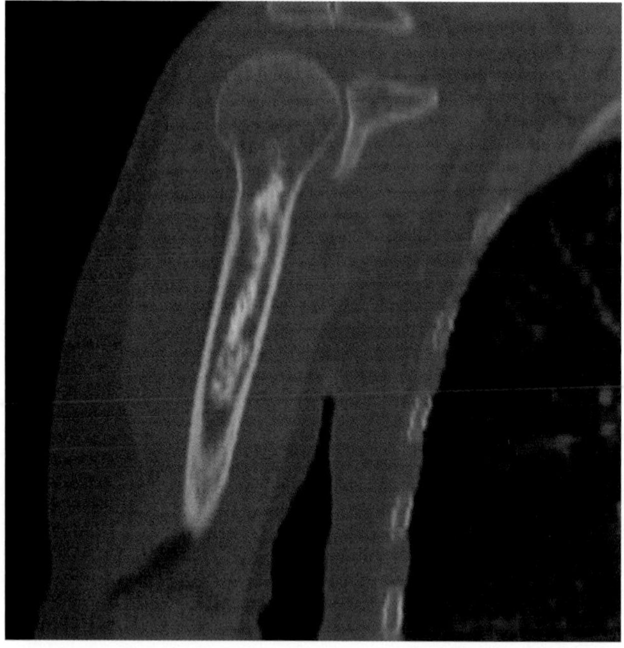

Fig. 2.32 Calcified lesion on coronal CT scan (enchondroma). (From Conrad EU. Orthopaedic Oncology: Diagnosis and Treatment. New York: Thieme; 2008. Reprinted with permission.)

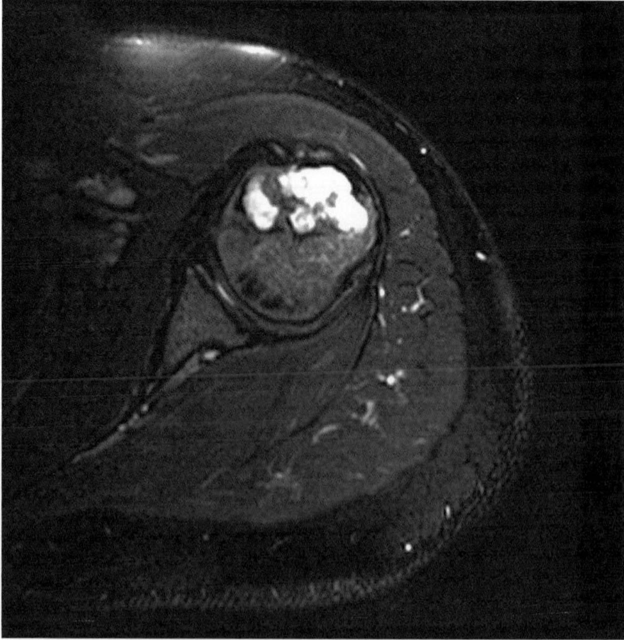

Fig. 2.33 Heterogeneous calcified lesion on axial MRI (enchondroma). (From Conrad EU. Orthopaedic Oncology: Diagnosis and Treatment. New York: Thieme; 2008. Reprinted with permission.)

- Demographic: age > 20 years
- Presentation: incidental, painless; may present as pathologic fracture, such as in the metacarpal/phalanx
- Location: diaphysis and metaphysis in hand, metaphyseal proximal humerus, distal femur

• Most common benign skeletal lesion in hand

- Imaging: well-defined, lucent, medullary lesions with stippled/mottled calcified appearance, popcorn calcification
  a. Can expand and thin cortex (common)
  b. Differential: low-grade chondrosarcoma, bone infarct ("smoke up chimney")
  c. Present in 3% of knee MRIs
- Histology: mature hyaline cartilage lobules separated by normal marrow, hypocellular
- Treatment: observation with serial radiographs (most common)
  a. Curettage and graft only after pathologic fracture has healed or prior to a fracture occurring if noted incidentally on X-ray (in the hand)
  b. Enchondromas of the hand generally treated surgically after fracture to prevent repeat fractures **(Fig. 2.35)**
- Syndromes
  a. Ollier's: multiple enchondromas, particularly unilateral, 30% lifetime risk of malignancy
  b. Maffucci's: multiple enchondromas, associated soft tissue hemangiomas, increased risk of visceral malignancies, 100% risk of transformation to chondrosarcoma

3. Osteochondroma **(Figs. 2.36, 2.37, 2.38)**
   - Benign surface lesions (35% benign lesions), typically associated with tendon insertions
   - May be single or multiple (multiple hereditary exostosis)
   - Demographic: ages 10–30 years
   - Presentation: incidental or painful (if overlying bursae, irritating tendon, joint capsule)
   - Location: metaphyseal—knee, proximal femur, proximal humerus
   - Imaging: surface lesion with cortex of the lesion and underlying cortex continuous with medullary cavity
     a. Sessile versus pedunculated
     b. Cartilage cap grows away from physis
     c. Stops growing with skeletal maturity
     d. Obtain MRI or CT to evaluate thickness of cartilaginous cap and presence of soft tissue mass if suspicious for chondrosarcoma in an adult with an enlarging lesion.

CT scan will demonstrate that the lesion is in continuity with the medullary cavity.

   - Histology: similar to that of enchondroma
     a. If cartilage cap > 2 cm, raise concern about conversion to chondrosarcoma
     b. Hyaline cartilage cap with cortical and trabecular bone comprising stalk, endochondral ossification
   - Treatment: observation (asymptomatic) versus excision (soft tissue irritation)
     a. New change in pain should be worked up to address concern about conversion to chondrosarcoma (order an MRI).

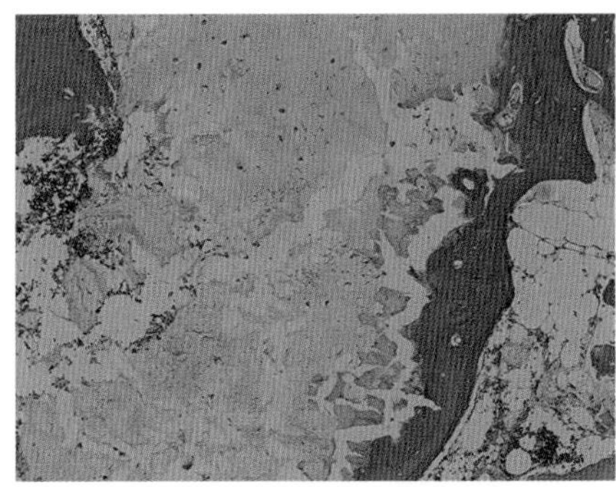

Fig. 2.34 Enchondroma abutting the cortex. There is no invasion into the bone but rather a "pushing" border against the bone. [Histo 4.2 (100×).]

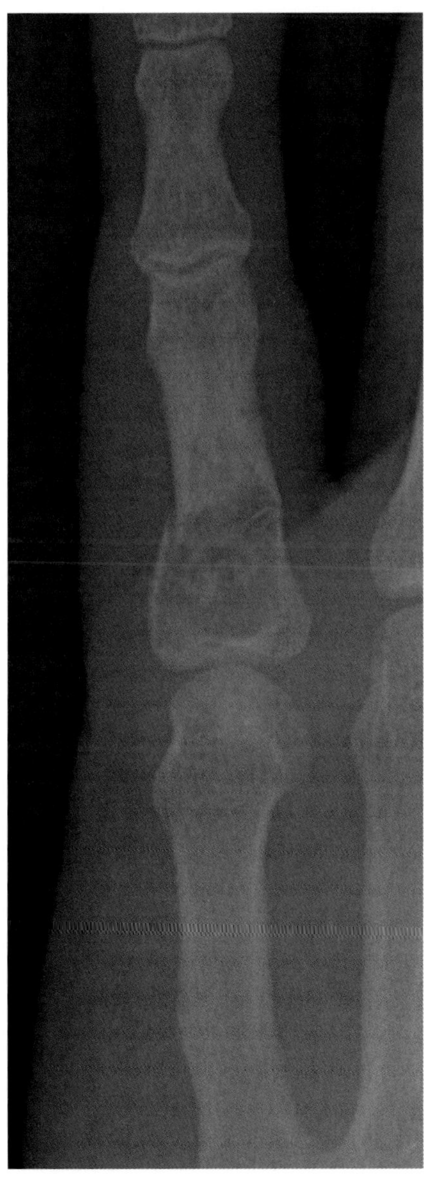

Fig. 2.35 **(Figure Enchondroma)** Fracture through an enchondroma of the proximal phalanx.

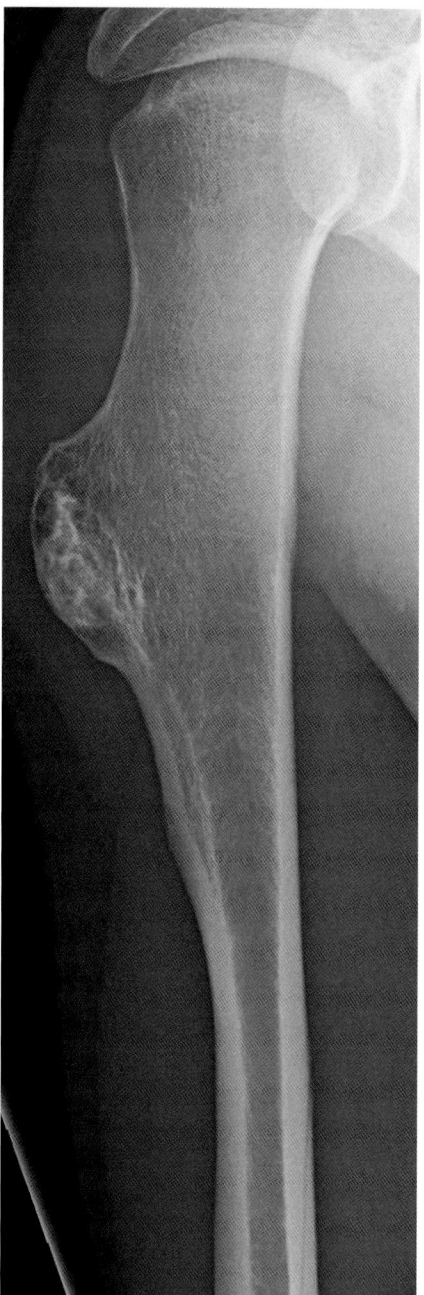

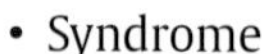

Fig. 2.36 **(Figure Osteochondroma 1)** Benign-appearing surface lesion extending from the medullary cavity of the humerus

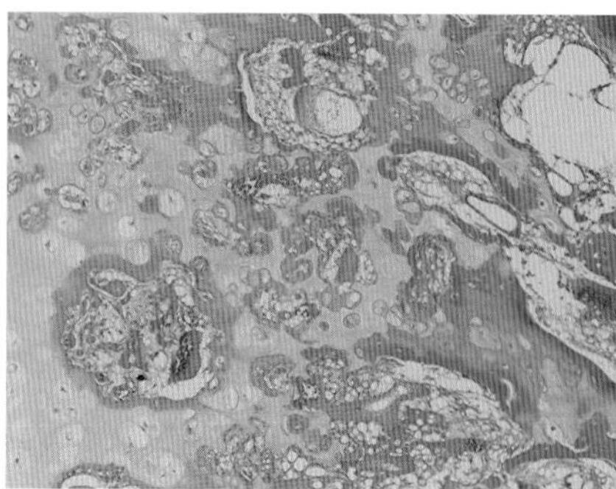

Fig. 2.37 The deep portion of the cartilage cap of an osteochondroma with endochondral ossification and deposition of woven bone on the surface of cartilage cores. This field is identical to that of a normal epiphyseal growth plate because the cartilage cap is really a displaced epiphyseal growth plate. [Histo 80.1 (400×).]

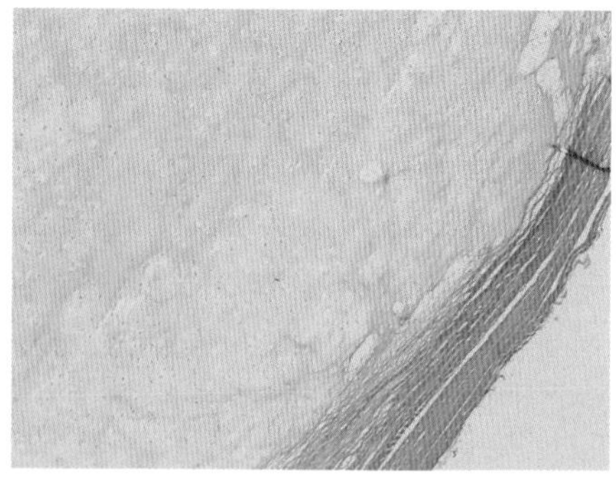

Fig. 2.38 The cartilage cap of an osteochondroma is covered by the dense collagenous perichondrium. Histologically the two diagnostic features are the presence of the perichondrium covering the hyaline cartilage cap and the direct communication of the bony stalk with the marrow space of the parent bone. There is no cortex separating the two. [Histo 80.11 (40×).]

- Syndrome
    a. Multiple hereditary exostosis **(Fig. 2.39)**
        - Gene: *EXT1*, *EXT2*, *EXT3*, autosomal dominant
            - Mutation affects prehypertrophic chondrocytes of the growth plate
        - 5–10% develop secondary chondrosarcoma, *EXT1* > *EXT2*
        - Primarily sessile lesions large in size
        - May cause progressive skeletal deformities including short stature, limb-length discrepancies, valgus

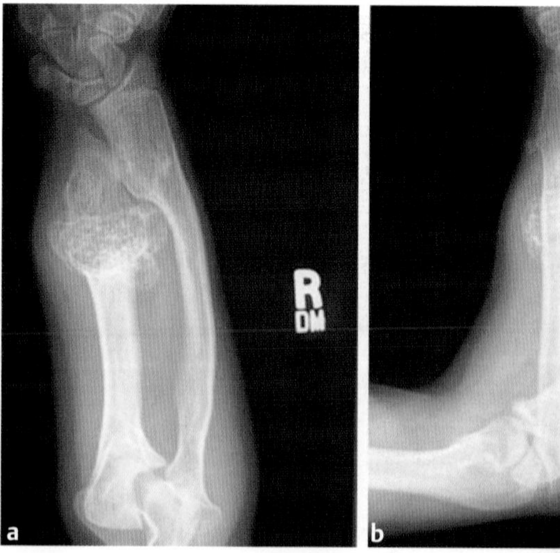

Fig. 2.39 **(a)** Anteroposterior X-ray of the forearm showing a typical exophytic lesion with classic ulnar shortening and secondary radial bowing. **(b)** Lateral forearm view showing a large exostosis extending into the flexor volar compartment. (From Conrad EU. Orthopaedic Oncology: Diagnosis and Treatment. New York: Thieme; 2008. Reprinted with permission.)

deformity or knee and ankle, asymmetry of pectoral and pelvic girdle, bowing of radius with ulnar deviation, subluxation of radiocapitellar joint
   - Metaphyseal widening

4. Bizarre parosteal osteochondromatous proliferation (BPOP)(Nora's tumor)
   - Reactive heterotopic ossification
   - Demographic: age > 20 years, males = females
   - Location: hands or feet
   - Imaging: bony mass with well-defined margins, may be pedunculated
   - Histology: cartilage, bizarre fibroblasts, disorganized bone
   - Treatment: wide margin resection, may recur locally
5. Chondroblastoma **(Figs. 2.40, 2.41, 2.42)**
   - Benign, aggressive, cartilage tumor
   - Genetics: mutation in specific histone 3.3 (giant cell tumors of bone as well); possible chromosomal abnormalities in chromosomes 5 and 8
   - Demographic: age in second decade, male-to-female ratio = 2:1
   - Presentation: mildly painful mass increasing in size
   - Location: epiphysis of distal femur, proximal tibia, proximal humerus (Codman tumor), femoral head, triradiate cartilage; also present in apophysis
   - Imaging: central region of bone destruction with thin rim of surrounding sclerotic bone and edema
     a. Typically epiphyseal but may extend to metaphysis
     b. Differential: giant cell tumor, osteomyelitis, clear cell chondrosarcoma
   - Histology: polygonal chondroblasts with scattered multinucleated giant cells, chicken wire calcification, "cobblestone pattern," coffee-bean nuclei
     a. Mononuclear cells S100+ staining
   - Treatment: curettage and bone grafting; 2% risk of metastasis to lungs
6. Chondromyxoid fibroma **(Figs. 2.43** and **2.44)**
   - Rare benign cartilage tumor containing chondroid, fibromatoid, myxoid elements

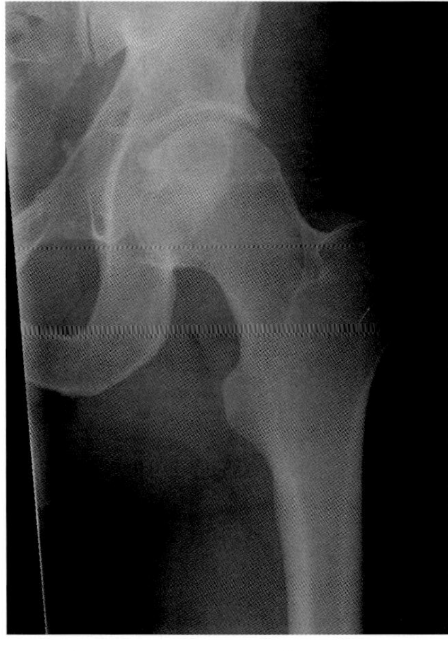

Fig. 2.40 Epiphyseal lesion with surrounding rim of sclerotic bone.

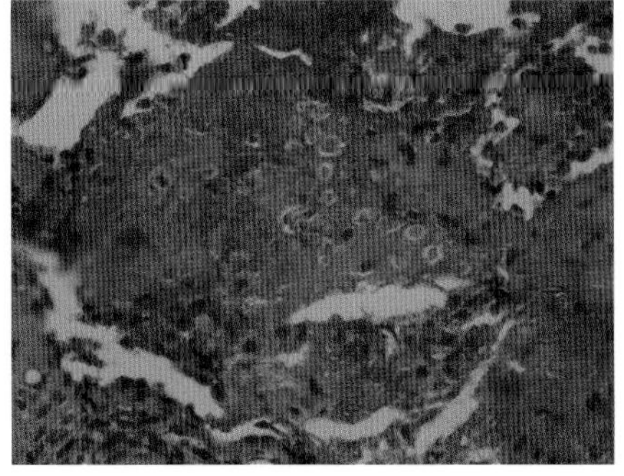

Fig. 2.41 Chondroblastoma with individual cell calcification producing the cyclone-fence or chicken-wire pattern.

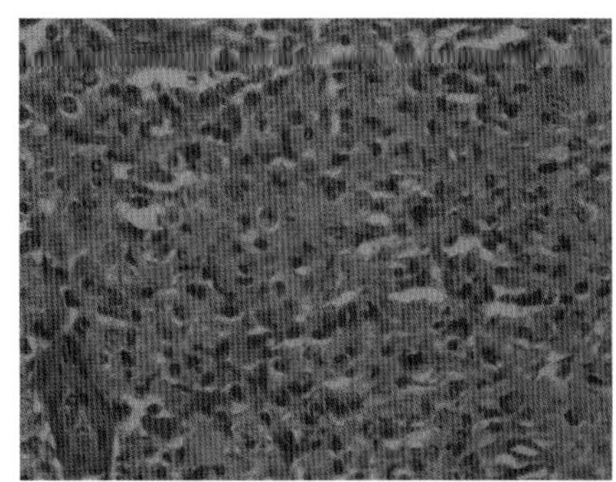

Fig. 2.42 Chondroblastoma with oval or round cells with good cytoplasmic borders.

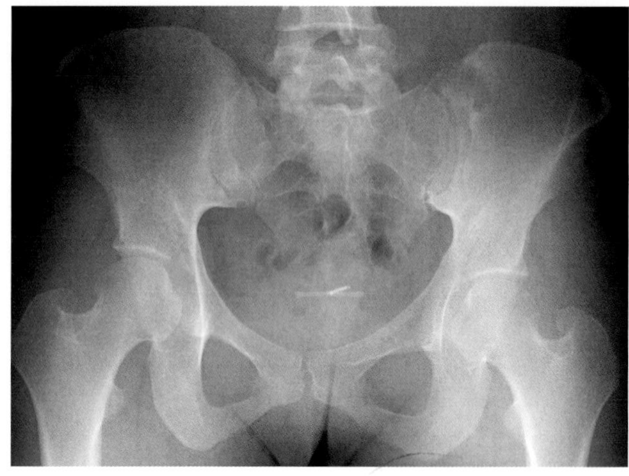

Fig. 2.43 Destructive lesion in the ilium with a scalloped rim.

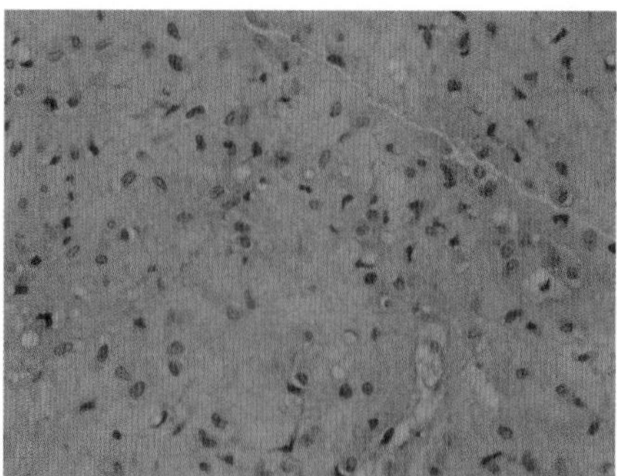

Fig. 2.44 Chondromyxoid fibroma with stellate cells, each with a single small round nucleus, embedded in a clear slightly bubbly matrix with scant vascularity. No hyaline cartilage is present.

- Demographic: ages 20–30 years
- Presentation: pain/swelling
- Location: long bones (tibia), pelvis, distal femur, feet
- Imaging: radiolucent, destructive, eccentric lesion in metaphysis
  a. Thinning and expansion of cortex with scalloped rim
  b. Differential: ABC
- Histology: stellate-appearing cells with hyperchromatic nuclei in lobules, chondroid, fibromatoid, myxoid lobules
- Treatment: curettage and bone grafting; risk of recurrence 10–25%

E. Malignant Cartilage Producing Lesions

1. Chondrosarcoma **(Figs. 2.45, 2.46, 2.47)**

For lesions in patients older than 40 years, consider metastatic disease, multiple myeloma, lymphoma, chondrosarcoma, and MFH/undifferentiated pleomorphic sarcoma (UPS).

- Cartilage producing bone tumor; may be primary or secondary
- Demographics: older adults (> 50 years), more common in males
- Presentation: pain or mass; pain may differentiate low-grade chondrosarcoma from enchondroma
- Risks for secondary chondrosarcoma: multiple hereditary osteochondromas, Ollier disease (30%), Maffucci disease (100%)
- Location: pelvis, proximal femur, spine, scapula
  a. Clear cell chondrosarcoma: epiphysis of long bones, most commonly proximal femur, proximal humerus **(Fig. 2.48)**
- Imaging: lytic lesion, thickened and expanded cortex with endosteal scalloping in more than two thirds of the cortical thickness, mineralization consistent with cartilage; "rings and arcs" in low-grade lesions; high-grade lesions with increased cortical destruction and soft tissue mass on MRI; bone edema on short tau inversion recovery (STIR) imaging
  a. Clear cell chondrosarcoma: round, well-defined lesion often confused with chondroblastoma; may occur in younger adults
  b. Clear cell chondrosarcoma and chondroblastoma are both epiphyseal lesions.

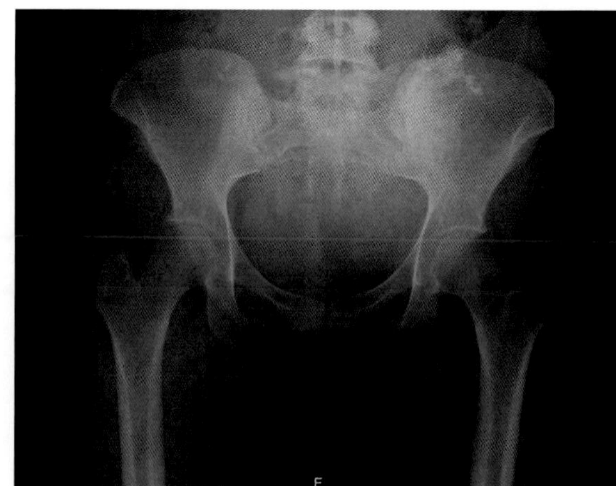

Fig. 2.45 X-ray showing a large calcified pelvic lesion. (From Conrad EU. Orthopaedic Oncology: Diagnosis and Treatment. New York: Thieme; 2008. Reprinted with permission.)

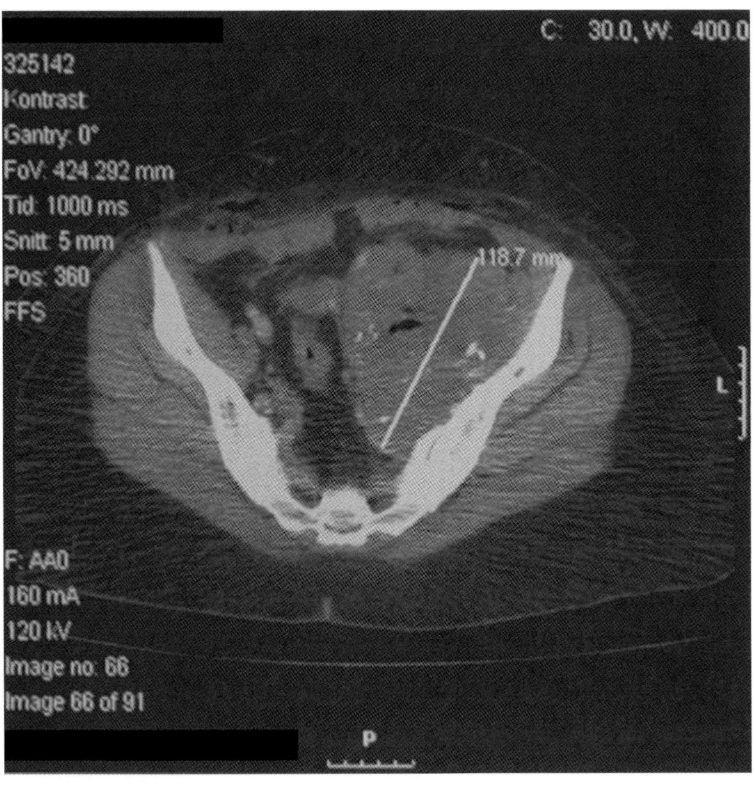

Fig. 2.46 Left pelvic tumor with large intrapelvic soft tissue extension. (From Conrad EU. Orthopaedic Oncology: Diagnosis and Treatment. New York: Thieme; 2008. Reprinted with permission.)

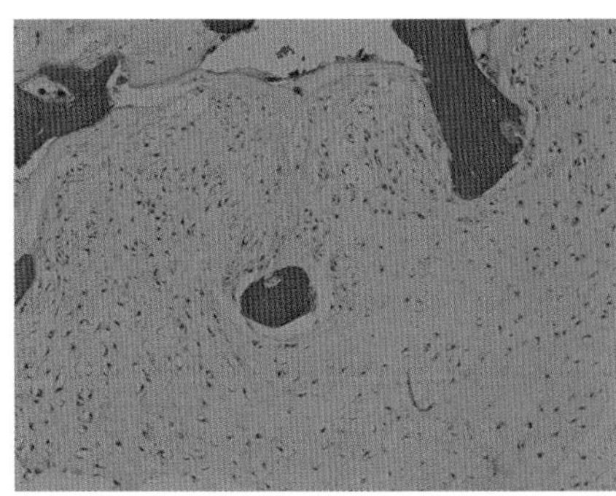

Fig. 2.47 Chondrosarcoma with hyaline cartilage surrounding and trapping dead lamellar bone trabeculae. This infiltrative pattern is characteristic of chondrosarcoma.

- Histology: enlarged, pleomorphic chondrocytes with increased cellularity, mitotic figures, multiple cells per lacunae, myxoid changes
  a. Clear cell chondrosarcoma: chondrocytes with clear vacuolated cytoplasm in chondroid matrix
- Treatment: grade 1 extremity—curettage; grade 2/3—no chemotherapy or radiation indicated, require wide excision
  a. All pelvic lesions, including low grade, require resection
  b. Recurrence rate related to increased telomerase activity and positive margins

2. Dedifferentiated chondrosarcoma **(Figs. 2.49** and **2.50)**
   - 5-year survival: 5–10%
   - Most malignant cartilage lesion
   - 50% with pathologic fracture
   - Presentation: pain
   - Location: distal, proximal femur, proximal humerus
   - Histology: high-grade sarcoma (UPS, fibrosarcoma, osteosarcoma) adjacent to low-grade or benign cartilage lesion
   - Treatment: chemotherapy, resection, chemotherapy, although controversial

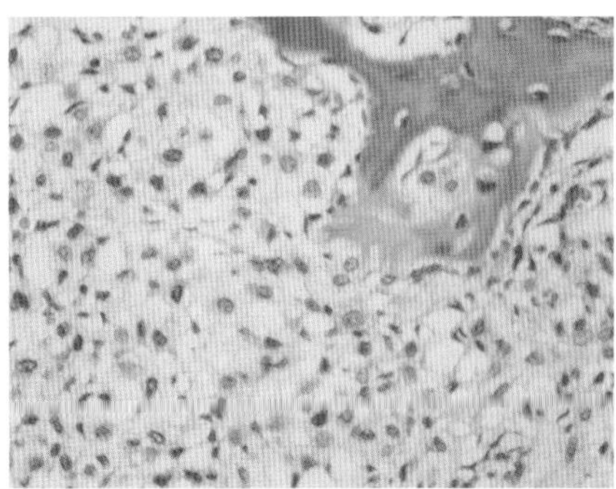

Fig. 2.48 Clear cell chondrosarcoma with large round cells filling up the marrow space each with clear cytoplasm and a round nucleus. Large, thin-walled vessels are present. There is always standard or conventional low-grade chondrosarcoma present in other parts of the tumor, but the diagnostic cells are the foci of chondrocytes with clear cytoplasm, containing glycogen and stain positively for S100 protein. Often, woven bone in admixed with zones of clear cells.

F. Fibrous and Histiocytic Lesions of Bone

1. Metaphyseal fibrous defect/nonossifying fibroma (NOF) **(Figs. 2.51** and **2.52)**
   - Common skeletal lesion related to faulty ossification

Metaphyseal fibrous defect/NOF is often found incidentally on radiographic workup after an injury that is unrelated to the lesion.

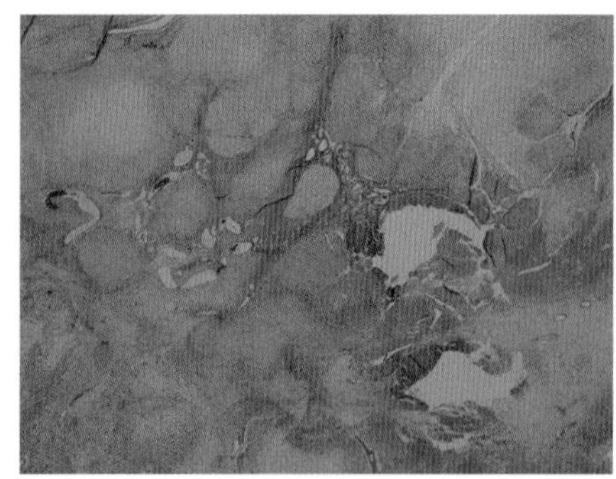

Fig. 2.49 Dedifferentiated chondrosarcoma has lobules of well-defined cartilage and areas of high-grade tumor cells without discernible cartilage differentiation.

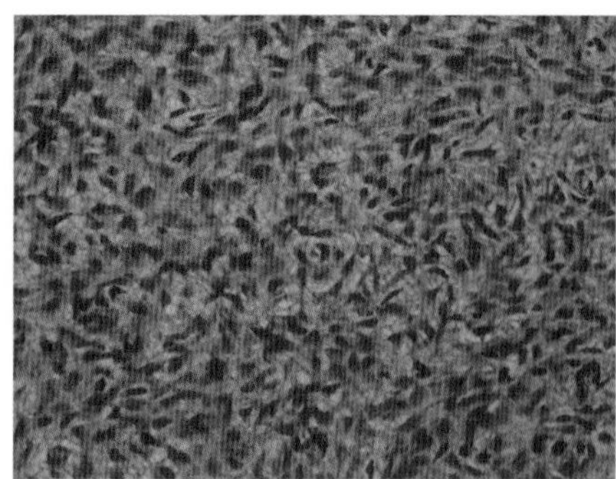

Fig. 2.50 Dedifferentiated chondrosarcoma with a focus of pleomorphic spindle and round cells with no cartilage differentiation.

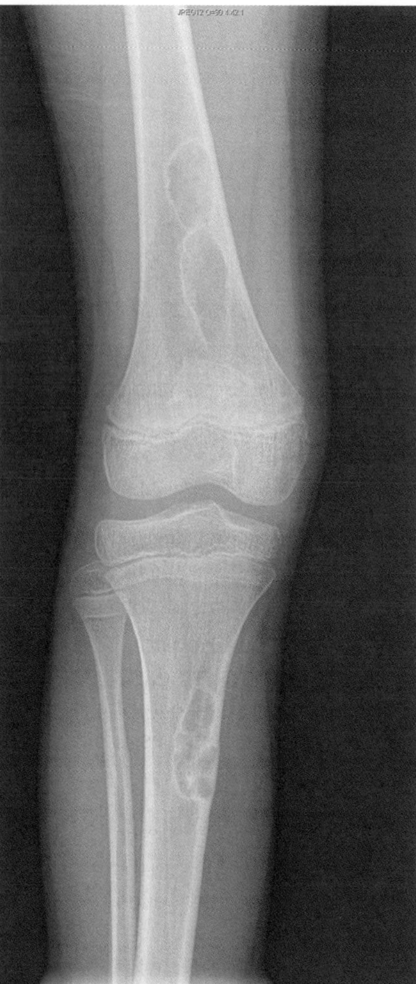

Fig. 2.51 Eccentric distal femoral and proximal tibia "cystic" lesions. (From Conrad EU. Orthopaedic Oncology: Diagnosis and Treatment. New York: Thieme; 2008. Reprinted with permission.)

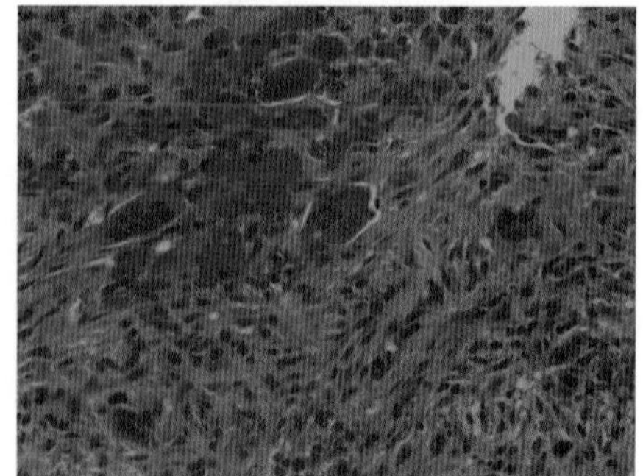

Fig. 2.52 Nonossifying fibroma with a focus of osteoclast-like giant cells and some lymphocytes in an area of hemorrhage.

- Demographic: young patients (ages 5–15 years)
- Location: distal femur, distal tibia, proximal tibia
- Presentation: incidental, occasional fracture
- Imaging: metaphyseal, lucent lesion, eccentric, surrounded by sclerotic, scalloped rim; cortex may be expanded and thinned
- Histology: whorled bundles, giant cells, hemosiderin
- Treatment: observation or curettage/bone graft (if risk for pathologic fracture)
  a. Lesions ossify at skeletal maturity and regress.

2. Desmoplastic fibroma
   - Rare, low grade, aggressive (equivalent to soft tissue desmoids); likely originates from myofibroblasts
   - Demographics: ages 10–30 years
   - Genetics: loss of 5q21–22, loss of 4p, rearrangement of 12q12–13, trisomy 8, trisomy 20 reported
   - Imaging: lytic lesion centrally located in metaphysis
   - Histology: abundant collagen, mature fibroblasts, no cellular atypia
   - Treatment: wide resection, aggressive curettage, high local recurrence rate
3. Malignant fibrous histiocytoma of bone/fibrosarcoma
   - Malignant tumor with proliferating cells with histiocytic quality, no osteoid production
   - MFH and fibrosarcoma now considered the same entity
   - Demographics: ages 20–80 years, more common in males
   - Presentation: pain, swelling, limp; may have fever, leukocytosis, hypoglycemia
   - Locations: metaphyseal, distal femur, proximal tibia, proximal femur, ilium, proximal humerus
   - Imaging: lytic or mixed lytic/blastic
     a. Differential: metastases, all malignant bone tumors
   - Histology: proliferating cells with histiocytic quality with indented nuclei, abundant cytoplasm, large nucleoli, giant cells, storiform appearance, herringbone pattern
   - Treatment: same as that for osteosarcoma; wide excision and radiation, with or without chemotherapy (high grade)
   - Metastasis: lung and bones

G. Tumor-Like Lesions of Bone

1. Langerhans cell histiocytosis **(Figs. 2.53, 2.54, 2.55)**
   - Called eosinophilic granuloma (EG) when in bone
   - Proliferation of Langerhans cells of dendritic system
   - Demographic: age < 30 years, male-to-female ratio = 2:1
   - Presentation: pain, swelling
   - Location: most common in long bones, skull, ribs, clavicle, scapula, vertebra; commonly causes vertebra plana (ages 2–6 years)
     a. **Single vertebra plana: EG, Ewing's sarcoma, ABC, osteomyelitis**
     b. **Multiple vertebra plana: mucopolysaccharidosis, Gaucher's disease, osteogenesis imperfecta (OI), lymphoma, metastatic disease**
   - Imaging: lytic lesion with well-defined margins; cortical thinning with periosteal reaction
     a. Differential: osteomyelitis, Ewing's sarcoma, leukemia
   - Histology: proliferating Langerhans cell with coffee bean indented nuclei, usually eosinophils in large numbers, giant cells
     a. Electron microscopy (EM): Birbeck granules (tennis racquet)
     b. Stain CD1A positive, S100+
   - Treatment: typically self-limiting, but may use methylprednisolone acetate injection, curettage/bone graft; can brace for vertebra plana; radiation for spinal cord compression/neurologic symptoms
   - **Can use steroids to treat UBC and EG.**
   - Syndromes (continuum from EG):
     a. Hand-Schuller-Christian disease
        - Multiple bone lesions and visceral involvement
        - **Classic triad: diabetes insipidus (pituitary involvement), exophthalmos, lytic lesions (often skull)**
     b. Letterer-Siwe: fatal, fulminating histiocytosis
2. Paget's disease **(Fig. 2.56)**
   - Disorder characterized by abnormal bone remodeling caused by osteoclastic dysfunction.
   - Genetics: autosomal dominant (40%)
   - Demographic: age > 50 years
   - Presentation: pain, high output cardiac failure (rare)

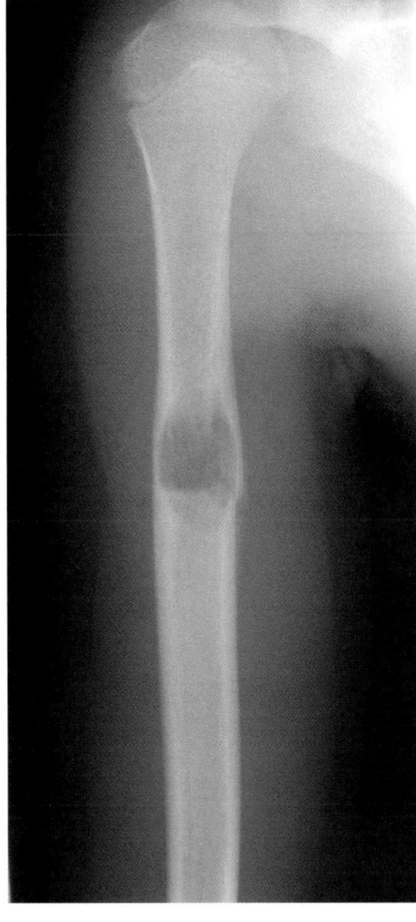

Fig. 2.53 Cystic diaphyseal lesion in a 10-year-old. (From Conrad EU. Orthopaedic Oncology: Diagnosis and Treatment. New York: Thieme; 2008. Reprinted with permission.)

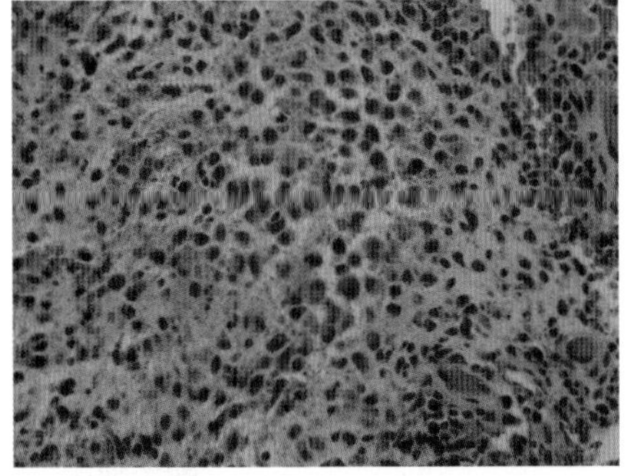

Fig. 2.54 Langerhans cell histiocytosis (LCH) is a cellular lesion composed of large kidney-shaped histocytes as a background cell with aggregations of eosinophils, leukocytes, and lymphocytes. The diagnostic cell is the histiocyte.

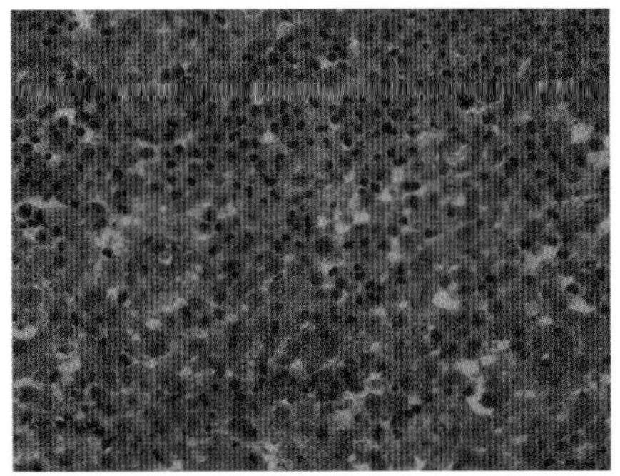

Fig. 2.55 Langerhans cell histiocytosis (LCH) with prominent eosinophils and a background of histiocytes.

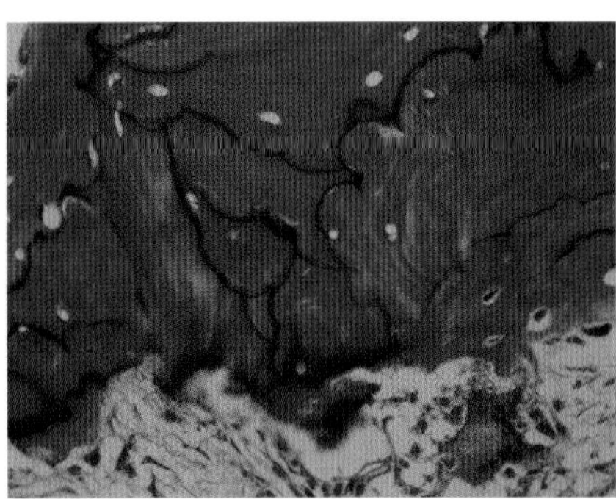

Fig. 2.56 Paget disease with the mosaic pattern of lamellar bone caused by the abnormal arrangement of units of lamellar fastened together along the prominent cement lines.

- Location: monostotic or polyostotic; femur, pelvis, tibia, skull, spine
- Labs: elevated hydroxyproline, increased urinary N- and α-C-telopeptides, elevated alkaline phosphatase
- Imaging: coarse trabeculae (blastic appearance of bone), thickened cortex, enlargement of bone; shepherd's crook deformity of proximal femur, tibial bowing
  a. Three radiographic stages of disease: lytic, mixed, sclerotic
  b. Bone scan: increased uptake
  c. MRI: thickened trabeculae with normal marrow signal
- Histology: irregular, broad trabeculae, prominent cement lines, osteoclasts, fibrous vascular tissue
- Treatment: bisphosphonates (decrease osteoclast activity), calcitonin
- 1% risk of malignant degeneration to sarcoma within Paget lesion
  a. Abrupt onset pain and swelling, soft tissue mass

New onset of pain requires a workup for possible malignant transformation.

  b. Treatment: surgery + chemotherapy or palliative radiation
  c. Survival at 5 years: < 5%

3. Tumoral calcinosis
   - Rare disorder, uncertain etiology involving phosphate metabolism dysfunction
   - Demographic: African descent, females
   - Associated with metabolic defects, collage vascular disorders, trauma
   - Presentation: slow growing mass
   - Location: soft tissue lesions well demarcated over extensor surfaces of large joints, typically hip, elbow, shoulder, foot, wrist
   - Histology: loculated calcific debris in fibrous stroma
   - Treatment: surgical removal if symptomatic; risk of recurrence
4. Synovial herniation pits
   - Tumor simulator
   - Common in femoroacetabular impingement

H. Fibrous Dysplasia, Osteofibrous Dysplasia, Adamantinoma

1. Fibrous dysplasia **(Figs. 2.57, 2.58, 2.59)**
   - Developmental abnormality, monostotic or polyostotic.
   - Failure of production of normal lamellar bone
   - Genetics: activating mutation of GSα surface protein; increased cyclic adenosine monophosphate (cAMP)
     a. High expression of fibroblast growth factor-23 (FGF-23)
   - Demographic: age < 30 years, females > males
   - Presentation: asymptomatic, incidental, occasionally painful
   - Location: any bone, proximal femur most common
   - Imaging: central lytic lesion in diaphysis or metaphysis, ground glass
     a. Can cause shepherd's crook deformity in proximal femur
     b. Fibrous dysplasia appears similar to low-grade osteosarcoma or osteomyelitis, but they all have a significantly different histology.
   - Histology: abundant fibroblasts, trabeculae of osteoid and bone within fibrous stroma without osteoblastic rimming (differentiate from osteofibrous dysplasia)
     a. "Alphabet soup," disorganized bone fragments

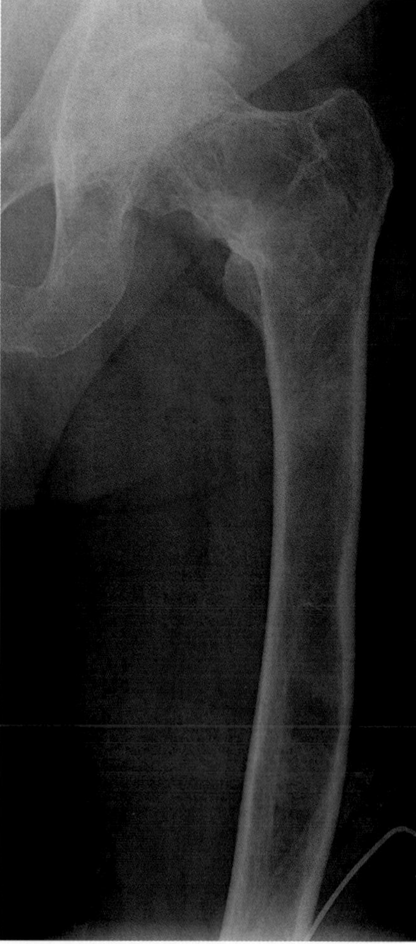

Fig. 2.57 Classic proximal femur cystic lesion with ground-glass appearance, and varus deformity causing a "shepherd's crook" deformity.

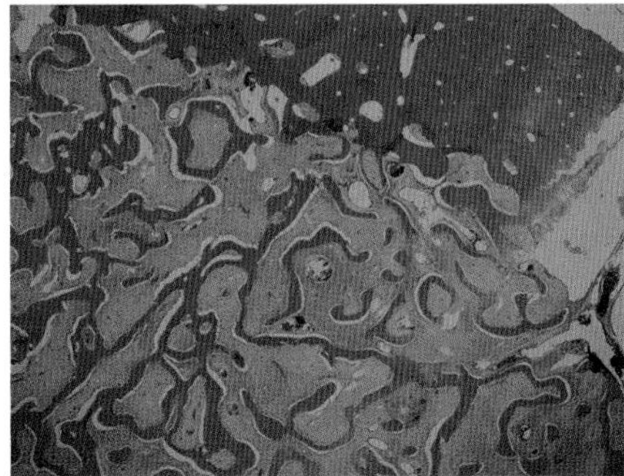

Fig. 2.58 Fibrous dysplasia (low power) replacing the entire marrow cavity but sparing the cortex. Irregular curvilinear woven bone spicules embedded in fibrous tissue can be seen.

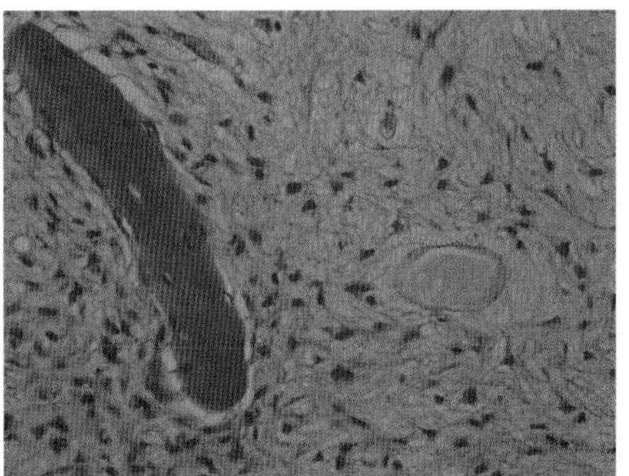

Fig. 2.59 Fibrous dysplasia with woven bone spicules, lacking prominent osteoblastic rimming, embedded in fibrovascular tissue.

- Treatment: observation or internal fixation if painful, pathologic or impending fracture, deformity
  a. Bisphosphonates shown to decrease pain associated with skeletal lesions
  b. Must use cortical or cancellous allografts for fixation because autogenous bone will be transformed to FD
- **Bisphosphonates used for treatment of fibrous dysplasia, metastatic disease, multiple myeloma, Paget's disease.**
- < 1% malignant transformation
- Syndromes:
  a. McCune-Albright: café-au-lait spots (with jagged coast of Maine borders), polyostotic fibrous dysplasia, endocrine abnormalities (precocious puberty)
  b. Mazabraud: polyostotic fibrous dysplasia with intramuscular myxomas

2. Osteofibrous dysplasia (**Figs. 2.60** and **2.61**)
   - Demographic: age < 10 years, males > females
   - Presentation: painless swelling over anterior tibia
   - Location: anterior tibial cortex
   - Imaging: eccentric, well-defined, lytic lesion of anterior tibia, often with cortical expansion
     a. Frequently causes bowing, can cause pathologic fracture
   - Histology: fibrous tissue stroma, osteoid, giant cells, osteoblastic rimming
   - Treatment: typically regress, may require bracing; may recur if removed prior to skeletal maturity
3. Adamantinoma (**Figs. 2.62** and **2.63**)
   - Rare, low-grade malignant tumor
   - Demographic: young adults (age > 20 years)
   - Presentation: insidious pain (months to years)
   - Location: anterior tibia most commonly, can affect other long bones
     a. Differential diagnosis: osteofibrous dysplasia; differentiate by histology as location and radiology are similar
   - Imaging: multiple, sharply circumscribed lucent defects, sclerotic bones, "soap bubble" appearance
   - Histology: nests of epithelial cells in benign stroma with palisading/glandular pattern
     a. Epithelial membrane antigen (EMA) and keratin positive

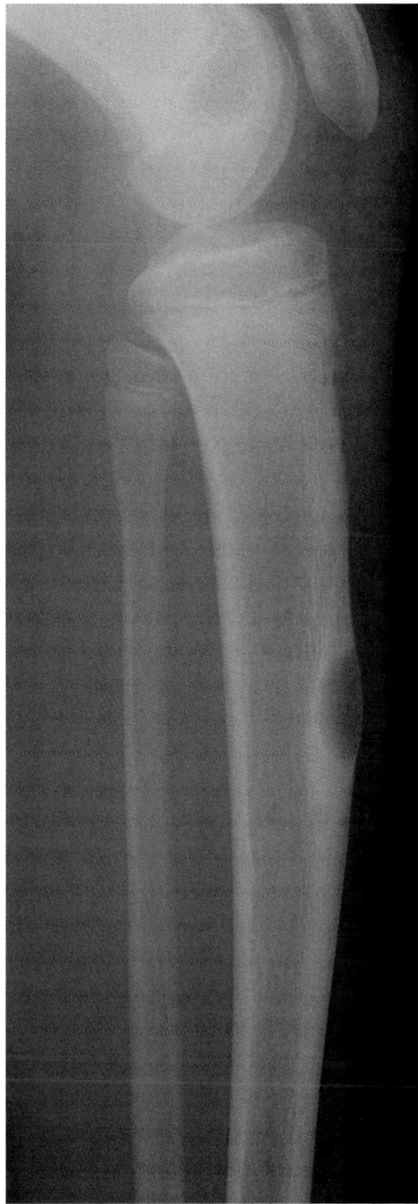

Fig. 2.60 Eccentric, lytic lesion of the anterior tibia seen in osteofibrous dysplasia.

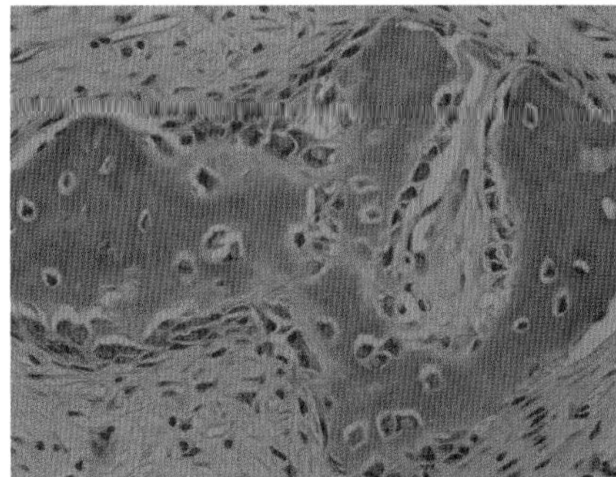

Fig. 2.61 Osteofibrous dysplasia with irregular woven bone spicules surrounded or rimmed by prominent osteoblasts.

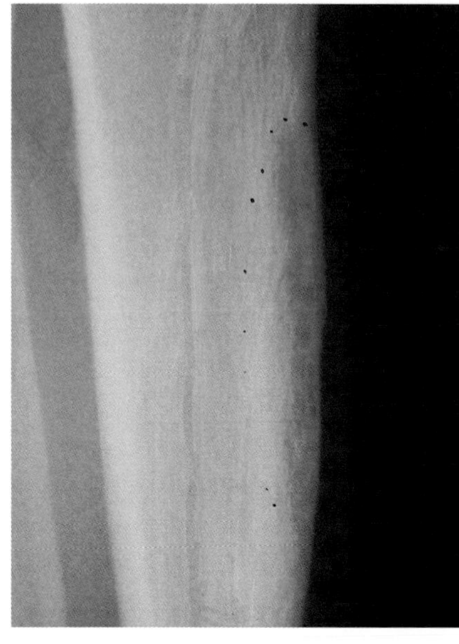

Fig. 2.62 Subtle lesion of the proximal anterior tibial cortex. (From Conrad EU. Orthopaedic Oncology: Diagnosis and Treatment. New York: Thieme; 2008. Reprinted with permission.)

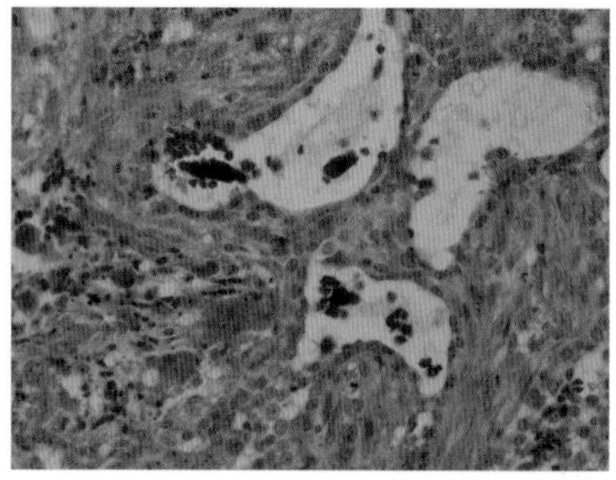

Fig. 2.63 Adamantinoma of the long bone with nests and islands of epithelial cells.

- Treatment: wide resection, risk of metastasis (2–3%); not chemotherapy or radiation sensitive

I. Hematopoietic Tumors

1. Lymphoma **(Figs. 2.64, 2.65, 2.66)**
   - Proliferation of B or T lymphocytes most commonly presenting as nodal disease that may metastasize to skeleton; rarely primary lymphoma of bone
   - Primary, metastatic foci, or in association with other osseous sites
   - Most commonly non-Hodgkin's B-cell lymphoma
   - Demographic: all ages, most commonly 35–55 years, males > females
   - Presentation: pain, soft tissue mass, pathologic fracture; B-symptoms: fever, weight loss, night sweats; may have neurologic symptoms from spinal metastasis
   - Workup: bone marrow biopsy, CT chest/abdomen/pelvis, bone biopsy if primary bone lesion
   - Location: distal femur, proximal tibia, pelvis, proximal femur, vertebra, shoulder girdle
   - Imaging: bone destruction, mottled appearance, often with reactive bone formation and thickened cortex; hot on bone scan
     a. Differential diagnosis: metastatic disease, myeloma, osteomyelitis
   - Histology: mixed cellular infiltrate with round blue cells of varying shapes and sizes
     a. Immunohistochemistry: CD20+, CD45+, CD99–, leukocyte common antigen (LCA)
   - Treatment: chemotherapy (cyclophosphamide, doxorubicin, prednisone, vincristine), ± radiation
   - Prognosis: primary lymphoma of bone with better prognosis than secondary involvement

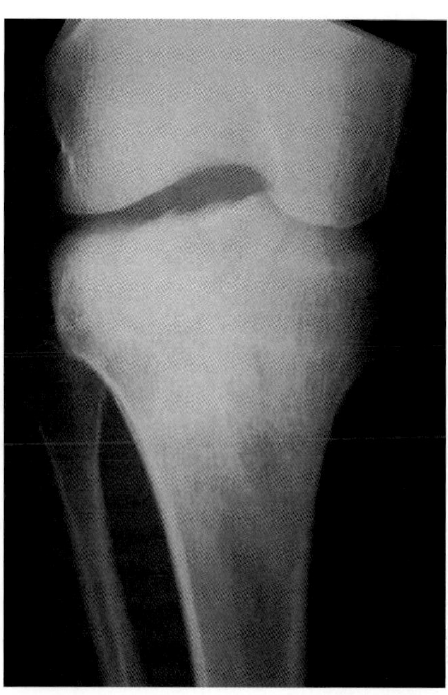

Fig. 2.64 Osteoblastic lesion of the proximal tibia in a 46-year-old. (From Conrad EU. Orthopaedic Oncology: Diagnosis and Treatment. New York: Thieme; 2008. Reprinted with permission.)

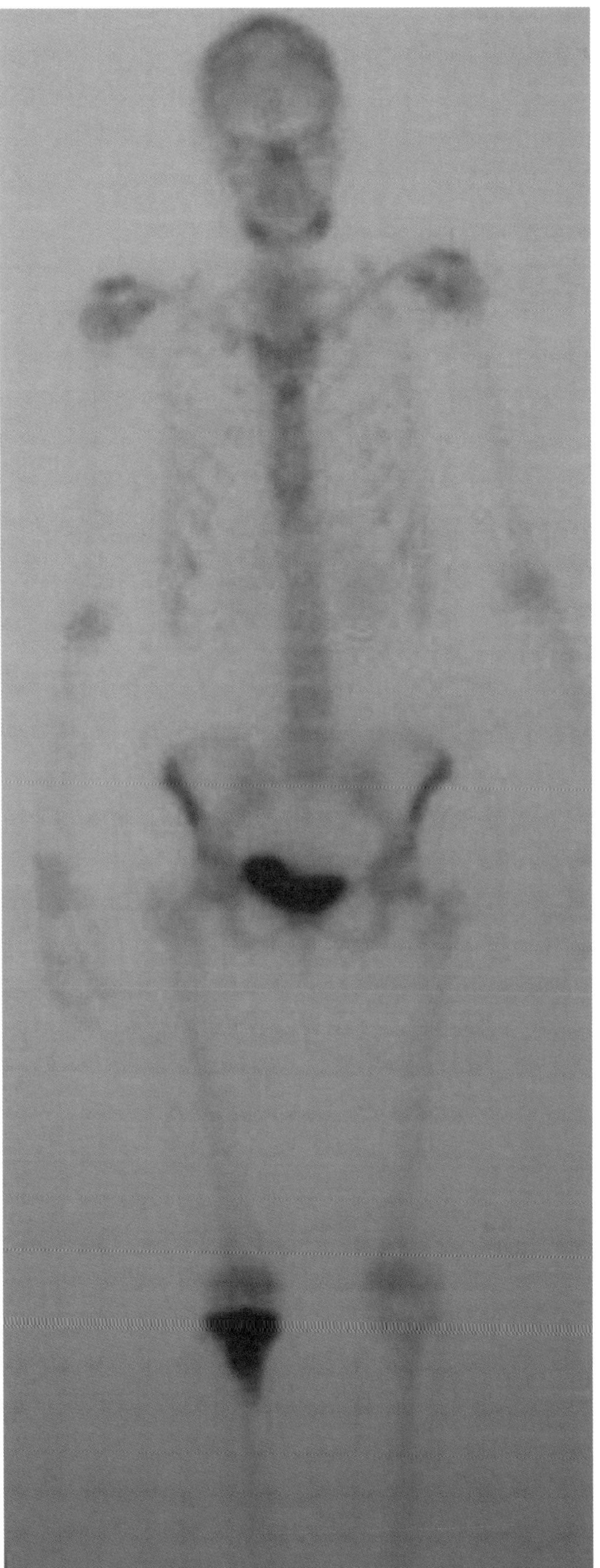

Fig. 2.65 Bone scan. (From Conrad EU. Orthopaedic Oncology: Diagnosis and Treatment. New York: Thieme; 2008. Reprinted with permission.)

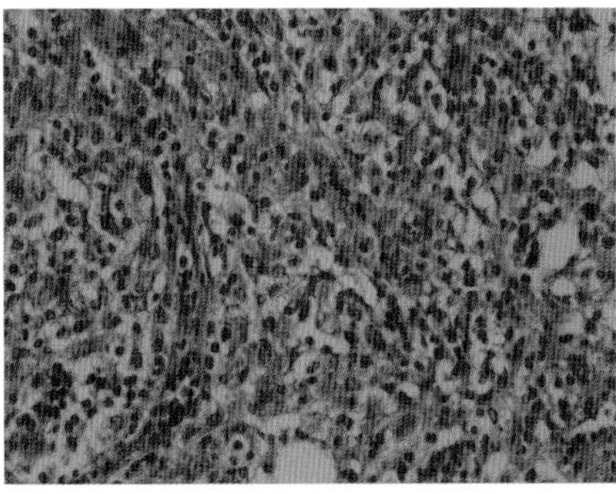

Fig. 2.66 Hodgkin's lymphoma is composed of atypical or bland histocytes admixed with lymphocytes, plasma cells, and large cells with a bilobed nucleus called a Reed-Sternberg cell.

2. Multiple myeloma (**Figs. 2.67** and **2.68**)
   - Malignant plasma cell disorder in which plasma cells produce immunoglobulins
   - **Most common primary malignant bone tumor**
   - Demographic: ages 50–80 years, males > females; black/white ratio = 2:1
   - Presentation: bone pain (spine/ribs), pathologic fracture, fatigue
   - Labs: serum protein electrophoresis (SPEP)/urine protein electrophoresis (UPEP), hypercalcemia (33%), elevated creatinine (Cr) (50%), normochromic, normocytic anemia, elevated erythrocyte sedimentation rate (ESR)
     a. Urine: Bence Jones proteins
        - **Bence Jones protein is a measure of immunoglobulin light chains in the urine.**

     b. UPEP: monoclonal light chain immunoglobulin
   - Imaging: punched-out lesions most commonly in skull, spine, long bones containing plasma cells
     a. Bone scan negative (30%) when there is minimal osteoblastic response
   - Histology: sheets of plasma cells with eccentric nucleus ("clock face") and perinuclear clear zone (Hoffa's clear zone)
     a. CD38+
   - Treatment: bisphosphonates to control osteoclast activity, reduce pain, decrease fracture risk; chemotherapy, radiation (for neurologic symptoms and pain relief)
   - Survival: 10% at 10 years
3. Solitary plasmacytoma
   - Must differentiate from multiple myeloma (more favorable prognosis in solitary form)
   - Imaging: solitary punched-out lesion
     a. A solitary punched-out lesion as opposed to multiple lesions seen in multiple myeloma
   - Labs: bone marrow plasmacyte count 10% or less, negative SPEP/UPEP
   - 50–75% will progress to multiple myeloma
   - Treatment: radiation
4. Osteosclerotic myeloma
   - Bone lesions associated with chronic inflammatory demyelinating polyneuropathy (CIDP)
   - Sensory symptoms first, then motor symptoms, spread distal to proximal
   - Painless
   - **POEMS syndrome: polyneuropathy, organomegaly, endocrinopathy, M-spike, skin changes**
   - Treatment: chemotherapy, radiation, plasmapheresis. Neurologic symptoms may not improve.

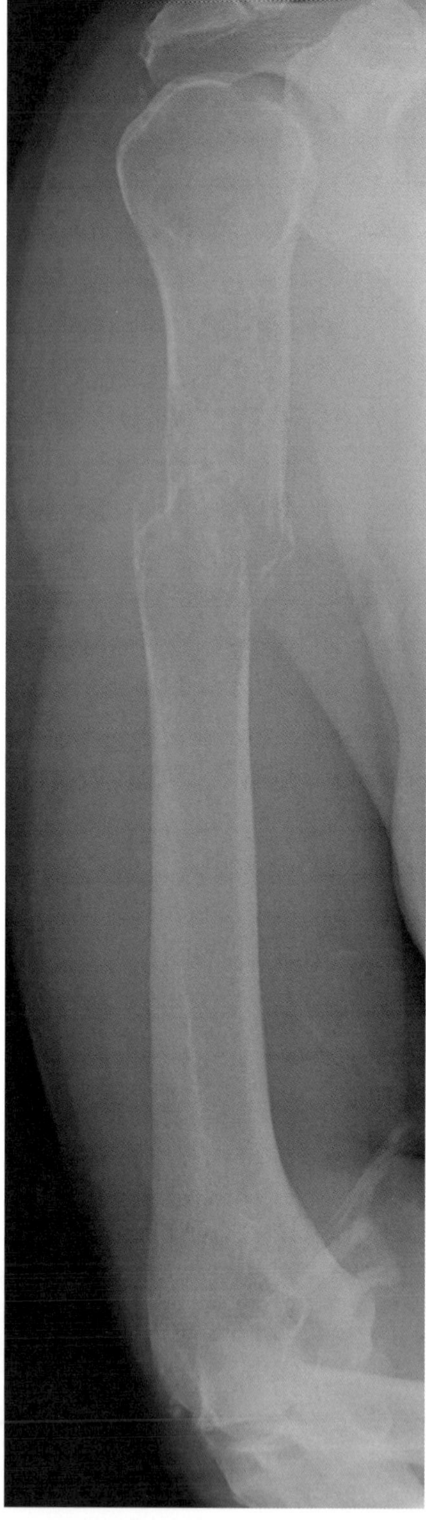

Fig. 2.67 Lytic lesion in a humeral shaft. Biopsy confirmed multiple myeloma.

J. Vascular Tumors

1. Hemangioma (**Fig. 2.69**)
   - Benign vascular tumor of bone
   - Location: vertebral bodies and craniofacial bones
   - Imaging:
     a. Spine: lytic destruction, vertical striations or honeycomb appearance; "jail bar" vertebrae
     b. MRI: heterogeneous lesion with numerous vessels and fatty infiltration; "bag of worms"; increased signal on T1 suggestive of fat in lesion

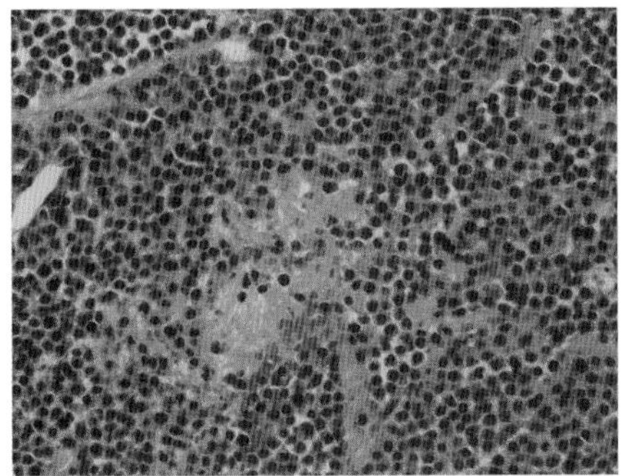

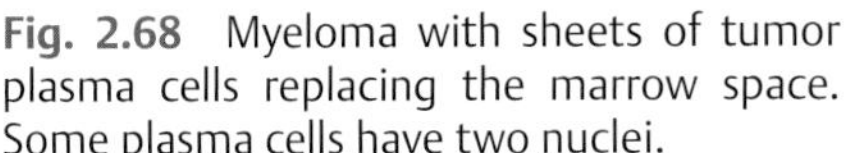

Fig. 2.68 Myeloma with sheets of tumor plasma cells replacing the marrow space. Some plasma cells have two nuclei.

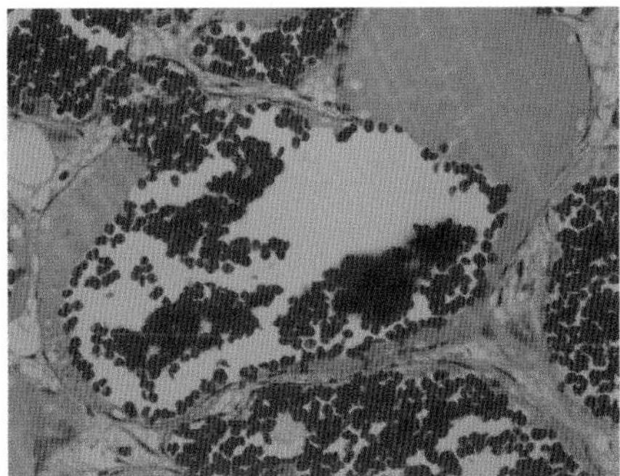

Fig. 2.69 Hemangioma of bone with thin-walled vessels, and endothelial-lined spaces lacking muscular coats in the vessel wall.

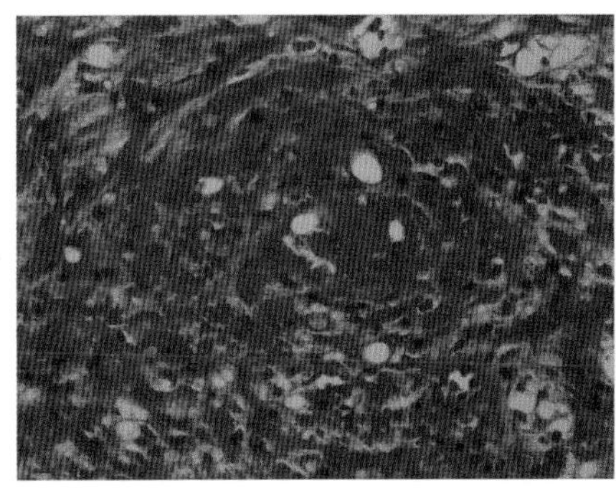

Fig. 2.70 Hemangiosarcoma with extensive endothelial cell pleomorphism.

- Histology: cavernous lesions with thin-walled vessels
- Treatment: observation, curettage and bone graft (if lesion accessible), low-dose radiation if inaccessible

2. Hemangioendothelioma/hemangiosarcoma **(Fig. 2.70)**
   - Rare malignant vascular tumor of bone
   - Demographic: all age groups
   - Presentation: pain
   - Location: multifocal involvement of same limb (30%)
   - Imaging: oval lytic lesion, no reactive bone formation
   - Histology: vascular spaces, varying in differentiation
   - Treatment: radiation (low grade) versus wide resection and radiation (high grade)

K. Notochordal Lesions of Bone

1. Chordoma **(Figs. 2.71, 2.72, 2.73)**
   - Malignant bone tumor originating from primitive notochordal rests, occurring in spine
   - Demographics: age > 40 years, male-to-female ratio = 3:1
   - Presentation: low back or sacral pain, typically without neurologic deficit but with bowel/bladder symptoms
   - Location: 50% sacrococcygeal, 30% spheno-occipital; 50% can be identified on rectal exam
   - Imaging: midline anterior soft tissue mass and sacral involvement on MRI
     a. Differential: chondrosarcoma, multiple myeloma, metastatic disease, giant cell tumor, lymphoma
   - Histology: physaliferous cell (pathognomonic), containing vacuoles and with bubbly appearance to cytoplasm
   - **Recognize the histological appearance of physaliferous cells as they are pathognomonic for chordoma.**
     a. S100+
   - Treatment: wide resection, with or without radiation for local recurrence, positive margins, inoperable tumor; very high local recurrence rate
   - Metastasis: to lungs in 30–50%
   - Survival: 25–50%

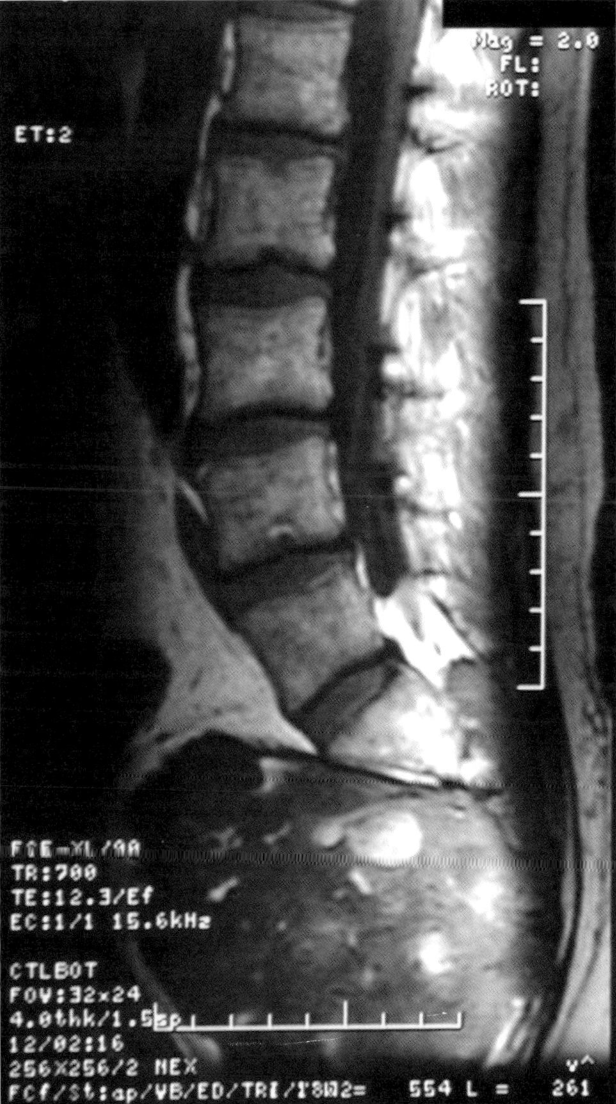

Fig. 2.71 Sagittal MRI showing large lesion with extension to S1 and into the epidural space. (From Conrad EU. Orthopaedic Oncology: Diagnosis and Treatment. New York: Thieme; 2008. Reprinted with permission.)

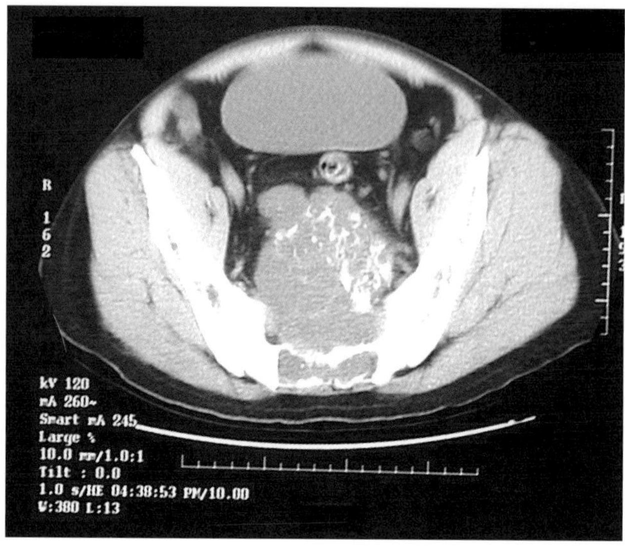

Fig. 2.72 CT of large central S1 tumor. (From Conrad EU. Orthopaedic Oncology: Diagnosis and Treatment. New York: Thieme; 2008. Reprinted with permission.)

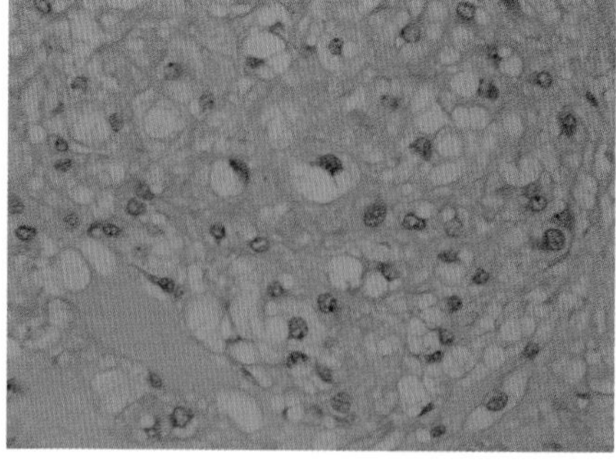

Fig. 2.73 Chordoma with characteristic large cells with bubbly cytoplasm (physaliphorous cell) embedded in clear to pink matrix.

L. Tumors of Unknown Origin

1. Metastatic bone disease (**Figs. 2.74** and **2.75**)

- **Lytic lesion most commonly occurs at age > 40 years.**
- **Five carcinomas likely to metastasize to bone: breast, lung, thyroid, kidney, prostate; mnemonic: BLT sandwich and a Kosher Pickle**
- **Renal cell metastases to undergo arterial embolization prior to surgery**
- **Hypercalcemia: breast cancer, multiple myeloma, lymphoma**

- Demographic: age > 40 years
- Presentation: increasing and progressive pain, constitutional symptoms, known primary cancer
- Laboratory studies (**Fig. 2.1**): complete blood count (CBC), basic metabolic panel, lactate dehydrogenase (LDH), alkaline phosphatase, urinalysis; may order specific tumor markers, such as prostate-specific antigen (PSA) for prostate, carcinoembryonic antigen (CEA) for colon/pancreas, cancer antigen (CA)-125 for ovarian
- Location: pelvis, vertebral bodies, ribs, proximal limb girdles
  a. Most common location of pathologic fracture: proximal femur
  b. Most common site of metastasis: spine, most commonly thoracic; spares intervertebral disk
  c. Metastasis distal to elbows and knees: most commonly from lung
  d. Lesser trochanter avulsion fracture indicates impending fracture of femoral neck
- Metastasis to lung: MFH, synovial sarcoma, GCT, chondroblastoma
- Pathogenesis:
  a. Batson's venous plexus
     ◦ Venous flow from breast, lung, prostate, kidney, thyroid into vertebral vein plexus

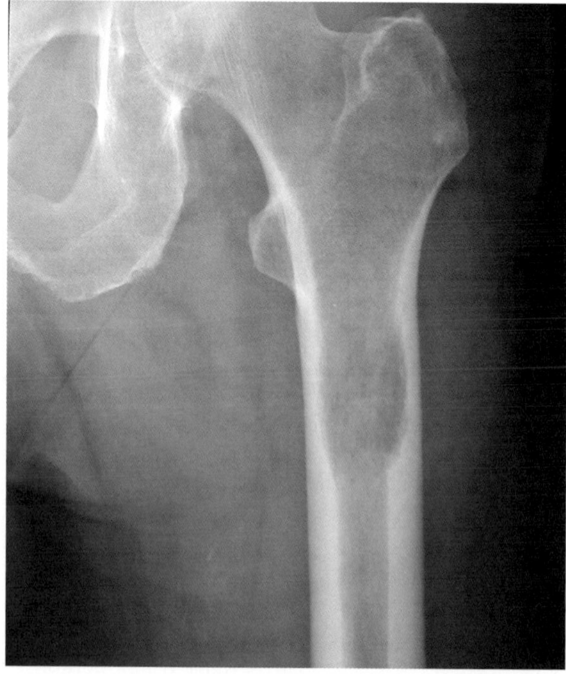

Fig. 2.74 Central "lytic" lesion of proximal femur. (From Conrad EU. Orthopaedic Oncology: Diagnosis and Treatment. New York: Thieme; 2008. Reprinted with permission.)

   b. Parathyroid hormone–related protein (PTHrP): secreted by tumor cells, activates the receptor activator of nuclear factor kappa B ligand (RANKL), upregulates osteoclasts
      - Release of transforming growth factor-β (TGF-β) and calcium (Ca) with bone destruction; stimulates tumor cells to release more PTHrP
- Imaging: destructive lesion (lytic, mixed lytic/bone forming, sclerotic)
   a. Lytic: lung, thyroid, kidney, gastrointestinal (GI) tract
   b. Blastic: prostate, bladder
   c. Mixed osteolytic/osteoblastic: breast
   d. Differential diagnosis: multiple myeloma, lymphoma, Paget's sarcoma, hyperparathyroidism, primary bone tumor
   e. Occult lytic metastatic disease with no known source after bone scan and CT chest/abdomen/pelvis most likely to be occult lung cancer or adenocarcinoma with unknown primary.
- Histology: epithelial cells in fibrous stroma
- Treatment:
   a. If concern that a lesion is pathological, biopsy first. Do not ream or stabilize lesion without a diagnosis. If known primary cancer presents with lytic lesion, must biopsy to prove metastasis unless patient has known metastatic bone lesions.
   b. Bisphosphonates (pamidronate, zoledronic acid) for pain control and to reduce skeletal events
   c. Isolated metastatic lesion to bone: consider wide resection with or without radiation, especially renal cell carcinoma and lesions of the proximal femur
   d. Multiple metastatic bony lesions: treat with internal fixation if risk of impending fracture, with or without radiation
   e. Criteria for impending fracture:
      - > 50% cortical destruction, subtrochanteric location, > 50–75% metaphyseal destruction, pain after radiation, pain with weightbearing
      - Mirel's criteria (**Table 2.7**); consider prophylactic fixation
   f. Goals of prophylactic fixation: limit pain, minimize time in hospital, improve quality of life
- Prognosis: lung cancer metastases entail the lowest life expectancy; lung < renal < breast < prostate < thyroid

2. Giant cell tumor (GCT) (**Figs. 2.76, 2.77, 2.78**)
   - Benign but aggressive bone tumor of mononuclear cells
   - Demographic: ages 30–50 years (uncommon with open physes), females > males
   - Presentation: pain, swelling
   - Location: epiphysis and metaphysis long bones: 50% around knee, vertebral body, sacrum, distal radius
   - **Radial side of distal radius for GCT. If ulnar side, think telangiectatic osteosarcoma (OS).**

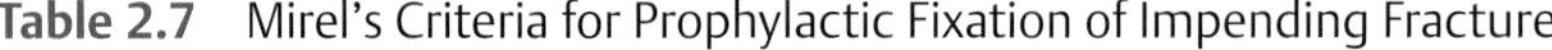

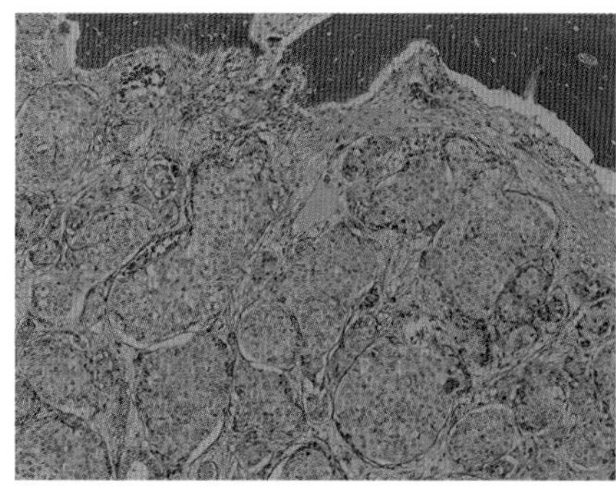

Fig. 2.75 Metastatic carcinoma arranged in nests surrounded by wisps of fibrovascular tissue.

Table 2.7 Mirel's Criteria for Prophylactic Fixation of Impending Fracture

Score	1	2	3
Site	Upper limb	Lower limb	Peritrochanteric
Pain	Mild	Moderate	Severe
Lesion	Blastic	Mixed	Lytic
Size (cortical involvement)	< ⅓	⅓–⅔	> ⅔

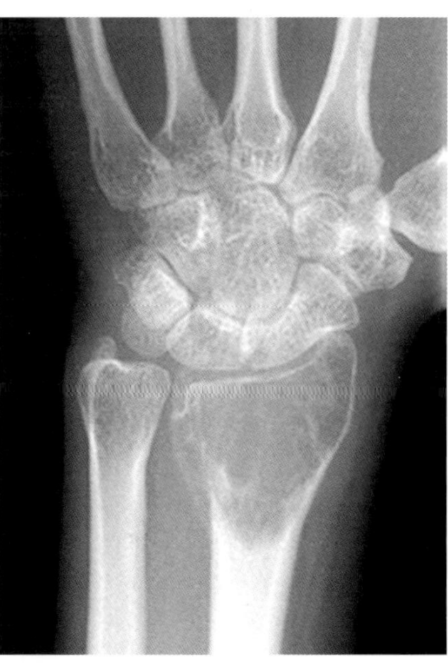

Fig. 2.76 Cystic lesion in a 39-year-old. (From Conrad EU. Orthopaedic Oncology: Diagnosis and Treatment. New York: Thieme; 2008. Reprinted with permission.)

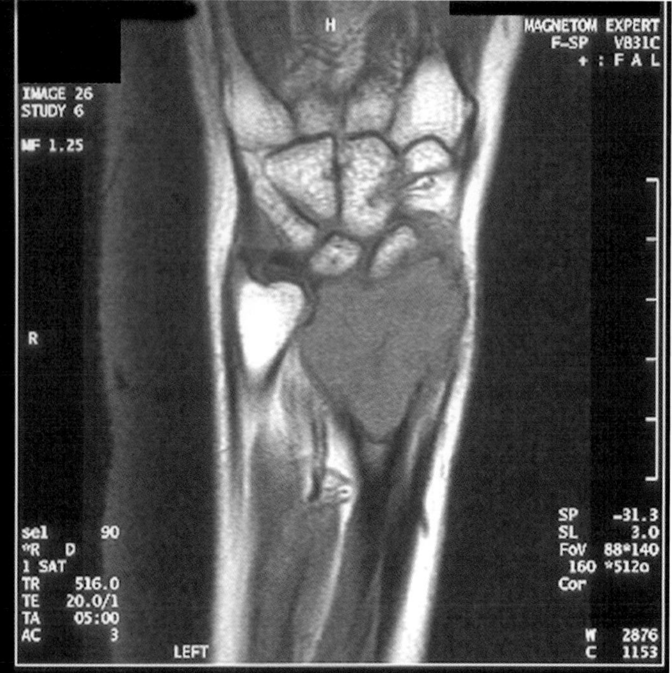

Fig. 2.77 Coronal MRI showing osseous “containment.” (From Conrad EU. Orthopaedic Oncology: Diagnosis and Treatment. New York: Thieme; 2008. Reprinted with permission.)

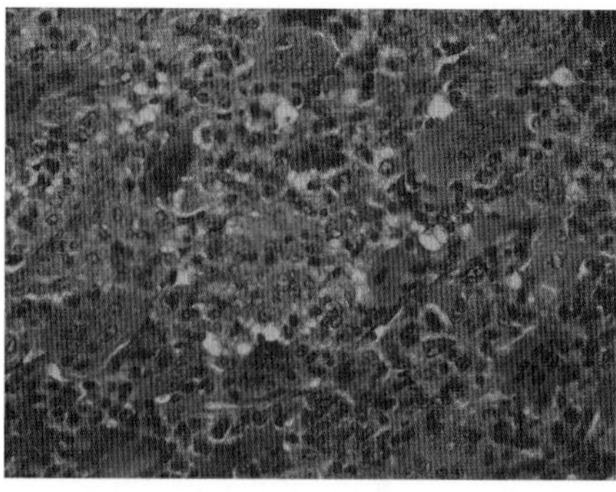

Fig. 2.78 Giant cell tumor with the three characteristic findings of oval or round mononuclear cells, random distribution of the giant cells, and similarity of the mononuclear cell nuclei to the nuclei of the giant cells.

- Imaging: lytic, eccentric, destructive lesion in metaphysis that extends to epiphysis, well demarcated without sclerosis
  a. Hot on bone scan
  b. MRI sometimes shows cortical disruption with soft tissue mass.
- Histology: sheet of giant cells and proliferating round/oval/spindle shaped cells
  a. Stromal cells are the neoplastic cells.
- Mechanism: activation of osteoclasts by tumor cells
- Treatment: Curettage with graft [methylmethacrylate (MMA) or bone graft], with or without adjuvant therapy (phenol, liquid nitrogen, hydrogen peroxide, sterile water); 10% risk recurrence
- Metastasis:
- **2–5% risk of metastasis to lungs**
  a. Risk factors for metastasis: local recurrence, location in distal radius, proximal femur, sacrum, immunocompromised
- Malignant: primary (sarcoma existing in GCT), secondary (after radiation for GCT, 3–50 years after treatment)
- **Benign tumors that can metastasize to lung: chondroblastoma and giant cell tumor**

3. Ewing’s sarcoma (**Figs. 2.79** and **2.80**)
   - Primitive neuroectodermal tumor (PNET) containing small blue cells
   - Demographic: ages 5–25 years, males > females
   - **Second most common sarcoma of bone**
   - **If age < 5 years, consider leukemia, neuroblastoma; if age > 30 years, consider lymphoma versus metastasis.**
   - Genetics: chromosomal translocation: t(11;22); fusion protein: EWS-FLI1
   - Presentation: pain, fever

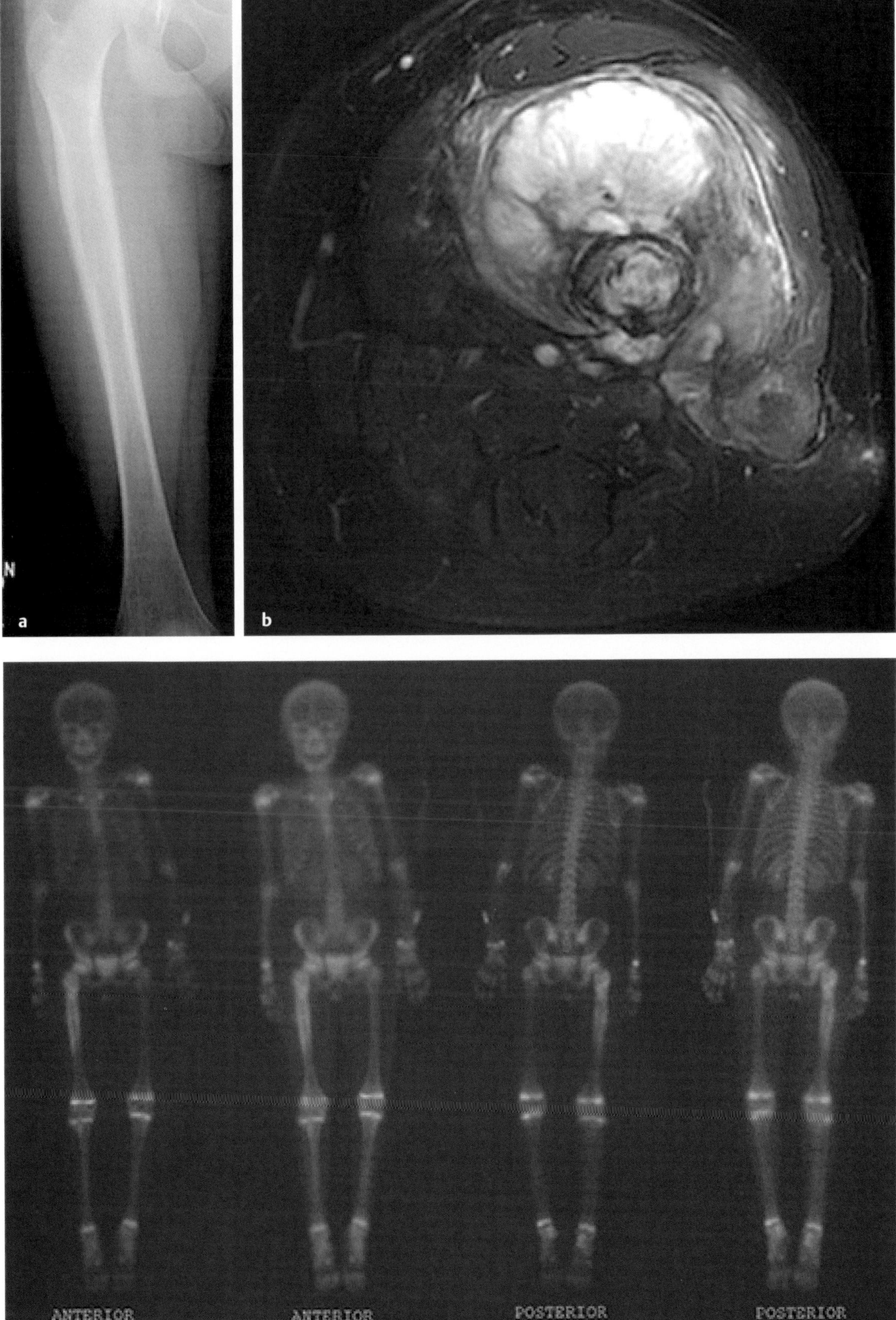

Fig. 2.79 **(a)** X-rays showing permeative lesion in the diaphysis of a femur. The periosteal reaction shows an "onion-skin" pattern that is classic for Ewing's sarcoma. Ewing's 2. **(b)** T2 axial MRI demonstrating the large soft tissue mass associated with this lesion. Ewing's 3. **(c)** Bone scan showing uptake within the femur.

- Location: flat bones—pelvis/scapula; long bones—metaphysis or diaphysis
- Labs: increased ESR, increased LDH, leukocytosis, anemia
- Imaging: destructive lesion in metaphysis or diaphysis with lytic or variable bone formation
- **May have onionskin appearance with periosteum lifted off bone in multiple layers**
  a. MRI: soft tissue mass
- Histology: sheet of small round blue cells, pseudorosettes (true rosettes: neuroblastoma)
  a. Immunohistochemistry: CD99 positive, vimentin stain positive, PAS positive, reticulin negative, MIC-2 positive
- **Lymphoma histology looks similar to Ewing's sarcoma; however, lymphoma is CD34+ (LCA) and CD99–, whereas Ewing's is CD99+ and CD34– (LCA).**
- Workup: requires bone marrow biopsy for marrow metastasis (worse prognosis), CT chest, bone scan
- Treatment: chemotherapy (vincristine, doxorubicin, cyclophosphamide dactinomycin), ± radiation, ± resection; use of radiation decreasing because of secondary sarcoma risk
  a. May radiate if unresectable tumor, positive margins
- Poor prognostic factors: spine/pelvic location, > 100 cm^3, poor response to chemotherapy (< 90% necrosis), elevated LDH, nonpulmonary metastasis, p53 mutation
- Survival: 65–70% with isolated extremity involvement; 5-year survival with metastatic disease < 20%

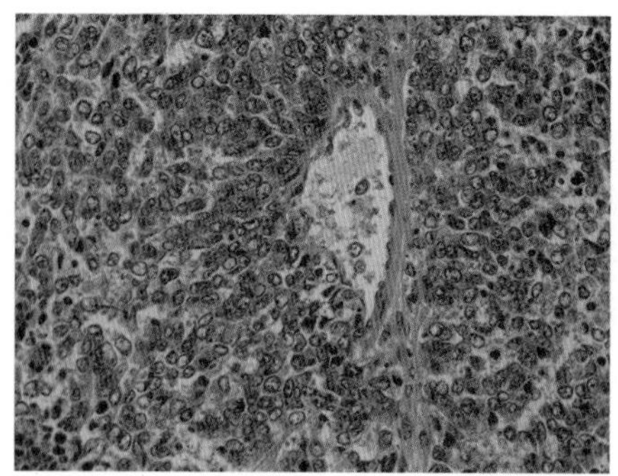

Fig. 2.80 Ewing's sarcoma is composed of sheets of small blue oval cells with little or no cytoplasm (naked nuclei), which are surrounding a central vessel. Mitoses are not prominent.

M. Other

1. Osteomyelitis **(Figs. 2.81** and **2.82)**
   - **Osteomyelitis can disguise itself as any tumor, so clinicians must always keep it in mind when considering the differential diagnosis.**
   - Presentation: pain, fever, draining sinus
   - Involucrum (reactive bone surrounding necrosis) and sequestrum (necrosis)
   - Risk of chronic infection and sinus undergoing transformation to squamous cell carcinoma
   - Labs: elevated ESR, C-reactive protein (CRP)
   - Histology: polymorphonuclear and plasma cells
   - **Marjolin's ulcer: squamous cell carcinoma developed in patients with burn scars or chronic osteomyelitis with sinus tract formation**
2. Multifocal culture negative osteomyelitis
   - Thought to be inflammatory disease of bone
   - Etiology: unknown
   - Workup: cultures negative
   - Treatment: anti-inflammatory medications
3. Osteopetrosis
   - Metabolic bone disease characterized by failure of osteoclastic resorption with formation of dense bone and loss of medullary cavity
   - Genetics: autosomal recessive (infantile or fatal in first few years of life) or autosomal dominant (AD).
     a. AD: associated with defects in carbonic anhydrase II, α3-subunit of vacuolar proton pump or chloride channel 7
   - Presentation: fracture, anemia, hearing loss

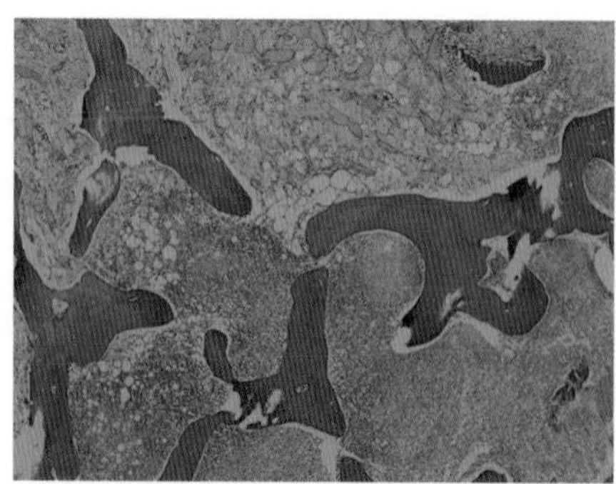

Fig. 2.81 Osteomyelitis with the marrow replaced by inflammatory cells. Large areas of necrosis *(upper half, pink)* and necrotic lamellar bone are present.

- Imaging: symmetric increase in bone mass with thickened bone and lack of medullary cavity and widened metaphyses (Erlenmeyer flask deformity)
- Histology: inactive osteoclasts
- Treatment: interferon gamma-1β (autosomal dominant form), bone marrow transplant, high-dose calcitriol (for autosomal recessive form)

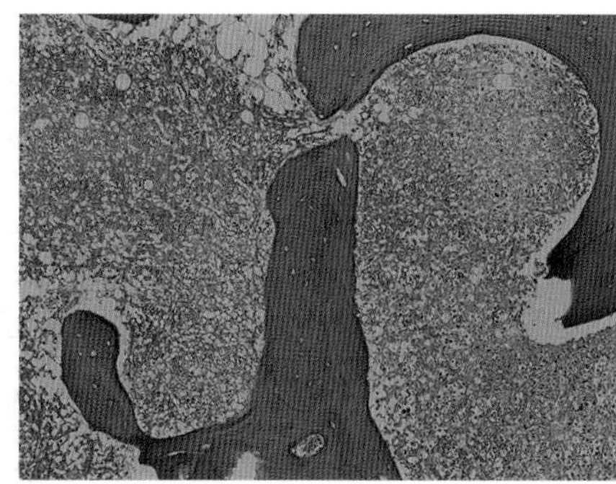

Fig. 2.82 Osteomyelitis with dead lamellar bone (empty osteocyte lacunae) called a sequestrum surrounded by pus.

III. Soft Tissue Tumors

A. Introduction: Benign Versus Malignant

1. Sarcoma: malignant tumors of mesenchymal origin
   - Demographic: age < 15 years, 15%; 15–55 years, 45%; > 55 years, 40%; males > females
   - Presentation: enlarging painless or painful soft tissue mass
   - Workup: radiographs, MRI for defining anatomy and characterizing lesion, CT chest for metastasis, CT chest/abdomen/pelvis for liposarcoma
     a. Any large, deep, heterogeneous mass on MRI in the extremities must be biopsied (assume sarcoma); may use needle or open biopsy
   - Staging: AJCC soft tissue sarcoma staging **(Table 2.3)**
   - Imaging: MRI: low signal on T1, bright on T2, heterogeneous
   - Treatment:
     a. Surgery: wide resection
     b. Radiation therapy for high grade (preoperative, perioperative, brachytherapy). Radiation decreases the risk of local recurrence but does not increase overall survival.
        - Brachytherapy: flexible catheters placed directly on tumor bed, loaded with radiation for 48–96 hours
     c. Superficial tumors any grade or low-grade sarcoma able to undergo wide resection may not need radiation
   - Outcome most dependent on initial tumor stage
   - Poor prognostic factors: metastases, high grade, > 5 cm (increased recurrence), location beneath deep fascia
   - Metastasis
     a. Sarcomas most commonly metastasize to lung (second most common: to lymph nodes). Should perform resection of lung metastases when possible.
     b. Rhabdomyosarcoma, clear cell sarcoma, synovial sarcoma, epithelioid sarcoma, angiosarcoma—lymphatic metastasis; may require sentinel node biopsy
     c. Sarcomas with lymphatic metastases: SCARE acronym: Synovial sarcoma, Clear cell sarcoma, Angiosarcoma, Rhabdomyosarcoma, Epithelioid sarcoma

B. Soft Tissue Tumors of Fibrogenic Origin

1. Calcifying aponeurotic fibroma
   - Demographic: age 3–30 years
   - Presentation: slow growing, painless mass
   - Location: hands and feet
   - Imaging: faint mass with stippling
   - Histology: fibrous tumor, central calcification and cartilage formation
   - Treatment: local excision (50% risk of recurrence), resolves with maturity
2. Fibromatosis **(Fig. 2.83)**
   - Benign aggressive fibrous lesion

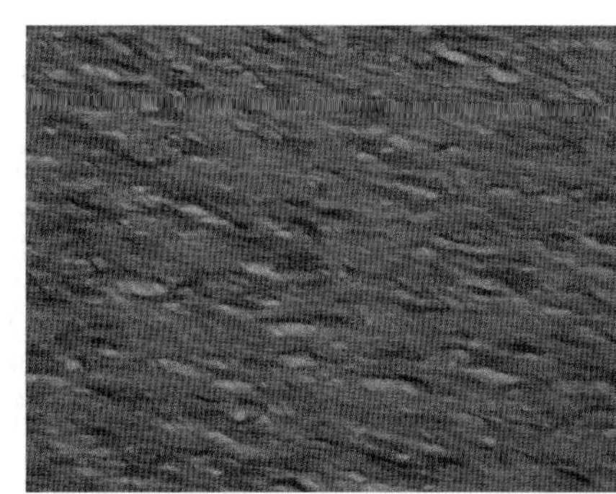

Fig. 2.83 Fibromatosis with wavy bland spindle cells. No pleomorphism or mitoses are present.

- Demographic: ages from puberty to 40s, females > males
- Location: proximal limbs or trunk (extra-abdominal desmoid tumor)
- Presentation: mass, deep and firm causing little if any pain
- Imaging: isointense to hypointense on MRI, significant enhancement with gadolinium
- Histology: infiltrates local normal tissue, spindle cells surrounded by abundant collagen without cell-to-cell contact
- Treatment: wide resection; frequently recurs; adjuvant radiation can prevent recurrence if marginal excision

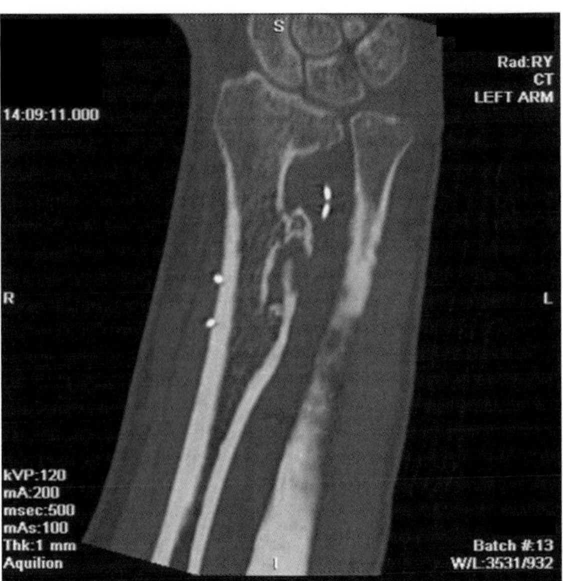

Fig. 2.84 CT of soft tissue desmoids of the distal forearm/wrist eroding into the adjacent radius and ulna. (From Conrad EU. Orthopaedic Oncology: Diagnosis and Treatment. New York: Thieme; 2008. Reprinted with permission.)

3. Extraabdominal desmoid tumor **(Fig. 2.84)**
   - Most locally invasive of benign soft tissue tumors; fibrous neoplasm
   - Demographic: ages 15–40 years, females > males
   - Desmoid tumors in family with other fibromatoses including Dupuytren's contracture and Ledderhose disease (contracture of palm and plantar fascia, respectively)
   - Presentation: "rock hard" character on palpation; may have multiple in same extremity
   - Location: 50% extra-abdominal, 50% abdominal
   - Imaging: infiltrative within muscles, low T1 signal, medium intensity T2; enhanced with gadolinium
   - Histology: well-differentiated fibroblasts, abundant collagen, infiltrating adjacent tissues
     a. Immunohistochemistry: estrogen receptor β positive
   - Treatment: wide resection if possible, radiation to prevent recurrence. Observation is an option because recurrence rate is high. Can use chemotherapy, NSAIDs, or tamoxifen for inoperable or recurrent lesions.
     a. Gardner syndrome: familial adenomatous polyposis with 10,000-fold increased risk of desmoid tumor
4. Nodular fasciitis
   - Common reactive lesion, self-limited, often mistaken for malignant fibrous neoplasm
   - Demographic: ages 20–40 years, males = females
   - Presentation: painful, rapidly enlarging mass, typically 1–2 cm
   - Location: 50% upper extremity
   - Imaging: MRI: typically superficial, nodular with extension along fascial planes; enhances with gadolinium
   - Histology: plump fibroblasts organized in short, irregular bundles/fascicles, dense reticulum network
   - Treatment: excision, marginal
5. Elastofibroma
   - **If MRI shows a scapular lesion, always consider elastofibroma in the differential.**
   - Unusual, tumor-like reactive process
   - Demographic: ages 60–80 years, females > males
   - Presentation: typically asymptomatic, may have snapping scapula
   - Location: between scapula and chest wall deep to the inferior wall of scapula, 10% bilateral
   - Imaging: mixed signal on T1 and T2
   - Histology: elastic fibers with beaded appearance
     a. Stains positive for elastin
   - Treatment: observation or excision if symptomatic

6. Malignant fibrous histiocytoma (MFH)/undifferentiated pleomorphic sarcoma (UPS) **(Fig. 2.85)**
   - MFH and UPS of soft tissues now considered same entity
   - Soft tissue sarcoma of fibroblasts
   - Demographic: ages 30–80 years, males > females
   - Presentation: slow-growing, painless mass
   - Location: anywhere
   - Imaging: lytic, metaphyseal lesion; MRI: low signal on T1, high signal T2
     a. Differential diagnosis: pleomorphic undifferentiated sarcoma (PUS)
   - Histology: fasciculated growth pattern with spindle cells, interwoven collagen fibers, herringbone pattern
   - Treatment: wide margin resection, radiation (when tumor > 5 cm)
   - Metastasis: 50% of high-grade lesions will metastasize
7. Dermatofibrosarcoma protuberans
   - Rare, nodular, cutaneous tumor
   - Demographic: early to middle adulthood, peak age 30s, males > females
   - Presentation: slow growing but progressive mass; pink or violet-red plaques surrounded by telangiectatic skin early; may progress to ulceration
   - Location: foot, upper/lower extremities
   - Imaging: MRI helpful to determine depth of lesion
   - Histology: uniform fibroblasts in storiform pattern around inconspicuous vasculature
   - Treatment: wide-margin resection; tendency to recur locally

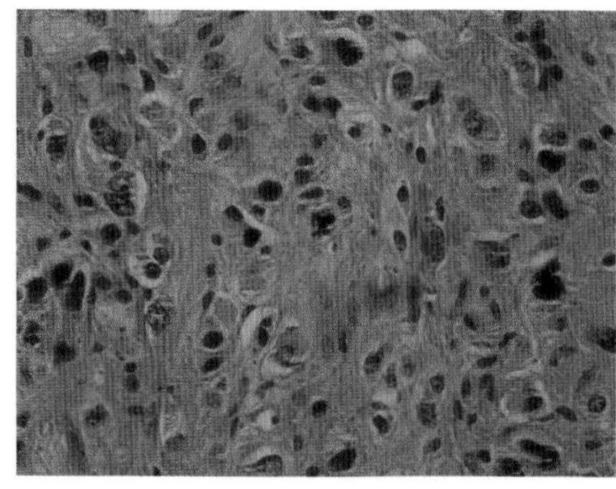

Fig. 2.85 High-power, undifferentiated pleomorphic sarcoma (UPS) in bone; however, the soft tissue primary can have the identical histology. The tumor is composed of swirls of pleomorphic spindle cells with scattered tumor giant cells, hyperchromatic nuclei, abundant mitoses, and collagen production.

C. Soft Tissue Tumors of Lipogenic Origin

1. Lipoma **(Fig. 2.86)**
   - **Lipoma accounts for 50% of soft tissue neoplasms.**
   - Common benign tumors of mature fat, occur subcutaneously, intra- and intermuscular
   - Demographic: ages 40–60 years, males > females
   - Presentation: painless mass, long duration, can have multiple lesions, sense of "fullness"
   - Location:
     a. Superficial lipomas: upper back, shoulders, arms, buttocks, proximal thigh
     b. Deep lipomas: typically larger, fixed, intramuscular; located in thigh, shoulder, calf
   - Imaging: radiolucent lesion in soft tissue
     a. MRI: well-demarcated lesion, identical signal to fat (bright on T1, moderate T2); low signal on fat-suppression sequences; if septations present, may be atypical lipoma or liposarcoma

Low signal on fat-suppression sequences without septations distinguishes lipoma from liposarcoma.

   - Histology: mature fat cells, moderate vascularity, often with a capsule
   - Treatment: observation if asymptomatic. If painful or increase in size, excision with marginal resection. May consider biopsy if increased septations on MRI.
   - Variations
     a. Spindle cell lipoma:
        - Demographic: men of ages 45–65 years
        - Presentation: solitary, painless, firm nodule

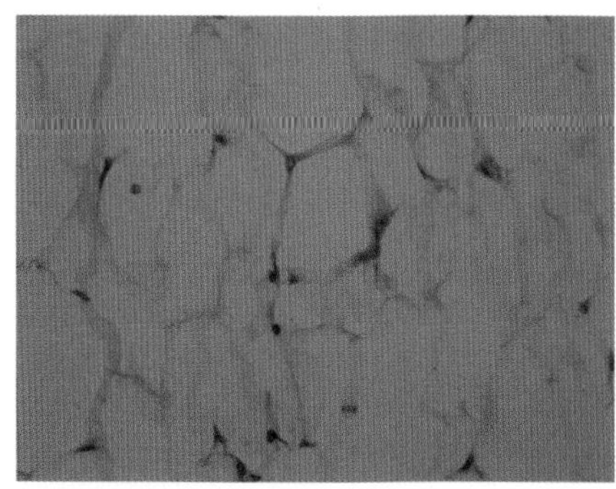

Fig. 2.86 Lipoma is composed of mature fat cells (lipocytes) with each cell nucleus pushed to the periphery, forming a signet-ring shape.

- Histology: mixture of fat cells and spindle cells with mucoid matrix
- Treatment: excision with marginal resection

b. Pleomorphic lipoma
- Demographic: middle-aged patients
- Presentation: slow-growing mass
- Histology: lipocytes, spindle cells, bizarre giant cells
- **Can be confused with liposarcoma.**
- Treatment: excision with marginal resection

c. Angiolipoma
- Presentation: Small nodules in upper extremity that are very painful when palpated
- **The only lipoma that is painful when palpated.**
- Imaging: small, fatty nodule or normal appearance
- Histology: mature fat cells, arborizing vessels
- Treatment: excision with marginal resection

d. Atypical lipoma
- Low-grade malignancy of mature adipocytes with focal atypia
- Demographic: ages 40–60 years
- Location: typically in lower limbs
- Imaging: appears similar to lipoma, may have increased number of septations
- Histology: cytological atypia of lipoblasts
- Treatment: excision with marginal resection

2. Liposarcoma **(Figs. 2.87, 2.88, 2.89)**
- Demographic: ages 50–80 years, males > females
- Location: usually deep tumor
- Presentation: slow-growing mass, lower extremities > upper extremities
- Low grade (well differentiated) versus intermediate grade (myxoid) versus high grade (dedifferentiated, round-cell, pleomorphic)

a. Metastasis occurs in the following frequencies based on grade:
- **Low grade: < 10%**

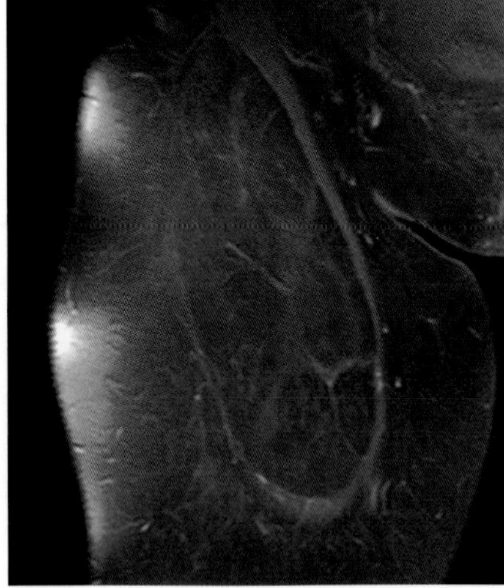

Fig. 2.87 T1 MRI showing a large, deep fatty tumor with septations.

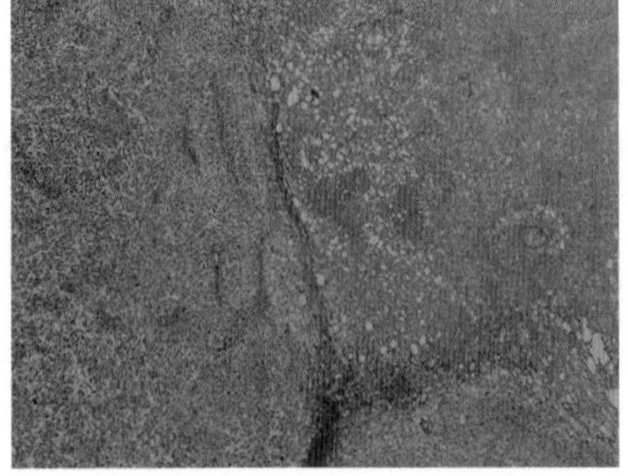

Fig. 2.88 Liposarcoma with large areas of necrosis *(pink)* and scattered vacuolated cells in both viable and necrotic areas.

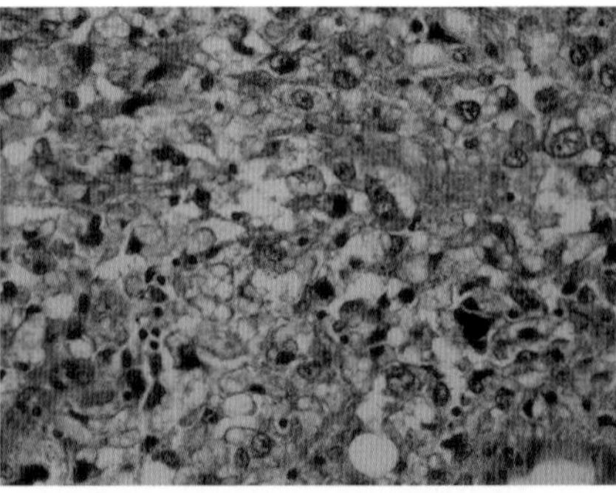

Fig. 2.89 Liposarcoma with large vacuolated or bubbly cells deforming and scalloping the nuclear borders (lipoblasts). Such cells are characteristic of liposarcoma. Many tumor cells are pleomorphic.

- **Intermediate: 10–30%**
- **High grade: > 50%**

- Most common type: myxoid (50%)
  a. Translocation: t(12;16)
  b. Age: 40s
  c. May metastasize to abdomen: requires CT chest/abdomen/pelvis
- Imaging: soft tissue mass on X-ray; may have foci of calcification if well differentiated
  a. MRI: heterogeneous mass, dark on T1, bright on T2; remains bright on fat-suppression sequences
  b. Must obtain a CT abdomen/pelvis in myxoid liposarcoma to monitor for metastases
- Histology:
  a. Myxoid: proliferating lipoblasts, myxoid matrix with interlacing network of small vessels, differentiating from myxoma
  b. Round cell: poorly differentiated, small round cells
  c. Pleomorphic: high-grade, pleomorphic appearance, giant lipoblasts
  d. Dedifferentiated: high-grade sarcoma adjacent to lipoma
- Treatment: wide surgical resection, radiation
- Metastasis: increasing lung metastasis with higher grade tumor

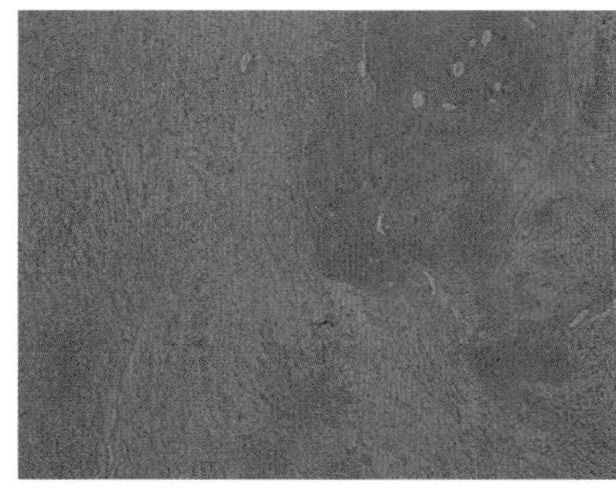

Fig. 2.90 Neurilemoma (schwannoma) as seen in this low-power field has Antoni A *(right)* and B *(left)* areas. Antoni A foci have dense spindle cells often with palisading (Verocay bodies), whereas Antoni B foci are loosely arranged spindle cells with abundant histocytes and thick-walled blood vessels.

D. Soft Tissue Tumors of Neural Origin

These tumors may present with neurologic symptoms.

1. Neurilemmoma (benign schwannoma) **(Figs. 2.90 and 2.91)**
   - Benign nerve sheath tumor, composed of Schwann cells, with true capsule of epineurium
   - Demographic: ages 20–50 years, males = females
   - Presentation: asymptomatic mass, may wax/wane in size; may cause a positive Tinel's sign
   - Location: flexor surfaces, head/neck, pelvis
   - Imaging: MRI: eccentric mass arising from peripheral nerve or indeterminate soft tissue mass; low signal T1, high signal T2, enhanced with gadolinium
     a. String sign: attenuation of nerve above and below tumor
     b. Differential diagnosis: neurofibroma
   - Histology:
     a. Antoni A: compact spindle cells with nuclear palisading, Verocay bodies
     b. Antoni B: less orderly and cellular, haphazardly matrix, large vessels irregularly spaced
     c. S100+
   - Treatment: observation or marginal excision, leaving nerve intact
2. Neurofibroma **(Fig. 2.92)**
   - Benign neural tumor involving multiple cell types
   - Demographic: ages 20–40 years, males = females
   - Presentation: superficial, slow growing; may be solitary or multiple; may have positive Tinel sign; may be exquisitely painful; may cause paresthesias
   - Imaging: low signal on T1, high T2 signal with dumbbell-shaped lesion that can expand neural foramen
   - Histology: interlacing bundles of elongated cells in wavy collagen bundles
     a. May be S100+

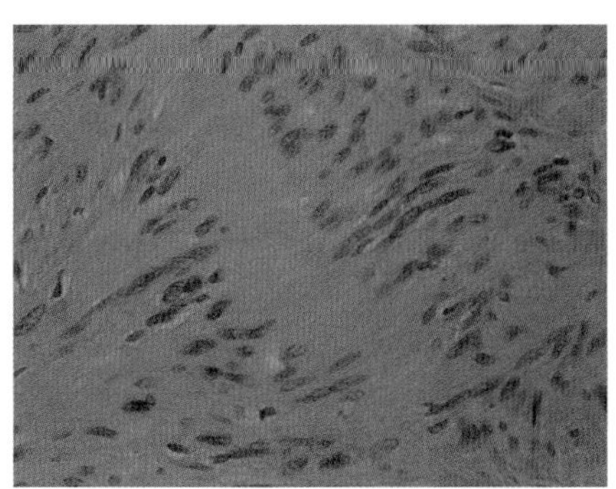

Fig. 2.91 Schwannoma with a Verocay body with palisading spindle cells.

- Treatment: excision with marginal margin or debulking with preservation of nerve fascicles
- Syndrome: neurofibromatosis (NF)—multiple neurofibromas
  a. Autosomal dominant, NF1 (chromosome 17)
  b. Café-au-lait spots
  c. Lisch nodules (hamartoma in iris)
  d. Optic glioma
  e. Axillary freckles
  f. Variable skeletal abnormalities (NOF, scoliosis, anterolateral bowing of tibia)
  g. 5–30% undergo malignant transformation to malignant peripheral nerve sheath tumor (MPNST): pain and increasing size

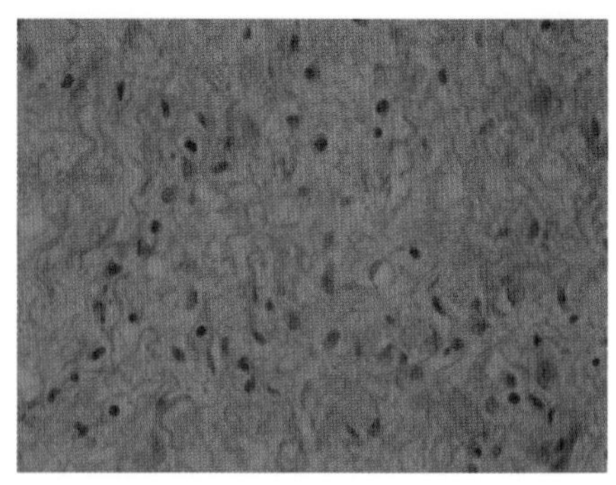

Fig. 2.92 Neurofibroma with thin, curved, elongated cells, some comma shaped, and collagen. No mitoses are present.

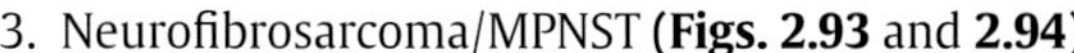

3. Neurofibrosarcoma/MPNST **(Figs. 2.93 and 2.94)**
   - Sarcoma arising de novo from peripheral nerve or neurofibroma
   - Demographic: ages 30–55 years if arising from solitary peripheral nerve, ages 20–40 years if arising from NF
   - 50% cases associated with NF1
   - Presentation: slow or rapid enlargement of soft tissue mass, with or without pain
   - Location: typically arise from large nerves (sciatic, brachial plexus)
   - Imaging: fusiform appearance within nerve, low intensity on T1, high intensity on T2
   - Histology: resembles fibrosarcoma with spindle cells with wavy nuclei
     a. S100 positive, keratin negative
   - Treatment: wide surgical resection (including nerve), radiation
4. Glomus tumor **(Fig. 2.95)**
   - Benign tumor of glomus body
   - Demographic: ages 20–40 years, males = females

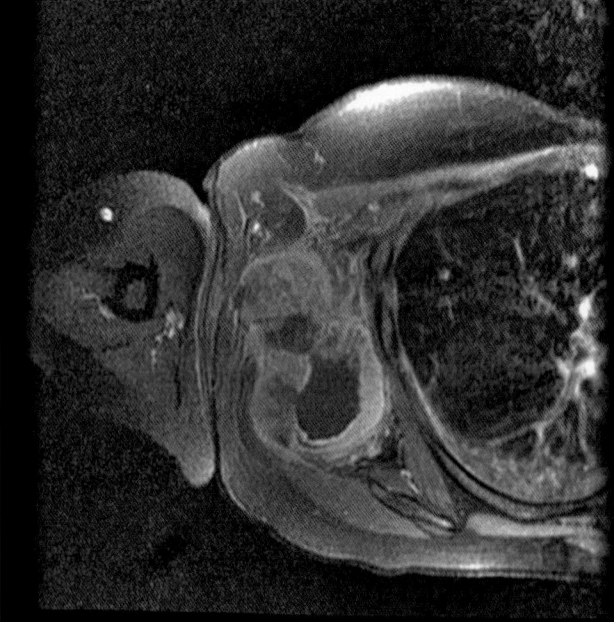

Fig. 2.93 MRI of large axillary soft tissue tumor with obvious central necrosis. (From Conrad EU. Orthopaedic Oncology: Diagnosis and Treatment. New York: Thieme; 2008. Reprinted with permission.)

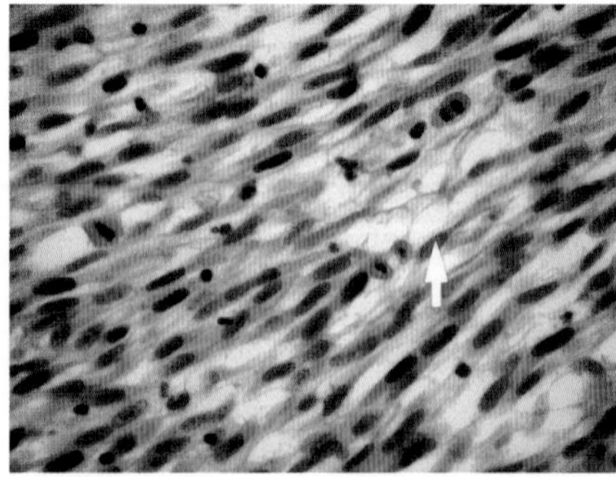

Fig. 2.94 Pyknotic, dividing nuclei with Antoni cell typical for malignant peripheral nerve sheath tumor (MPNST) *(arrow)*. (From Conrad EU. Orthopaedic Oncology: Diagnosis and Treatment. New York: Thieme; 2008. Reprinted with permission.)

- Presentation: small (< 1 cm) mass, typically subungual at proximal nail plate; may cause nail abnormalities; typically painful (usually very specific spot on nail plate or fingertip, sensitive to cold; 10% multiple; may have a "bluish" hue at the site of tumor in the nail plate

If patient presents with a bluish lesion at the fingertip that is painful to palpation, always think glomus tumor.

- Imaging: best identified on MRI (but imaging not necessary)
- Histology: small blue nodule on gross pathology; vessels and glomus cells in hyaline or myxoid stroma; periodic acid-Schiff (PAS) stain positive
- Treatment: marginal excision

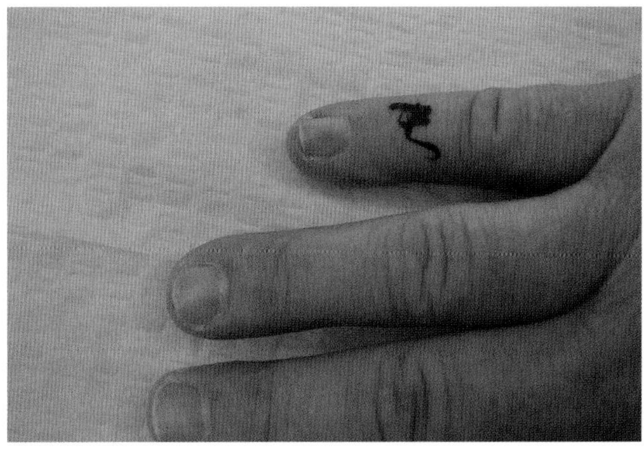

Fig. 2.95 A glomus tumor deep to the nail. Note the blue hue.

E. Soft Tissue Tumors of Muscle

1. Leiomyosarcoma **(Fig. 2.96)**
   - Presentation: small nodule or large extremity mass
   - Low or high grade
   - Histology: positive for vimentin, actin, desmin
   - Treatment: chemotherapy, resection
2. Rhabdomyosarcoma **(Fig. 2.97)**
   - Sarcoma of mesenchymal origin
   - Most common soft tissue sarcoma in children (ages < 10 years)

   - **Infants and children: embryonal rhabdomyosarcoma**
   - **Adolescents/young adults: alveolar rhabdomyosarcoma**
   - **Rhabdomyosarcoma is most common soft tissue sarcoma; osteosarcoma is most common bone tumor in children**

   - Subtypes: embryonal, alveolar, botryoid, pleomorphic (adults)
     a. Most common subtype: embryonal
     b. Genetics: alveolar rhabdomyosarcoma t(2;13)
   - Demographic: first and second decades, males > females
   - Presentation: 15% occur in extremities, typically rapidly enlarging, painless
   - Imaging: indeterminate, low signal on T1, high signal on T2

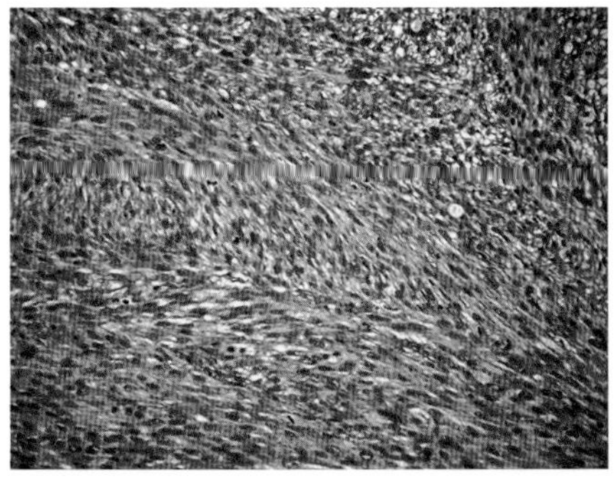

Fig. 2.96 Myxoid and eosinophilic spindle cells arranged in bundles, typical for leiomyosarcomas. (From Conrad EU. Orthopaedic Oncology: Diagnosis and Treatment. New York: Thieme; 2008. Reprinted with permission.)

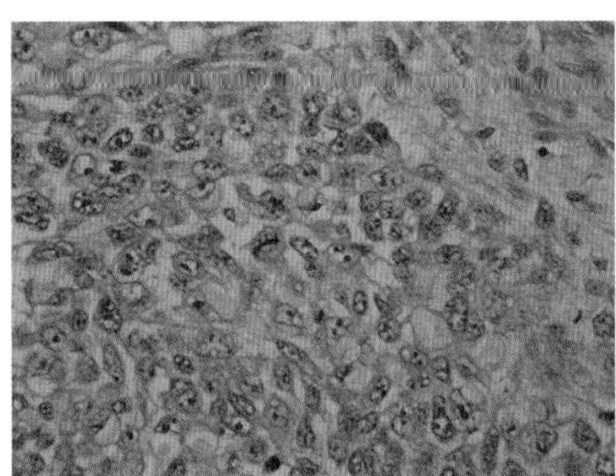

Fig. 2.97 Rhabdomyosarcoma with spindle and round pleomorphic tumor cells with scattered mitoses.

- Histology: spindle cells in parallel bundles, giant cells, racquet-shaped cells; rhabdomyoblasts entail cross-striations within tumor cells
  a. Stains positive for desmin, myoglobin
- Treatment: chemotherapy, resection, radiation (for unresectable lesions or positive margins); chemotherapy not effective in pleomorphic subtype in adults
- **Rhabdomyosarcoma is one of the few sarcomas in which chemotherapy is effective.**
- Metastasis: to regional lymph nodes and bone marrow; sentinel node biopsy required as part of staging

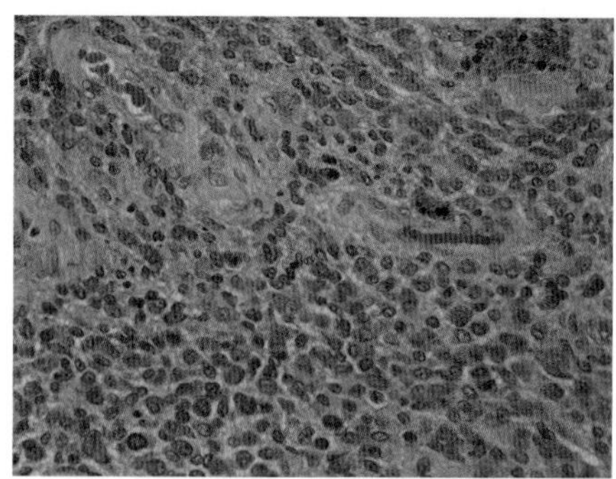

Fig. 2.98 Pigmented villonodular synovitis (PVNS) with prominent hemosiderin pigment in some tumor cells. The diagnostic cell is the round or oval neoplastic synovial lining cell.

F. Soft Tissue Tumors of Synovial Tissue

1. Ganglion
   - Out-pouching of synovial lining of adjacent joint
   - Locations: wrist, foot, knee; in distal interphalangeal (DIP) joint of fingers is secondary to osteoarthritis and is called a mucous cyst
   - Filled with mucoid, gelatinous material
   - Imaging: low T1 signal, bright T2, nonenhancing
   - Treatment: marginal resection if fails conservative management. In the DIP joint, it requires removal of the mucous cyst with debridement of osteophytes.
2. Pigmented villonodular synovitis (PVNS) **(Fig. 2.98)**
   - Reactive condition characterized by exuberant proliferation of synovial villi and nodules
     a. Localized or diffuse subtypes
   - Demographic: ages 30–50 years, males = females
   - Presentation: pain, swelling, recurrent atraumatic hemarthrosis
   - Location: knee (most common), hip, shoulder, ankle; anterior knee is most common location of localized form
   - Imaging: nodular findings both anteriorly and posteriorly (intra- or extracapsular) in the knee
     a. MRI: hypointense on both T1 and T2 because of significant hemosiderin deposition
   - Arthroscopy: deep red synovial fronds, hemosiderin deposition
   - Histology: highly vascular villi, plump hyperplastic synovial cells, hemosiderin-stained giant cells, chronic inflammatory cells
     a. Analogous to giant cell tumor of tendon sheath in extraarticular location with same histology
   - Treatment:
     a. Localized: excision
     b. Diffuse: complete synovectomy (arthroscopic or open)
     c. Recurrence common
3. Giant cell tumor of tendon sheath **(Fig. 2.99)**
   - Yellow/brown nodular tumors along tendon sheaths
   - **The most common solid soft tissue mass in the hand**
   - Presentation: painless mass, firm; frequently out of the "midline" of the finger
   - Location: hands and feet
   - Histology: lobulated on pathology, with moderately cellular zones (sheets of polygonal cells), hypocellular zones, multinucleated giant cells, xanthoma cells, histiocytes containing abundant hemosiderin
   - Treatment: Marginal excision; recurrence common

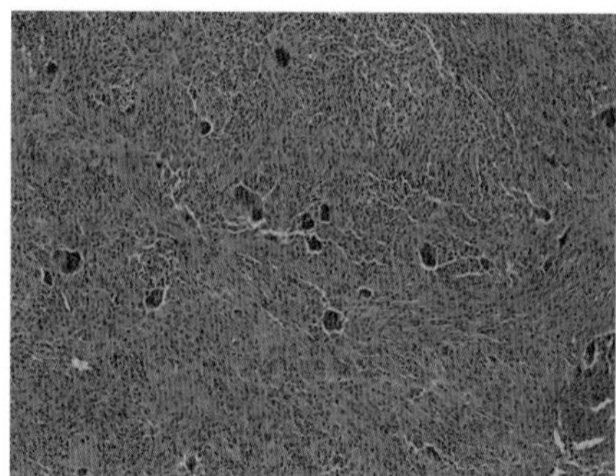

Fig. 2.99 Giant cell tumor of synovium or tender sheath, localized, with prominent collagen bands, multinucleate osteoclast-type giant cells, usually aggregated around hemorrhage, and the background tumor synovial cells.

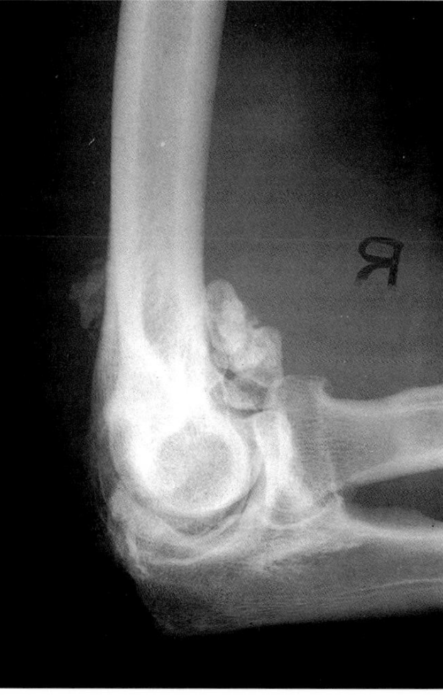

Fig. 2.100 Synovial chondromatosis with soft tissue calcifications. (From Conrad EU. Orthopaedic Oncology: Diagnosis and Treatment. New York: Thieme; 2008. Reprinted with permission.)

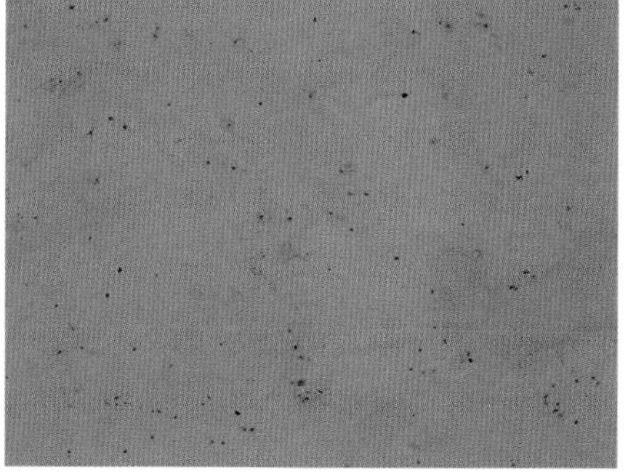

Fig. 2.101 Synovial chondromatosis with benign hyaline cartilage formation. Each chondrocyte has a dot-like nucleus with little or no atypicality.

4. Synovial chondromatosis **(Figs. 2.100** and **2.101)**
   - Synovial proliferative disorder occurring within joints or bursa
   - Demographic: ages 30–50 years, male-to-female ratio = 2:1
   - Presentation: joint pain, stiffness, swelling
   - Location: knee (most common), hip, shoulder, elbow, ankle
   - Imaging: fine stippled calcifications or calcified loose bodies
     a. CT demonstrates multiple loose bodies.
     b. Can cause joint destruction
   - Histology: discrete metaplastic hyaline cartilage nodules, undergoing ossification; ossifies from the periphery inward
   - Treatment: symptomatic treatment, removal of loose bodies, synovectomy
5. Synovial sarcoma **(Figs. 2.102, 2.103, 2.104)**
   - Highly malignant, high-grade tumor
   - **Does not arise from synovium and is usually extra-articular**
   - **Most common sarcoma of foot**
   - Genetics: t(X:18); gene fusion products: SYT-SSX1 and SYT-SSX2
   - Demographic: ages 15–40 years
   - Presentation: slow growing or rapidly enlarging; pain
   - Location: knee most common, foot, shoulder, arm, elbow
   - Imaging: calcification or ossification within lesion (25%), irregular contour.
     a. MRI: typical sarcoma appearance (low signal on T1, high signal on T2), areas of cyst formation (20%)
   - Histology: biphasic population of epithelial (glands/nests) and spindle cell components with glandular differentiation or monophasic
     a. Positive for keratin, epithelial membrane antigen, and vimentin
   - Treatment: wide margin resection, radiation, with or without chemotherapy

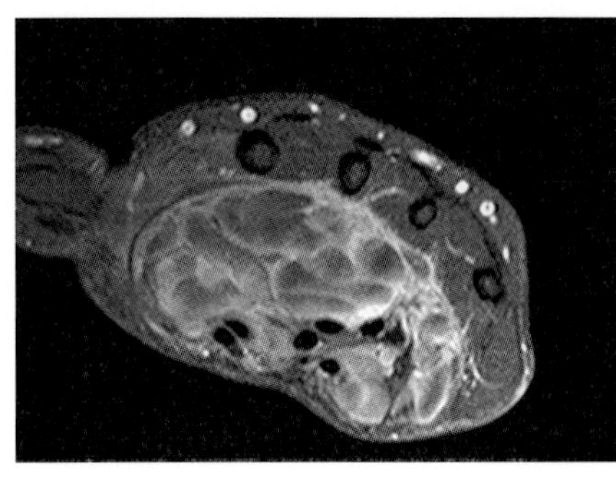

Fig. 2.102 Axial MRI of the mid-hand showing large mass. (From Conrad EU. Orthopaedic Oncology: Diagnosis and Treatment. New York: Thieme; 2008. Reprinted with permission.)

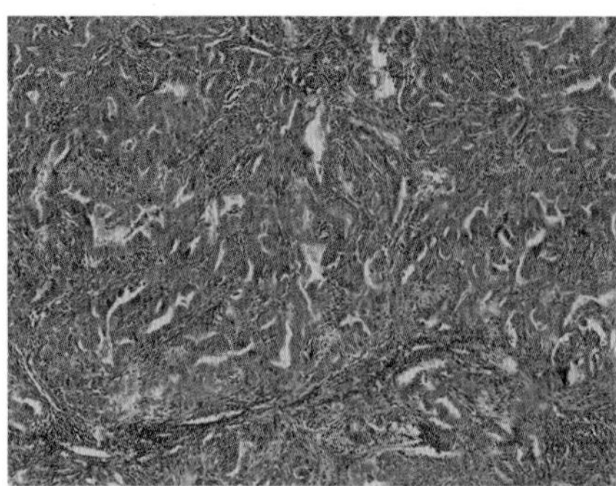

Fig. 2.103 Synovial sarcoma with a biphasic pattern; gland-like areas and spindle areas.

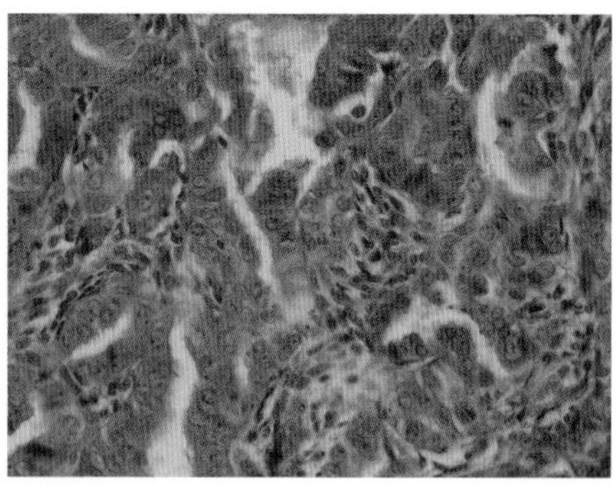

Fig. 2.104 A biphasic synovial sarcoma with a spindle area and gland-like area. All the cells in this field are malignant.

- **Size and patient survival**
  - **a. < 5 cm: 100% survival**
  - **b. 5–10 cm: 75% survival**
  - **c. 10 cm: 20% survival**
- Metastasis: 30–60% of cases, increased risk if tumor > 5–10 cm; metastasizes to lymph nodes

G. Soft Tissue Tumors of Vascular Origin

1. Hemangioma (**Figs. 2.105** and **2.106**)
   - Benign vascular tumor occurring in deep tissues
   - Demographic: children and adults, age often < 30 years
   - Presentation: aching, heaviness, swelling if large, varies in size with activity and position
   - Location: cutaneous, subcutaneous, or intramuscular
   - Imaging: soft tissue: phleboliths (plain films); intraosseous: lytic lesion with coarsened trabeculae, common in vertebral body
   - Histology: multiple lumens/vessels, no cellular pleomorphism
   - Treatment: NSAIDs, compression stockings, activity modification; vascular coiling/embolization
2. Angiosarcoma (**Fig. 2.107**)
   - Highly malignant, infiltrative
   - Presentation: pain, overlying skin changes
   - Histology: resemble endothelium of blood vessels, CD31 positive
   - Imaging: eccentric, purely lytic, metaphyseal and diaphyseal lesions with calcifications; MRI recommended to evaluate soft tissue invasion
   - Treatment: wide surgical resection with high risk of recurrence, may require amputation
   - Metastasis: pulmonary metastases common
   - **Lesions with calcifications: angiosarcoma, hemangioma, synovial sarcoma, epithelioid sarcoma, tumoral calcinosis**

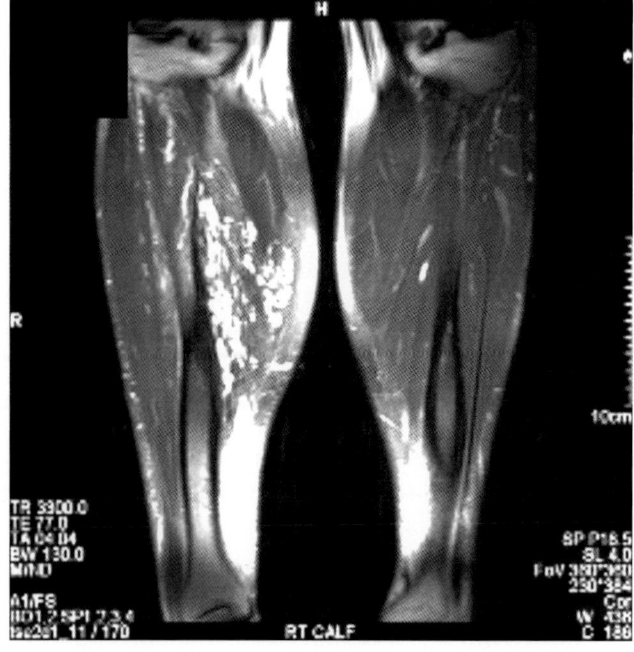

Fig. 2.105 Coronal MRI of anterior-medial soft tissue mass. (From Conrad EU. Orthopaedic Oncology: Diagnosis and Treatment. New York: Thieme; 2008. Reprinted with permission.)

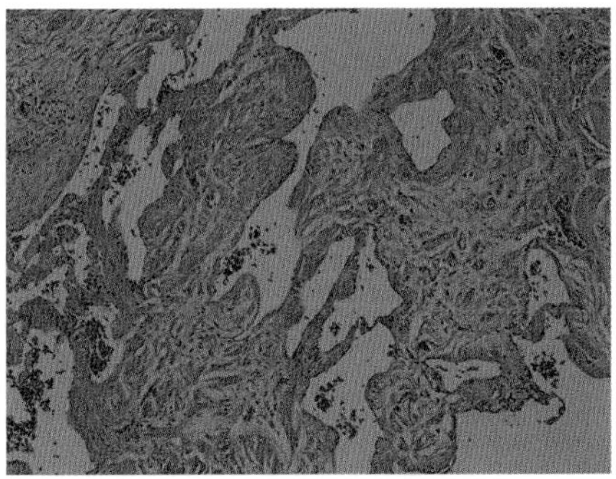

Fig. 2.106 Hemangioma has endothelial-lined spaces forming disorganized vascular channels.

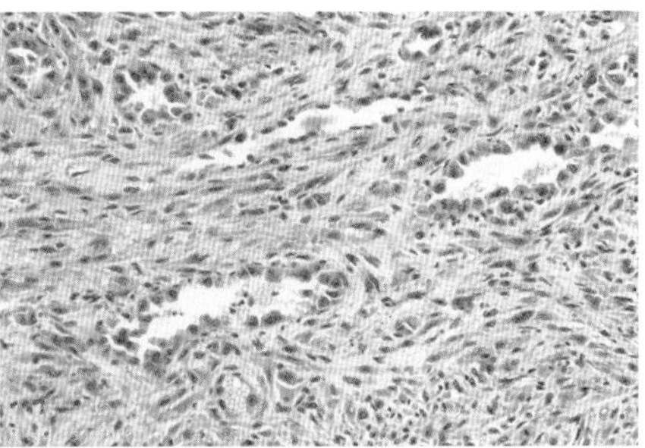

Fig. 2.107 Ovoid cells seen with eosinophilic cytoplasm. (From Conrad EU. Orthopaedic Oncology: Diagnosis and Treatment. New York: Thieme; 2008. Reprinted with permission.)

H. Other Soft Tissue Lesions

1. Epithelioid sarcoma
   - Frequently mistaken for benign granulomatous process
   - Demographics: young adults (ages 10–35 years), males > females
   - Presentation: small, slow-growing mass; painless, but may ulcerate if superficial
     a. Differential diagnosis: rheumatoid nodule, granuloma
   - Location: upper extremity (hand, forearm, fingers), buttock/thigh, knee, foot; multinodular mass
   - **Most common sarcoma of hand**
   - Imaging: may have calcification within lesion
     a. MRI: nodule along tendon sheath; low signal on T1, high signal on T2
   - Histology: ovoid to polygonal cells, eosinophilic cytoplasm, central necrosis within granulomatous pattern
     a. Stains positive for keratin, vimentin, CD34
   - Treatment: wide-margin resection, radiation; may require sentinel node biopsy; frequently excised with inadequate margins secondary to misdiagnosis
   - Metastasis: to lymph nodes
   - Prognosis: poor
2. Clear cell sarcoma
   - Soft tissue sarcoma with distinct ability to produce melanin
   - Genetics: 12:22 chromosomal translocation
   - Demographics: young adults (ages 20–40 years), females > males
   - Presentation: slow-growing mass in association with tendons or aponeuroses
   - Location: foot and ankle, then knee, thigh, hand
   - Imaging: nonspecific, may appear nodular on MRI
   - Histology: compact nests or fascicles or rounded/fusiform cells with clear cytoplasm, giant cells
     a. Stains positive for melanin, S-100, HMB45
   - Treatment: wide margin resection, radiation
   - Metastasis: lungs
   - Prognosis: poor with pulmonary metastasis
3. Alveolar soft parts sarcoma
   - Demographic: ages 15–35 years
   - Presentation: slow-growing, painless mass

- Location: anterior thigh
- Histology: dense, fibrous trabeculae dividing tumor into nest-like arrangement; cells large and rounded with one or more vesicular nuclei
  a. Translocation: t(X;17)
- Treatment: wide-margin surgical resection, radiation

3

Trauma

Melissa A. Christino, Peter Kaveh Mansuripur, and Roman Hayda

I. General Trauma Principles

1. Primary survey: airway, breathing, circulation (ABCs)
2. Shock
   - Hemorrhagic shock classes I–IV **(Table 3.1)**
   - Compensated shock patients have relative hypoperfusion with preferential perfusion to heart and brain; may have normal heart rate/blood pressure and urine output but are at increased risk of systemic inflammatory response
   - Neurogenic
     a. Hypotension combined with bradycardia
   - Septic: etiology is a drop in systemic vascular resistance due to infection-driven inflammation
     a. Hypotension, tachycardia, fever
3. Resuscitation
   - **Fluid bolus challenge of three to four times the estimated blood loss; if inadequate response, transfuse at plasma/platelets/packed red blood cells (PRBCs) ratio of 1:1:1**
   - Interleukin-6 (IL-6) associated with systemic inflammatory response after trauma/musculoskeletal injury and correlates with injury severity and outcome
   - End points: base deficit (normal –2 to 2), lactate (normal < 2.5), gastric intramucosal pH (normal > 7.3, indicates normal tissue oxygenation) are best predictors of resuscitation status, risk of death, and multisystem organ failure; time it takes to correct these parameters can predict survival
   - **Base deficit is best predictor of resuscitation in the first 6 hours following insult**
   - Hypothermia less than 95°F (35°C) is associated with increased mortality in trauma patients.
4. Trauma scoring systems
   - Injury Severity Score (ISS): calculated as the sum of the squares of the three highest Abbreviated Injury Scale (AIS) scores from the six body regions; score over 18 is considered polytrauma; mortality correlated with age and higher score
   - Revised Trauma Score: calculated from systolic blood pressure (SBP), respiratory rate (RR), and Glasgow Coma Scale (GCS)
   - Trauma and Injury Severity Score (TRISS): survival probability calculator, combining above scores and weighting by age (< 55 years greater survival, ≥ 55 years lower survival) and mechanism (lower survival for blunt trauma, higher for penetrating trauma)
5. Damage control orthopaedics (DCO)
   - Technique of external fixation of bony injuries in the polytrauma patient

Table 3.1 Stages of Hemorrhagic Shock

Class	Blood Loss	MS	UOP	Cardiac	Other
I	< 15%	Anxiety	Normal	Normal	
II	15–30%	Confusion	Decreased	Tachycardic |PP	éRR
III	30–40%	Irritability	Decreased	Hypotensive	
IV	> 40%	Lethargy	Minimal	Hypotensive	

Abbreviations: MS, mental status; PP, pulse pressure; RR, respiratory rate; UOP, urinary output.

- Inflammatory surge 2–5 days after trauma in polytrauma patients; surgery in this window can lead to "second-hit" phenomenon, increase risk of acute respiratory distress syndrome (ARDS); if patient cannot be adequately resuscitated for definitive treatment in first 12–24 hours, DCO restricts surgery to life- and limb-saving procedures
- Consider if: ISS > 40, ISS > 20 with thoracic trauma, multiple injuries with severe pelvic/abdominal trauma and hemorrhagic shock, bilateral femoral fractures, pulmonary contusion noted on radiographs, hypothermia of less than 35°C, head injury
- External fixation for acute stabilization of long bone fractures can decrease overall inflammatory burden and leads to less multisystem organ failure and ARDS than if patient is left untreated.
- Head injury: not a contraindication for acute intramedullary nailing (IMN) of long bone fractures; no worsened GCS in patients with early nailing as long as there is no intraoperative hypotension or hypoxia

6. Compartment syndrome:
   - **Remember the five P's: pain out of proportion to injury, paresthesias, pallor, pain with passive stretch, pulselessness**
   - Clinical diagnosis with use of objective measures to assist in diagnosis; permanent damage to muscle and nerve can occur after 6 hours
   - Mechanism: blunt extremity soft tissue injury, associated with fracture, particularly lower extremity (tibia)
   - Presentation: most reliable symptom is pain out of proportion to injury; most reliable sign is pain with passive stretch ; external compression, vascular compromise.
   - Diagnosis: clinical diagnosis; needle compartment pressure monitoring can assist in diagnosis; objective measure of intracompartmental pressure, positive result if:
     a. Difference between diastolic blood pressure and compartment pressure (Delta P) < 30 mm Hg; corollary to perfusion pressure to tissue
     b. Absolute compartment pressure > 30 mm Hg
   - **Pressure monitoring is used as an adjunct; compartment syndrome is a clinical diagnosis**
   - Treatment: fasciotomy to decrease intracompartmental pressure to improve perfusion; delayed closure
7. Open fractures
   - AO/OTA open fracture classification: evaluates 5 areas for degree of injury
     a. Skin
        - Edges that approximate
        - Edges that do not appoximate
        - Extensive degloving
     b. Muscle
        - No appreciable muscle necrosis

- Partial muscle loss
  - Transected or dead muscle unit with loss of function

c. Arterial
  - No major vessel disruption
  - Vessel injury without ischemia
  - Vessel injury with ischemia

d. Contamination
  - Minimal contamination
  - Superficial contamination
  - Embedded contamination in muscle or bone

e. Bone loss
  - None
  - Bone loss but with remaining contact between bone ends
  - Segmental bone loss

- Gustilo and Anderson classification: energy of mechanism is more important than wound size but is more difficult to quantify. Example: comminuted femoral shaft fracture is type III regardless of wound size.
  a. Type I: wound < 1 cm
  b. Type II: wound 1–10 cm
  c. Type IIIA: wound > 10 cm or significant comminution or periosteal stripping
  d. Type IIIB: requires flap coverage (best outcomes and lowest infection rate with early coverage; goal < 7 days)
     - Coverage options in tibia fractures:
       - ♦ Proximal third: gastrocnemius flap or free tissue transfer
       - ♦ Middle third: soleus flap or free tissue transfer
       - ♦ Distal third: fasciocutaneous or free tissue transfer
       - ♦ Risk of infection in type IIIB open tibia coverage is related to timing of soft tissue coverage
  e. Type IIIC: associated vascular injury requiring repair, irrespective of wound size
- Treatment:
  a. Debridement: removal of contaminants and devitalized tissue
     - Best irrigation technique in open injuries: saline, low-flow gravity
  b. Antibiotics: time to first dose important predictor of infection
       - ♦ First generation cephalosporin for types I and II, add aminoglycoside for type III, add penicillin for heavy contamination/farm wounds; tetanus prophylaxis for all
- Limb salvage versus amputation: most important factor in success of limb salvage in open tibia fractures is extent of soft tissue injury, whereas amputation level is determined by soft tissue available for coverage
- Lower Extremity Assessment Project (LEAP) study: compares amputation to limb salvage; most important predictors of patient satisfaction at 2 years after injury include the ability to return to work, absence of depression, faster walking speed, and decreased pain
- Sickness Impact Profile (SIP) scores and rate of return to work not significantly different between groups at 2 years; self-efficacy (defined as one's belief in one's ability to succeed; part of the SIP) as well as social support thought to be two most important predictors in both groups

8. General fracture complications
   - Deep venous thrombosis (DVT): 5% develop pulmonary embolus
   - Fat embolus: can occur at time of fracture, reduction, or during intramedullary instrumentation; usually manifested in 48–72 hours of injury

a. Presentation: hypoxia (Pa_{O_2} < 60 mmHg), tachycardia, petechial rash
b. Treatment: supportive pulmonary care

- Nonunion
 a. Definitions
  - Delayed union: fracture not completely healed in usual timeframe (varies with type and location)
  - Nonunion: no radiographic evidence of healing over 3 months following expected union or lack of progression of healing or no healing by 6 months
 b. Classification **(Fig. 3.1)**
  - Hypertrophic: adequate biology, inadequate stability
  - Oligotrophic: adequate biology, fracture displaced (i.e., overdistracted during nailing)
  - Atrophic: compromised biology (vascularity), adequate stability
  - Infected

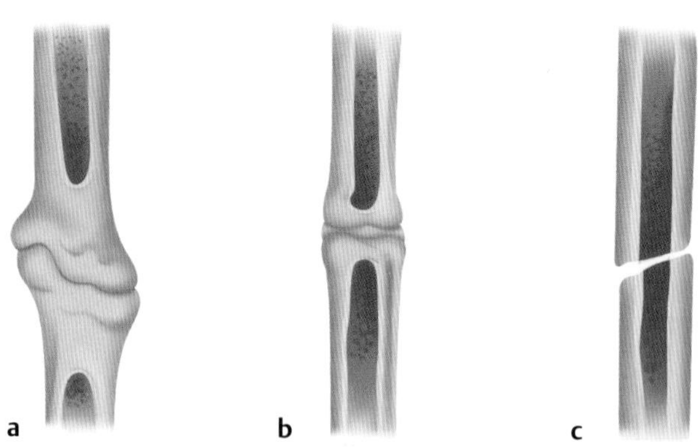

Fig. 3.1 Types of nonunion. **(a)** Hypertrophic (hoof-like appearance). **(b)** Oligotrophic. **(c)** Atrophic.

 c. Treatment
  - Hypertrophic: improved stabilization (cast/brace vs operative)
  - Oligotrophic: reduce displacement/interposition
  - Atrophic: augment biology [bone graft, bone morphogenic protein (BMP), bone stimulation, vascularized graft]
   - ♦ Bone graft materials (see Chapter 1)
  - Infected: treatment of infection with or without removal of hardware acutely or in a delayed fashion after union
- Segmental bone loss
 a. Treatment options: bone transport (Ilizarov, spatial frame), vascularized interposition graft (defect size > 10 cm), nonvascularized graft
  - Masquelet technique: an option for large defects where bone cement is interposed in defect for 4–6 weeks while a biologically active pseudomembrane is induced, and then cement is removed and cancellous autograft placed at 4–6 weeks

 b. Growth factors shown to be at highest concentration in membrane around 4 weeks

- Heterotopic ossification (common around acetabulum/ elbow)
 a. Risk factors: extensive muscle damage, head injury
 b. Prophylaxis within 72 hours of surgery
  - Indomethacin: 75 mg/day for 4–6 weeks
  - Radiation: single 700 cGy (rad) dose
- Infection/osteomyelitis
 a. Presentation: pain, fevers, draining wound, erythema, edema, inability to ambulate
 b. Diagnosis: elevated erythrocyte sedimentation rate (ESR), C-reactive protein (CRP); on X-ray, lytic region is often seen surrounded by sclerotic bone; bone loss
  - Sequestrum: necrotic bone that serves as a nidus for infection
  - Involucrum: new bone around an area of necrotic bone
  - CRP increases within 6 hours, peaks at 2–3 days, normalizes 5–21 days; ESR peaks on days 4–11, remains elevated longer (up to 90 days) in noninfected cases; both are nonspecific markers of infection/inflammation
 c. Treatment: castile soap irrigation (nonsterile liquid soap additive) is as effective as bacitracin irrigation in terms of postoperative infection and fracture healing and entails fewer problems with wound healing

- Long-term intravenous (IV) antibiotics; may require multiple debridements and removal of any hardware; amputation for uncontrolled infection

9. Gunshot wounds
   - High energy: hunting rifles, assault weapons, close-range shotguns—treated as open fractures
   - Low energy: handguns—treated as closed fractures, with antibiotics and wound care unless deformity and instability require surgery
10. Fracture biomechanics
    - Fracture pattern based on direction of energy load **(Fig. 3.2)**
    - Strain: change in fracture gap/overall length of fracture gap (delta L/L)
    - Absolute stability (strain < 2%): rigid fixation, compression plating, lag screw
      a. No motion at fracture site; leads to primary bone healing; no callus formation
    - Relative stability (strain 2–10%): intramedullary nailing, bridge plating
      a. Micromotion at fracture site; leads to secondary bone healing; callus formation
    - Fixation that leads to strain ranging from 11–20% leads to fibrous union
    - Fixation that leads to strain > 20% leads to nonunion and pseudoarthrosis
11. Fixation biomechanics **(Fig. 3.3)**
    - External fixation: the biggest influence on construct stiffness is pin diameter; other factors increasing stiffness: pin spread ("near-near-far-far"), bar to bone distance, bar number, out of plane pin; circular frames more stable than uniplanar frame, with wires tensioned at 90 degrees giving best angular and torsional stability
    - Lag screws
      a. Interfragmentary compression, absolute stability; neutralization plate to protect screw from torsion
    - Compression plating
      a. Pre-bend to convex shape to eliminate gap on opposite side of the fracture at the cortex

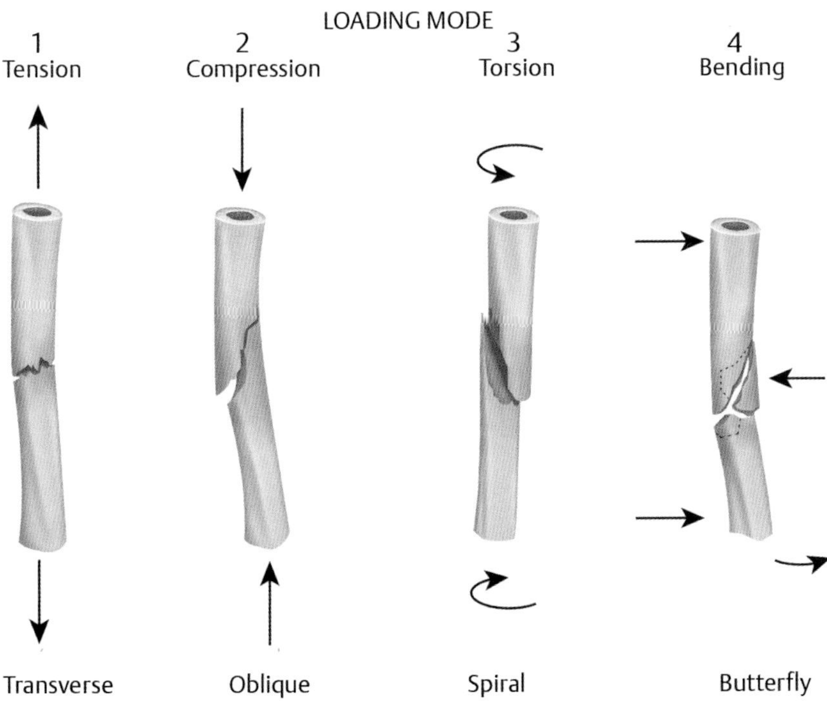

Fig. 3.2 Fracture type is based on the direction of energy load. 1, a transverse fracture is created when bone fails in tension (patella fracture for example). 2, in compression, an axial load creates an oblique fracture 45 degrees to the axis. 3, because bone is stronger in compression than in tension, when a transverse (direct blow) or bending load is applied, bone first fails in tension, and then fails in compression; there is a butterfly fragment on the compression side of the fracture. 4, in a torsional or twisting energy load, a spiral fracture is created 45 degrees to the long axis

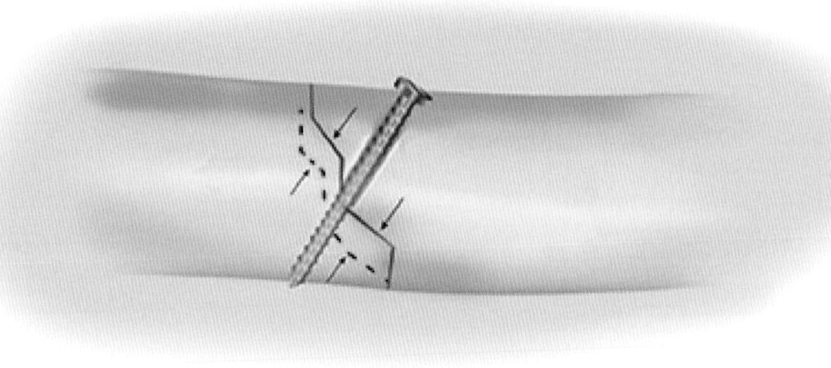

a

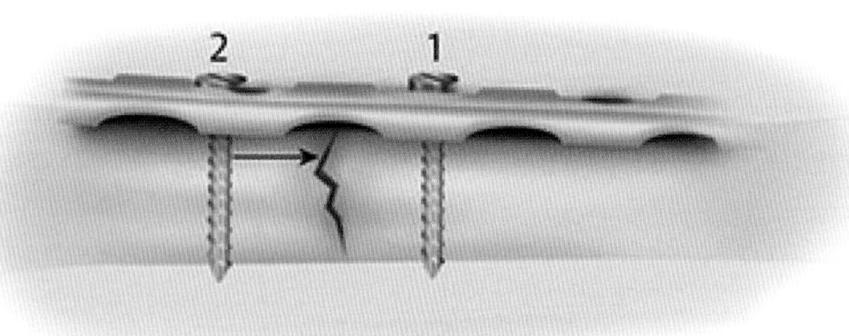

b

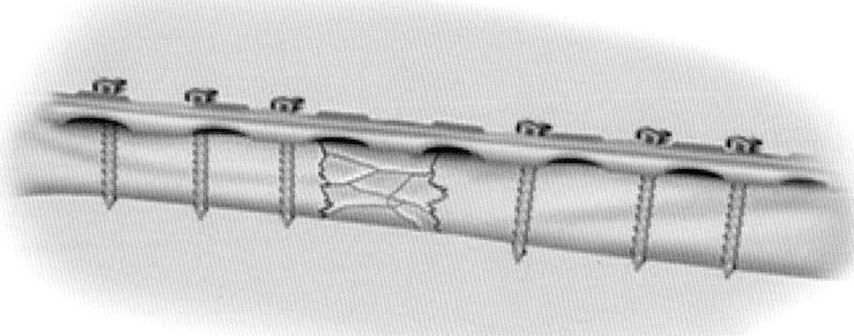

c

Fig. 3.3 Fixation techniques. **(a)** Lag screw. Note the overdrilled near cortex and countersunk screw head. The angle of the screw bisects the angle between the lines normal to the bone surface and fracture plane. **(b)** Compression plate. A neutral screw *(1)* is placed first centrally, forming an axilla between the plate and the proximal fragment; a compression screw *(2)* is placed in the distal fragment in the distal aspect of the hole. **(c)** A bridge plate spanning the area of comminution. Fixation is performed away from the fracture to protect the biology.

  b. Screw order: neutral, compression, lag; strongest construct is lag screw through plate
  c. Absolute stability
- Bridge plating
  a. Comminuted fractures, hypertrophic nonunion
  b. Relative stability
  c. Submuscular plating: respects fracture and soft tissue biology
- Locked plating
  a. Fixed angle construct; absolute stability
  b. Short metaphyseal fractures, osteoporotic bone
  c. In hybrid plating of osteoporotic bone with both nonlocked and locked screws, biomechanically creating a stiffer construct requires placing at least three locked screws on each side of the fracture. If a locked screw is placed between the fracture and a nonlocked screw, the locked screw serves to protect the nonlocked screw (place a locked screw nearest to the fracture on each side).

d. Locking plates do not provide buttress support when used in pure locking mode.

- Intramedullary nails
  a. Relative stability
  b. Nail stiffness proportional to nail cross-sectional radius to the third power (r^3) in bending and radius to the fourth power (r^4) in torsion
  c. Radius of curvature: less than anatomic for improved interference fit
    - Mismatch can induce fracture
    - Larger radius of curvature risks breaching anterior cortex in femur fractures

  d. Nail with a larger radius of curvature is straighter than one with a smaller radius of curvature; therefore, it has less "bow" to it and it can breach the anterior cortex in a femur, for example.

II. Upper Extremity

1. Shoulder
   - Sternoclavicular (SC) dislocation
     a. Presentation: localized SC joint pain and swelling; in posterior dislocations can present with tachypnea, dysphagia, and stridor
     b. Associated injuries: compression of thoracic structures in 30% of posterior dislocations
     c. Imaging: X-ray demonstrates 40-degree cephalic tilt to evaluate direction of dislocation (serendipity view); axial CT typically required to identify vessel or tracheal compression
       - **Cephalic tilt of X-rays from medial to lateral: 40 degrees for SC (serendipity), 30 degrees for clavicle, and 10 degrees for acromioclavicular (AC) (Zanca view)**
     d. Pathology: clavicle either anteriorly or posteriorly dislocated on sternum
     e. Treatment
       - Conservative: anterior dislocations, though can attempt closed reduction; chronic dislocations (> 3 weeks old) and in ligamentously lax
       - Surgical: posterior dislocations, closed or open reduction in operating room (OR) with thoracic surgeon available
   - Clavicle fractures
     a. Mechanism: fall onto upper extremity or direct injury to shoulder
     b. Associated injuries: rib fractures, rarely brachial plexus injury
       - Open clavicle fractures are high-energy injuries and are associated with closed head injury, pulmonary injuries, or spine fractures.
     c. Imaging: AP and 30-degree cephalad oblique X-rays
     d. Classification by location: medial, middle (most common), distal third
     e. Treatment (middle clavicle fractures)
       - Conservative: equivalent healing in sling versus figure-of-eight brace, higher incidence of contralateral nerve compression with figure-of-eight brace; closed treatment of displaced midshaft fracture leads to decreased (20%) strength and endurance, with higher nonunion rate
       - Surgical: open fractures, vascular injury, skin compromise due to fracture displacement, 100% displaced middle third with comminution or > 2 cm shortening
     f. Outcomes: fixation of displaced clavicle fractures leads to decreased nonunion/malunion and has better functional outcomes up to 1 year compared with conservative treatment.

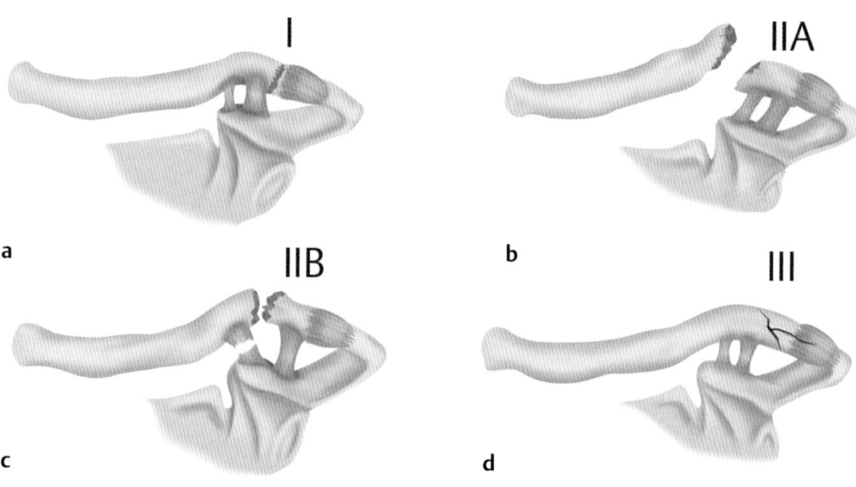

Fig. 3.4 Distal clavicle fractures. **(a)** Type I: fracture between coracoclavicular (CC) and acromioclavicular (AC) ligaments, nondisplaced. **(b)** Type IIA: fracture proximal to CC ligaments, displaced. **(c)** Type IIB, fracture between conoid and trapezoid ligaments with torn conoid, displaced. **(d)** Type III, fracture extends into AC joint.

g. Distal third clavicle fractures **(Fig. 3.4)**
   - Type I: nondisplaced; between coracoclavicular (CC) and AC ligaments
   - Type IIA: displaced; conoid and trapezoid attached to distal fragment; high rate of nonunion
   - Type IIB: displaced; conoid torn, trapezoid attached to distal fragment; high rate of nonunion
   - Type III: fracture extends into AC joint
   - Treatment: indications similar to middle clavicle fractures; open, displaced, or extending into AC joint
   - Outcomes: fixation leads to decreased nonunion/delayed union rates; however, nonunion may be clinically asymptomatic without effects on function.

- Acromioclavicular (AC) dislocations
  a. Classified by displacement magnitude and direction, determined by involvement of CC and AC ligaments
  b. Types I-VI **(Fig. 3.5)**
  c. Imaging: X-ray, Zanca view (10 degrees cephalad, 50% penetrance)
  d. Treatment:
     - **Types I, II, and III AC dislocations treated conservatively**
     - Types I and II: sling
     - Type III: sling is treatment of choice; some have suggested surgery in athletes and laborers (Weaver-Dunn)
     - Types IV to VI: surgery
- Scapula fractures
  a. Mechanism: high energy; fall from height, motor vehicle accident, motorcycle crash
  b. Associated injuries: polytrauma; head injury, hemo/pneumothorax, rib/sternum fracture, brachial plexus injury
  c. Imaging: anteroposterior (AP) chest X-ray, AP/lateral shoulder X-rays, computed tomography (CT), Stryker notch view (coracoid)
  d. Zdravkovic and Damholt anatomic fracture classification:
     - Type I: body
     - Type II: coracoid and acromion
     - Type III: scapular neck and glenoid
  e. Treatment
     - Nonoperative: isolated scapular body fracture and minimally displaced glenoid neck fractures; sling and early range of motion (ROM)

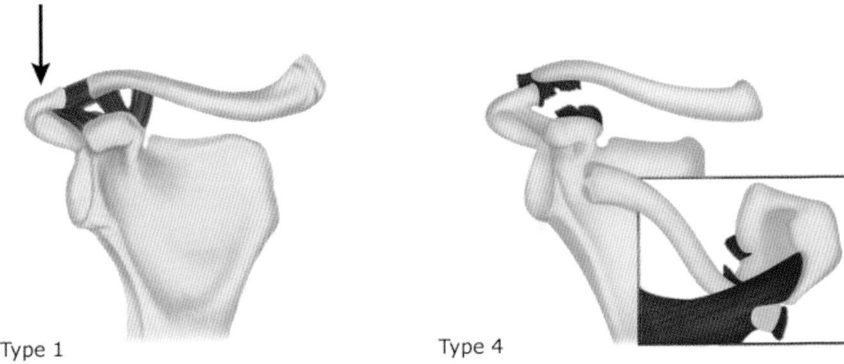

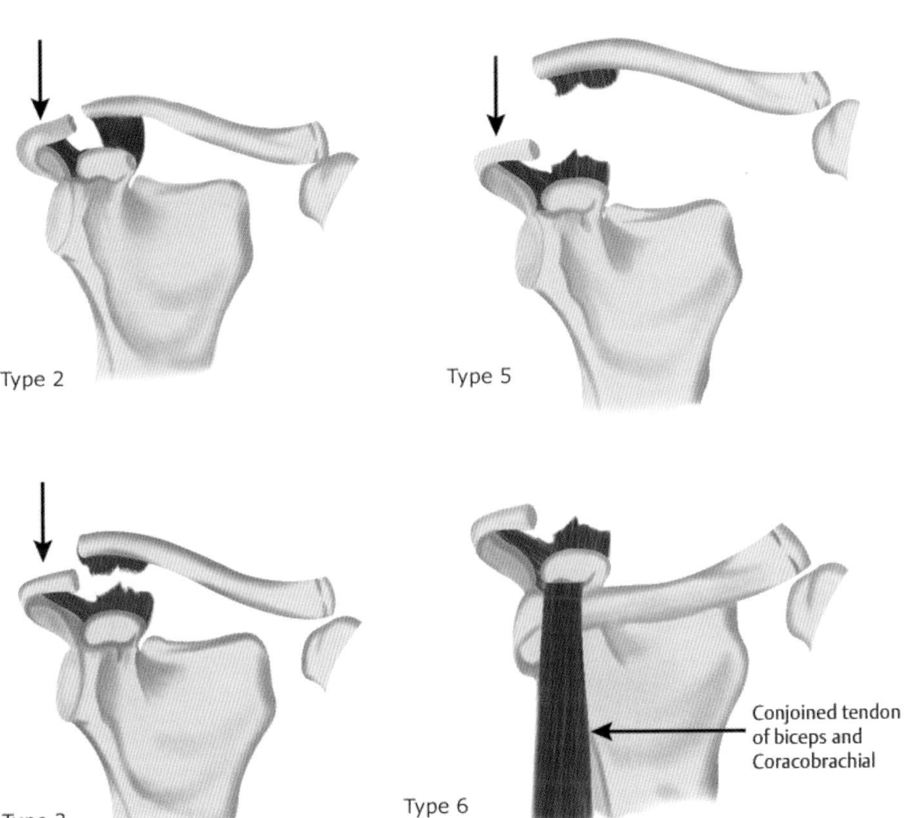

Fig. 3.5 Acromioclavicular (AC) ligament complex injuries, type I to VI. Type I: AC sprain. Type II: AC tear, CC sprain. Type III: AC/CC tear, less than 100% superior displacement. Type IV: clavicle posterior, sometimes buttonholes trapezius. Type V: Clavicle displaced more than 100% superiorly. Type VI: Clavicle inferior, caught under conjoined tendon. Mnemonic: Four out the Trap Door (trapezius), High Five, Deep Six.

   - Operative indications: humeral head instability, glenoid rim fracture involving > 25% articular surface, glenoid fossa fracture with > 3–5 mm displacement, significant anterior/medial displacement of glenoid neck (> 1 cm) or angulation > 40 degrees; some suggest injury to both scapula and clavicle (double disruption of superior shoulder suspensory complex)
   - Treatment: fixation through posterior approach through interval between infraspinatus and teres minor; Judet approach elevates entire infraspinatus for sub-infraspinatus approach **(Fig. 3.6)**

f. Complications: suprascapular nerve and artery, and circumflex scapular artery at risk during posterior approach

- Scapulothoracic dissociation: lateral displacement of > 1 cm of scapula on AP chest X-ray compared with spinous process (can also use axial CT scan)
  a. High frequency of brachial plexus and vascular injury (subclavian)
  b. 10% mortality, 90% neurologic injury

c. Management contingent on success of vascular repair
d. Forequarter amputation in severe cases

2. Proximal humerus fracture
   - Mechanism: direct fall on upper extremity
   - Imaging: trauma shoulder series (X-rays: AP, axillary lateral, and scapular Y)
   - Neer classification **(Fig. 3.7)**
     a. One- to four-part fractures; separate parts defined by displacement—45-degree angulation or 1 cm displacement (5 mm for greater tuberosity)
     b. Parts: head, shaft, greater and lesser tuberosities
   - Treatment
     a. One-part fracture: none of the parts is displaced
        - Treatment: sling and early ROM
        - Age predicts outcome in conservative management of displaced fractures
     b. Two-part fracture: one part displaced
        - Treatment: percutaneous pinning or open reduction and internal fixation (ORIF)
     c. Three-part fracture; two parts displaced
        - Treatment: ORIF (young) or hemiarthroplasty or reverse total shoulder arthroplasty (elderly); good results with low avascular necrosis (AVN) rates in ORIF of valgus impacted fractures
     d. Four-part with or without head splitting fracture: three parts displaced
        - Treatment: ORIF (young) or hemiarthroplasty or reverse total shoulder arthroplasty (elderly)
        - In hemiarthroplasty, pectoralis major tendon insertion is the best landmark to assess prosthesis height and version; superior aspect of tendon is 5.6 cm distal to top of humeral head
   - Complications:
     a. Most common complication following ORIF is screw penetration of articular surface (15–30%)
   - Hemiarthroplasty or reverse total shoulder arthroplasty (elderly) is salvage procedure of choice; total shoulder arthroplasty (TSA) if glenoid damaged
        - Decreased cut-out rate with use of inferomedial calcar screw
     b. Humeral head AVN
        - Predictors of AVN: four-part fractures with disrupted medial hinge, angular displacement (> 45 degrees), tuberosity displacement > 10 mm, glenohumeral dislocation, head-split components
        - **Having 8 mm of the posterior medial calcar attached to the articular segment is a good prognostic indicator for head vascularity (via posterior humeral circumflex artery).**
     c. Complications: axillary nerve, musculocutaneous nerve, cephalic vein at risk; axillary nerve at higher risk during anterolateral approach to the shoulder versus deltopectoral (usually emerges anteriorly 5 cm distal to lateral aspect of acromion)

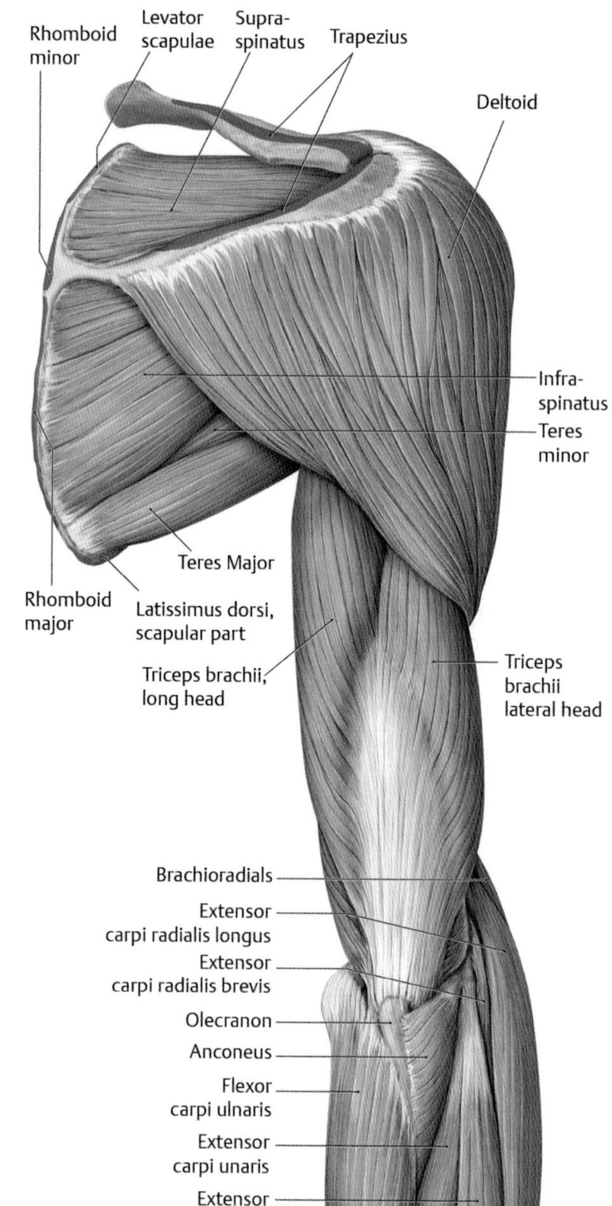

Fig. 3.6 The posterior muscles of the shoulder joint and arm. Muscles of the right shoulder and right arm from the posterior view after removal of the deltoid and forearm muscles. (From Schuenke M, Schulte E. General Anatomy and the Musculoskeletal System: Thieme Atlas of Anatomy. New York: Thieme; 2005. Illustration by Karl Wesker.)

3. Glenohumeral dislocation (also see Chapter 7)
   - Mechanism: direct/indirect trauma, seizures/electrocution (posterior dislocations)

- Associated injuries: axillary nerve injury, rotator cuff tears (elderly patient), labral tears, bony injury (Hill-Sachs, Bankart), shoulder instability
  a. Anterior dislocation associated with rotator cuff tears in patients of ages > 40 years, and labral tears in patients of ages < 20 years
- **Posterior dislocations present with the inability to externally rotate the shoulder.**
- Imaging: shoulder trauma series (axillary lateral most revealing)
- Treatment
  a. Conservative: closed reduction; sling, early ROM
  b. Surgical: irreducible dislocation; labral/capsular procedures for multiple dislocations, refractory instability (capsular shift in multidirectional instability), young overhead athlete

4. Humeral shaft fracture
   - Treatment
     a. Conservative: accept 20-degree angulation in AP plane, 30-degree varus/valgus angulation, 3-cm shortening; treat in fracture brace or coaptation splint
     b. Surgical: open fractures, floating elbow, polytrauma, segmental fracture, articular extension, short transverse pattern in active individual (relative)
        - ORIF: lower reoperation rate, no rotator cuff injury/shoulder impingement pain, allows immediate postoperative weight bearing
        - Intramedullary nailing (IMN): for segmental or pathologic fracture, polytrauma patient
        - No difference between ORIF and IMN in terms of infection, nonunion, or radial nerve issues
   - Complications:
     a. IMN distal interlocking screws: radial nerve injury with lateral to medial screw, musculocutaneous nerve injury with AP screw; shoulder pain
     b. Radial nerve palsy: most common with distal third spiral fracture (Holstein-Lewis lesions), 92% resolve with observation; following closed fracture or ORIF, wait 3 months before ordering electromyogram (EMG); exploration indicated for open fractures (transection more common) or after workup after 3 months of deficit; consider tendon transfers for the wrist and fingers if no improvement
     c. Atrophic nonunion: bone graft/compression plate
5. Distal humerus fracture
   - Single-column fractures (lateral or medial condyle)
     a. Conservative: immobilization in supination or pronation for nondisplaced fractures
     b. Surgical: ORIF for displaced fractures
     c. Complications: loss of motion (most common), cubitus valgus/varus, ulnar nerve injury
     d. Radial nerve crosses posterior to anterior roughly 10 cm proximal to radiocapitellar joint and at risk in this area; therefore, the region within 7.5 cm of the radiocapitellar joint is considered the "safe zone" for posterior approach to distal humerus
   - Two-column fractures
     a. Jupiter classification: describes common patterns of comminution **(Fig. 3.8)**
     b. Treatment: bicolumn plate fixation versus total elbow arthroplasty (TEA) for age > 65 years
        - Low demand and elderly patients with comminuted distal humerus fracture, consider TEA, especially in setting of osteoporosis, steroid use, or rheumatoid arthritis (RA)

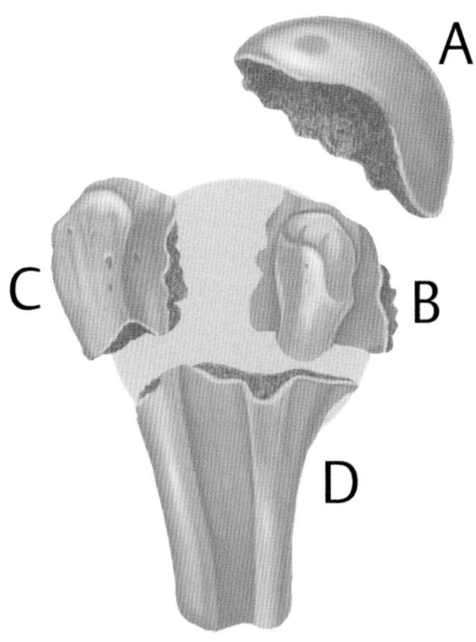

Fig. 3.7 Four parts of proximal humerus in the Neer classification: A, head; B, greater tuberosity; C, lesser tuberosity; D, shaft.

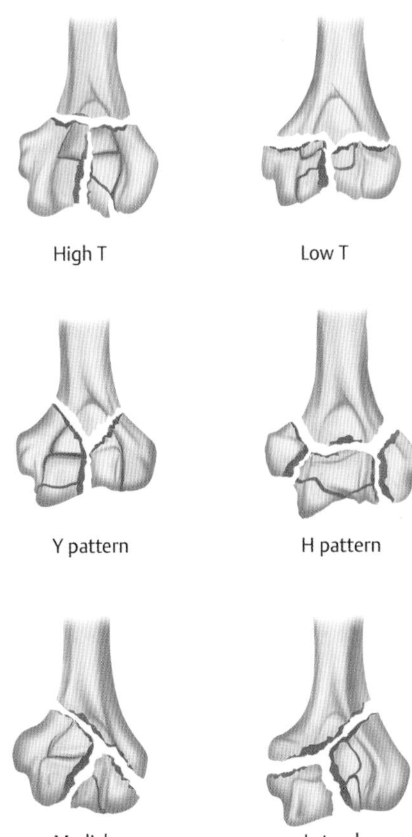

Fig. 3.8 Jupiter classification of distal humerus fractures.

- ORIF of displaced intra-articular distal humerus fractures; regaining full motion is rare and patients can expect a residual loss of elbow flexion strength of 25%

c. Complications:
   - Stiffness most common (treat with static progressive splinting), loss of strength, arthritis, ulnar nerve injury (transpose if in direct contact with metal hardware)

6. Olecranon fracture
   - Classification: by fracture orientation and comminution
   - Treatment

     a. Conservative: 1–2 mm displacement or with greater displacement in elderly/infirm patient; immobilization and early ROM

     b. Surgical
        - Tension band: simple transverse fractures without comminution; anteriorly prominent Kirschner wires (K-wires) decreases forearm rotation, associated with anterior interosseous nerve (AIN) injury
        - Plating: fractures involving coronoid, oblique, comminuted, or associated with dislocation
        - Excision/triceps advancement for low demand, elderly patients (stability possible in up to 50–70% posterior articular surface excision if anterior structures intact)
   - Complications: symptomatic hardware

7. Coronoid fracture
   - Classification: types I-III **(Fig. 3.9)**

     a. Suggestive of elbow instability; shear injury of distal humerus against coronoid
   - Associated injuries

     a. Posteromedial rotatory instability; coronoid anteromedial facet fracture with lateral collateral ligament (LCL) injury from posteromedial rotation; secondary to varus force and leads to varus instability if not addressed

     b. Posterolateral rotatory instability; coronoid fracture with LCL injury and radial head fracture; leads to instability with supination and valgus stress if not addressed

     c. Terrible triad (see 9. Elbow dislocation, below)
   - Operative indications: must address in setting of elbow instability, or must address associated injuries until elbow stable
   - Treatment: suture lasso technique using suture to fix coronoid through bone tunnels through olecranon, ORIF
   - Complications: elbow instability, late degenerative change

8. Radial head fracture
   - Classification: Mason types I-IV **(Fig. 3.10)**
   - Associated injuries

     a. Essex-Lopresti injury-radial head fracture with disruption of the interosseous membrane; must examine wrist in setting of radial head fracture to rule it out; treatment with radial head resection leads to shortening of the radius, and distal radioulnar joint (DRUJ) injury/chronic wrist pain

     b. Posterolateral rotatory instability (see 7. Coronoid fracture, above)

     c. Terrible triad (see 9. Elbow dislocation, below)

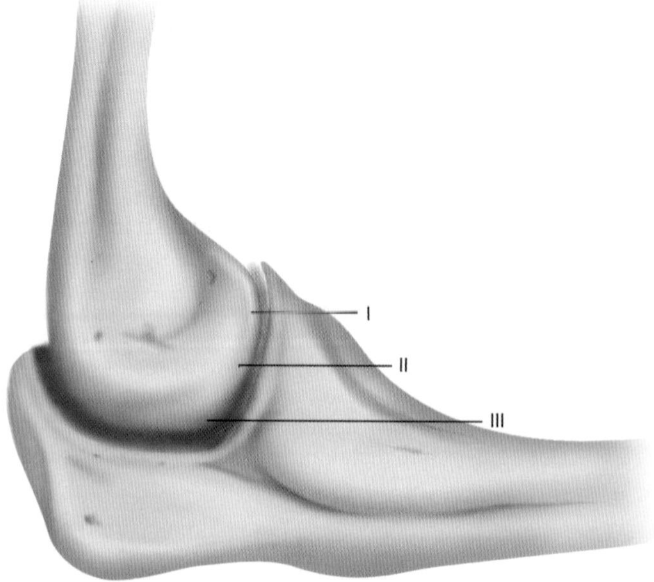

Fig. 3.9 Coronoid fracture classification. I: Tip of coronoid. II: Less than 50% of coronoid height. III: Greater than 50% of coronoid. Useful landmark: on a lateral film, the coronoid and olecranon are roughly the same height.

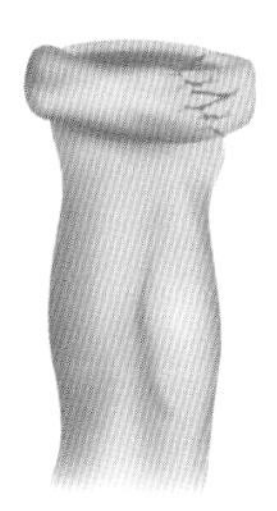
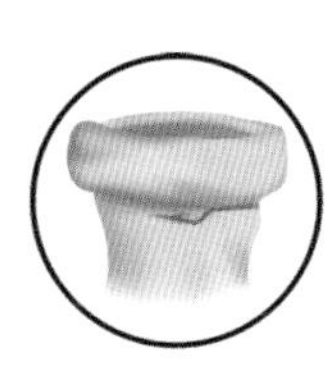

Type I

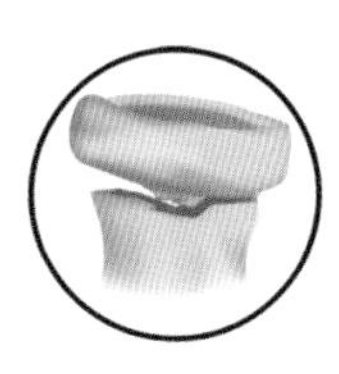
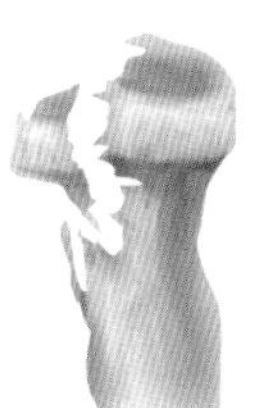

Type II

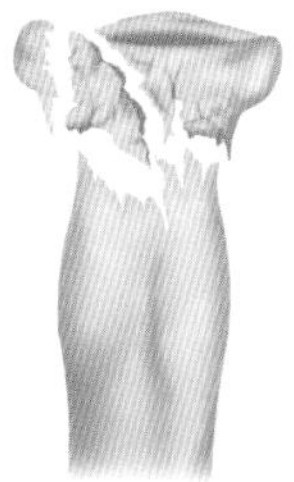
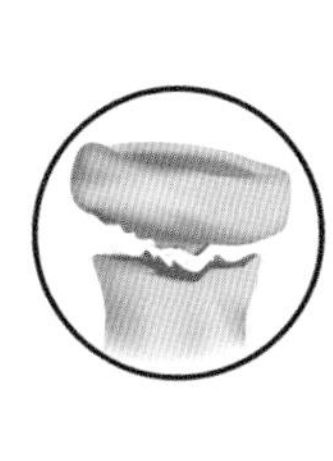

Type III

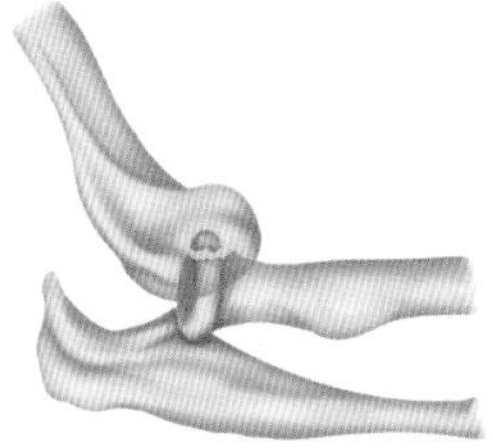

Type IV

Fig. 3.10 Mason classification of radial head fractures. Type I: Nondisplaced. Type II: Some displacement, articular involvement. Type III: Comminution involves entire head. Type IV: Associated dislocation.

- Treatment:
  a. Type I- early ROM
     - **Minimally displaced fractures without block to motion should undergo immediate elbow range of motion as tolerated.**
  b. Type II: early ROM unless mechanical block, in which case ORIF indicated
  c. Type III: ORIF or replacement; if > 3 fragments, replacement has better short-term outcomes than fixation (long-term outcomes still unknown)
  d. Type IV: ORIF or radial head replacement; head resection contraindicated, as dislocation implies marked ligamentous injury
  e. 25% of the radial head, defined as the 90-degree arc between the radial styloid and Lister's tubercle, does not articulate with the ulna and is the "safe zone" for placement of fixation
  f. Kocher approach (anconeus/extensor carpi ulnaris [ECU]) to radial head: forearm held in pronation to protect posterior interosseous nerve (PIN)
- Complications: stiffness, PIN injury (pronate to move nerve out of field), shortening (in excisions with Essex-Lopresti injury)

9. Elbow dislocation **(Fig. 3.11)**

- Classification: by direction (posterolateral, posterior, anterior, medial, lateral, divergent) and presence/absence of fracture (complex versus simple)
- Pathology:
  a. Primary stabilizers: joint articulation, lateral ulnar collateral ligament (LUCL), anterior band of medial collateral ligament (MCL)
  b. Secondary stabilizers: radial head, capsule, mobile wad and surrounding musculature
  c. Pattern of ligament failure from lateral to medial; only LUCL failure required for dislocation
- Treatment
  a. Conservative: simple dislocation; brief immobilization (1–2 weeks), then ROM
  b. Surgical: complex; address fracture with ORIF

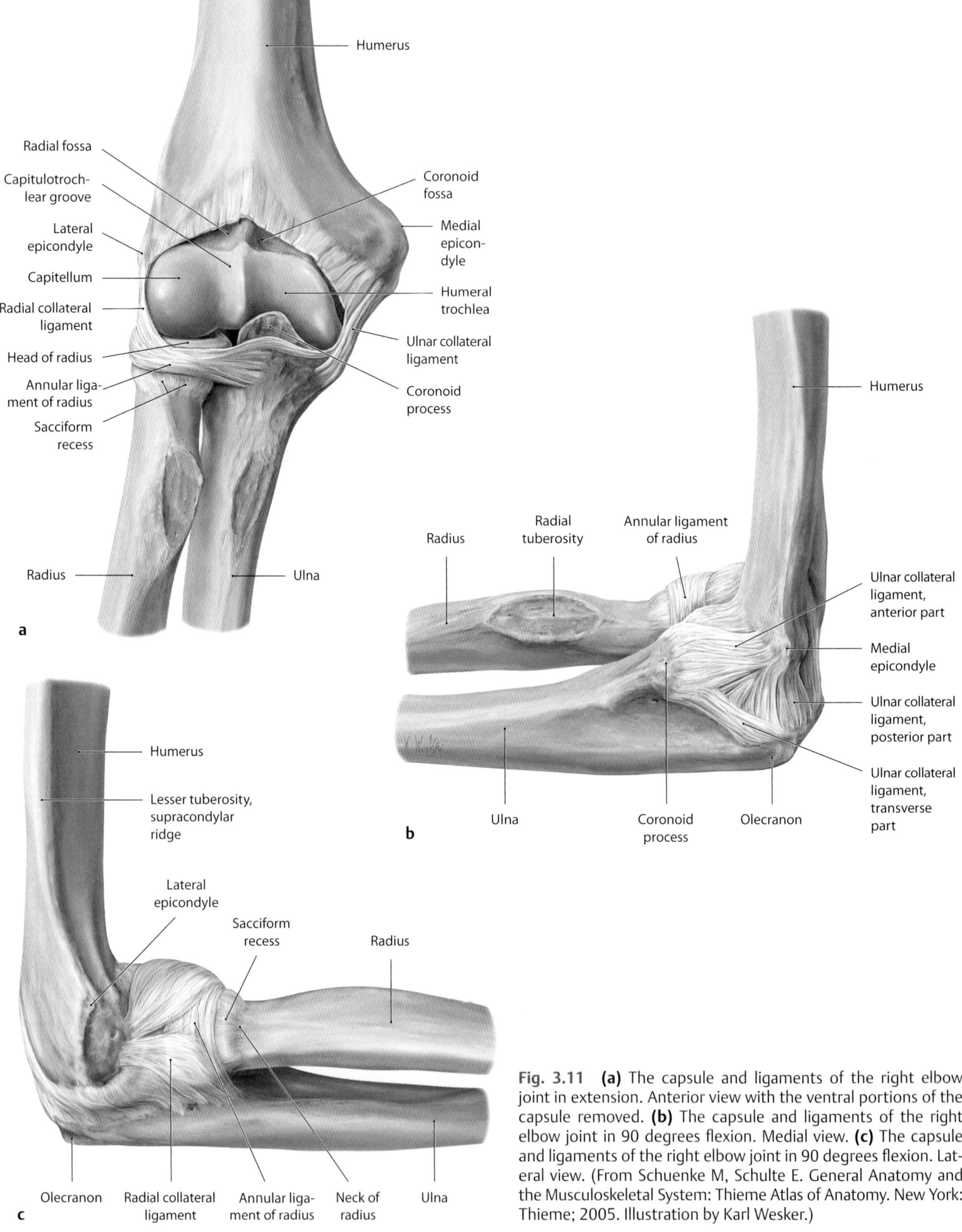

Fig. 3.11 **(a)** The capsule and ligaments of the right elbow joint in extension. Anterior view with the ventral portions of the capsule removed. **(b)** The capsule and ligaments of the right elbow joint in 90 degrees flexion. Medial view. **(c)** The capsule and ligaments of the right elbow joint in 90 degrees flexion. Lateral view. (From Schuenke M, Schulte E. General Anatomy and the Musculoskeletal System: Thieme Atlas of Anatomy. New York: Thieme; 2005. Illustration by Karl Wesker.)

c. Terrible triad: elbow dislocation, coronoid fracture (tip), radial head fracture
   - Mechanism: valgus and supination force
   - Treatment: surgical management with coronoid fixation, radial head replacement or fixation, and LUCL repair to humeral origin
     - If elbow is unstable after above repairs, then must repair MCL
     - If unstable after medial ligamentous repair, requires hinged external fixator to ensure elbow stability
     - LUCL avulsion from humerus is most common mode of failure

- Complications
  a. Stiffness (most common); posttraumatic arthritis
  b. Heterotopic ossification (HO): can resect after maturation; use prophylactic radiation in head-injured patients; Indocin may have some effect in prevention
  c. Neurovascular injury: brachial artery, ulnar/median nerve

10. Forearm fracture
- Monteggia: proximal ulna fracture with radial head dislocation
  a. Classification: Bado **(Fig. 3.12)**
  b. Treatment: ORIF of ulna; radial head reduces when ulna fixed anatomically; if radiocapitellar joint nonconcentric, usually due to annular ligament interposition requiring open reduction of radial head
  c. Complications
     - PIN injury: most resolve; observe
     - Bado type II Monteggia fracture (posterior) has a higher nonunion rate and poorer outcomes compared with other Monteggia fractures.
- Radius and ulna fracture
     - Restoration of radial bow important for pronation/supination
  a. Treatment: ORIF with compression plating
  b. Complications: stiffness, loss of rotation (related to restoration of radial bow), nonunion, synostosis (higher with single incision approach), PIN injury
     - Refracture risk after plate removal (12–18 months); highest with diaphyseal location of initial fracture; other risks are removal before 12 months, high initial comminution/displacement, and immediate full weight bearing
- Ulna fracture (nightstick)
  a. Classification: stable if < 25–50% displacement, < 10- to 15-degree angulation; otherwise considered unstable
  b. Treatment
     - Stable: reduce and cast
     - Unstable: ORIF
- Radial shaft fracture with DRUJ instability (Galeazzi)
  a. Treatment: ORIF fracture, assess DRUJ; if unstable, pin DRUJ in position of concentric reduction (usually supination)
     - If irreducible, assess for muscle interposition (usually ECU); the closer the radius fracture is to DRUJ, the more likely it is unstable.

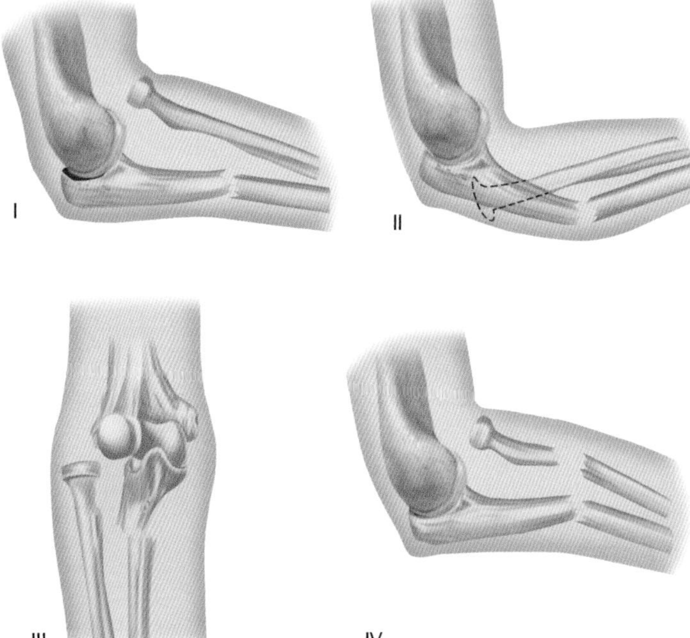

Fig. 3.12 Bado classification of Monteggia fractures. Classified by direction of ulnar angulation/radial head dislocation. I: Anterior. II: Posterior. III: Lateral. IV: Associated proximal radius fracture. (Medial not possible as the ulna blocks the radial head.)

11. Distal radius fracture (also see Chapter 9)
   - Classification: multiple systems; Fernandez classification based on mechanism and treatment **(Table 3.2)**
   - Common eponyms:
     a. Colles': low-energy, extra-articular, dorsally displaced fracture
     b. Smith's: low-energy, extra-articular, volarly displaced fracture
     c. Chauffer's: radial styloid fracture (high association with scapholunate ligament tear)
     d. Die punch: impaction fracture of lunate fossa, typically with coronal and sagittal split
     e. Barton's: coronal intra-articular shear fracture leading to radiocarpal dislocation (either volar or dorsal)
   - Treatment
     a. Conservative: extra-articular fracture with <5-degree loss of radial inclination, < 5 mm loss of radial height, neutral to 5-degree dorsal angulation; closed reduction and cast
     b. Surgical: percutaneous pinning, external fixation, ORIF (volar or dorsal)
        - Operative indications: > 3–5 mm loss of radial height (normal 13 mm), > 5-degree loss of radial inclination, > 2 mm articular stepoff, > 0- to 10-degree dorsal angulation
        - Volar distal radius locking plates resist radial shortening, dorsal angulation, and buttress the distal radius (biomechanically stronger than dorsal plating).
          - ♦ Volar plating does not allow for visualization of the articular surface through a capsulotomy; the dorsal approach does.
        - Elderly patients (> 65 years) can be treated conservatively beyond these criteria with successful outcome compared with surgical management.
        - Acute carpal tunnel syndrome persisting after closed reduction: requires ORIF and carpal tunnel release
        - Fix ulnar styloid if associated with DRUJ instability
   - Complications:
     a. Complex regional pain syndrome (CRPS): American Academy of Orthopaedic Surgeons (AAOS) guidelines recommend vitamin C supplementation to prevent CRPS
     b. Malunion/nonunion; arthritis present if > 2 mm residual stepoff, symptoms variable
     c. Extensor pollicis longus (EPL) rupture: 3% of nonoperative cases treated with cast; treatment with extensor indicis proprius (EIP) or palmaris tendon transfer; occurs with minimally displaced or non-displaced fractures
     d. Flexor pollicis longus (FPL) most commonly ruptured tendon after volar plate fixation (up to 12% at 10 months); treatment with interposition graft or flexor digitorum superficialis (FDS) transfer
     e. Extensor tendon irritation: dorsal plating; requires removal of hardware at times

III. Pelvis/Acetabulum

1. Anatomy of pelvis/acetabulum
   - Pelvis: composed of the sacrum attached to two innominate bones (made up of the fused ilium, ischium, and pubis) connected anteriorly by the pubic symphysis **(Fig. 3.13)**

Table 3.2 Fernandez Classification of Distal Radius Fractures

Type	Image	Description	Mechanism	Treatment
I	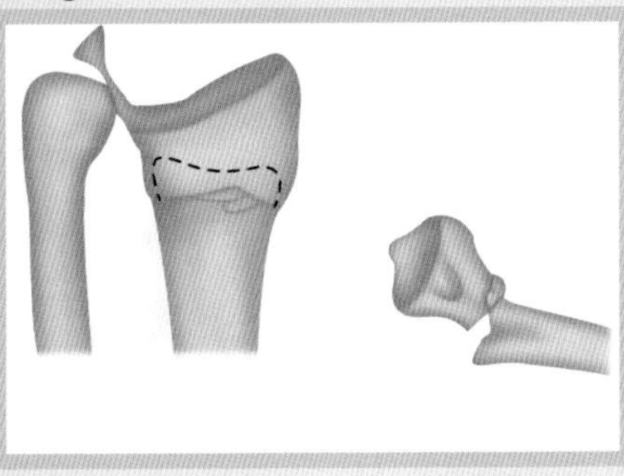	Extra-articular, metaphyseal	Bending	Cast if stable, CRPP/ORIF if unstable
II	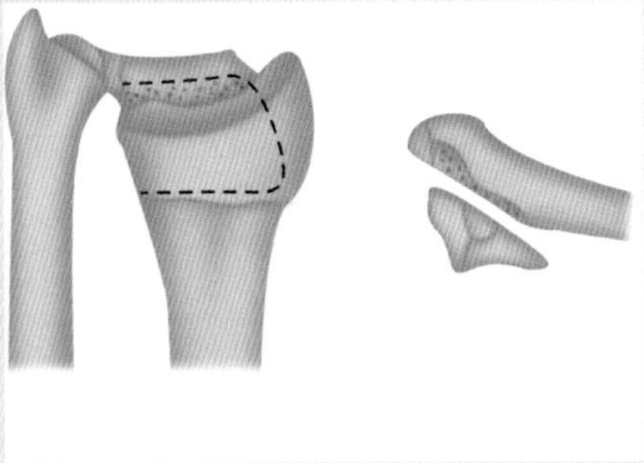	Volar or dorsal lip shear, usually unstable	Articular shear	ORIF
III	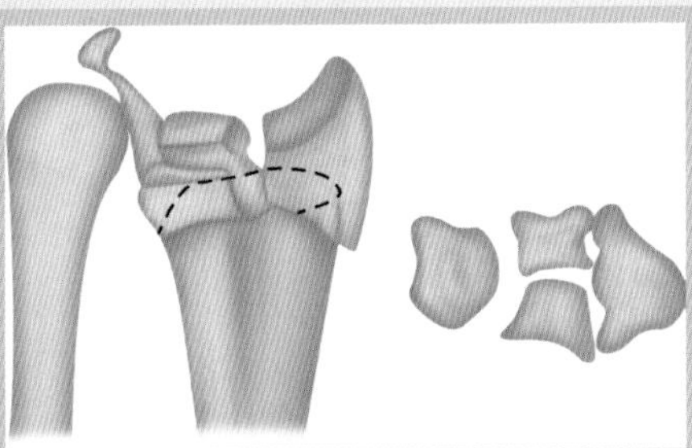	"Die punch," impacted articular surface	Compression	Cast if nondisplaced, tamp up and back graft if depressed
IV	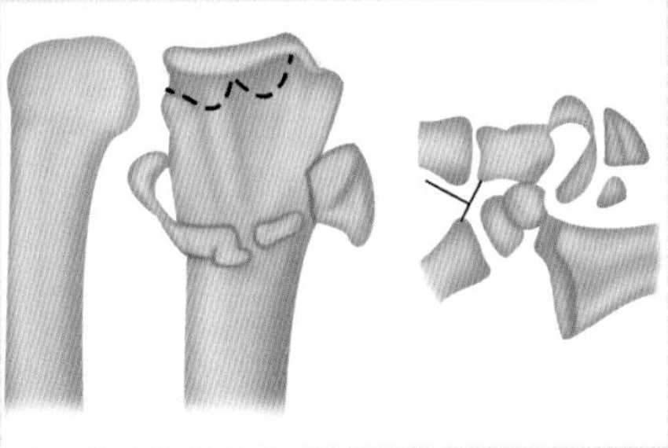	High energy	Fracture- dislocations	Styloid repair often increases stability
V	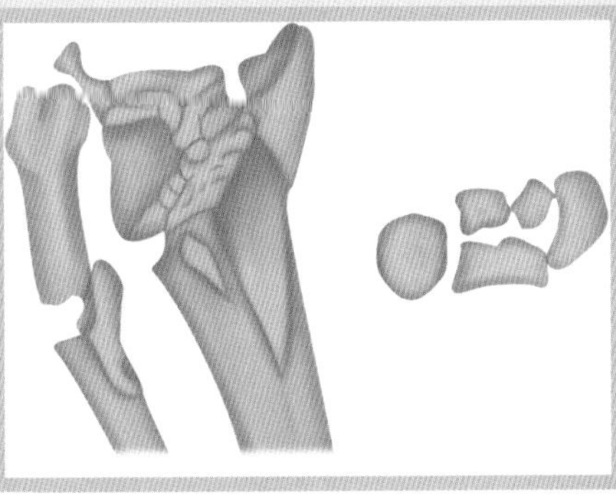	High energy	Combined	Multiple techniques

Abbreviations: CRPP, closed reduction and percutaneous fixation; ORIF, open reduction and internal fixation.

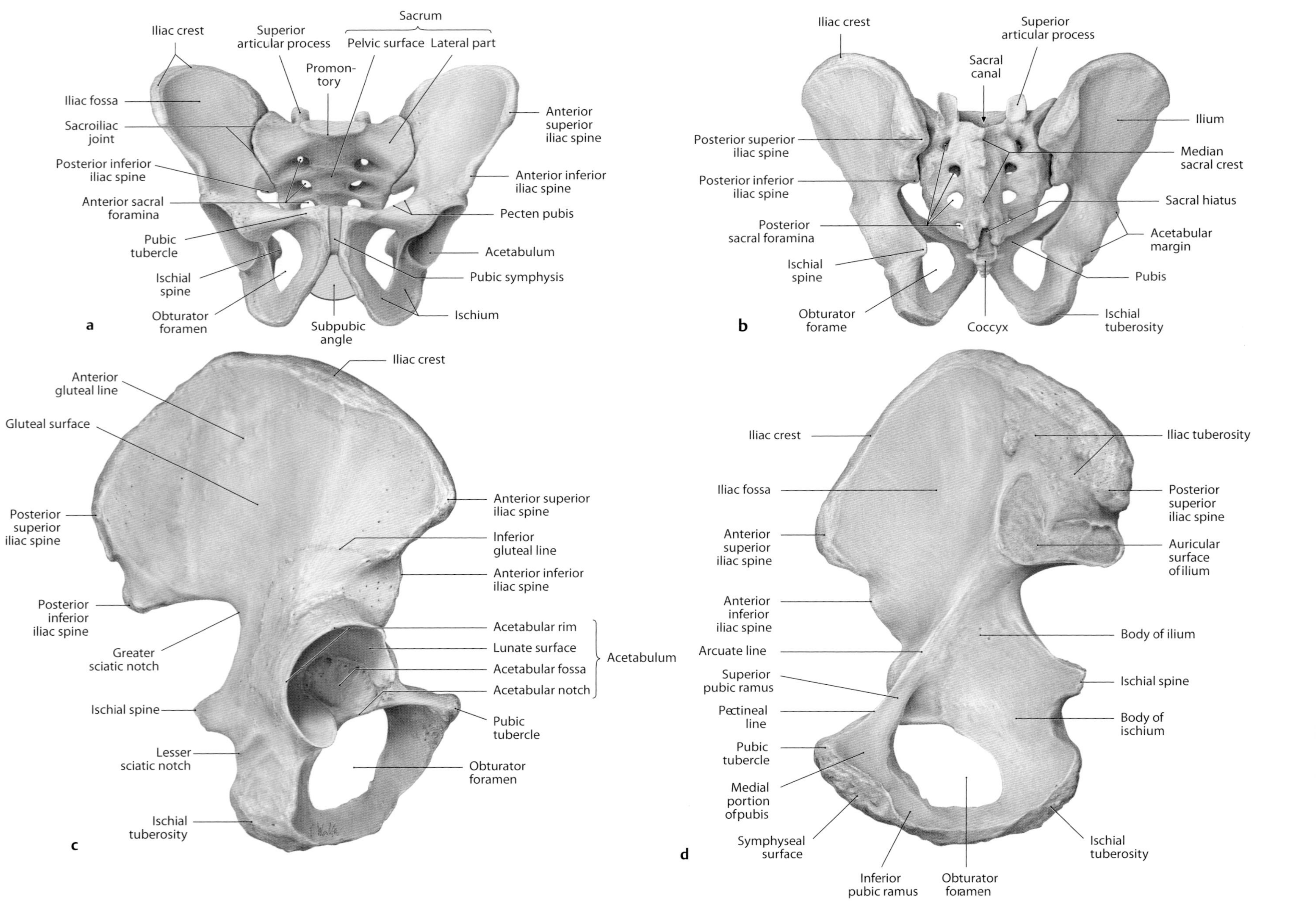

Fig. 3.13 **(a,b)** The male pelvis: **(a)** anterior view, **(b)** posterior view. **(c,d)** The right hip bone: **(c)** lateral view, **(d)** medial view. (From Schuenke M, Schulte E. General Anatomy and the

a. Bony landmarks
   - Anterior superior iliac spine (ASIS): origin of sartorius, abdominal muscles (internal/transverse), and inguinal ligament
   - Anterior inferior iliac spine (AIIS): origin of rectus femoris and iliofemoral ligament
   - Posterior superior iliac spine (PSIS): at level of S2 spinous process
   - Iliopectineal eminence: represents union of the ileum to the pubis; iliopsoas passes between the iliopectineal eminence medially and the AIIS laterally

b. Musculature: pelvis and proximal thigh **(Table 3.3)**

c. Important Ligaments **(Fig. 3.14)**
   - Sacroiliac ligaments: stabilize the sacroiliac joint, anterior and posterior (stronger) ligaments
   - Sacrospinous ligament: anterior sacrum to ischial spine, marks the inferior border of greater sciatic notch and separates the greater notch from the lesser notch; provides rotational stability
   - Sacrotuberous ligament: posterolateral sacrum to ischial tuberosity, marks the inferior border of lesser sciatic notch; provides vertical stability
   - Pubic ligaments: superior and arcuate ligaments stabilize the two hemipelvises anteriorly with a fibrocartilaginous disk between pubic bones
   - Iliolumbar ligaments: ileum to L5 transverse process

d. Greater sciatic notch: exiting structures include piriformis, sciatic nerve, superior gluteal artery/nerve/vein, inferior gluteal artery/nerve/vein, pudendal artery/nerve/vein, nerve to obturator internus, posterior femoral cutaneous nerve, nerve to quadratus femoris **(Fig. 3.15)**
   - Piriformis is the key structure; superior gluteal nerve, artery, and vein exit above it; all other structures come out below; sciatic nerve is anterior (deep) to piriformis and exits just below it, lying posterior (superficial) to the short external rotators; in 2% of cases, the sciatic nerve passes through the piriformis
   - Nerve to obturator internus and pudendal nerve reenter the pelvis via the lesser sciatic notch
   - **Use mnemonic POPS IQ for the order of nerves exiting the greater sciatic notch below piriformis: Pudendal, Obturator internus, Posterior femoral cutaneous, Sciatic, Inferior gluteal, Quadratus.**

e. Lesser sciatic notch: exiting structures include short external rotators of hip

f. Important nerves **(Fig. 3.16)**
   - Genitofemoral nerve pierces psoas and lies on its anteromedial surface.
   - Femoral nerve lies between the iliacus and psoas and travels with the iliopsoas.
   - Lateral femoral cutaneous nerve exits the pelvis under the inguinal ligament's lateral attachment on the ASIS.
   - Sciatic nerve (L4-S3): peroneal division is the most lateral, thereby making it the most susceptible to injury with pelvic/hip surgery; peroneal branch runs on the deep surface of the long head of biceps and innervates the short head of biceps femoris and distal musculature
   - Obturator nerve: anterior division supplies obturator externus, pectineus, adductor longus/brevis, gracilis, medial thigh skin sensation; posterior division supplies only obturator externus, adductor brevis, and knee joint (referred pain); can be injured when retractors are placed behind the transverse acetabular ligament
   - L5 nerve root lies on the superior/anterior sacral ala [2 cm medial to sacroiliac (SI) joint] and can be damaged when SI screws are placed too anterior or superior

Table 3.3 Pelvis and Thigh Musculature

Muscle	Origin	Insertion	Nerve
Pelvis Musculature			
Iliacus	Iliac fossa, AIIS, anterior hip capsule	Iliopsoas tendon to lesser trochanter of femur, linea aspera	Femoral nerve
Psoas	Vertebral bodies/disks T12–L4, Transverse processes L1–L4	Iliopsoas tendon to lesser trochanter of femur, linea aspera	L1–L3
Pectineus	Pubis, superior pubic ramus	Pectineal line of femur	Femoral nerve (obturator nerve)
Gluteus maximus	Ilium, sacrum, coccyx	IT band, femoral gluteal tuberosity	Inferior gluteal
Gluteus medius	Ilium, gluteus aponeurosis	Femur greater trochanter	Superior gluteal
Gluteus minimus	Ilium	Femur greater trochanter, hip joint capsule	Superior gluteal
Piriformis	Sacrum anterior surface	Femur greater trochanter	Nerve to piriformis
Superior gemellus	Ischial spine	Femur greater trochanter	Nerve to obturator internus
Obturator internus	Obturator foramen	Femur greater trochanter	Nerve to obturator internus
Inferior gemellus	Ischial tuberosity	Femur greater trochanter	Nerve to quadratus femoris
Quadratus femoris	Ischial tuberosity	Posterior femur, intertrochanteric crest	Nerve to quadratus femoris
Anterior Thigh Musculature			
Tensor fascia lata	Iliac crest, ASIS	Anterior IT band, which inserts on Gerdy's tubercle on anterolateral tibia	Superior gluteal
Rectus femoris	AIIS, reflected head to ilium just above acetabulum	Quadriceps tendon to the patella, terminally inserts on tibial tuberosity via patellar tendon	Femoral nerve
Vastus lateralis	Femur greater trochanter	Quadriceps tendon to the patella, terminally inserts on tibial tuberosity via patellar tendon	Femoral nerve
Vastus intermedius	Anterolateral femoral shaft	Quadriceps tendon to the patella, terminally inserts on tibial tuberosity via patellar tendon	Femoral nerve
Vastus medialis	Femoral intertrochanteric line, linea aspera	Quadriceps tendon to the patella, terminally inserts on tibial tuberosity via patellar tendon	Femoral nerve
Posterior Thigh Musculature			
Semitendinosus	Ischial tuberosity	Medial proximal tibia, pes anserine	Sciatic nerve
Semimembranosus	Ischial tuberosity	Posteromedial tibia, popliteal ligament	Sciatic nerve
Biceps femoris	Long head: ischial tuberosity Short head: linea aspera, intermuscular septum	Fibular head	Long head: sciatic nerve Short head: common peroneal nerve
Medial Musculature			
Adductor magnus	Ischial tuberosity, ischial ramus, inferior pubic ramus	Medial epicondyle at adductor tubercle, linea aspera	Posterior fibers: sciatic nerve Anterior fibers: obturator nerve
Adductor longus	Pubis	Linea aspera	Obturator nerve
Adductor brevis	Inferior pubic ramus	Linea aspera	Obturator nerve
Gracilis	Pubis, inferior pubic ramus	Medial proximal tibia, pes anserine	Obturator nerve
Obturator externus	Obturator foramen	Femoral trochanteric fossa	Obturator nerve

Abbreviations: ASIS, anterior superior iliac spine; AIIS, anterior inferior iliac spine; IT, iliotibial.

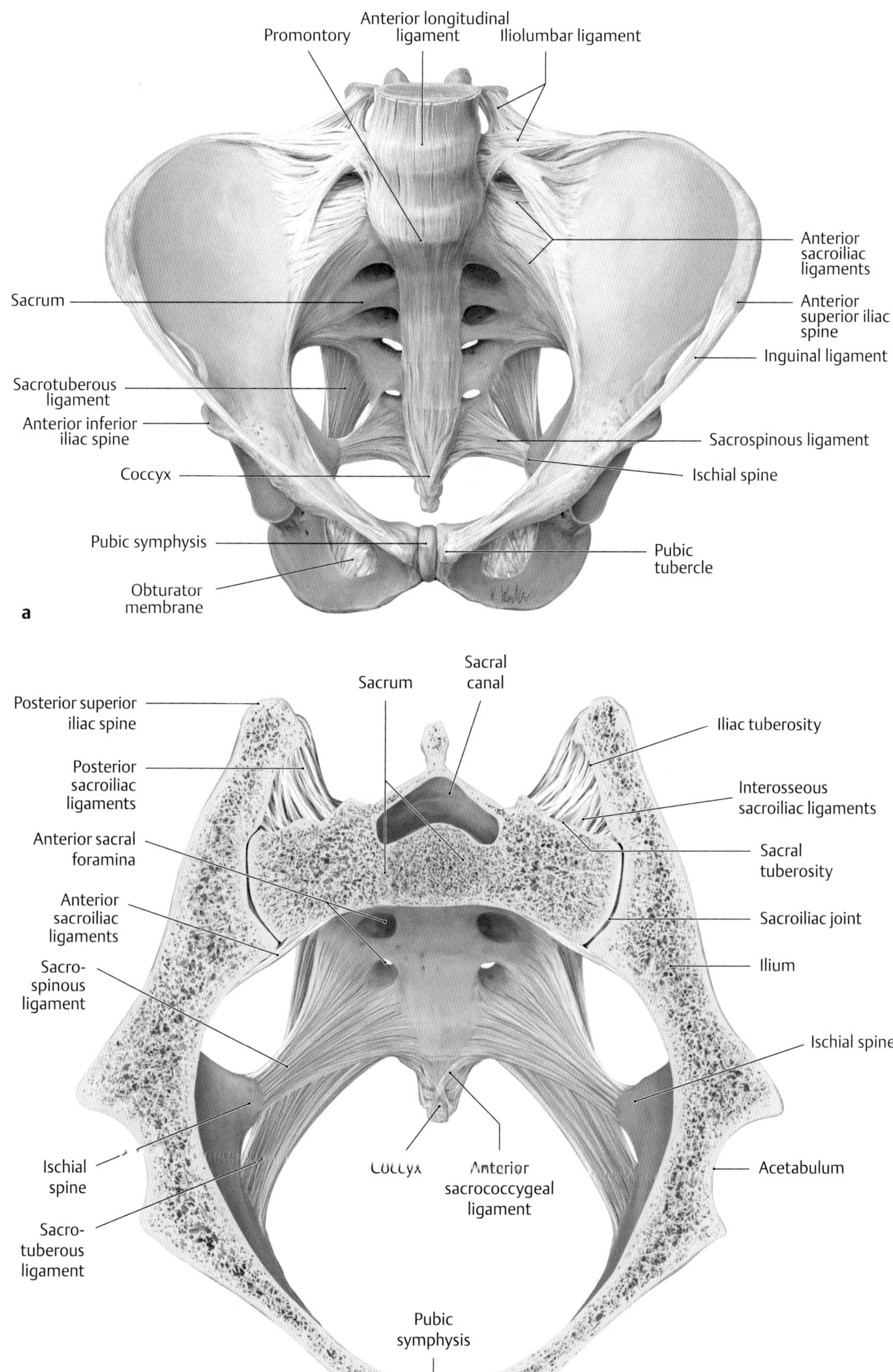

Fig. 3.14 Ligaments of the male pelvis. **(a)** Anterosuperior view. **(b)** Ligaments of the sacroiliac joint. Oblique section through the pelvis at the level of the pelvic inlet plane, superior view.

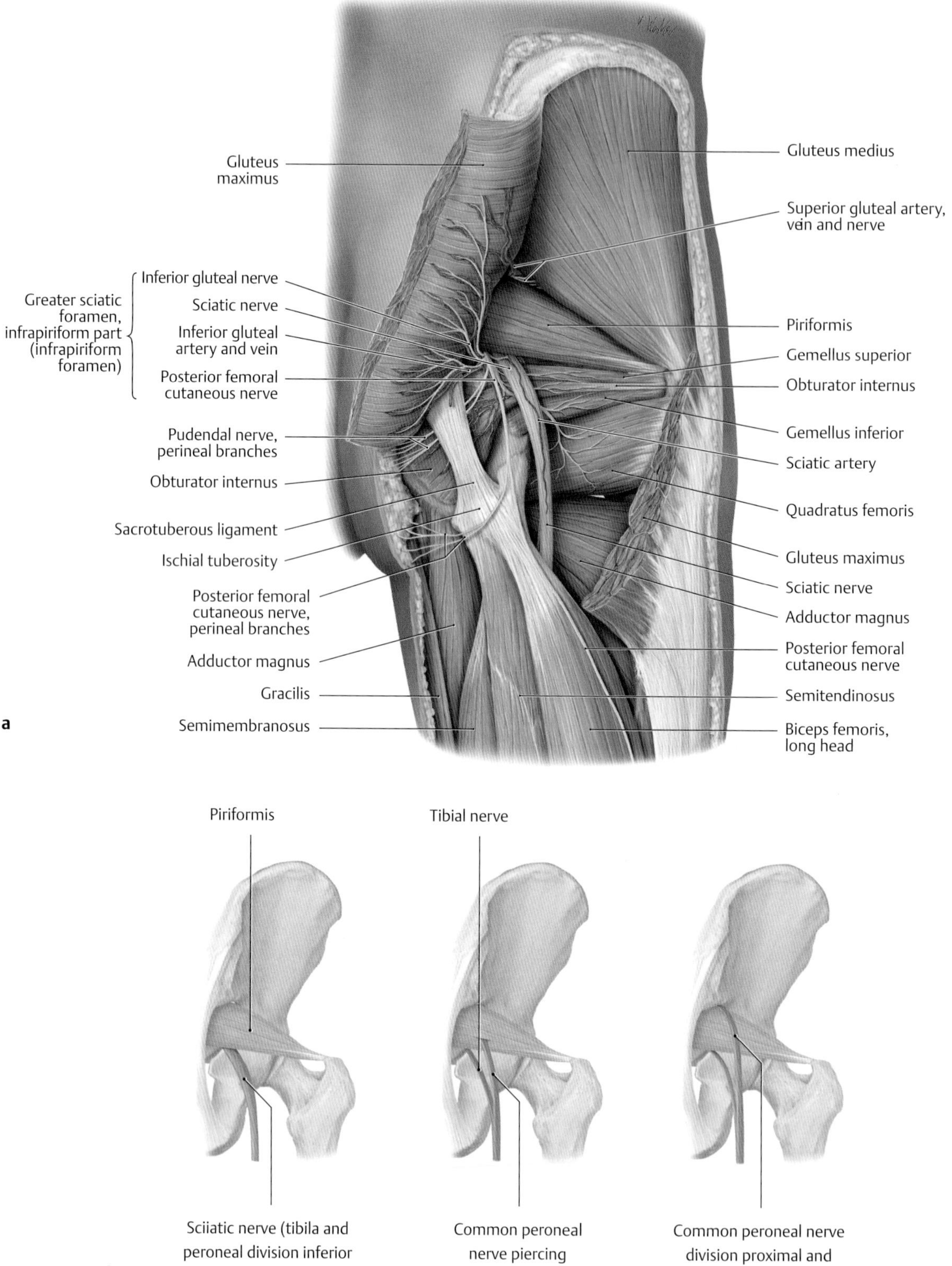

Fig. 3.15 Greater sciatic notch structures and the relationship of the sciatic nerve to the piriformis. **(a)** Vessels and nerves of the deep gluteal region. **(b)** Posterior view, with the gluteus maximus partially removed. Variations of the course of the sciatic nerve relative the piriformis muscle. (From Schuenke M, Schulte E. General Anatomy and the Musculoskeletal System: Thieme Atlas of Anatomy. New York: Thieme; 2005. Illustration by Karl Wesker.)

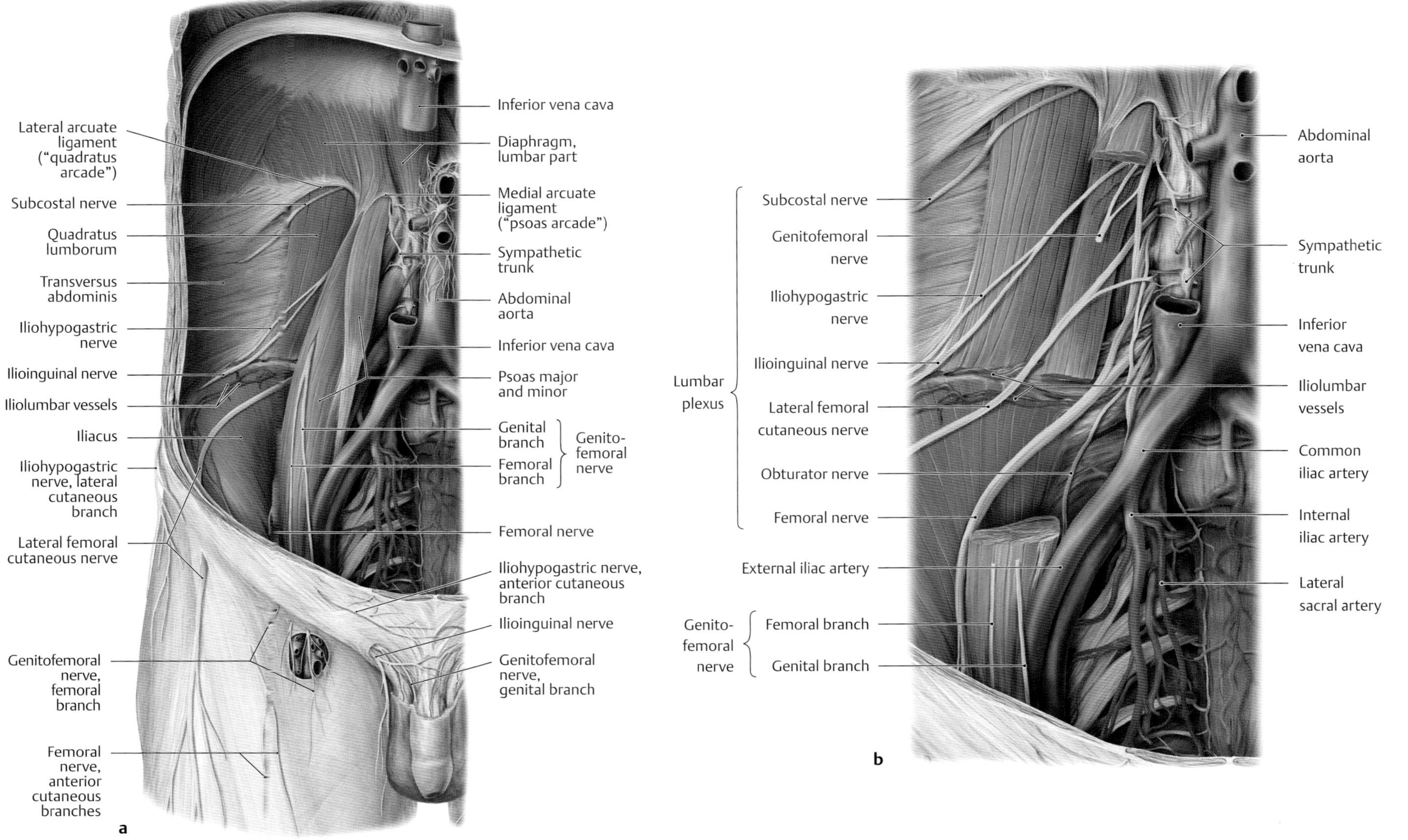

Fig. 3.16 Important pelvic nerve locations. Neurovascular structures on the anterior side of the posterior trunk wall, anterior view. **(a)** Lumbar fossa on the right side after removal of the anterior and lateral trunk wall, the intra- and retroperitoneal organs, the peritoneum, and all the fasciae of the trunk wall. The inferior vena cava has been partially removed. **(b)** Lumbar fossa with the lumbar plexus of the right side after removal of the superficial layer of the psoas major. The lumbar plexus is formed by the ventral branches of the T12–L4 nerves lateral to the lumbar spine and is partially covered by the psoas major muscle. The nerves run laterally and obliquely downward to the abdominal wall and thigh, except for the obturator nerve, which runs through the lateral wall of the lesser pelvis and the obturator foramen (not visible here) to the medial part of the thigh. (From Schuenke M, Schulte E. General Anatomy and the Musculoskeletal System: Thieme Atlas of Anatomy. New York: Thieme; 2005. Illustration by Karl Wesker.)

g. Vessels **(Fig. 3.17)**
   - Aorta branches to the common iliac arteries at the L4 level.
   - Common iliac arteries divide into the internal/external iliacs at the S1 level.
   - External iliac artery passes under the inguinal ligament to become the femoral artery.
   - Internal iliac artery becomes the obturator artery and gives branches to the superior/inferior gluteal and pudendal arteries.
   - Posterior venous plexus: large collection of veins that drain into the internal iliac vein, commonly the source of bleeding in pelvic injuries
   - Corona mortis: anastomotic connection between the external iliac arterial system (inferior epigastric branch) and the obturator artery; lies on pelvic brim approximately 6 cm lateral to pubic symphysis; must identify and ligate during surgical approaches (Stoppa and ilioinguinal)
   - Deep external pudendal artery: at risk during percutaneous tenotomy of adductor longus

h. Femoral triangle: lateral border is sartorius, medial border is pectineus, and superior border is inguinal ligament; floor consists of iliacus, psoas, pectineus, and adductor longus (from lateral to medial) **(Fig. 3.18)**
   - Contents: femoral nerve (which travels with iliopsoas muscle) and the femoral sheath with includes the femoral artery, femoral vein, and the femoral canal (lymphatics)
   - **Use mnemonic NAVeL for order of femoral structures from lateral to medial: *N*erve, *A*rtery, *V*ein, and *L*ymphatic vessels.**
   - Saphenous nerve branches off of the femoral nerve at the apex of the triangle and travels under the sartorius.

- Acetabulum

a. Supported by two columns of bone in an inverted-Y pattern **(Fig. 3.19)**
   - Anterior column: iliac wing to pubic symphysis
   - Posterior column: greater sciatic notch through the middle of the acetabulum to the inferior pubic ramus

b. Normal anatomy: anteverted 15 degrees and abducted 45 degrees

c. Labrum provides increased coverage for, and stability of, the femoral head.

d. Superior gluteal artery (branch of internal iliac artery) can be injured in posterior column fractures; internal pudendal can also be injured.

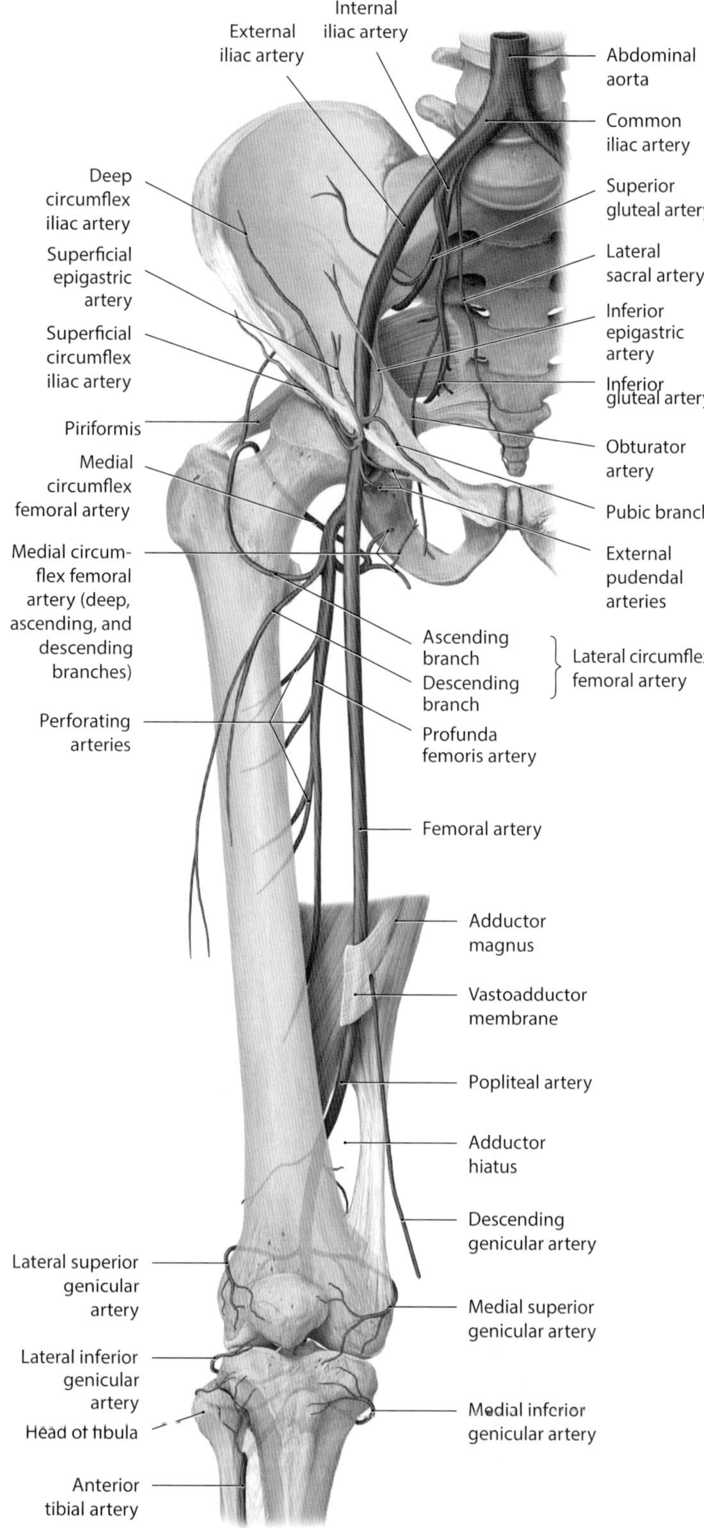

Fig. 3.17 Pelvic vasculature. Course and branches of the femoral artery. The femoral artery, the distal continuation of the external iliac artery, runs along the medial side of the thigh to the adductor canal, through which it passes to the back of the leg. After emerging from the adductor hiatus, it becomes the popliteal artery. In clinical parlance the femoral artery is often called the superficial femoral artery because of its superficial course down the front of the thigh, distinguishing it from the more deeply placed profunda femoris artery that arises from it. (From Schuenke M, Schulte E. General Anatomy and the Musculoskeletal System: Thieme Atlas of Anatomy. New York: Thieme; 2005. Illustration by Karl Wesker.)

2. Pelvic imaging
   - Radiographic cardinal lines **(Fig. 3.20)**
     a. Iliopectineal line corresponds to the anterior column.
     b. Ilioischial line corresponds to the posterior column.
   - X-ray views **(Fig. 3.21)**
     a. AP pelvis
     b. Inlet view: shows AP displacement of the pelvic ring, axial view of S1, beam directed 60 degrees caudally
     c. Outlet view: shows vertical translation of pelvic ring, true AP of sacrum, beam directed 45 degrees cephalad
     d. Judet views
        - **Judet views show iliac oblique of one side while showing the obturator oblique of the other side.**
        - Iliac oblique: shows posterior column and anterior wall, external rotation view
        - Obturator oblique: shows anterior column and posterior wall, internal rotation view; shows obturator foramen en face
          - ♦ Spur sign for both column acetabular fractures seen best on this view (represents the intact ilium without any acetabular surface connected) **(Fig. 3.22)**
          - ♦ **Use mnemonic IOWA: Iliac Oblique—Wall Anterior**

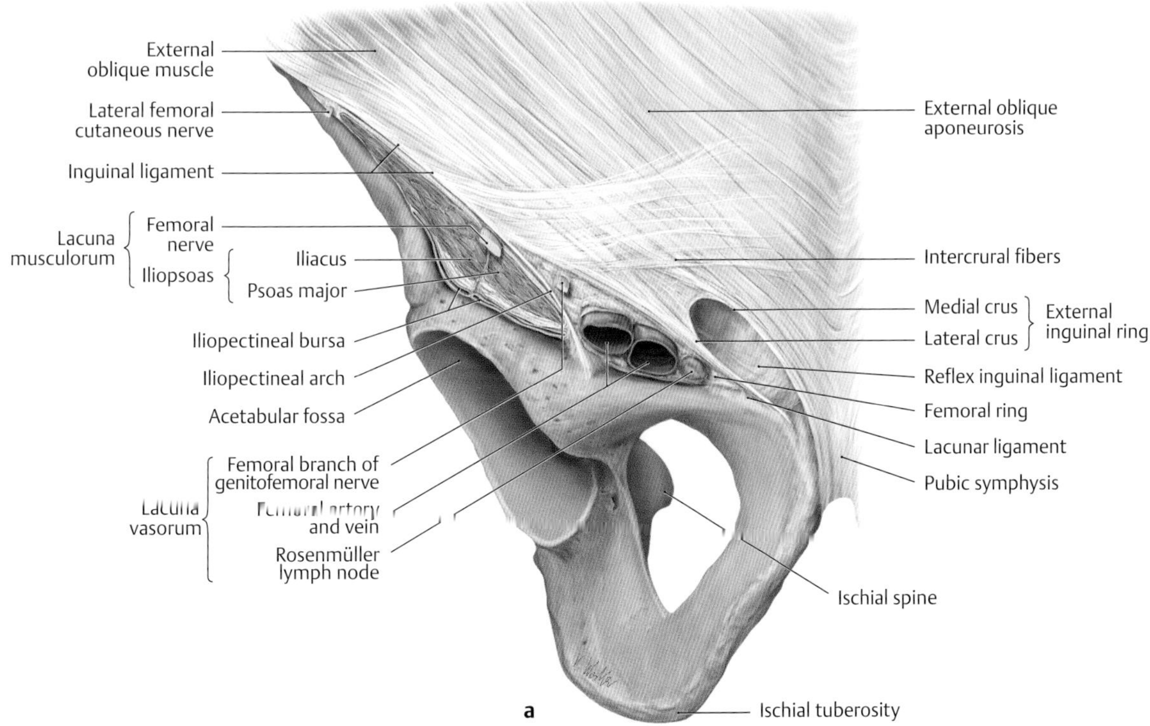

Fig. 3.18 Femoral canal anatomy**.** Inguinal region and the contents of the lacuna musculorum and lacuna vasorum, anterior view. **(a)** A portion of the right hip bone and the adjacent anterior inferior abdominal wall with the external inguinal ring and the contents of the lacuna musculorum and lacuna vasorum below the inguinal ligament. The site of emergence of the muscles and vessels, bounded by the inguinal ligament and the superior pelvic rim, is subdivided by the fibrous iliopectineal arch into a lateral muscular port(lacuna musculorum) and a medial vascular port (lacuna vasorum). (*continued on page 108*)

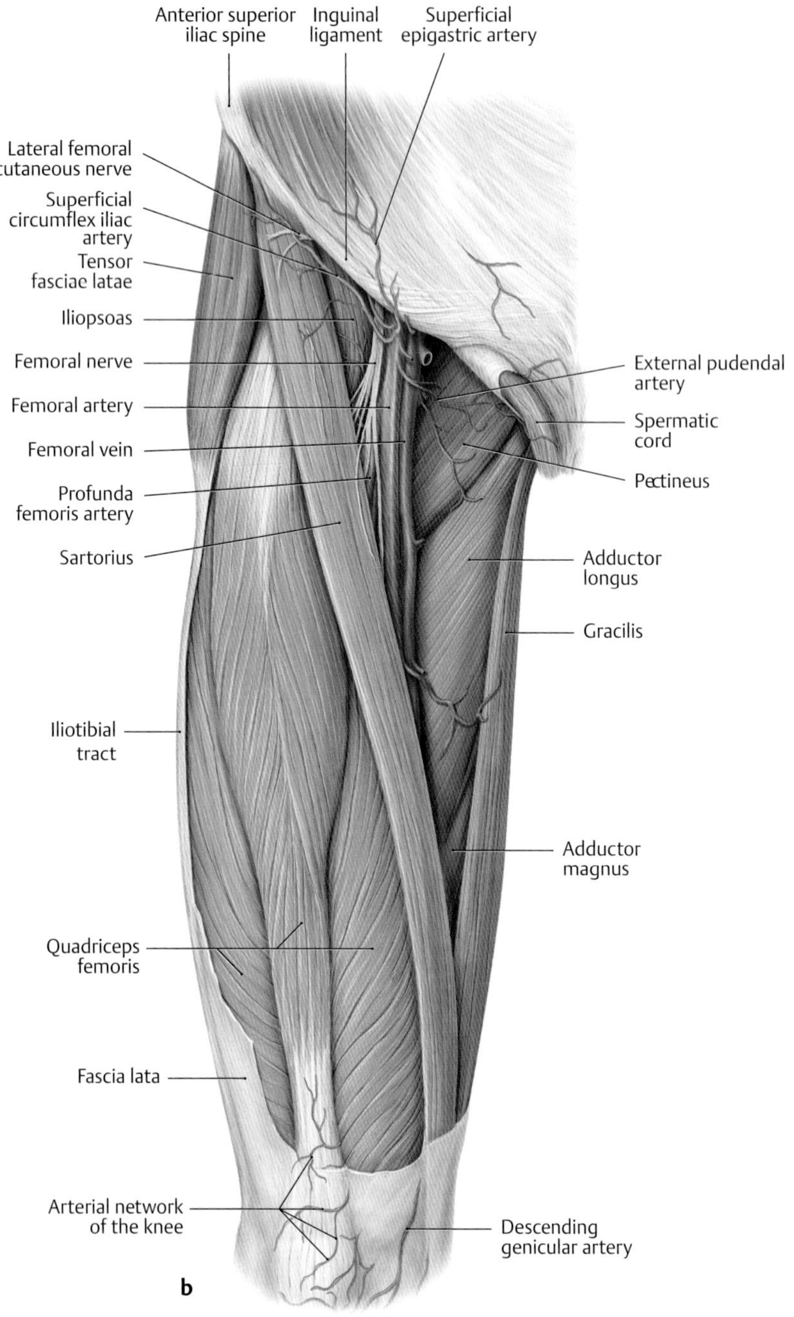

Fig. 3.18 (*continued*) **(b)** The femoral triangle: right thigh, anterior view. The skin, subcutaneous tissue, and fascia lata have been removed to demonstrate the neurovascular structures in the femoral triangle. The femoral triangle is bounded superiorly by the inguinal ligament, laterally by the sartorius muscle, and medially by the adductor longus. It contains the neurovascular structures that emerge from the pelvis and pass below the inguinal ligament to the anterior side of the thigh through the lacuna musculorum and lacuna vasorum. The posterior muscular wall of the femoral triangle is formed from lateral to medial by the iliopsoas and pectineus. (From Schuenke M, Schulte E. General Anatomy and the Musculoskeletal System: Thieme Atlas of Anatomy. New York: Thieme; 2005. Illustration by Karl Wesker.)

e. Key combination views:
    - Inlet iliac oblique: avoids guidewire or screw penetration of the inner cortex of superior pubic ramus
    - Inlet obturator oblique: best shows the position of supra-acetabular screws in ilium and helps avoid intra-articular penetration
    - Outlet obturator oblique: used to identify starting point for external fixation pins placed in the AIIS
    - **Outlet obturator view required to see the column of supracetabular bone to place the pin**

3. Surgical approaches to the pelvis/acetabulum **(Table 3.4)**
    - Anterior and posterior approaches to iliac crest

- Ilioinguinal
  a. Incision from 2 cm proximal to pubic symphysis to ASIS along iliac crest
  b. Working windows
     - Medial: medial to the external iliac vessels
     - Middle: between external iliac vessels and iliopsoas
     - Lateral: lateral to iliopsoas (lateral window can be used in combination with other approaches such as Stoppa)
  c. Iliopectineal fascia separates femoral nerve and external iliac artery (separates lateral and middle windows).
     - **Iliopectineal fascia is the key structure that separates the lateral and medial windows during dissection.**
  d. Lowest incidence of HO
- Kocher-Langenbeck
  a. Incision is curved from 5 cm anterior to PSIS to greater trochanter and femoral shaft, gluteus maximus is split, piriformis and short external rotators tendons are divided 1 cm from insertion, quadratus femoris remains intact to protect the femoral head blood supply.
  b. Trochanteric osteotomy increases superior exposure.

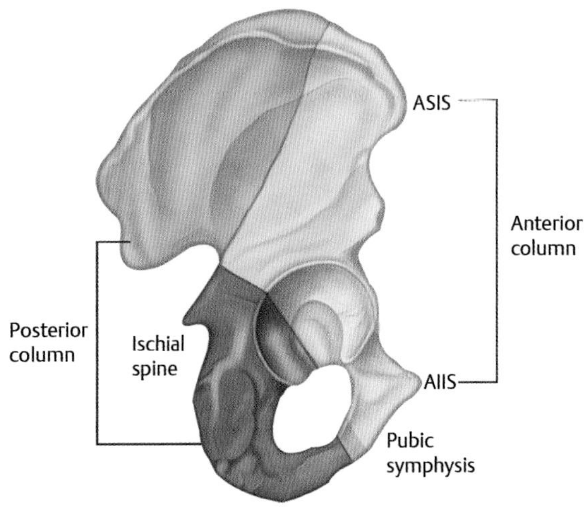

Fig. 3.19 Anterior and posterior columns of acetabulum. ASIS, anterior superior iliac spine; AIIS, anterior inferior iliac spine.

- Iliofemoral
  a. HO is common; prophylactic radiation dose is 700 cGy (rad) and should be given within 48–72 hours of surgery or chemical prophylaxis with indomethacin 25 mg t.i.d. for 4–6 weeks
- Stoppa: Pfannenstiel incision 1–2 cm proximal to pubic symphysis
  a. Add lateral window of ilioinguinal approach for additional exposure
  b. Structures at risks: corona mortis, obturator nerve
- Extended iliofemoral and triradiate approaches have high complication rates (infection, HO) but are used for complex fractures.

4. Pelvic ring injuries
   - Mechanism: high energy, blunt trauma
   - Associated injuries: chest/head injuries, polytrauma, shock
     a. Leading cause of death is hemorrhage; superior gluteal artery is most common artery to be damaged by a pelvic fracture; internal pudendal artery yields the most symptomatic bleeds.
     b. Suspect urogenital injury with gross hematuria, high-riding prostate, or blood at meatus; workup with cystogram for bladder injury or retrograde urethrogram for urethral injury; peritoneal bladder rupture requires surgical repair.
     c. Inspect perineum and perform vaginal speculum exam and rectal exam in setting of pelvic fractures to rule out overt and occult open fracture; open pelvic fractures usually require diverting colostomy and have high mortality rate.
     d. Age, shock, and transfusion amount in first 24 hours are predictors of mortality after pelvic trauma.
     e. Morel-Lavallee lesion: internal degloving injury where subcutaneous tissue is avulsed from underlying fascia leaving a cavity that is at high risk for poor healing and infection; surgical treatment/debridement is indicated.
   - Imaging: X-rays—AP pelvis, inlet view, outlet view, iliac oblique, obturator oblique; CT with pelvic reconstructions (see 1. Anatomy of Pelvis/Acetabulum, above)

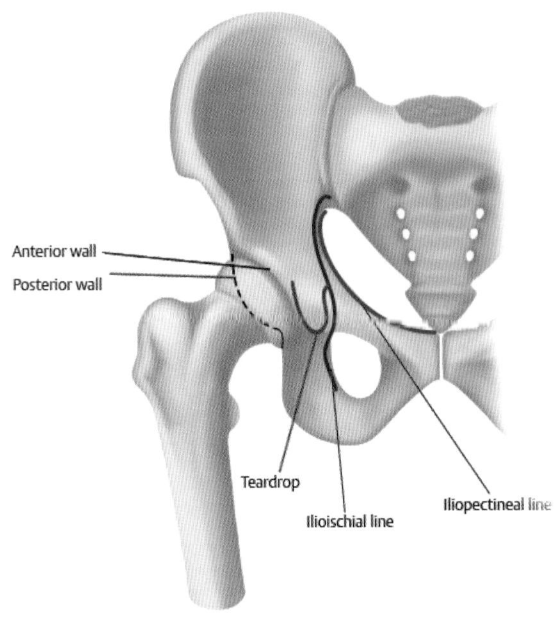

Fig. 3.20 Radiographic cardinal lines/landmarks.

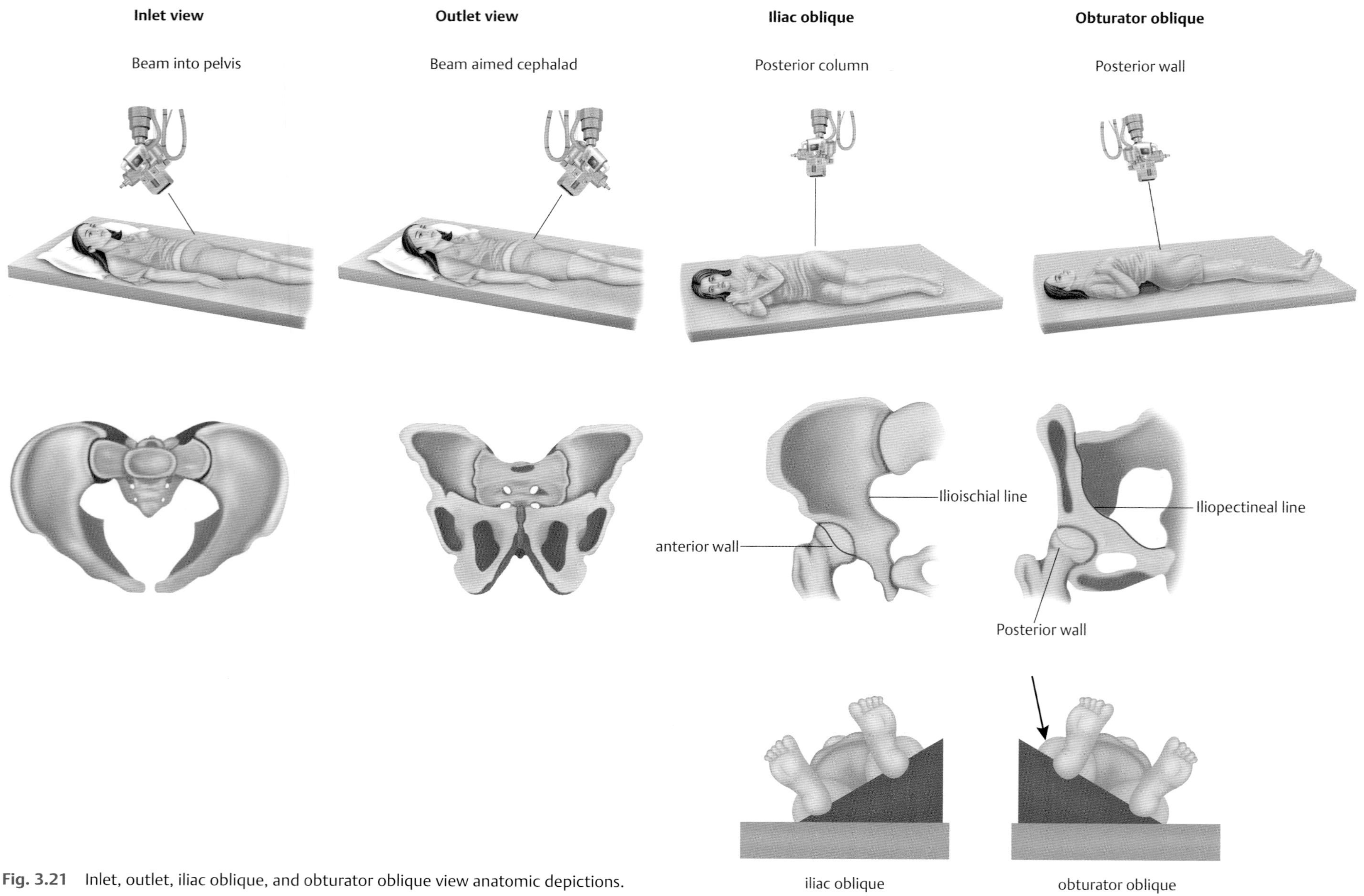

Inlet view

Beam into pelvis

Outlet view

Beam aimed cephalad

Iliac oblique

Posterior column

Obturator oblique

Posterior wall

Ilioischial line

anterior wall

Iliopectineal line

Posterior wall

iliac oblique

obturator oblique

Fig. 3.21 Inlet, outlet, iliac oblique, and obturator oblique view anatomic depictions.

- Avulsion injuries
  a. Hamstring: ischial tuberosity avulsion
  b. Rectus: AIIS avulsion
  c. Sartorius: ASIS avulsion
- Fracture classifications
  a. Young and Burgess **(Table 3.5, Fig. 3.23)**
    - Anteroposterior compression (APC): associated with retroperitoneal hemorrhage
      - **APC type 3 injuries have the highest rate of blood loss and urogenital injury, are associated with abdominal trauma and shock, and require the most blood transfusions.**
    - Lateral compression (LC) pelvic fractures: associated with head, chest, abdominal trauma; most common cause of death is closed head injury
    - Vertical sheer: due to vertically applied force, highly unstable in cephaloposterior direction; associated with intrapelvic hemorrhage/neurologic injury
      - Treatment: traction provisionally if superior displacement; anterior and posterior ORIF definitively
  b. Tile classification
    - Type A: stable fracture patterns

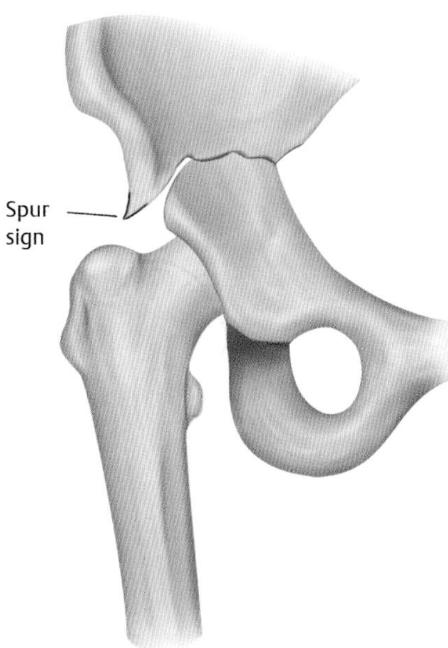

Fig. 3.22 Spur sign for both column acetabular fracture. Best seen on obturator oblique X-ray.

Table 3.4 Quick Reference to Pelvic/Acetabular Approaches

Approach	Access	Acetabular Fracture Indications	Risks
Ilioinguinal	Indirect access to acetabulum Inner table of ilium Quadrilateral plate Superior pubic ramus Medial window: medial to external iliac vessels Middle window: between iliopsoas and ext. iliacs Lateral window: lateral to iliopsoas	Both column Anterior column Anterior wall Anterior column-posterior hemitransverse Transverse	Obturator artery/nerve Corona mortis Femoral nerve/vessels Lateral femoral cutaneous nerve, Spermatic cord/round ligament
Kocher-Langenbeck	Outer table of ilium Sciatic notch Ischium Posterior wall	Posterior Column Posterior Wall Transverse T-type	Sciatic nerve Superior gluteal artery Medial femoral circumflex artery Heterotopic ossification
Iliofemoral	Extensile approach Direct access to posterior and anterior acetabulum Inner and outer table of ilium	High anterior column Both column, T-type, fractures more than 3 weeks old	Heterotopic ossification High complication rates
Stoppa	Pubic symphysis Pelvic brim Quadrilateral plate Lateral window (from ilioinguinal): gives additional access to inner table of ilium, anterior sacroiliac joint	Anterior column Anterior wall fractures, Transverse T-type Both column Anterior column-posterior hemitransverse	Corona mortis Obturator nerve
Anterior iliac crest	Iliac crest	N/A	Lateral femoral cutaneous nerve
Posterior iliac crest	Iliac crest	N/A	Cluneal and superior gluteal nerves

Abbreviation: N/A, not applicable.

3 Trauma

Table 3.5 Pelvic Fractures: Young and Burgess Classification

Type	Fracture Characteristics	Treatment	Key Concepts
Anterior-Posterior Compression (APC)			
APC 1	< 2.5 cm anterior diastasis Vertical fractures of pubic rami Stretched but intact anterior SI Sacrospinous/sacrotuberous ligaments Intact posterior SI ligaments	Nonsurgical Weight bearing as tolerated	Rotationally and vertically stable AO/OTA; Tile A
APC 2	≥ 2.5 cm symphyseal diastasis Widened SI joints but posterior SI ligament intact Disruption of the following: Anterior SI ligaments Sacrospinous ligament Sacrotuberous ligament Posterior SI ligaments intact	ORIF anterior pelvis	Rotationally unstable, vertically stable AO/OTA; Tile B
APC 3	Symphyseal widening SI joint diastasis (not connected to sacrum) Internal hemipelvectomy Disruption of the following: Anterior SI ligaments Posterior SI ligaments Sacrospinous ligament Sacrotuberous ligament	Urgent pelvic sheet or binder to stabilize the pelvis ORIF of anterior pelvis with posterior fixation (IS screws)	Rotationally and vertically unstable AO/OTA; Tile C Associated with retroperitoneal hemorrhage, shock, and abdominal injury Highest rate of blood loss/ transfusion Highest rate of urogenital injury
Lateral Compression (LC)			
LC 1	Transverse pubic rami fractures Sacral compression fracture on side of impact	Nonsurgical Weight bearing as tolerated	Rotationally and vertically stable AO/OTA; Tile A
LC 2	Transverse pubic rami fractures Crescent fracture of iliac wing on side of impact Variable disruption of posterior ligamentous structures	Non–weight bearing ORIF may be indicated	Rotationally unstable, vertically stable AO/OTA; Tile B
LC 3	LC1 or LC2 injury with contralateral open book pelvis "Windswept" pelvis	ORIF anterior and posterior pelvis	Rotationally and vertically unstable AO/OTA; Tile C Associated with head, chest, and abdominal trauma Most common cause of death is closed head injury
Vertical sheer	Complete disruption of the following: SI ligaments Sacrotuberus ligament Sacrospinous ligament Symphysis pubis	Traction initially ORIF anterior and posterior pelvis	Highly unstable, rotationally and vertically AO/OTA; Tile C Associated with intrapelvic hemorrhage and neurologic injury

Abbreviation: AO/OTA, *Orthopaedic Trauma Association;* IS, iliosacral; ORIF, open reduction and internal fixation; SI, sacroiliac.

- Type B: rotationally unstable, vertically stable
- Type C: rotationally and vertically unstable

- Treatment (provisional)

a. Stabilize pelvis: binder, sheet, C-clamp for APC injuries to stabilize and to allow clot to form; traction for vertical shear injuries

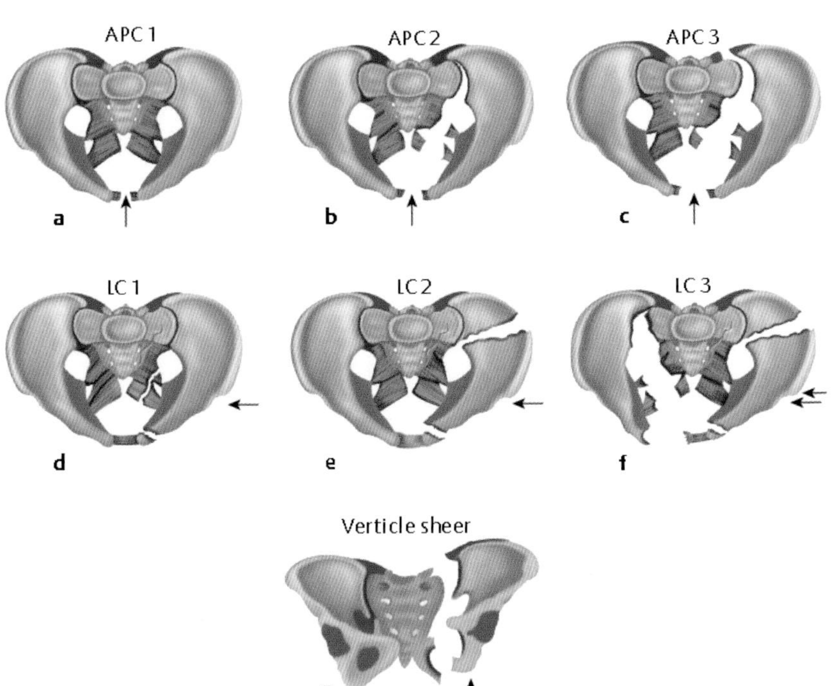

Fig. 3.23 Young and Burgess pelvic fracture classification. APC, anteroposterior compression; LC, lateral compression.

b. External fixation: indicated if going for exploratory-laparotomy with an unstable pelvic ring injury; half pins can be placed in iliac wing or in AIIS in the strong column of bone that runs from AIIS to the posterior iliac crest
   - **Starting point for AIIS pins is seen best on obturator outlet view.**

c. Pelvic packing: technique for hemodynamically unstable patients involving pelvic retroperitoneal packing via a midline subumbilical incision and possible pelvic external fixation

d. Angiography/embolization for active bleeding and hemodynamic instability following resuscitative efforts, initial pelvic stabilization, and ruled out thoracoabdominal sources

- Treatment (definitive)

  a. ORIF: pubic diastasis ≥ 2.5 cm, posterior diastasis/instability (APC types 2/3), vertical instability
     - Anterior plating versus external fixation with posterior percutaneous SI screws or open posterior SI fixation

- Complications

  a. DVT: most common complication following pelvic injury; without prophylaxis, DVT rates are as high as 70–80%; reduced to 10% with prophylaxis

  b. Lateral femoral cutaneous nerve injury, especially from external fixation (ex-fix) pins

  c. Nonunion and loss of fixation seen in vertical sacral fractures; pain seen after SI fracture/dislocation

  d. Death; transfusion requirement in first 24 hours most predictive

  e. Urologic; urethral stricture

  f. Pelvic trauma in women entails a higher incidence of sexual dysfunction/dyspareunia and cesarean section childbirth compared with the general population.

5. Sacral fractures
   - Mechanism: high energy, blunt trauma
   - Imaging: AP pelvis/inlet/outlet/lateral X-rays; CT is study of choice

- Classification: Denis **(Fig. 3.24)**
  a. Zone 1: alar fracture, L5 nerve root at risk, 6% neurologic injury
  b. Zone 2: transforaminal, L5/S1/S2 nerve roots at risk, 28% neurologic injury
  c. Zone 3: spinal canal, 57% neurologic injury associated with bowel/bladder/sexual dysfunction
  d. Fracture of lateral sacrum can be an avulsion of the sacrospinous/tuberous ligaments and is suggestive of an unstable pelvic injury
  e. U- or H-type sacral fractures have a high incidence of neurologic injury; best diagnosed on lateral sacral X-ray/CT sagittal reconstruction
- Treatment
  a. Conservative: minimal displacement (< 1 cm) with normal neurologic exam; protected weight bearing
  b. Surgical: displacement > 1 cm, neurologic deficits (foraminal or canal compromise
     - Neurologic deficit with zone 3 fracture needs decompression and anterior/posterior stabilization
     - Treat transverse fractures with lateral mass plates if displaced
     - Percutaneous SI screws (for fracture or SI disruption)–three key X-ray views:
       - Pelvic outlet view: visualize sacral foramina
       - Pelvic inlet view: visualize S1 and S2 body
       - Lateral sacral view: stay within body to avoid L5 root injury; safe zone on lateral for screw insertion is below the iliac cortical density, which parallels the sacral alar slope, caudad to the sacral end plate
     - Transiliac screws: can be placed percutaneously through both posterior iliac wings
     - Transiliac bars or plating: an alternative to SI screws/transiliac screws and placed via an open approach
     - Combined iliosacral and lumbosacral fixation is the most stable construct for unstable transforaminal sacral fractures and vertical shear injuries.
- Complications
  a. Neurologic injury: from initial injury or iatrogenic from suboptimal fixation technique (L5 nerve root)
  b. Cauda equina syndrome

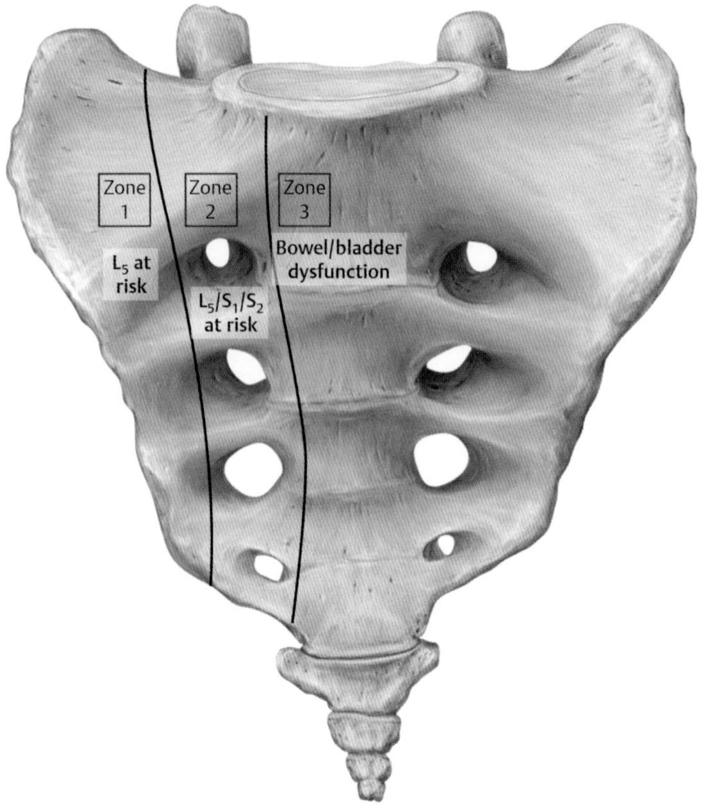

Fig. 3.24 Denis classification of sacral fractures. (From Schuenke M, Schulte E. General Anatomy and the Musculoskeletal System: Thieme Atlas of Anatomy. New York: Thieme; 2005. Illustration by Karl Wesker.)

6. Acetabular fractures
   - Mechanism: injury pattern is based on the position of the hip and direction of force applied at time of trauma
   - Imaging: X-ray—AP pelvis, Judet views (obturator and iliac oblique); CT to assess the articular surface, marginal impaction, loose bodies, and preoperative planning (see 1. Anatomy of Pelvis/Acetabulum, above)
   - Classification: Letournel **(Fig. 3.25)**
     a. Simple patterns: posterior wall, posterior column, anterior wall, anterior column, and transverse
     b. Associated patterns: posterior column/posterior wall, transverse with posterior wall, T type, anterior column/posterior hemitransverse, both column

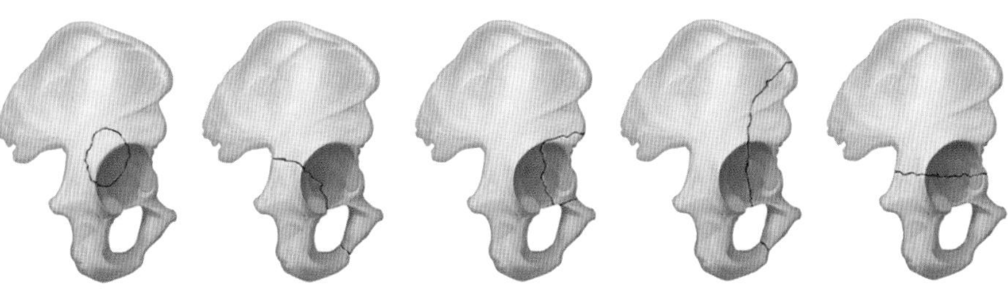

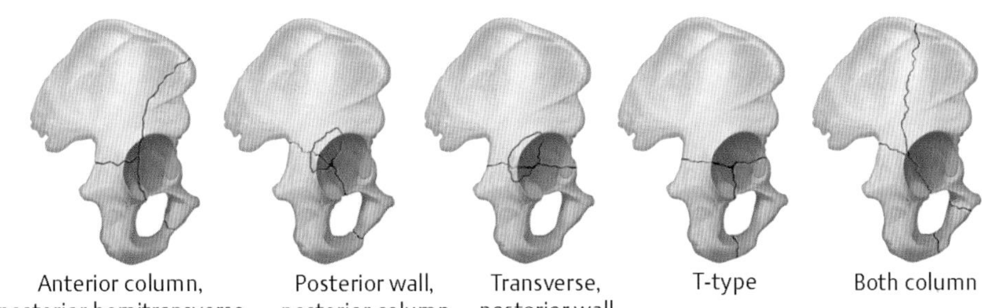

Fig. 3.25 Letournel classification of acetabular fractures.

- Both column fractures: articular surface of the acetabulum is completely dissociated from the ilium/axial skeleton; may have secondary congruence; "spur sign" is diagnostic on obturator oblique view and represents the intact posterior ilium **(Fig. 3.22)**
- **In both column fractures the articular surface is not attached to the axial skeleton.**

- Treatment
  a. Conservative: < 2 mm displacement, roof arc angles > 45 degrees on AP/Judet views, posterior wall fracture involving < 20% of wall, posterior wall fracture involving 20–40% of wall stable under stress exam under anesthesia (EUA), secondary congruence, high comminution in elderly patient with planned delayed total hip arthroplasty (THA)
  b. Operative: displacement > 2 mm, posterior wall fracture involving 20–40% of wall and unstable under stress EUA, posterior wall fracture involving ≥ 20% of wall **(Fig. 3.26)**, roof arc angle < 45 degrees, incongruity of hip joint, incarcerated fragments/loose bodies, marginal impaction, irreducible fracture-dislocation
     - Approaches: see 1. Anatomy of Pelvis/Acetabulum, above
     - Surgical management: ORIF and THA
       - "Gull sign" on X-ray represents superomedial dome impaction; elderly patients with this injury may benefit more from arthroplasty than from ORIF **(Fig. 3.27)**.
     - Acetabular fixation: likelihood of nonanatomic reduction increases with time to surgery (15 days for simple, 5 days for associated patterns)
     - Best determinant of operative versus nonoperative posterior wall fracture is a dynamic exam under anesthesia using an obturator oblique view; this exam may also be useful in some transverse and column fractures.

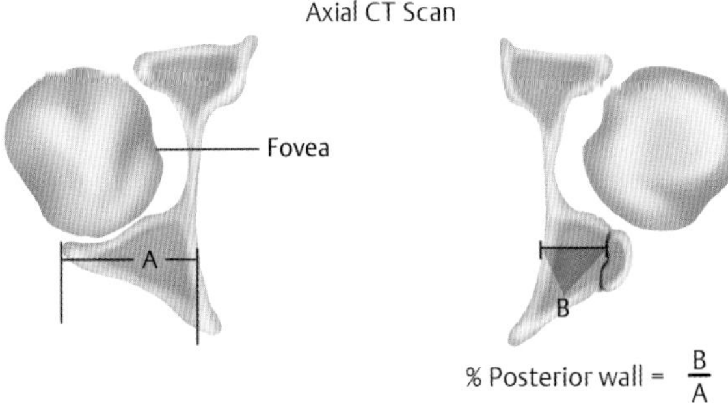

Fig. 3.26 Measurement of size of posterior wall fractures. Measurements done on axial computed tomography (CT) images at the level of the femoral fovea.

- Complications
  a. DVT
  b. HO: most common with iliofemoral approach
  c. Neurologic injury
  d. Posttraumatic arthritis: THA after acetabular fractures has worse outcomes compared with primary arthroplasty for osteoarthritis; worse outcomes also with femoral head articular injury, central impaction (gull sign)
  e. Malreduction: outcome correlates with accuracy of reduction

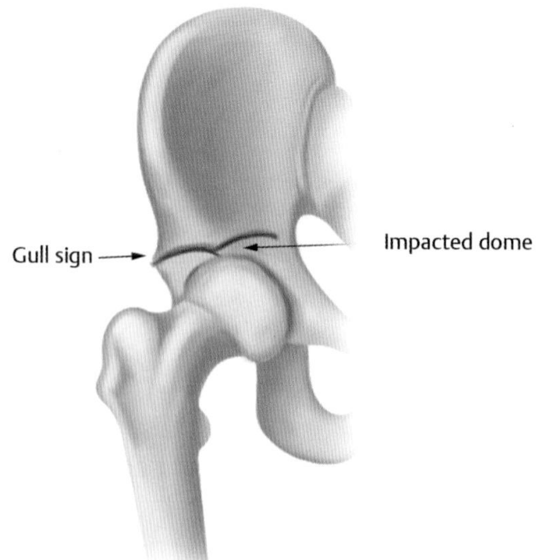

Fig. 3.27 Diagram of the "gull sign" that can be seen on radiographs and represents medial acetabular impaction.

IV. Lower Extremity

A. Hip Injuries

1. Avulsion injury
   - Psoas: lesser trochanter avulsion
     - Isolated lesser trochanter fracture in an adult is associated with metastatic disease and suggests a pathologic fracture.
     - Treatment: conservative; weight bearing as tolerated
   - Abductors: greater trochanter avulsion
     - Treatment: conservative with limited active hip abduction, weight bearing as tolerated
2. Hip dislocation
   - Mechanism: axial load
   - Presentation: posterior dislocation—hip flexed, internally rotated, and adducted; anterior dislocation—hip externally rotated and abducted
   - Associated injuries:
     - Posterior wall acetabular fracture: posterior dislocation
     - Femoral head fracture: posterior dislocation
     - Femoral neck fracture
     - Ipsilateral knee injury (dashboard injury)
       - ♦ 30% rate of meniscal tear
       - ♦ Posterior cruciate ligament (PCL) tear
     - Femoral artery/nerve injury: anterior dislocation
   - Imaging:
     - X-rays: AP/lateral of hip, Judet views
     - Postreduction CT should be performed in all patients to rule out fractures, loose bodies, nonconcentric reduction, and marginal impaction.
   - Classification: based on direction of dislocation
     - Posterior: most common; hip is flexed, adducted, internally rotated; can be associated with thoracic aorta injury
     - Anterior: hip extended, abducted, externally rotated
     - Obturator: dislocate into obturator foramen
   - Treatment:
     - Conservative
       - ♦ Emergent closed reduction within 6 hours, postreduction CT scan
       - ♦ Stability evaluation
   - If stable and isolated injury: weight bearing as tolerated
   - If unstable with associated injuries: traction/knee immobilizer/abduction pillow, exam under anesthesia with or without operative intervention
     - Surgical

- ♦ Open reduction if closed reduction unsuccessful (rare)
    - ♦ Open reduction and fixation of associated injuries as indicated (femoral head or neck fracture, acetabular fracture)
    - ♦ Hip dislocation with incarcerated fragments and nonconcentric reduction is best treated with urgent ORIF, as delay in treatment increases damage to the articular surface.
- Complications
  - Sciatic nerve injury: 20%; peroneal branch most affected
  - Osteonecrosis: 15%
  - Posttraumatic arthritis: correlated with reduction of articular surface
  - Instability/recurrent dislocation: uncommon, more associated with posterior wall acetabular fracture involving > 30–40% of wall

3. Femoral head fractures
   - Mechanism: axial load/dislocation shear injury
   - Associated injuries: hip dislocation
   - Imaging: AP/lateral X-rays of hip; CT evaluates fragment and acetabulum
   - Classification **(Fig. 3.28)**: Pipkin type I, infrafoveal; type II, suprafoveal; type III, femoral head fracture with associated femoral neck fracture; type IV, femoral head fracture with associated acetabular fracture
   - Treatment
     - Key principles: restoration of the articular surface of the weight-bearing surface of head, restoration of hip stability, protect femoral head blood supply
     - Conservative: Pipkin type I with minimal displacement, nondisplaced Pipkin type II; protected weight bearing for 4–6 weeks

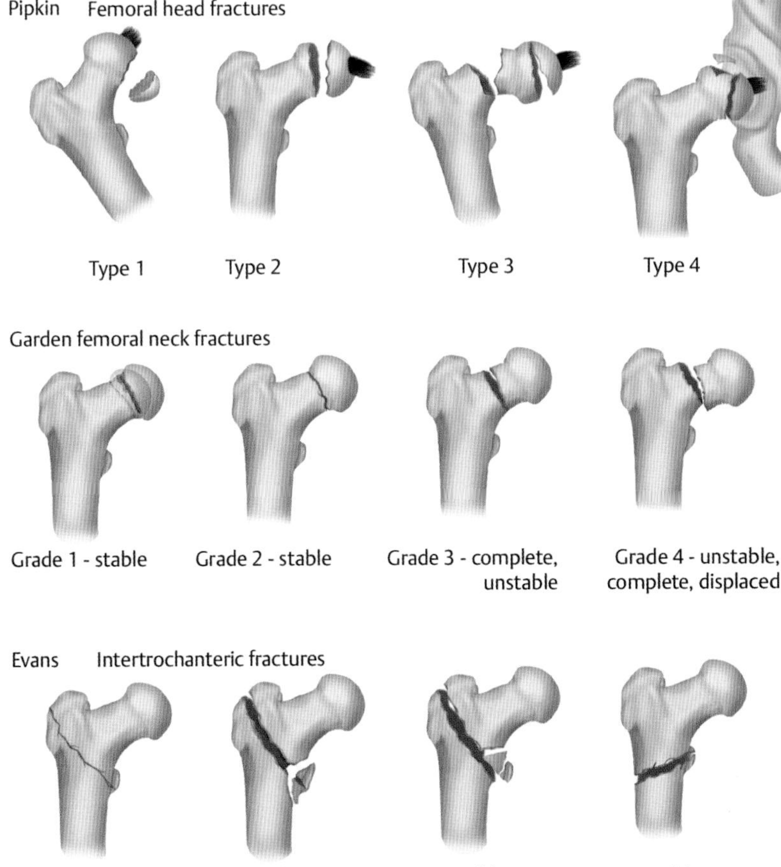

Fig. 3.28 Hip fracture classifications: femoral head, femoral neck, and intertrochanteric fractures.

- Surgical: > 1 mm stepoff, loose bodies, associated femoral neck/acetabular fracture requiring fixation, polytrauma patient
  - Anterior approach: Smith-Petersen approach for isolated femoral head fracture without acetabular fracture; interval: tensor fascia lata (superior gluteal nerve) and sartorius (femoral nerve)
  - Posterior approach: Pipkin type IV; interval: split gluteus maximus (inferior gluteal nerve)
  - Surgical hip dislocation can address femoral head fractures and posterior wall acetabular fractures
  - Fragment excision for comminuted irreparable Pipkin I fractures
- Fixation options: countersunk lag screws or variable pitch buried screws; THA or hemiarthroplasty for irreparable fractures

- Complications
  - Sciatic nerve injury: 20%, peroneal branch most affected
  - Osteonecrosis: 15%, most common after Pipkin type III injuries
  - Posttraumatic arthritis
  - Instability/recurrent dislocation

4. Femoral neck fractures
   - Mechanism: fall from standing position, high-energy trauma in young patients
   - Associated injuries: femoral shaft fractures
   - Imaging: AP/lateral X-rays of hip and femur, AP of pelvis; magnetic resonance imaging (MRI) most sensitive to rule out an occult femoral neck fracture
   - Classification

   a. Garden **(Fig. 3.28)**
      - Stable: Garden grade I, valgus impacted; Garden grade II, nondisplaced
      - Unstable: Garden grade III, incomplete/varus; Garden grade IV, complete/displaced

   b. Pauwels types I, II, III: ≤ 30 degrees, 31–70 degrees, > 70 degrees of vertical orientation of femoral neck fracture, respectively; more vertical fractures have more shear forces, which make them more unstable; higher nonunion and AVN rates associated with Pauwels type III

   - Treatment

   a. Key principles: decreased mortality in elderly patients with urgent surgery following medical optimization; timing is controversial but ideally within 72 hours

   b. Mobilize early

   - **Medical optimization is the most important step prior to surgery.**

   c. Conservative: high-risk surgical candidates, limited functional demands (non-ambulators)

   d. Surgical
      - Young or middle-aged patients < 50–65 years (based on functional level, not chronologic age): ORIF with decompression of hip capsule to decrease risk of AVN; younger women at higher risk for femoral head AVN with displaced femoral neck fractures
      - **Quality of reduction important for stability and head survival**
      - Elderly patients > 65 years: hemiarthroplasty versus THA
        - Hemiarthroplasty: elderly, low demand with displaced fractures, no evidence of preexisting arthritis; good for demented/Parkinson's patients as hemiarthroplasty has a low dislocation rate
          - Cementing: better in osteopenic bone with wide canals but more risk of cardiopulmonary complications; shown to have decreased mortality compared to uncemented patients

- Bipolar is equivalent to unipolar in terms of functional result but with increased cost
- ♦ THA: active elderly patients with displaced fractures, osteoarthritis (OA)/rheumatoid arthritis (RA); higher dislocation rate than hemiarthroplasty
- ♦ Fixation techniques:
  - Three percutaneous screws: indicated for Garden I/II fractures; screws are placed in an inverted-V pattern; do not start distal to lesser trochanter as this predisposes to subtrochanteric fracture
  - Sliding hip screw: basicervical and vertically oriented fractures with or without derotation screw
  - No study showing superiority of sliding hip screw versus percutaneous fixation

e. Complications
- Decreased mortality is associated with fixation compared to arthroplasty; however, there is a 30% failure rate of fixation requiring subsequent arthroplasty after ORIF/closed reduction and percutaneous fixation (CRPP).
- **Reoperation rate is higher in fixation of femoral neck fractures, although mortality rate is lower.**
- Osteonecrosis: main blood supply to the femoral head is the medial circumflex artery; AVN is more common with greater displacement, suboptimal reduction; it is controversial whether decreased time to reduction or decompression of hip capsule makes a difference in the incidence of AVN.
- Nonunion: 10–30%; no healing at 12 months; high risk with vertical fractures due to sheer stress and varus malalignment or malreduction; treat with arthroplasty or valgus intertrochanteric osteotomy to make the vertical fracture more horizontal and salvage the native femoral head.
- Infection
- Decreased functional status: 1-year mortality in elderly is 20–30%

5. Femoral neck stress fractures
- Mechanism: overuse injury, runners
- Imaging: MRI or bone scan (X-rays often negative)
- Classification:
  a. Compression type: on inferior femoral neck, usually stable
  b. Tension type: on superior femoral neck; predisposition to fracture completion and displacement
- Treatment:
  a. Conservative: compression type; can be treated with protected weight-bearing
  b. Surgical: tension type; unstable and likely to displace; should be treated acutely with percutaneous pinning and protected weight bearing

6. Intertrochanteric fractures
- Mechanism: fall from standing position in elderly, high-energy trauma in young
- Risks: osteoporosis, prior hip fracture, fall risk
- Imaging: AP/lateral X-rays of hip/femur, AP of pelvis; MRI if need to rule out occult fracture
- Classification: Evans **(Fig. 3.28)**
  a. Stable: posteromedial cortex intact or with minimal comminution; will withstand medial compressive load; two-part will reduce with medial compressive loads

b. Intermediate, three-part: large posteromedial fragments are unstable, lesser trochanter displacement suggests instability but may be converted to stable pattern with reduction
c. Unstable, comminuted four-part: highest risk for collapse into varus/shortening/nonunion, reverse obliquity fractures

- Treatment
  a. Key Principles: early mobilization
  b. Conservative: high-risk surgical candidates, limited functional demands, nondisplaced fracture in an infirm patient
  c. Surgical: any displaced fracture in an ambulatory patient; nondisplaced fracture in active patient
    - Sliding hip screw: contraindicated in reverse obliquity, subtrochanteric fracture, or fractures involving or threatening the lateral wall; more collapse and medialization when used for unstable fractures compared with IMN, lower perioperative peri-implant fracture rate than IMN, lag screw placed center-center with tip apex distance (TAD) < 25 mm is ideal **(Fig. 3.29)**; new literature suggests center-low may be the optimal position
    - **Tip apex distance (TAD) is the sum of the distance from the tip of the screw to the apex of the femoral head on AP and lateral X-rays.**
    - IMN: short nail for standard stable intertrochanteric fracture; long nail for stable and unstable patterns (reverse obliquity, subtrochanteric fractures, and standard intertrochanteric fractures)
- Starting point for trochanteric entry femoral nail is at tip or slightly medial to tip of greater trochanter to avoid varus malalignment or blowout of lateral wall
- Reduced collapse compared to sliding hip screw, higher risk of anterior cortex perforation at distal tip of nail due to femur/implant curvature mismatch; higher peri-implant fracture rate
  a. Comparison of IMN and sliding hip screw **(Table 3.6)**. No differences in infection, mortality, medical complications, blood loss, hospital stay, or functional outcomes have been found between the two fixation types.
  b. Fixed-angle blade plate, 95 degrees: reverse obliquity fracture, comminuted fracture, or nonunion
  c. Proximal femoral locking plate: reverse obliquity, comminuted fracture, or nonunion; caution: there is a risk of implant failure

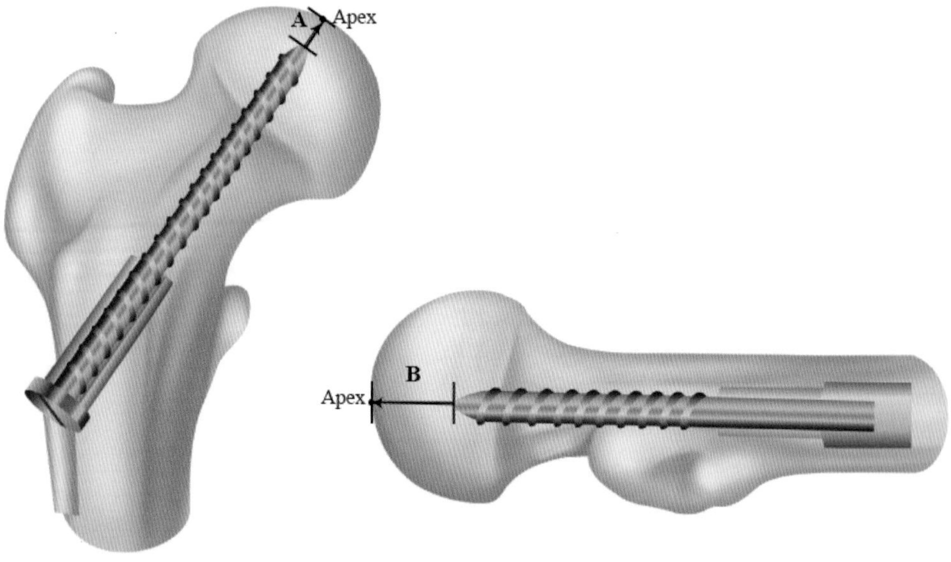

Fig. 3.29 The tip apex distance (TAD) is measured by taking the sum of the distance from the tip of the lag screw to the apex of the femoral head on anteroposterior (AP) and lateral X-rays.

Table 3.6 Cephalomedullary Nail Versus Sliding Hip Screw

	Cephalomedullary Nail	Sliding Hip Screw
Indications	Intertrochanteric, basicervical femoral neck, subtrochanteric, midshaft femur fractures	Basicervical femoral neck, intertrochanteric fractures
Contraindications	Short nails should not be used in reverse obliquity or subtrochanteric fractures Reconstruction nail contraindicated when the piriformis fossa is involved in fracture	Reverse obliquity fractures Subtrochanteric fractures Fracture that involves/threatens the lateral cortex
Advantages	Reduced collapse in unstable patterns	Lower perioperative peri-implant fracture rate
Disadvantages	Higher perioperative peri-implant fracture rate Higher risk of distal anterior cortex perforation	More collapse and medialization when used for unstable patterns

d. Arthroplasty: for severely comminuted fractures; usually require calcar-replacing stem

e. Complications
- Collapse: results in limb shortening and medialization of the shaft, decreases offset; abductor lever arm shortened; more collapse is seen with sliding hip screws
- Implant failure/cutout: TAD > 25 mm
- Peri-implant fracture: more common with IMN
- Infection
- Mortality: American Society of Anesthesiologists (ASA) classification predicts mortality; early surgery < 48 hours is associated with decreased 1-year mortality

B. Femur Fractures

1. Subtrochanteric fractures: within 5 cm of lesser trochanter
   - Mechanism: high-energy, insufficiency fractures from long-term bisphosphonate therapy
   - Imaging: AP/lateral X-rays of hip and femur; proximal segment is flexed, externally rotated, and abducted
   - Russell-Taylor classification: based on the involvement of the lesser trochanter and piriformis fossa
     a. Type I: piriformis fossa intact
        - Ia lesser trochanter intact; Ib lesser trochanter fractured.

     b. Type II: piriformis fossa involved
        - IIA/IIB for intact/fractured lesser trochanter
   - Treatment
     a. Operative: restore alignment/rotation/length
        - Deforming forces: flexion (iliopsoas), external rotation (short external rotators), abduction (abductors); leads to apex anterior and varus deformity
        - Reconstruction IMN: reconstruction mode if fracture involves lesser trochanter (Ib) (screws into femoral neck/head), antegrade mode if lesser trochanter intact (Ia) (screw into lesser trochanter)
          - ♦ Piriformis nail can be helpful to avoid varus deformity but contraindicated for fractures involving piriformis fossa (type II)
          - ♦ Alternatively, third-generation cephalomedullary nail may be used; lower reoperation rate at 1 year compared to fixed-angle construct
          - ♦ **Medial starting point on greater trochanter important in subtrochanteric femur fractures in order to keep the fracture out of varus**

- Fixed-angle blade plate, 95 degrees: indicated for comminution, nonunion, or type II fractures with involvement of the piriformis fossa
- Proximal femoral locking plate: consider use for comminution or nonunion

• Complications
  a. Nonunion
  b. Varus malalignment
  c. Implant failure
  d. Infection: increased risk with increased soft tissue dissection

2. Diaphyseal femur fractures: 5 cm distal to the lesser trochanter to 8 cm above the knee joint
   • Mechanism: high-energy trauma, atypical fractures of long-term bisphosphonate therapy
   • Associated injuries
     a. Ipsilateral femoral neck fracture: incidence is 2.5–5% but approximately 30% of these are missed; most commonly nondisplaced; some recommend fine-cut CT to evaluate all femoral necks in setting of high-energy femoral shaft fractures
     b. Closed head injury: avoid intraoperative hypotension
   • Imaging: AP/lateral X-rays of femur and hip including internal rotation view. CT with fine cuts is the gold standard to rule out femoral neck fracture.
   • Classification systems: Winquist-Hansen classification, Orthopaedic Trauma Association (OTA) classification (simple, wedge, complex)
   • Treatment
     a. Key principles: Restore length, alignment, and rotation. Early stabilization (< 24 hours) reduces morbidity and systemic complications of the polytrauma patient (pulmonary, thromboembolic).
     b. Conservative: long leg cast/brace for nondisplaced fractures, traction, pillow splint, rarely indicated; rare
     c. Surgical
        ◦ External fixator: used for patients with vascular injury, contaminated open injuries, polytrauma patients with planned delayed nailing (DCO); compared with other operative interventions, results in decreased blood loss, hypothermia, and release of inflammatory mediators; can be converted to IMN within 3 weeks with equal union/infection rates
        ◦ Plate fixation: periprosthetic fractures; has higher nonunion/infection/implant failure rate, and longer time to weight bearing compared with IMN
        ◦ IMN: high union rates
          ♦ Retrograde: obesity, ipsilateral tibia or femoral neck fractures, ipsilateral acetabular fracture, traumatic knee arthrotomy, bilateral femur fractures, polytrauma patient, associated spine fractures; can cause knee pain; obese patients have higher operative and fluoroscopy times with antegrade nailing
          ♦ Antegrade: standard technique; can cause hip pain; distal and proximal interlocking screws required
          ♦ Reamed nailing has higher union rates and higher incidence of fat embolization compared with unreamed but the clinical significance of this is unclear.
          ♦ Starting points:
            ▪ Piriformis entry: contraindicated when fracture extends to piriformis fossa; anterior starting point associated with increased hoop stress and risk of iatrogenic anterior cortical blowout
            ▪ Trochanteric entry: anterior starting point has minimal hoop stress, risks medial comminution of shaft, varus malalignment, or lateral wall blowout

- Ipsilateral femoral neck fracture: femoral neck takes priority; sliding hip screw or three parallel screws with either plate fixation or retrograde nail of femoral shaft; can also use reconstruction nail for nondisplaced femoral neck fractures but use of a single device is associated with increased risk of malreduction of one or more of the fractures (not recommended)
- Periprosthetic femur fractures: lateral plate for stable prosthesis; revision long stem arthroplasty for unstable prosthesis with lateral plate; allograft struts used for bone loss, overlap plates/prosthesis

- Complications
  a. Infection: rare; treat with nail removal and canal reaming after fracture healed
    - Overall infection rates are comparable between initial femoral nail and initial damage control orthopedics; external fixator transitioned to nail within 2–3 weeks

  b. Nonunion
    - Increased risk with postoperative nonsteroidal anti-inflammatory drugs (NSAIDs)
    - Nonunions after IMN are usually treated by reamed exchange nailing; after failed exchange nail, treatment should be compression plating with autograft

  c. Delayed union: dynamization less successful than exchange nailing

  d. Malalignment
    - Always compare rotation to contralateral side before leaving OR
    - **Know the malalignments that can occur with supine and lateral nailing.**
    - Supine nailing and using a fracture table: higher incidence of internal rotation malalignment
    - Lateral nailing: higher incidence of external rotation malalignment
    - Single implants for ipsilateral femoral neck/shaft fractures are associated with increased malreduction of one of the two fractures, putting it at risk for malunion/nonunion (not recommended)

  e. HO: most frequent complication; seen in antegrade nailing, rarely clinically important but occurs in abductor musculature from reaming

  f. Leg length discrepancy

  g. Hip pain/weakness: with antegrade nailing

  h. Pudendal nerve injury: from traction table using intramedullary nail

  i. Anterior cortex penetration: when nail has greater radius of curvature (is straighter) than the femur

  j. Osteonecrosis: adolescents with open physes treated with piriformis entry nail; blood supply to femoral head compromised in piriformis fossa

  k. Retrograde nailing: knee pain and patellar chondral injury; femoral nerve and deep femoral artery at risk from AP proximal interlocking screws if placed below the lesser trochanter

3. Distal femur fractures
- Mechanism: high energy in young, low energy in elderly
- Associated injuries: popliteal artery injury
- Imaging: AP/lateral X-rays of femur/knee; CT of knee if suspicion of intracondylar extension; angiography if no pulses after alignment is restored
  a. Hoffa fragment: coronal fracture line **(Fig. 3.30)**; most common site is the lateral femoral condyle; plain X-rays often miss this fragment; CT recommended for supracondylar/intercondylar fractures
- Classification: OTA classification: 33A, extra-articular—supracondylar; 33B, simple articular (unicondylar); 33C, complex articular

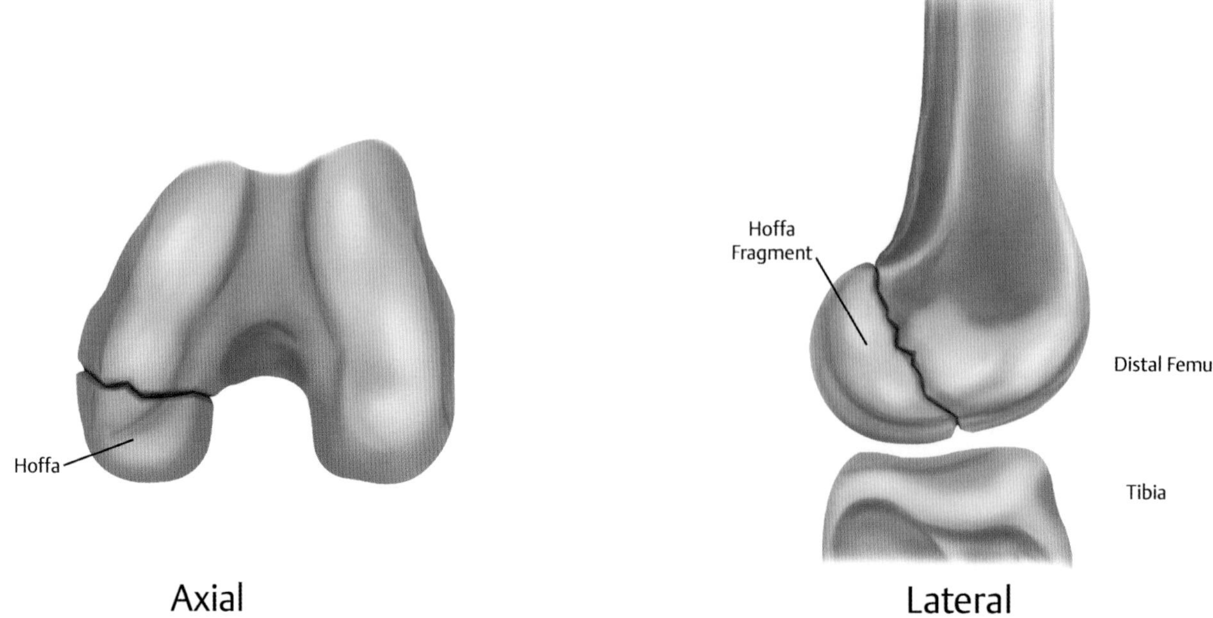

Fig. 3.30 Hoffa fragment. Diagram depicts appearance on axial and lateral views of the distal femur.

- Treatment
  a. Key principles: restore articular surface, rigid stabilization of articular fracture, and stable fixation of articular surface to rest of shaft
  b. Conservative: nondisplaced fractures, treat with hinged knee brace or knee immobilizer for 6–8 weeks; early ROM encouraged with closed chain ROM at 3–4 weeks; non–weight bearing for at least 6 weeks
  c. Surgical: displaced fractures and intra-articular fractures
     - Approaches: lateral approach with indirect reduction of articular components; arthrotomy for direct reduction of articular components
     - Hoffa fragments fixed with countersunk lag screws
     - **Beware of the Hoffa fragment in the coronal plane; requires CT scan of the distal femur and anatomic reduction**
     - Fixed-angle plates: less commonly used with newer devices available; indicated for metaphyseal comminution; non–fixed-angle plates are prone to varus collapse if there is metaphyseal comminution
     - Locked plates: multiple fixed-angle points of fixation
     - Retrograde supracondylar IMN: extra-articular fractures and simple intra-articular fractures, but need at least two screws in the articular block for secure fixation
     - Periprosthetic fractures: distal femoral locking plate or retrograde nail if cruciate retaining arthroplasty (nail can fit through intercondylar space)
     - Arthroplasty: usually distal femoral replacement if prior joint replacement or nonreconstructable fracture where stable fixation cannot be achieved; reduced longevity compared to ORIF but immediate weight bearing is possible
- Complications
  a. Nonunion: associated with rigid locking plates and medial fracture gap; treat with autologous bone graft and revision plating
  b. Malalignment: valgus malreduction with plate; varus collapse with nonlocking plates; malalignment is most common with IMN

c. Loss of fixation: varus collapse due to toggle on nonlocked distal screws or IMN, lack of rigid fixation or nonunion

d. Infection: highest in diabetics

e. Knee stiffness/pain: early ROM to prevent

f. Painful hardware: avoid long medial screws

C. Knee Injuries

1. Knee dislocation

- Mechanism: high energy or low energy in obese patients

  a. Direction: anterior, posterior, medial, lateral, posterolateral rotatory; 50% present as reduced; easily missed injury

- Associated injuries

  a. Vascular injury in up to 30%

  b. Peroneal nerve injury in up to 25%

- Exam: ankle-brachial index (ABI) is best to assess vascular status; ABI of > 0.9 is associated with an intact artery; selective arteriography based on physical exam should be considered

- Imaging: AP/lateral X-rays of knee; MRI to assess soft tissue injury; angiography for vascular concern

- Classification: Schenck classification of knee dislocation; not commonly used

- Treatment

  a. Key principles: emergent reduction and neurovascular reassessment, revascularize within 6 hours

  b. Conservative: immobilization in extension or protected motion for 6 weeks if knee stays reduced; delayed soft tissue reconstruction may be indicated if still unstable

  c. Surgical: external fixation provisionally; ligament repair or reconstruction (acute reconstruction may be better than delayed); early motion and possible hinged external fixator; unstable knee dislocation requiring vascular repair should have external fixation to protect the repair; fasciotomies indicated after vascular repair

- Complications

  a. Stiffness: arthrofibrosis is the most common complication

  b. Vascular injury: most at risk with fracture-dislocation

  c. Neurologic injury: 25%; peroneal nerve most common

  d. Ligamentous laxity/chronic knee instability

2. Patellar/quad tendon rupture

  a. Patellar tendon: patients aged < 40 years with overload of the extensor mechanism, most common with athletic activity

    - Risk factors: anabolic steroids, metabolic disorders, rheumatologic disease, renal failure, corticosteroids, patellar tendonitis, infection; most common site of rupture is an avulsion off of the distal pole of the patella or intrasubstance tear

  b. Quad tendon: patients aged > 40 years with medical problems; male-to-female ratio = 8:1; nondominant limb is 2× more commonly injured

    - **Picture the number 40 on the patella; above 40 you find quad tendon ruptures, and below 40 you find patellar tendon ruptures**

    - Risk factors: renal failure, diabetes mellitus (DM), RA, hyperparathyroid, connective tissue disorders, steroid use, intra-articular injections; most common location of rupture is at the osseotendinous junction, within 2 cm of proximal pole

- Exam findings: patient unable to perform straight leg raise; palpable defect in extensor mechanism
- Imaging: AP/lateral X-rays of knee showing patellar baja (quad tendon rupture) or patella alta (patellar tendon rupture) (see Lower Extremity Sports)
- Treatment
  a. Conservative: incomplete < 50% quad tendon rupture, with full active extension and no extensor deficit
  b. Surgical: inability to straight leg raise; direct primary repair with nonabsorbable suture through patellar drill holes; can supplement with semitendinosus autograft/allograft; quad tendon ruptures > 2 weeks old may be retracted, chronic quad tendon ruptures may require V-Y lengthening (Codivilla procedure) or quad lengthening
- Complications: extensor weakness and stiffness, inability to resume prior level of athletic/recreational activity

3. Patellar dislocation
   - Mechanism: lateral dislocation with injury to medial patellofemoral ligament
   - Exam: effusion, patellar instability
   - Treatment
     a. Key principles:
        - Conservative: reduce with extension and immobilize initially for 2–3 weeks followed by progressive motion and brace while ambulating, weight bearing as tolerated
        - Surgical: associated osteochondral fractures, loose bodies, recurrent instability requiring medial patella-femoral ligament (MPFL) reconstruction
   - Complications: redislocation is common (approximately 30%); osteochondral fractures
4. Patella fractures
   - Mechanism: direct blow to knee
   - Exam: effusion, usually inability to perform straight leg raise unless retinaculum intact and allow continuity of extensor mechanism
   - Imaging: AP/lateral X-rays of knee
   - Classification: transverse, vertical, comminuted (stellate), nondisplaced, proximal/distal pole
   - Treatment
     a. Key principles: preserve patella whenever possible; avoid complete patellectomy
     b. Conservative: vertical fractures rarely require surgery (able to straight leg raise); nondisplaced fractures with intact extensor mechanism; treat in extension for 2–3 weeks followed by gradual flexion in a hinged brace
     c. Surgical: displacement > 3 mm, articular stepoff > 2 mm, inability to straight leg raise
        - Tension band: cannulated screws biomechanically stronger than K-wires
        - Cerclage and tension band: minimally displaced stellate fractures/comminution
        - Partial patellectomy: attach tendon to anterior part of patella; extra-articular distal pole, severely comminuted fractures
     d. Complications: symptomatic hardware, loss of reduction, nonunion, infection, stiffness/arthrofibrosis, pain, arthritis
5. Floating knee: femoral and tibial shaft fractures
   - Treatment: retrograde IMN femur, antegrade IMN tibia

D. Tibia/Fibula Fractures

1. Tibia spine/tubercle fractures
2. Tibial plateau fractures
   - Mechanism: axial load
   - Schatzker classification **(Fig. 3.31)**: type I, lateral split; type II, lateral split-depression; type III, lateral depression; type IV, medial plateau (equivalent to knee dislocation); type V, bicondylar; type VI, metaphyseal-diaphyseal dissociation
   - Associated Injuries:
     a. Anterior cruciate ligament (ACL)/medial collateral ligament (MCL) injuries in 30–50%; MCL injury more common
     b. Meniscus tears in > 50%: lateral more common, mostly peripheral tears; Schatzker type II often has lateral meniscus pathology and may incarcerate; Schatzker type IV often has medial meniscus pathology
     c. Compartment syndrome
     d. Soft tissue injuries
   - Imaging: AP/lateral X-rays of knee; CT to assess intra-articular involvement, consider MRI for soft tissue injury (ligamentous or meniscal injuries)
   - Treatment
     a. Key principles: restore joint surface and normal alignment; restoration of mechanical axis more important than articular congruity in terms of posttraumatic arthritis
     b. Conservative: stable knees (< 10 degrees coronal instability with knee in extension) and < 3 mm articular stepoff; brace with early knee ROM and delayed weight bearing at least 4–6 weeks
     c. Surgical: articular stepoff > 3 mm, condylar widening > 5 mm, knee instability, all medial and bicondylar plateaus

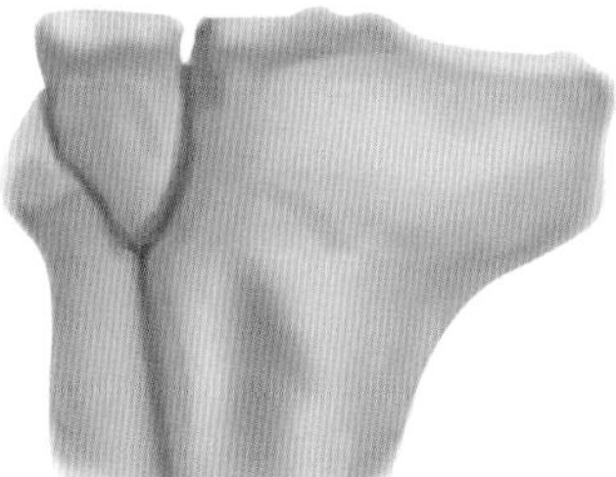

Type 1 : Lateral split

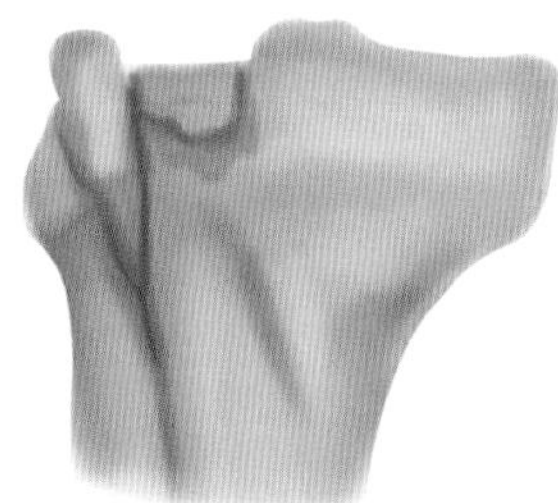

Type 2 : Lateral split depression

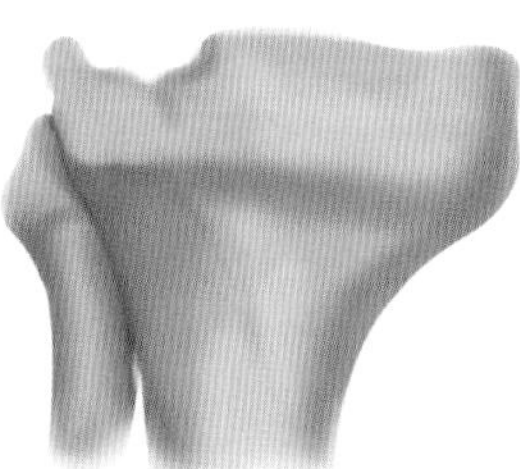

Type 3 : Lateral depression

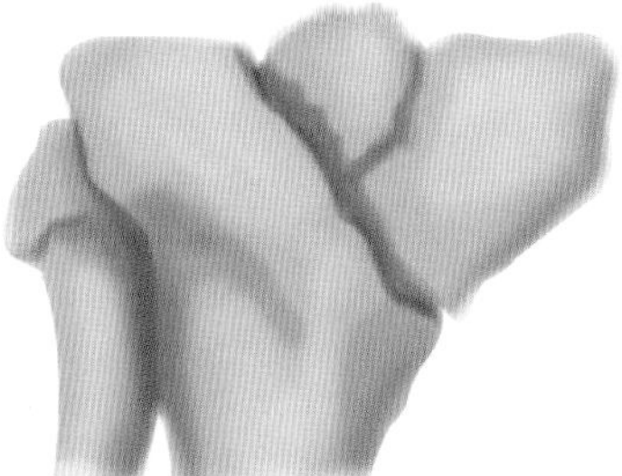

Type 4 : Medial plateau

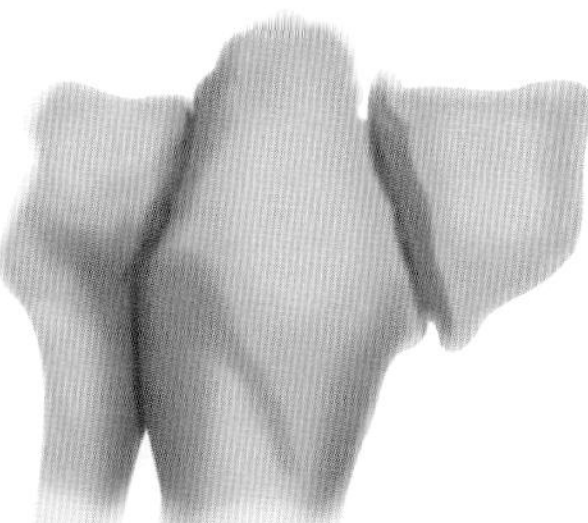

Type 5 : Bicondylar

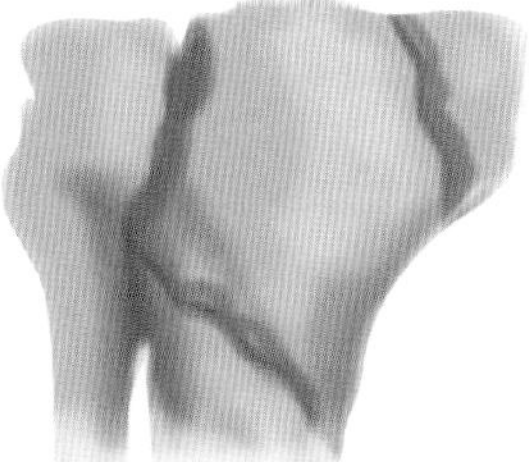

Type 6 : Bicondylar with shaft involvement

Fig. 3.31 Schatzker classification for tibial plateau fractures.

- Approaches
  - Lateral: approach through iliotibial (IT) band to Gerdy's tubercle with possible elevation of anterior compartment based on fracture pattern
  - Posteromedial: interval between semimembranosus and medial gastrocnemius
- External fixation: for bicondylar fractures, severe soft tissue injuries or unstable/high-energy injuries prior to definitive fixation; if using Ilizarov/hybrid fixator, wires should be ≥ 15 mm from joint to avoid septic joint
- **Knee capsule extends 14 mm below the subchondral bone on the posterolateral aspect of the proximal tibia; avoid intra-articular wires by placing ≥ 15 mm from joint**
- ORIF: lateral locked buttress plate versus screws for Schatzker I, II, and III; favor locked plating in osteoporotic bone
  - Posteromedial fragments are often not captured with a lateral plate; use separate posteromedial incision and buttress plate for medial fracture in Schatzker IV, V, and VI
- Bone void filler: calcium phosphate cement has highest compressive strength and lower subsidence compared to autogenous iliac crest bone graft (ICBG)
- Rehabilitation: early range of motion exercise is beneficial to cartilage healing; avoid shear forces and weight bearing
- **The best predictor of a good outcome is adequate mechanical alignment and restoration of knee stability.**

- Complications
  a. Posttraumatic arthritis (after 5–7 years)
  b. Infection
  c. Malunion often with varus collapse; alignment is the most important predictor of outcome after fixation of tibial plateau
  d. Ligament instability: predicts worse outcomes
  e. Wound complications: fewer complications if delay surgery 10–20 days
  f. Peroneal nerve injury
  g. Compartment syndrome

3. Tibial shaft fractures/tibial-fibular shaft fractures
- Mechanism: direct blow to leg; most common long bone fracture
  a. High energy: comminuted, tibia and fibula fractures at the same level, transverse pattern, extensive soft tissue injury, segmental
  b. Low energy: spiral fracture, tibia/fibula fractures at different levels
- Associated injuries: soft tissue injuries requiring extensive debridement (open fractures), compartment syndrome
- Imaging: AP/lateral X-rays of tibia-fibula, knee, ankle; CT for any intra-articular extension
- Treatment
  a. Key Principles
     - Soft tissue management critical to outcome
     - Restore alignment, length, rotation
     - Prompt antibiotics for open fractures
     - **Tibial shaft fracture with fibula fracture tends to fall into valgus; if fibula is intact, tibia tends to fall into varus.**
  b. Conservative: low-energy fractures, shortened < 1–2 cm, cortical apposition > 50%, varus-valgus < 5 degrees, sagittal plane angulation < 10 degrees, rotational alignment < 10 degrees; long leg cast/non–weight bearing 4–6 weeks

- Shortening and cortical apposition seen on injury X-ray are related to shortening at union; cortical apposition of < 50% is associated with higher reoperation rates

c. Surgical: open fractures, failed conservative management, fracture pattern that does not meet nonoperative criteria (see above), ipsilateral femoral fracture, polytrauma, morbid obesity
  - External fixation: DCO, highly contaminated open fractures; definitive treatment with external fixation for type IIIB open fractures entails longer time to union and poorer outcomes compared with IMN; can convert external fixator to IMN within 3 weeks
  - Plate fixation: extreme proximal or distal fractures; higher infection risk in open fractures compared to IMN; percutaneous less invasive stabilization system (LISS) plate puts the superficial peroneal nerve at risk for holes 11 to 13 when using a 13-hole plate [incision should be used here with blunt dissection for long lateral minimally invasive plate osteosynthesis (MIPO) plating].
  - IMN: reduced immobilization time compared with cast, earlier weight bearing, union rate > 80% for closed injuries; reamed nailing has higher union rates for closed fractures, but there is no difference in union rates in open fractures between reamed and unreamed nails; static interlocks can be used for stable and unstable patterns, dynamic interlocks should only be used for stable patterns.
    - Anterior knee pain is a common consequence (30–50%)
    - Compared with external fixation, IMN is associated with decreased malalignment, decreased reoperation rates, and decreased time to weight bearing
  - Proximal shaft fractures with IMN: avoid malreduction associated with valgus and apex anterior angulation (procurvatum) with the following tactics:
    - More lateral starting point
    - Blocking screws placed where the nail should not go—posteriorly and laterally (on the convexity of the deformity)
  - **Blocking screws, also known as Poller screws, are placed Posterior and Lateral (use mnemonic PoLler) in the proximal segment**
    - Provisional unicortical plate
    - Semi-extended position
    - Femoral distractor
  - Amputation for mangled, nonsalvageable extremity
    - Relative indications: warm ischemia time > 6 hours, severe ipsilateral foot trauma
    - Absent plantar sensation after severe type IIIB tibial fracture is not an indication for primary amputation and is not prognostic of functional outcome or future sensory status.
    - LEAP study (cited earlier): no difference in functional outcomes with limb salvage versus amputation both with significant disability related to self-efficacy, education, employment status

a. BMP-2 for type III open tibia fractures with IMN

b. BMP-7 for tibial nonunion

- Complications

a. Anterior knee pain (30–50%); most common

b. Ankle stiffness

c. Nonunion: rule out infection; dynamize IMN versus reamed exchange nailing; bone graft or BMP-7

d. Malunion: most common with proximal fractures (valgus/apex anterior); rotation malalignment common with distal-third fractures

e. Delayed union: risk factors within first year are transverse pattern, open fracture, cortical contact < 50%, distal third fracture

f. Infection: increased risk with more extensive soft tissue injury

g. Compartment syndrome

h. Osteonecrosis:

  - Overreaming the tibial canal to a larger size generates increased heat that can lead to osteonecrosis.
  - Tourniquet use during reaming leads to decreased heat dissipation and osteonecrosis.

4. Fibula fractures

- Mechanism: direct blow, twisting injury, high or low energy
- Associated injuries: tibial shaft fractures, syndesmotic injury, proximal tibia fractures, LCL avulsions
- Imaging: AP/lateral X-rays of tibia/fibula, knee, ankle
- Classification: proximal fibula fracture, fibular shaft fracture, distal fibula fracture
- Treatment

  a. Conservative: shaft fractures, minimally displaced proximal fibula fractures without knee instability, minimally displaced fractures not associated with ankle or syndesmotic instability

  b. Surgical: displaced proximal fibula fracture with knee instability, syndesmotic disruption

E. Ankle/Plafond Injuries

1. Pilon fractures

- Mechanism: high-energy axial load, motor vehicle accident, fall from height
- Associated injuries: extensive soft tissue injury
- Imaging: AP/lateral/oblique X-rays of ankle and foot, AP/lateral of tibia-fibula; CT for intra-articular involvement; obtain once fracture is reduced or in external fixator for better delineation of fracture fragments
- Classification

  a. Key fragments:

    - Medial: attached to deltoid ligament
    - Posterolateral/Volkmann: attached to posterior inferior tibiofibular ligament
    - Anterolateral/Chaput: attached to anterior inferior tibiofibular ligament

  b. Ruedi-Allgower: type 1 nondisplaced, type 2 simple displacement of articular surface, type 3 comminuted articular surface

- Treatment

  a. Key principles: restore joint surface, meticulous management of soft tissues

  b. Conservative: only for patients too ill or with significant wound healing risks (diabetes/vascular disease), nondisplaced fractures (rare)

  c. Surgical: displaced fractures

    - External fixation: commonly used for planned staged fixation of pilon fractures to maintain length/alignment while allowing soft tissue recovery; open fractures requiring further debridement or delayed ORIF; fractures with significant joint depression
    - Limited internal fixation with external fixation: proposed decreased infection rate, soft tissue breakdown, stiffness compared to ORIF; may use hybrid fixation
    - Internal fixation: restore length, reconstruct metaphyseal shell, bone graft, reattach metaphysis to diaphysis; high incidence of soft tissue

complications; need at least 7 cm skin bridge between incisions to minimize risk of wound breakdown

- **Open pilon fractures: staged treatment has better outcomes, beginning with irrigation/debridement and external fixation**

- Outcomes: patients can report functional improvements up to 2 years postoperatively; pilon fractures are significant injuries and patients report lower scores on the Short Form-36 (SF36) than patients with AIDS, polytrauma, pelvic fractures, diabetes, and myocardial infarction
- Complications: wound dehiscence, infection 5–15% with internal or external fixation (worse with diabetes), malunion, nonunion, posttraumatic arthritis (approximately 50%), chondrolysis, loss of ankle motion, neurovascular injury

2. Ankle fractures
- Mechanism: rotation, may or may not involve syndesmotic disruption/instability
- Imaging: AP/lateral/oblique X-rays of ankle and foot, AP/lateral of tibia-fibula; CT for intra-articular involvement
  - Normal ankle radiographs: medial clear space < 4 mm, talocrural angle 83 ± 4 degrees, talar tilt < 2 mm, syndesmotic tibial clear space < 5 mm (medial border of fibula and incisura), tibia-fibula overlap 10 mm or 42% width of fibula, continuous curve between lateral talus and tip of distal fibula
- Classifications **(Fig. 3.32)**
  a. Lauge-Hansen: descriptions derived from foot position (first word) and motion of talus relative to leg (second word)
  - Supination-adduction
  - Supination-external rotation: most common
  - Pronation-external rotation
  - Pronation-abduction
  - Pronation-dorsiflexion

  b. Danis-Weber: based on location of fibula fracture
  - Type A: infrasyndesmotic fibular fracture
  - Type B: fibular fracture at the level of the syndesmosis
  - Type C: suprasyndesmotic fibula fracture

  c. Maisonneuve fracture: ankle fracture or complete ligamentous disruption with a high fibula fracture; results from an external rotation force at the ankle that is transmitted through the interosseous membrane proximally and disrupts the syndesmosis and deltoid ligament **(Fig. 3.33)**
  - Routinely missed if tibia-fibula X-rays are not checked in addition to ankle films
  - Treatment: operative fracture that requires reduction/stabilization of syndesmosis

  d. Bosworth fracture/dislocation: distal fibula is entrapped behind the tibia and the posterolateral tibial ridge prevents reduction; mostly irreducible closed due to intact intraosseous membrane and requires open reduction
- Treatment
  a. Key principles: anatomic reduction of mortise, confirm syndesmotic stability; restoration of fibular length and rotation critical to stability

  b. Conservative: isolated lateral malleolus with intact deltoid ligament, isolated medial malleolus fracture

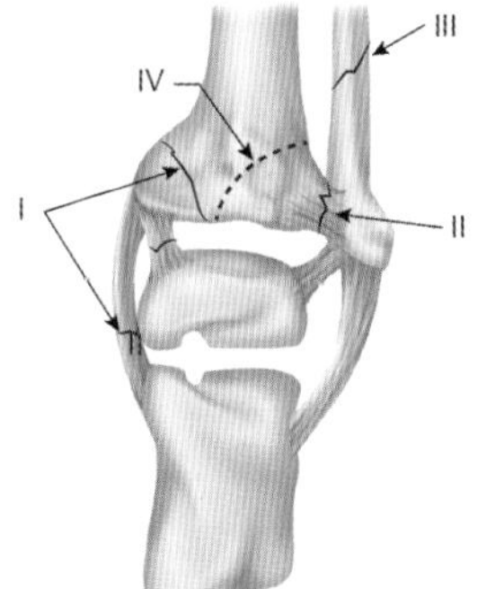

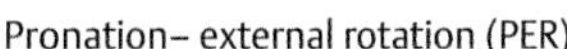
Pronation– external rotation (PER)

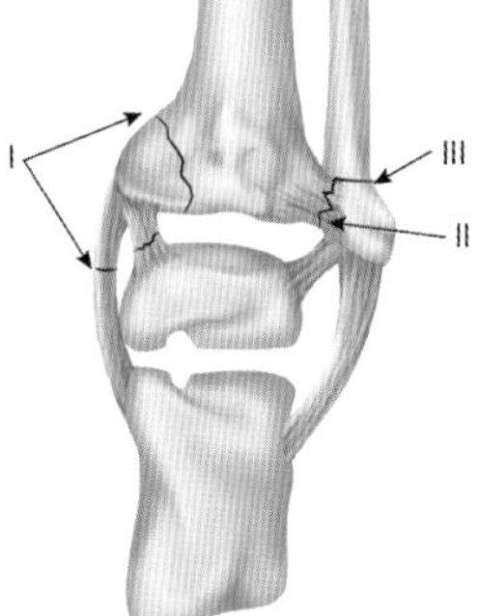

Pronation– abduction (PA)

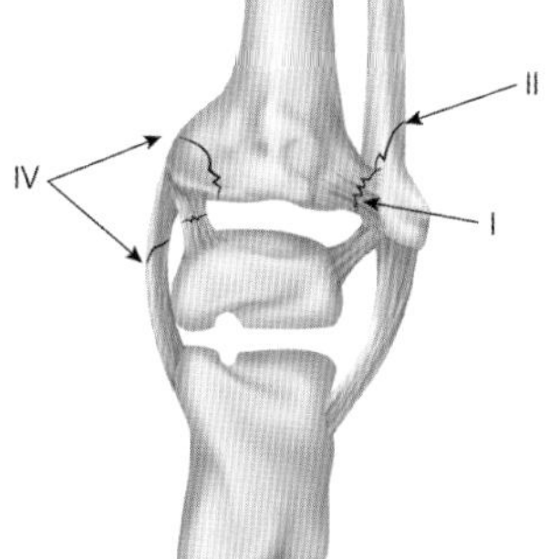

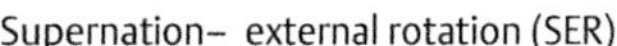
Supernation– external rotation (SER)

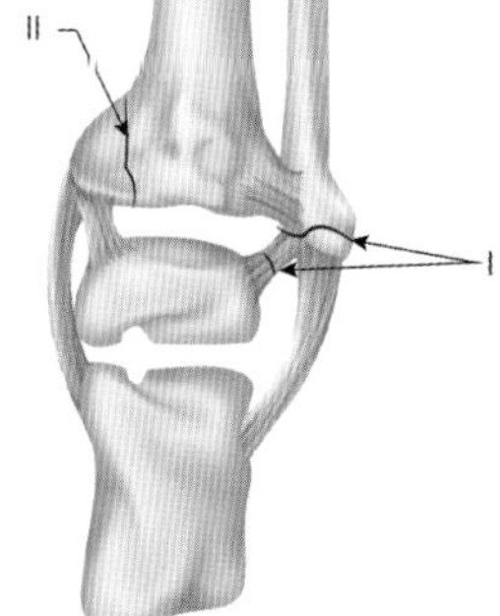

Supination abduction (SA)

Fig. 3.32 Lauge-Hansen ankle fracture classification.

that is nondisplaced or minimally displaced, nondisplaced bimalleolar fractures; immobilize for 6 weeks

c. Surgical: ORIF for displaced bimalleolar or trimalleolar fractures, displaced lateral malleolus fracture with incompetent deltoid, syndesmotic disruption, displaced medial malleolus fractures, posterior malleolus fractures > 25%, ankle instability; goal of ORIF is to restore anatomic reduction of the talus in the mortis
   - Fibular fixation with lag screws and a lateral neutralization plate for oblique patterns; has less peroneal irritation but a higher rate of articular screw penetration
   - Posterolateral anti-glide plate is more stable than a lateral plate but is associated with peroneal irritation.
   - Lateral and posterolateral plates have equivalent hardware removal rates.
   - Medial malleolus: lag screws or tension band for transverse fractures; buttress plate for vertical fractures (supination-adduction)
   - Posterior malleolus: if > 25% of plafond or associated with continued ankle instability; anterior to posterior lag screws or posterior buttress plate
   - Deltoid incompetence: isolated fibula fracture with stress radiographs showing medial clear space widening > 4 mm or lateral talar subluxation are indicative of deltoid incompetence and are supination external rotation (SER) type IV equivalent fractures; requires fibula fixation to keep ankle reduced

d. Syndesmotic instability: common with fibula fractures > 6 cm above ankle joint (Weber C and pronation injuries)
   - Fibula is most unstable in the anterior-posterior plane with syndesmotic injury.
   - Provocative tests: Cotton test—clamp fibula and pull laterally; or external rotation of foot at neutral ankle dorsiflexion (most accurate syndesmotic assessment)
   - Treatment: fix with two syndesmotic screws 3.5 mm or greater (three or four cortices); malreduction is associated with poor functional results; 30% risk of screw breakage with weight bearing; may remove screws at 3–6 months (optional)

e. Rehabilitation: postoperative immobilization or walker boot for 6 weeks; physical therapy for proprioceptive training

f. Driving after lower extremity trauma: braking time is reduced until 6 weeks after resumption of weight bearing

- Complications: wound complications and infection (worse for diabetic patients), stiffness, posttraumatic ankle arthritis; treatment is with ankle arthrodesis if arthritis is debilitating

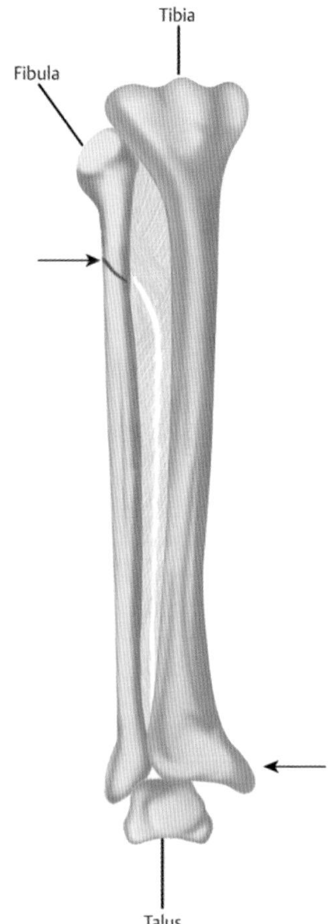

Fig. 3.33 Maisonneuve fracture.

4

Pediatrics

Philip McClure, Josh Vaughn, and Craig Eberson

I. Normal Growth/Development (Fig. 4.1), Appearance of Secondary Centers of Ossification, and Chronology of Physeal Closure (Fig. 4.2)

1. Diagram with expected growth rates/ratio **(Figs. 4.3, 4.4)**
2. Basic rules of growth rates
   - Females physes close at ages 14–16
   - Males physes close at ages 16–18
3. Annual growth of the leg
   - **3, 9, 6, and 3 mm are the average respective growth rates of the lower extremity long bones.**
   - Proximal femur: 3 mm
   - Distal femur: 9 mm
   - Proximal tibia: 6 mm
   - Distal tibia: 3 mm

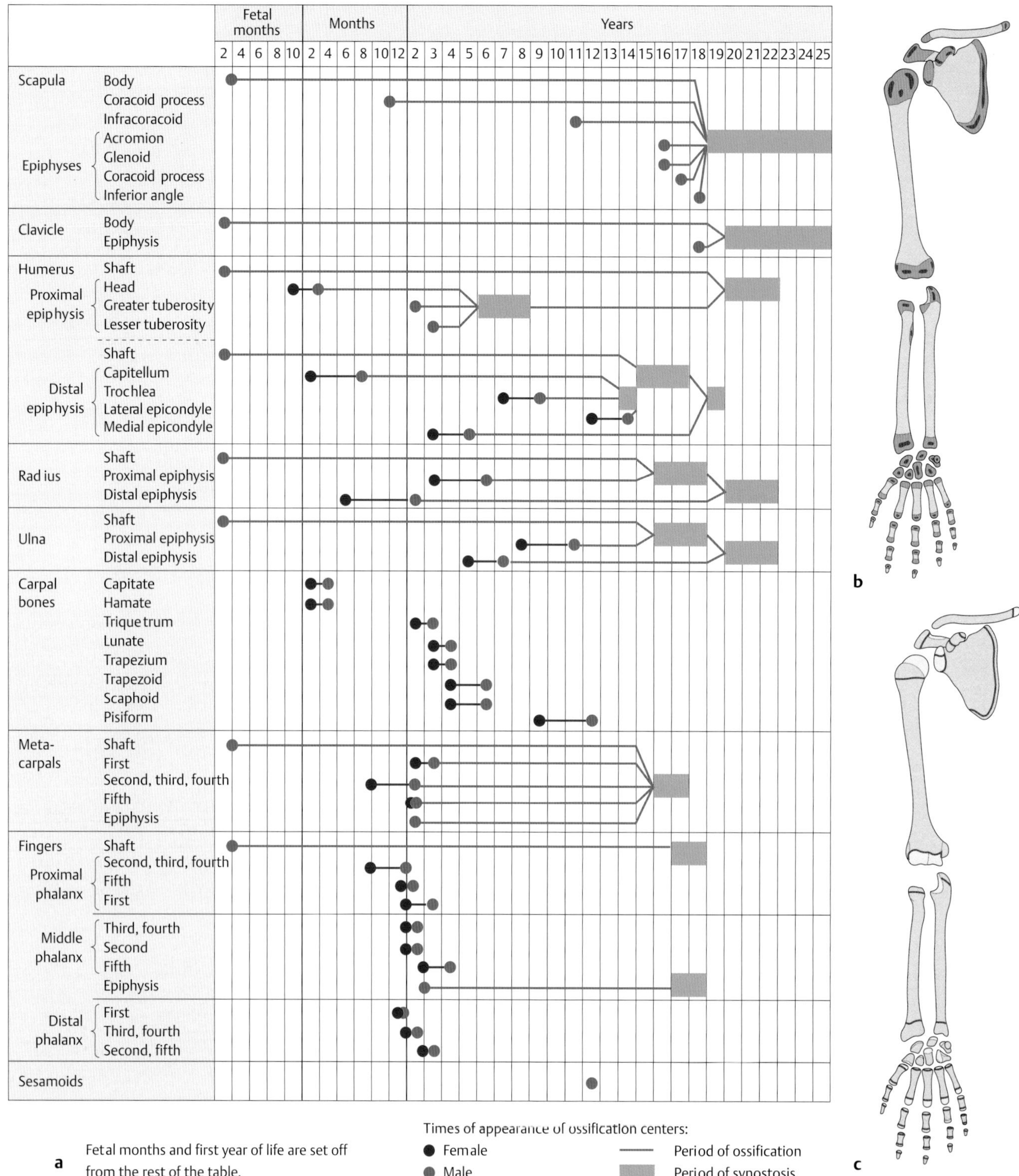

Fig. 4.1 **(a)** Ages at which the primary and secondary centers of ossification and physeal closure develop in the upper extremity, as shown by location. **(b)** and **(c)** represent schematics of the locations of secondary ossifcation centers. (From Niethard FU. Kinderorthopadie [Pediatric Orthopedics]. Stuttgart: Thieme; 1997.)

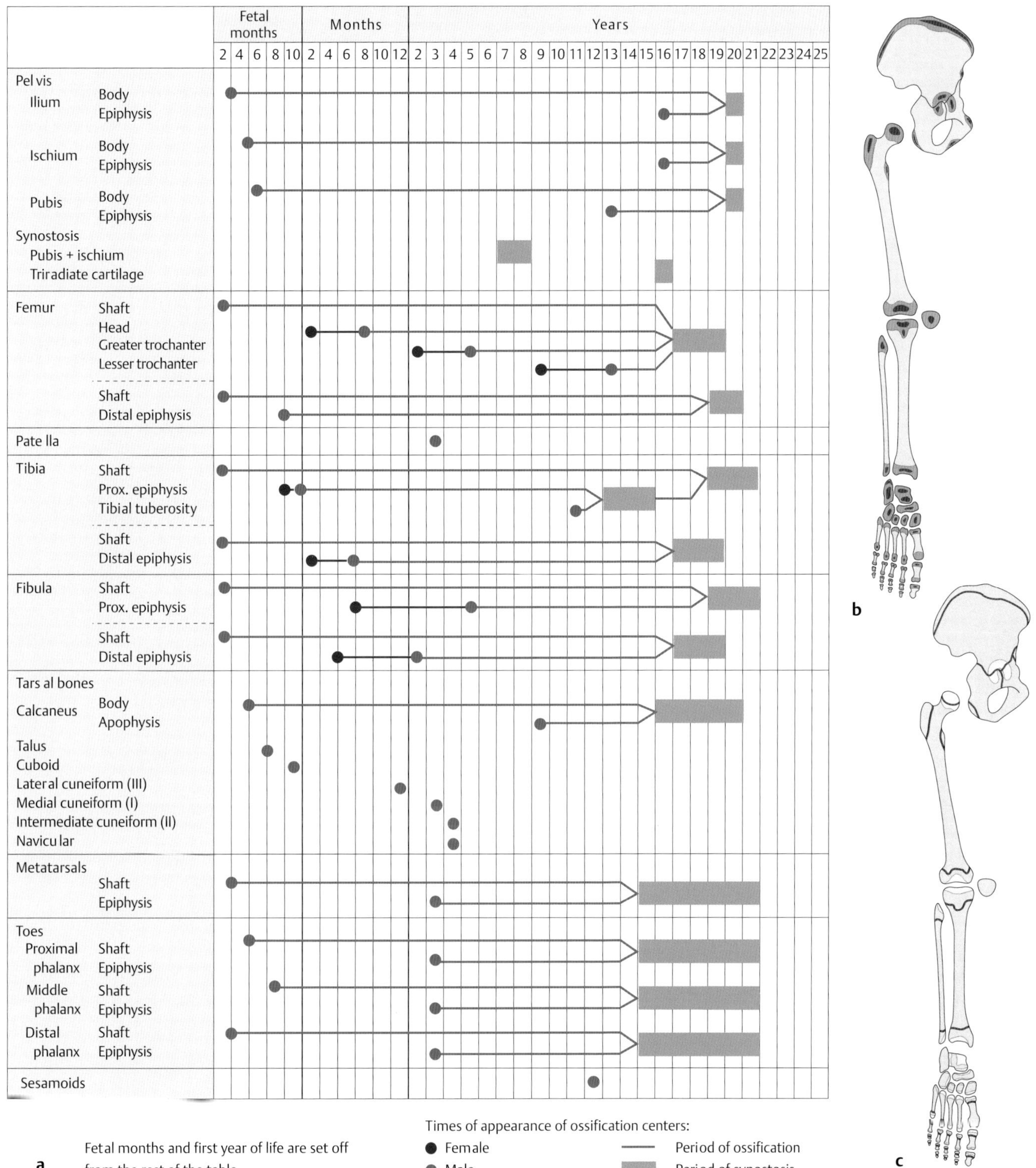

Fig. 4.2 **(a)** Ages at which the primary and secondary centers of ossification and physeal closure develop in the lower extremity, as shown by location. **(b)** and **(c)** represent schematics of the locations of ossifcation centers. (From Niethard FU. Kinderorthopadie [Pediatric Orthopedics]. Stuttgart: Thieme; 1997.)

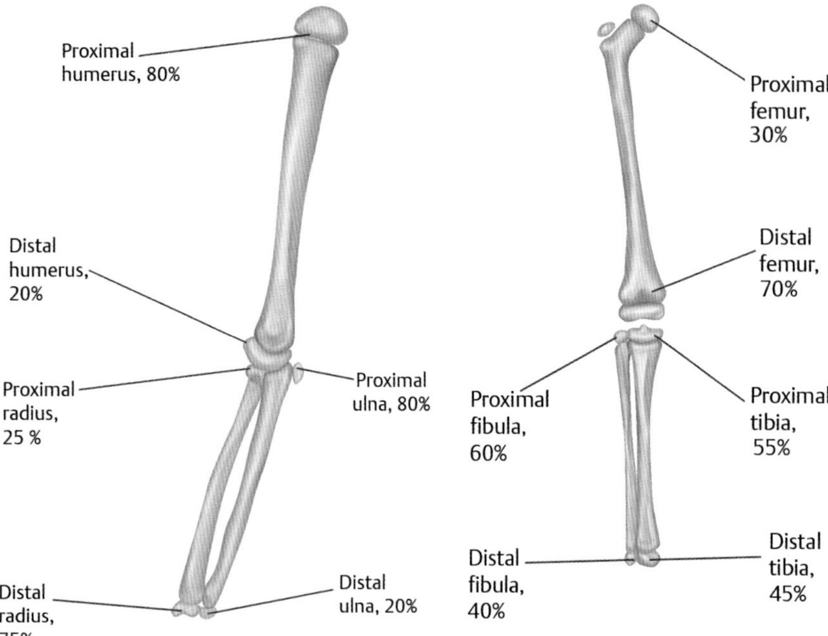

Fig. 4.3 Percentage of growth provided by each physis of the upper extremity.

Fig. 4.4 Percentage of growth provided by each physis of the lower extremity.

4. Can predict effect of epiphysiodesis/premature growth plate closure on leg length
   - Effect = Physis rate × Years of growth left **(Figs. 4.3** and **4.4)**
5. Normal developmental milestones
   - 3 months: head control; can lift head off the floor when prone
   - 6 months: rolls over
   - 6–9 months: sits up without support
   - 9 months: crawls
   - 12 months: walks with one hand support (cruising)
   - 12–17 months: walks independently
   - 2 years: ascends stairs and can run forward
   - 3 years: rides a tricycle
   - 4 years: balances on one foot
   - 5 years: hops on one foot
   - **Handedness develops between ages 2 and 3 years; an earlier preference may be pathological.**

II. Pediatric Imaging

1. General
   - Assess physeal closure and compare with the contralateral side if needed.
2. Elbow: Baumann's angle (normal 20 degrees; used to measure varus/valgus in supracondylar fracture), anterior humeral line (should pass through middle third of capitellum); radial head should align with capitellum in all views, though capitellum may not be visible in infants **(Fig. 4.5)**.

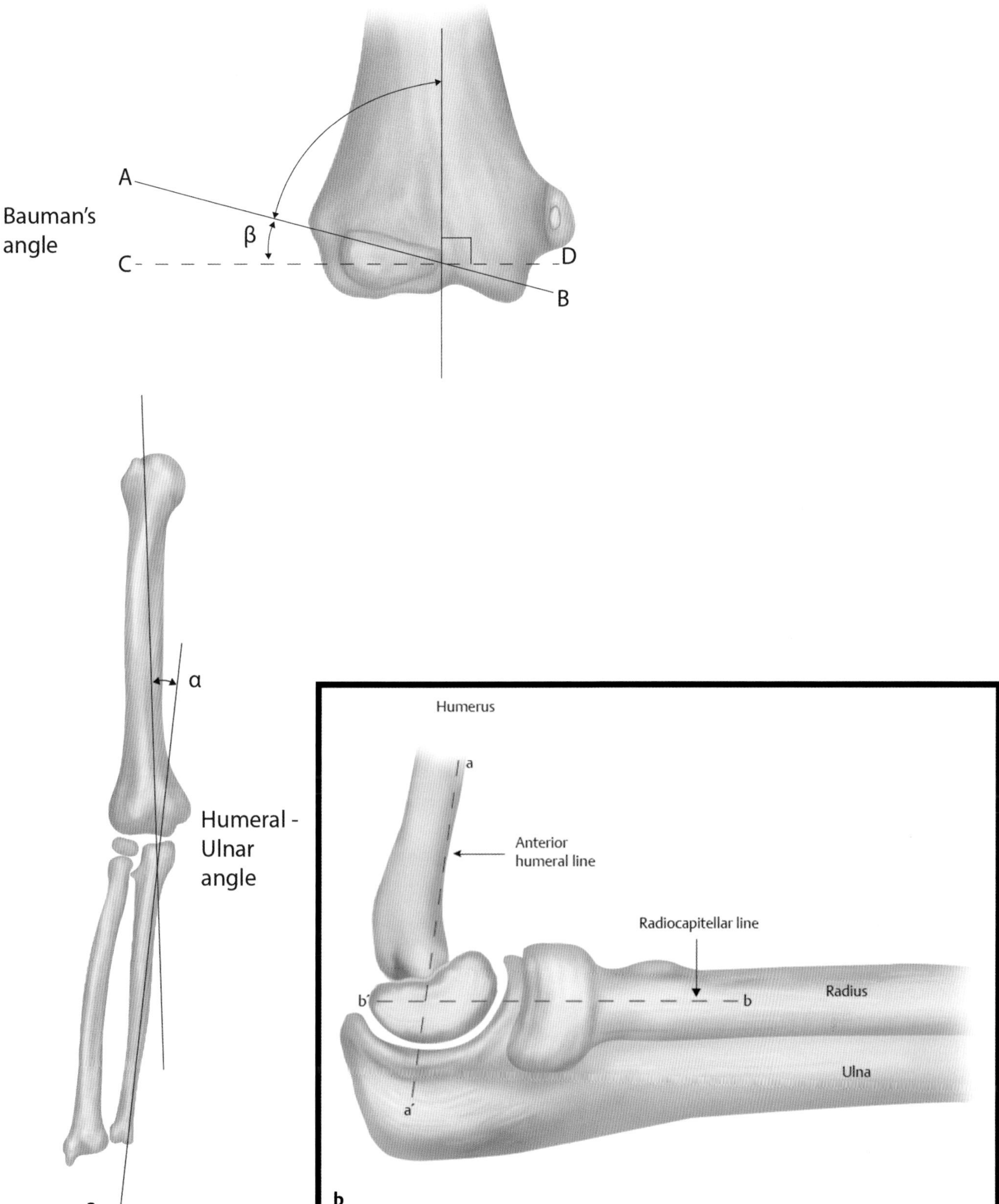

Fig. 4.5 **(a)** Examples of Baumann's angle, humerus-ulnar angle, and metaphyseal-diaphyseal angle of the distal humerus. **(b)** The normal relationship of the anterior humeral line. Note that this line intersects the central third of the capitellum. In type II supracondylar humerus fractures, the line will either intersect the anterior third of the capitellum or will not intersect at all, which is useful in judging the adequacy of the reduction.

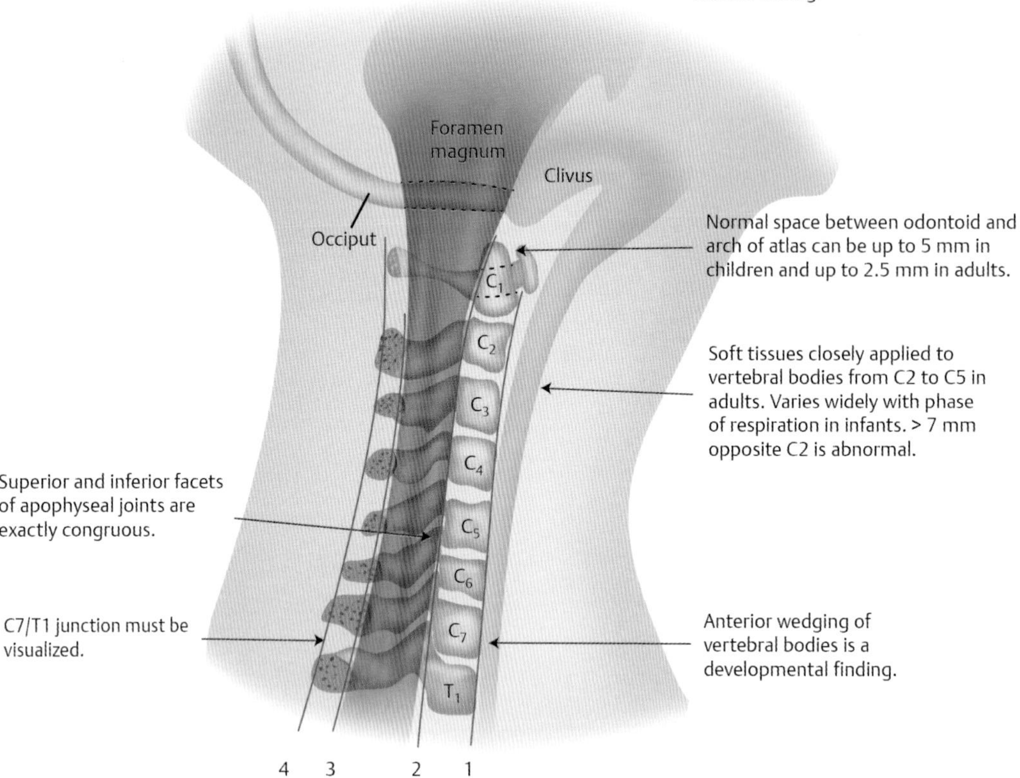

The four lines shown in the figure are :
1. Anterior vertebral line.
2. Posterior vertebral line (anterior wall of the spinal canal).
3. Spinolaminar line.
4. Spinous process line.

All lines should be smooth with no steps or angulation.
The spinolaminar line will continue to be smooth in the setting of pseudosubluxation.

Fig. 4.6 Diagram showing how to interpret a lateral cervical spine radiograph in a child younger than age 8. The spinolamellar line remains intact in pseudosubluxation (most common C2–C3 and C3–C4).

3. Cervical spine **(Fig. 4.6)**
4. Lumbar spine **(Fig. 4.7)**
5. Hip **(Fig. 4.8)**
6. Slipped capital femoral epiphysis (SCFE) **(Figs. 4.9** and **4.10)**
7. Knee: thigh–foot angle, anatomic axis/alignment **(Fig. 4.11)**
8. Foot: Kite's angle **(Fig. 4.12)**
   - **Increased parallelism of the talus and calcaneus constitutes clubfoot.**

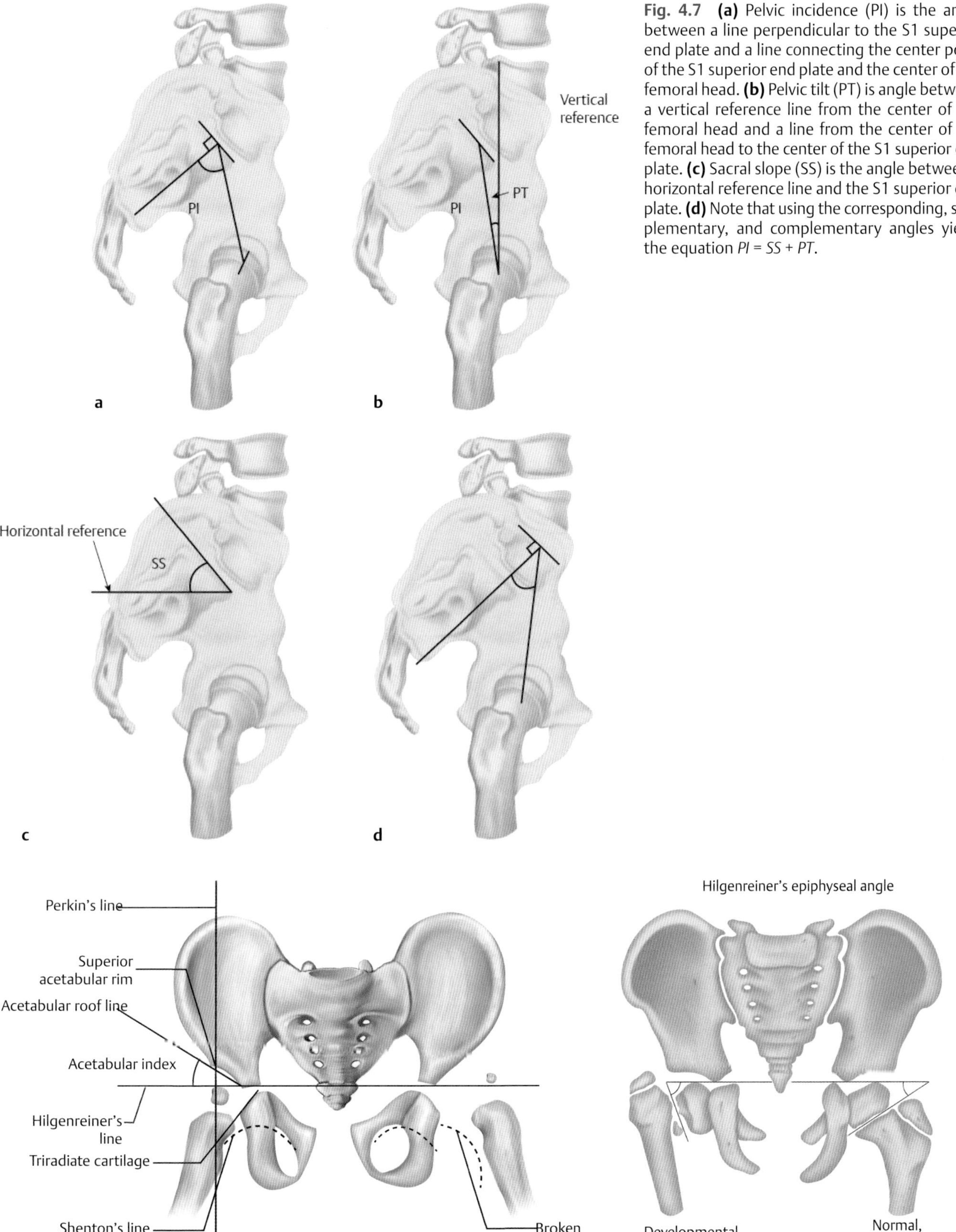

Fig. 4.7 **(a)** Pelvic incidence (PI) is the angle between a line perpendicular to the S1 superior end plate and a line connecting the center point of the S1 superior end plate and the center of the femoral head. **(b)** Pelvic tilt (PT) is angle between a vertical reference line from the center of the femoral head and a line from the center of the femoral head to the center of the S1 superior end plate. **(c)** Sacral slope (SS) is the angle between a horizontal reference line and the S1 superior end plate. **(d)** Note that using the corresponding, supplementary, and complementary angles yields the equation $PI = SS + PT$.

Fig. 4.8 Examples of Hilgenreiner's line, Perkin's line, Shenton's line, the acetabular index, the center edge angle, and Southwick's line. **(a)** The femoral head should be located medial to Perkin's line and inferior to Hilgenreiner's. Shenton's line should be unbroken. The acetabular index should be < 25 degrees. **(b)** Increased Hilgenreiner's–epiphyseal angle indicates coxa vara.

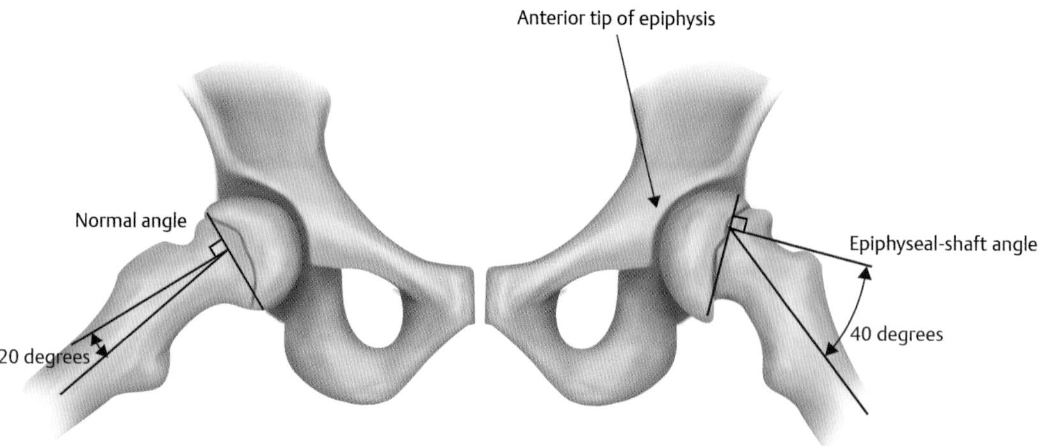

Fig. 4.9 Southwick slip angle: the angle between the femoral shaft and a line drawn along the physis (from one side to the other; may not go through the entire physis). It is used to determine the severity of slip: mild, < 30 degrees of increase compared with the contralateral side; moderate, 31–50 degrees; severe, > 50 degrees. The normal angle (to use for reference in bilateral slip) is 12 degrees.

III. Pediatric-Specific Anatomy

1. Developmental dysplasia of the hip (DDH) **(Fig. 4.13)**
2. Femoral head blood supply: artery of ligamentum teres plays significant role until age 4
3. Blood supply to epiphysis comes through muscular attachments; no blood vessels cross the physis **(Fig. 4.14)**

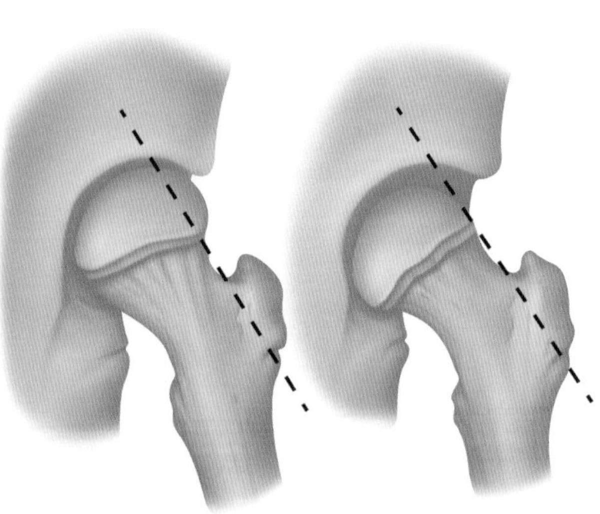

Fig. 4.10 Klein's line (drawn along the superior border of the femoral neck) should contact the epiphysis on both anteroposterior (AP) and lateral images. If it does not, slipped capital femoral epiphysis (SCFE) is diagnosed. The lateral X-ray is more sensitive, but is not necessary if the AP X-ray is positive.

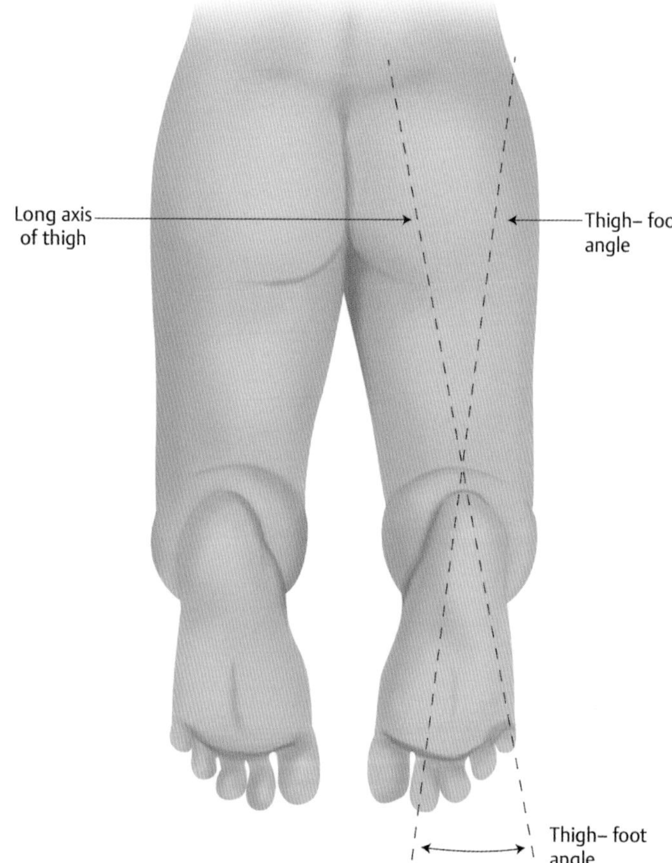

Fig. 4.11 Thigh–foot angle is used to determine the source of in-toeing. If the foot is internally rotated relative to the thigh, tibial torsion is present. However, metatarsus adductus can lead to misinterpretation of the thigh–foot angle. A normal thigh–foot angle would indicate that excessive anteversion is present.

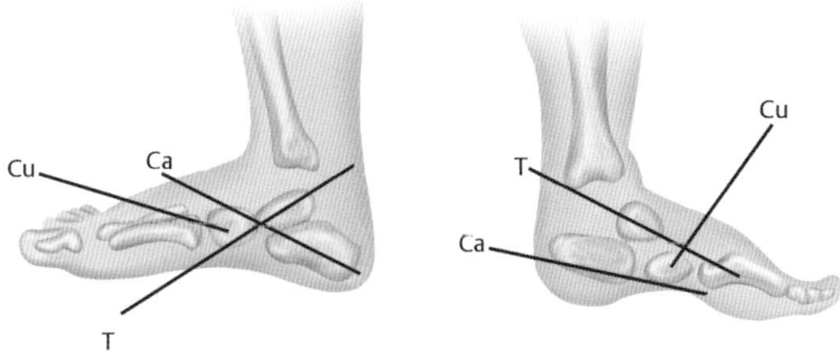

Fig. 4.12 Examples of Kite's angle: 20–40 degrees, normal, < 20 degrees, clubfoot. Ca, calcaneus; Cu, cuboid; T, talus.

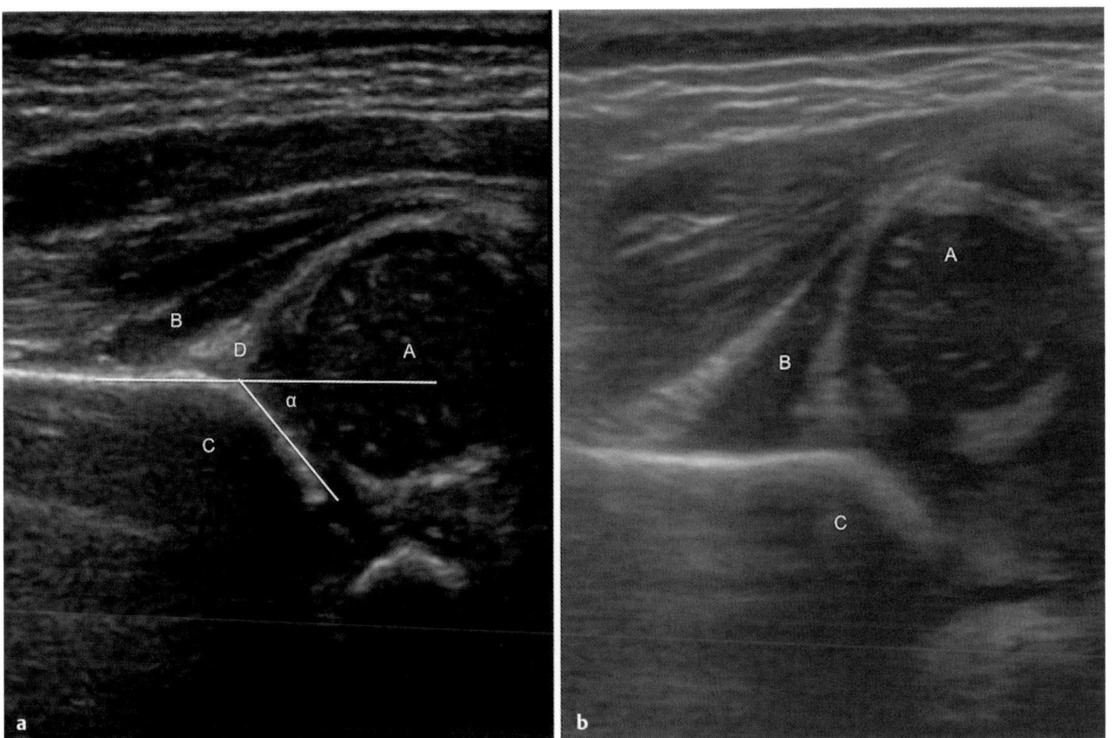

Fig. 4.13 Example of dysplastic hip ultrasounds. *A*, femoral head; *B*, abductor muscles; *C*, bony acetabulum; *D*, cartilaginous acetabulum/labrum. **(a)** Ultrasound of a dysplastic hip that is not dislocated. **(b)** Ultrasound of a dysplastic hip that is dislocated. α is the angle between the acetabular roof and the extension of the ilium.

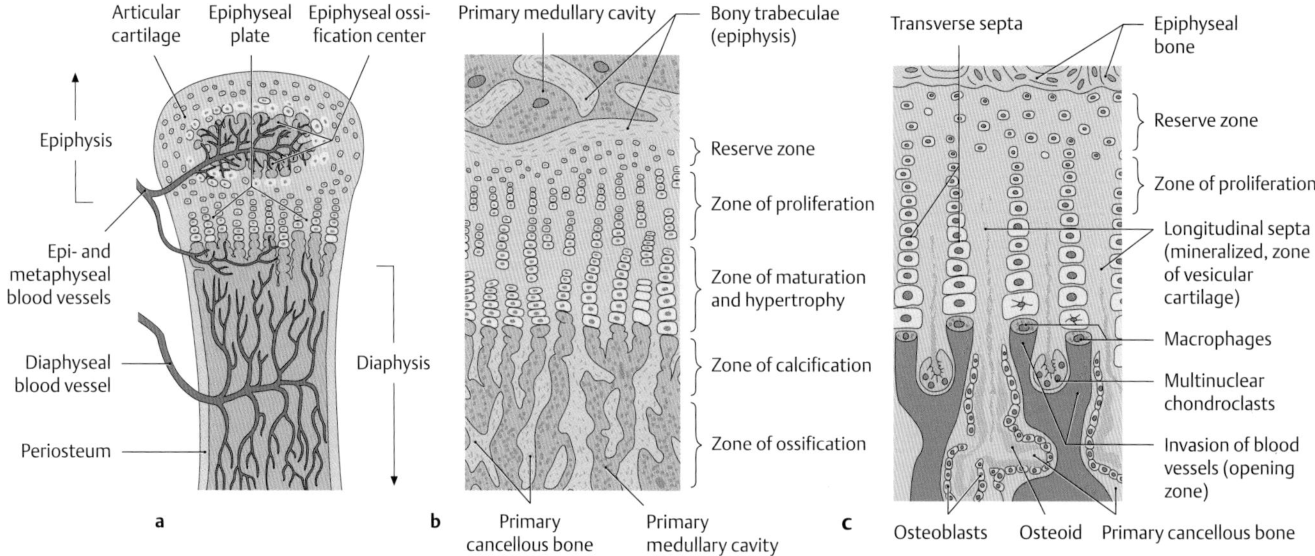

Fig. 4.14 **(a)** Example of the blood supply to the femoral head. **(b)** The different zones of the physis. **(c)** The proliferating physis in more detail. (From Schuenke M, Schulte E. General Anatomy and the Musculoskeletal System: Thieme Atlas of Anatomy. New York: Thieme; 2005. Illustration by Marcus Voll.)

IV. Pediatric Physical

1. Focus on normal growth and development.
2. Limb alignment is often of significant parental concern.
3. All joints should be checked for range of motion; asymmetry or lack of full motion can be the first clue to underlying orthopaedic disease.
   - Decreased hip abduction in an infant should prompt evaluation for hip dysplasia.
4. Evaluate ligamentous laxity.
   - Recurvatum of knees/elbows
5. Evaluate muscular tone.
   - An infant should never "slip through" the examiners hands when placed under the axillae; indicates hypotonia.
6. Neurologic exam
   - Some variability exists in resolution of primitive reflexes, but persistence of primitive reflexes should prompt further evaluation.

V. Syndromes with Growth Disturbance

1. Achondroplasia: quantitative defect in proliferative zone resulting in disproportionate dwarfism
   - **Most common cause of dwarfism is a mutation in fibroblast growth factor receptor-3 (FGFR-3), which results in achondroplasia**
   - Pathology: autosomal dominant (AD); FGFR3 mutation, 80% spontaneous
   - Enchondral ossification more affected than appositional growth
   - Presentation: rhizomelic (short limb), hypotonia (results in delayed motor milestones), small nasal bridge with frontal bossing, trident hands, radial head subluxation, frontal bossing, thoracolumbar kyphosis in infancy
   - **Not prone to early osteoarthritis like pseudoachondroplasia**
   - Short pedicles and decreased interpedicular distance result in spinal stenosis, which often leads to disability. Foramen magnum stenosis may lead to

death. Excessive kyphosis in infancy, often spontaneously resolves. Excessive lumbar lordosis after infancy.

- Imaging: pelvic X-ray shows "champagne glass" with increased width/height ratio; spine with decreased interpedicular distance
- Treatment: neurologic deficit with lumbar decompression/fusion, progressive kyphosis with anteroposterior (AP) fusion (greater than 60 degrees at age 5 if refractory to bracing); lower extremity treatment of angular deformities

2. Pseudoachondroplasia
   - Pathology: AD; mutation in collagen oligomeric protein (COMP); normal facies; disproportionate dwarfism
   - Presentation: normal facies
   - **Normal facies and cervical instability are seen in pseudoachondroplasia**
   - Cervical instability (different from achondroplasia), scoliosis/lumbar lordosis, early osteoarthritis
   - Imaging: radiographs demonstrate flaring of metaphysis, and delayed appearance of secondary centers of ossification.
3. Multiple epiphyseal dysplasia (MED)
   - Pathology: AD; defect in COMP, or type IX collagen
   - Presentation: late-onset dwarfism; MED and spinal epiphyseal dysplasia involve all extremities
   - Pulmonary and ocular (retinal detachment) complications common
   - Irregular, delayed ossification of multiple epiphyses (similar stage differentiates from Perthes); valgus knees that may require osteotomy for correction
   - Imaging: skeletal survey should be obtained to search for multiple sites (coxa vara, valgus knees, early degenerative joint disease).
     a. Irregular appearance of epiphysis with late appearance (consider this in differential of bilateral Perthes)
     b. **Diagnosis is MED if bilateral at same stage, with acetabular involvement; diagnosis is Perthes if asymmetric with normal acetabulum (early)**
4. Spondyloepiphyseal dysplasia (SED)
   - Pathology
     a. Congenital form: AD; defect in type II collagen
     b. Tarda form: X-linked; *SEDL* gene
   - Presentation: involves all extremities (like MED) but also involves the spine (scoliosis with sharp curve)
     a. Congenital form: cleft palate, platyspondyly
     b. Tarda form: kyphosis, hip dysplasia
   - Hypoplastic dens may lead to C1-C2 instability.
5. Kniest syndrome
   - Pathology: AD; type II collagen defect (*COL2A1* gene): osteopenia and dumbbell-shaped bones
   - Presentation: short trunk, dumbbell femurs, joint contractures, scoliosis, kyphosis, hypoplastic pelvis/spine
   - Often with skull abnormality leading to hearing loss and otitis media
6. Metaphyseal chondrodysplasia
   - Normal epiphysis, abnormalities in proliferative and hypertrophic zones of physis
   - Waddling gate, genu varum, hyperlordosis, short dwarfism, mental retardation
   - Irregular vascular invasion in zone of provisional calcification, resulting in nests of cartilage in metaphysis

Table 4.1 Clinical Characteristics of Metaphyseal Chondrodysplasias

Jansen	Schmidt	McKusick
PTHrp mutation	Type X collagen	Autosomal recessive
Autosomal dominant	Autosomal dominant	Fine hair
Bulbous metaphyses	Coxa vara/genu varum	Amish and Finnish
Most severe	Often late diagnosis, most common	Atlantoaxial instability
Rare	Proximal femur most striking	Prone to malignancy

- Jansen's
  a. Pathology: AD; parathyroid hormone (PTH) receptor abnormality
  b. Presentation: mental retardation, bulbous metaphyseal expansion of long bones, rounded epiphyses, short-limb dwarf
- Schmidt's
  a. Pathology: AD; type X collagen abnormality
  b. Presentation: Coxa vara, genu varum
  c. Can be confused with rickets but has normal laboratory findings
- McKusick's
  a. Pathology: autosomal recessive (AR)
  b. Presentation: small-diameter hair, C1-C2 instability; seen in Amish and Finish population **(Table 4.1)**

7. Mucopolysaccharidosis **(Table 4.2)**
   - Differentiated by urinary excretion by-product and clinical manifestations
   - **Associated with carpal tunnel syndrome and trigger finger**
   - **Hunter's syndrome patients see clearly and shoot toward the X; Hurler's syndrome patients do poorly; Morquio syndrome patients have spine instability with normal intelligence**
8. Diastrophic dysplasia
   - Pathology: AR; sulfate transport defect leads to undersulfation of cartilage proteoglycan
   - Presentation: severe cervical kyphosis, scoliosis, cleft palate, rigid clubfoot, cauliflower ears, hitchhiker thumb
   - **Hitchhiker (thumb) lacks adequate (sulfate) transporter.**
   - Spinal deformity can lead to neurologic defects.
9. Cleidocranial dysplasia
   - **Leads to absent clavicles**
   - Pathology: *CBFA-1 (RUNX-2)* defect (AD)

Table 4.2 Clinical Characteristics of Mucopolysaccharidoses

Syndrome	Cornea	Marker Sulfate	IQ	Genetics	Prognosis	Consider
Sanfillipo	Clear	Heparin	Decreased	AR	Regressive development (age 2)	Bone marrow transplant
Morquio	Cloudy	Keratan	Normal	AR	Most common	Spinal instability C1-C2
Hunter	Clear	Dermatan/heparin	Decreased	X-linked recessive		
Hurler	Cloudy	Dermatan/heparin	Decreased	AR	Worst	Bone marrow transplant

Abbreviation: AR, autosomal recessive.

- Presentation: proportionate dwarf, absent clavicles, coxa vara, shoulder hypermobility, skull abnormalities pubic diastasis
- Affects membranous ossification

VI. Syndromes of skeletal muscle

1. Duchenne muscular dystrophy
   - Pathology: X-linked recessive; dystrophin protein absent
   - Presentation: high creatine phosphatase due to muscle breakdown, proximal muscle weakness predominant (Gower's sign), calf pseudohypertrophy
   - Treatment: knee–ankle–foot orthoses and contracture release can prolong walking (usually lost by age 10 years); wheelchair-dependent in teenage years, death by age 20
     a. Steroids may delay progression of disease.
   - Scoliosis does not respond to bracing; operative treatment before 30 degrees indicated
     a. Operative timing more determined by pulmonary and cardiac status than by curve degree. If pulmonary function test (PFT) < 35% of normal, more likely to require tracheostomy and to fail to wean from vent.
2. Becker muscular dystrophy
   - Pathology: X-linked recessive, decreased dystrophin levels
   - Presentation: later onset and milder than Duchenne
3. Fascioscapulohumeral muscular dystrophy
   - **These patients can't whistle.**
   - Pathology: AD
   - Presentation: scapular winging, inability to whistle; normal creatine phosphokinase (CPK) levels

VII. Syndromes of Collagen/Connective Tissue

1. Ehlers-Danlos syndrome
   - Pathology: connective tissue disorder
   - Presentation: generalized ligamentous laxity, skin hyperelasticity, pathological collagen defect, poor wound healing, DDH, clubfoot
2. Marfan syndrome
   - **Optic lens dislocation (ectopia lentis): usually bilateral & superotemporal**
   - Pathology: AD, defect in fibrillin
   - Presentation: tall stature, thin limbs, myopia, dural ectasia, pectus excavatum, superior lens dislocation, cardiac abnormality, ligamentous laxity, aortic dilatation/rupture and mitral valve prolapse, scoliosis
   - Cardiopulmonary assessment should be done preoperatively. Order magnetic resonance imaging (MRI) to look for dural ectasia, increased pseudarthrosis rate with spinal instrumentation
3. Osteogenesis imperfecta (OI)
   - Pathology: qualitative (type III/IV) defect of type I collagen more severe; quantitative (type I) defect less severe; *COL1A1/2* mutation from glycine substitution
   - Presentation: prone to fracture, blue sclera, olecranon avulsion fracture pathognomonic, basilar invagination, scoliosis
   - Normal fracture healing, but limited remodeling

- Treatment: routine fracture treatment; chronic bisphosphonate administration (may decrease skeletal events and generate multiple radiodense lines)
- Bracing ineffective for scoliosis in OI, operate on angle > 50 degrees

4. Larsen syndrome
   - Presentation: multiple dislocated joints, scoliosis, foot deformity, cervical kyphosis (could be lethal), clubfoot, accessory ossification center on calcaneus
   - Can also have airway problems, heart valve lesions, aorta, hyperelasticity, hypotonia, late myelopathy

VIII. Neurologic Syndromes

1. Charcot-Marie-Tooth (CMT) syndrome
   - Pathology: AD; duplication on chromosome 17 creating mutation of peripheral myelin protein (PMP)-22; diagnose with DNA testing
   - Presentation: predominant weakness of distal muscle groups; cavovarus foot deformity (weak tibialis anterior, peroneus longus/brevis) and acetabular dysplasia
2. Friedreich's ataxia
   - Pathology: frataxin gene abnormality (repeat)
   - Presentation: onset in preteen/teen years; gait instability (wide-based gait), cardiomyopathy, cavus foot, scoliosis, decreased deep tendon reflexes
   - **Cardiomyopathy seen in Friedreich's ataxia, neurofibromatosis (NF), and Holt-Oram syndrome**
   - **Cavus feet seen in Friedreich's ataxia and CMT, but acetabular dysplasia with CMT**
   - Loss of α motor neurons
   - Death in fifth decade
   - Treatment: scoliosis treated at 50 degrees with surgery, bracing ineffective
3. Neurofibromatosis (NF)
   - **Causes of hemihypertrophy: *Proteus*, Beckwith-Wiedemann syndrome, Klippel-Trenaunay syndrome, NF**
   - Pathology: AD; defect in neurofibromin
   - Presentation: neurofibromas and café au-lait spots (smooth; coast of California borders)
     a. Anterolateral tibia bowing (bracing prior to fracture), pseudarthrosis (debride, fix)

     Can see renal abnormalities in NF, Klippel-Feil syndrome

     b. Cutaneous neuromas, axillary freckling, Lisch nodule
   - Treatment:
     a. Check renal ultrasound (US), cardiac echocardiogram, and MRI of spine for other abnormalities.
     b. Short dystrophic scoliosis; dural ectasia decreases pedicle size (requires MRI); fuse if any progression or over 40 degrees (may require anterior/posterior in young patient to prevent crankshaft phenomenon); high incidence of pseudarthrosis
   - No scoliosis in NF2
4. Spinal muscular atrophy
   - Pathology: AR, defect in survival motor neuron gene
   - Decreased protein levels in anterior horn cells of the spine cause cell death.

- Presentation: muscle weakness, atrophy; consider if delay or loss of motor milestones, scoliosis
- Electromyogram (EMG) shows fibrillations; muscle biopsy shows denervation.
- Disease severity correlates with ability to produce survival of motor neuron (SMN) protein from the number of functioning *SMN II* genes remaining (all *SMN I* genes are nonfunctional in affected individuals).
- Treatment: hip subluxation: treat nonoperatively and keep dislocated; scoliosis, bracing not tolerated

5. Arthrogryposis
   - Pathology: decreased anterior horn cells
   - Presentation: nonprogressive; myopathic or neuropathic; normal intelligence and facial appearance; multiple joint contractures without skin creases; rigid clubfeet or vertical talus
   - Treatment: may require muscle transfers or release; fusions if refractory to soft tissue work alone (triple arthrodesis)
     a. Bilateral hip dislocations often left alone (can reduced bilaterally through medial approach in young patients), unilateral dislocation reduced (medial approach)
     b. Triceps transfer with posterior elbow release to obtain elbow flexion
     c. Knee contractures treated with hamstring lengthening

IX. Other Syndromes

1. Osteochondroses
   - Navicular (Kohler's)
     a. Treatment: non–weight bearing with cast for initial treatment
   - Scaphoid (Preiser's)
   - Femoral head (Chandler's)
   - Capitellum (Panner's)
2. Osteopetrosis: AR, defect in carbonic anhydrase
3. McCune-Albright syndrome
   - Pathology: Defect in GS-α subunit of cyclic adenosine monophosphate (cAMP) second messenger pathway
   - Presentation: polyostotic fibrous dysplasia, precocious puberty, café-au-lait spots (coast of Maine borders)
   - Fibrous dysplasia leads to varus proximal femoral deformity (shepherd's crook deformity); correct with valgus osteotomy

X. Cerebral Palsy

1. Static nonprogressive encephalopathy with progressive manifestations
2. Multiple causes [all with central nervous system (CNS) injury before age 2]
3. Three classification systems with varying criteria (descriptive and severity based) **(Table 4.3)**
4. Independent sitting by age 2 predicts ambulation; persistence of more than one primitive reflex makes ambulation less likely.
   - Moro reflex normally gone by 6 months (pathological if persists longer)
   - Parachute reflex normally gone by 12 months (pathological if persists longer)
5. In hip dislocation, posterosuperior quadrant is deficient
6. Highest risk for scoliosis with spastic quadriplegia
7. Treatment:

Table 4.3 Classification of Cerebral Palsy

Physiological Classification					
	Spastic	Athetoid	Ataxic	Mixed	
Anatomic	Hemiplegia	Diplegia (lower extremities)	Quadriplegia		
Functional (GMFCS)	Level 1: speed and coordination impaired	Level 2: difficulty on uneven surfaces/ crowds rail to climb stairs	Level 3: unable to walk on uneven surface, wheelchair for long distance	Level 4: short distance walking in the home with assistance only	Level 5: difficulty maintaining head posture, no independent mobility

Abbreviation: GMFCS, Gross Motor Function Classification System.

8. Spasticity: Botox, baclofen [γ-aminobutyric acid (GABA) agonist]; transfer of spastic muscles can improve flexible deformities
   - Toe walking: if ankle is able to dorsiflex past neutral, stretching and AFO; if unable to reach neutral, consider Achilles or gastroc lengthening
   - Crouched gait: multilevel releases
   - Stiff knee gait: rectus femoris transfer due to its firing out of phase; hamstring lengthening
   - Equinovarus foot: split posterior tibial tendon transfer due to overpull of this tendon (or the anterior tibialis tendon), which can contribute to varus deformity (but not equinus). Achilles tendon is involved and correction is required to address equinus. Address whichever tendon is spastic during stance and swing.
   - Hip subluxation: may require adductor release; varus producing osteotomy, acetabuloplasty
     a. In young patients, maximize therapy and range of motion prior to releases and lengthenings
     b. Hip at risk (age < 5 years) with < 45 degrees hip abduction: adductor and psoas release
     c. Hip subluxation: tenotomies with or without femoral or acetabular osteotomies for valgus femoral neck or acetabular dysplasia
     d. Spontaneous dislocation: open reduction, varus derotation osteotomy (VDRO), pelvic osteotomy
     e. Windswept pelvis: bilateral varus osteotomies of hips
     f. Scoliosis: curves with marked pelvic obliquity, require anterior and posterior fusion; spinal fusion indicated for curve > 50 degrees, progressive pelvic obliquity, sitting problems
     g. Fusion to pelvis indicated in nonambulatory patients with pelvic obliquity
     h. Hallux valgus: orthotics; metatarsophalangeal (MTP) fusion if patient fails conservative management

XI. Birth Injuries and Related Abnormalities

1. Brachial plexus injury (see Chapter 9)
   - More common with large babies, shoulder dystocia, forceps delivery, breech position
   - No biceps motion at 6 months is a poor prognostic indicator.
   - Horner's syndrome indicates lower trunk root avulsion and poor prognosis.
   - Maintain passive range of motion (ROM) while awaiting potential recovery **(Table 4.4)**.

Table 4.4 Classification and Prognosis of Brachial Plexus Injury

Type	Roots	Prognosis
Complete	C5-T1	Worst
Erb-Duchenne	C5-C6	Best
Klumke	C7-T1	Poor

2. Torticollis
   - Pathology: secondary to intrauterine compartment syndrome or positional contracture of the sternocleidomastoid
   - Treatment: involves stretching and possible release
   - 12–20% associated with DDH
3. Congenital pseudarthrosis of the clavicle
   - Can be mistaken for fracture but has resorbed edges
   - Enlarging painless mass
   - If functional symptoms may treat at age 3–5 with open reduction and internal fixation (ORIF)

XII. Spine

1. Spondylolysis: stress fracture of pars
   - Physical exam: pain with lumbar extension
   - Imaging: oblique X-ray of questionable utility; computed tomography (CT) and MRI more sensitive; single photon emission computed tomography (SPECT) most sensitive imaging study
   - Acute treatment: bracing
   - Surgery if refractory versus pars repair
2. Spondylolisthesis
   - Pathology: anterior translation of proximal vertebral segment
   - Presentation: most common at L5-S1
     a. Lytic subtype from spondylolysis
     b. Dysplastic from abnormal anatomy, higher progression
   - Graded by percentage of anterior translation (quartiles)
   - Treatment
     a. Low-grade translation treated with brace/therapy
     b. Higher grade (3–4) treated with fusion (l4-S1)
     c. Return to play with spondylolisthesis
        - Grade 1: return after pain resolves
        - Grade 2: no gymnastics or football; slip angle greater than 10 degrees or greater than 30 degree with sacral inclination may progress
        - Grade 3 and 4: usually cause neurologic symptoms; require prophylactic fusion (posterolateral)
3. Scoliosis (**Fig. 4.15** and **Table 4.5**)
   - Indications for MRI: left thoracic curve, thoracic kyphosis, congenital or juvenile disease, rapid progression, child with other syndrome, neurologic abnormality
   - General
     a. Cervical stability views for Morquio or Down syndromes; cardiology and pulmonary for muscular dystrophy; hematology if associated radial deficiency
   - Juvenile
     a. Growing rods: indicated if thoracic size needs to increase prior to definitive treatment; increasing force required for subsequent distractions, with less correction obtainable
   - Adolescent idiopathic
     a. Progression of curve can be minimized with brace wear greater than 12 hours/day (actual wear), (82% successful)

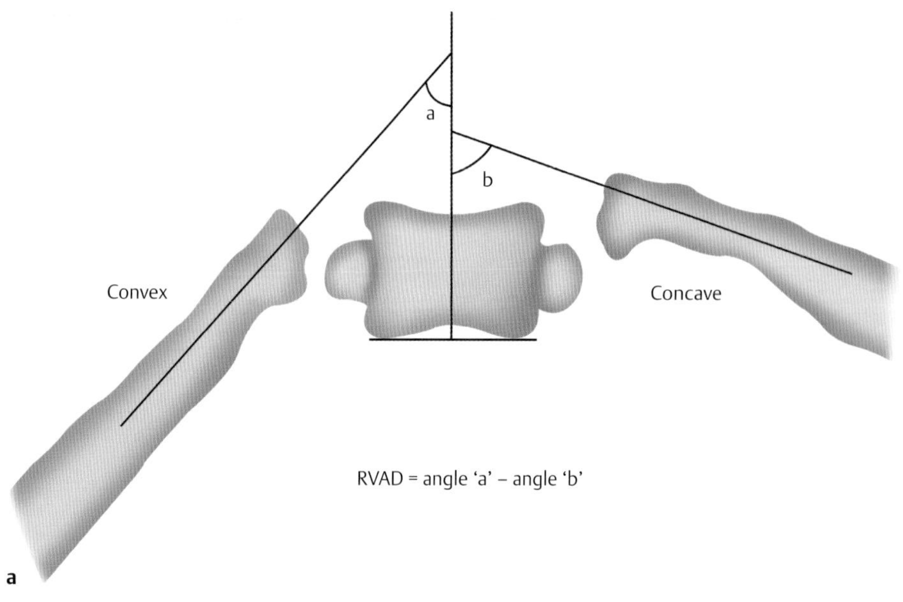

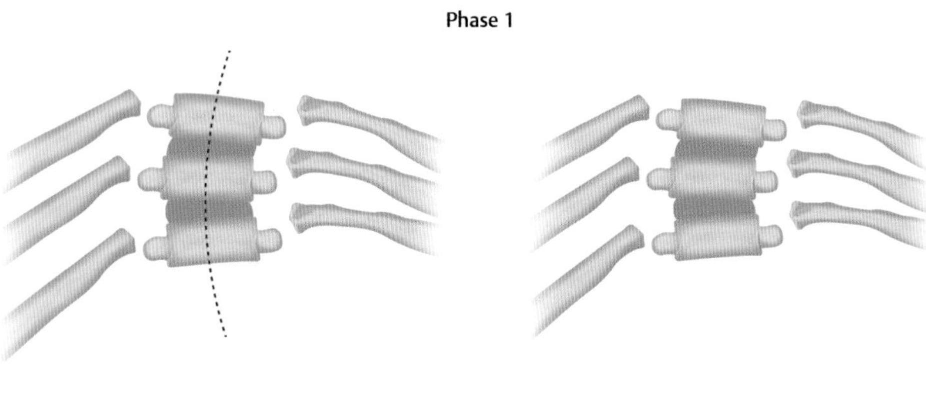

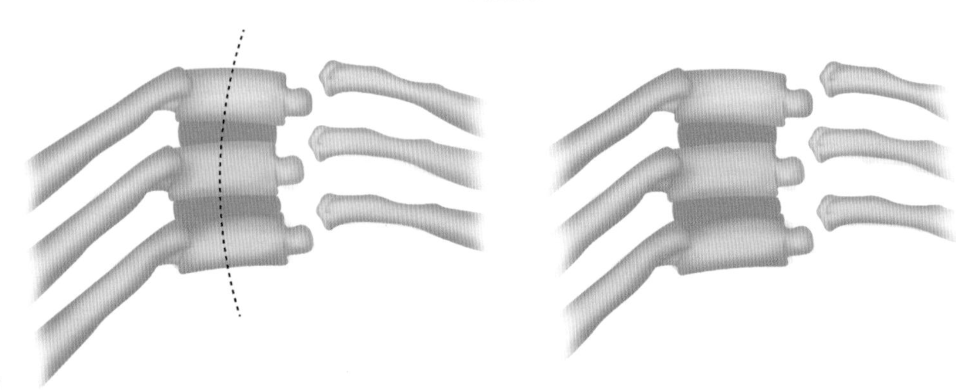

Fig. 4.15 **(a)** Example of the rib vertebral angle difference (RVAD). **(b)** Example of the rib phase used in infantile scoliosis, measured on the concave side of the curve. Phase 1, the rib does not overlap the vertebral body; phase 2, the rib overlaps the vertebral body.

b. Risser stages:
   - Stage 0: no apophysis visible
   - Stage 1: anterior ¼ visible
   - Stage 2: anterior ½ visible
   - Stage 3: anterior ¾ visible
   - Stage 4: all visible but unfused
   - Stage 5: fused

c. Curve progression most rapid at peak height velocity, which occurs during Risser stage 0 and before menarche

Table 4.5 Scoliosis in the Pediatric Patient

Subtype	Age (Years)	Sex	Thoracic Pattern	Bracing	Surgery	Typical Course
Congenital	–	–	–	Ineffective	Excision of abnormality	Failure of formation or segmentation; hemivertebra with contralateral bar worst prognosis, block vertebra best; order MRI; treat L5 hemivertebrae with oblique takeoff with hemivertebrectomy
Infantile idiopathic	< 3	M	Left	Casting followed by bracing for flexible curves with RVAD > 20 degrees	Growing rods (proximal/distal fusion only) for RVAD > 40 degrees (preoperative MRI) Delay full fusion to age 10	Spontaneous resolution in general, progression predicted by rib overlap, RVAD < 20 degrees (observe); order MRI
Juvenile idiopathic	3–10	F	Right	< 45 degrees	Growing rods if < 10, PSF after	70% need treatment, 50% surgery; order MRI
Adolescent idiopathic	≥ 11	F	Right	> 25–30 degrees if growth remaining	> 50 degrees	If > 50 degrees at maturity, progresses 1 degree per year
Neuromuscular	–	–	Left, long curve	For seating in wheelchair	DMD: 25–30 degrees CP > 50 degrees T2–pelvis if nonambulatory	Varies with disease; in DMD pulmonary/cardiac compromise must be considered, ambulatory status important in CP, infection rate increased

Abbreviations: CP, cerebral palsy; DMD, Duchenne muscular dystrophy; MRI, magnetic resonance imaging; PSF, posterior spinal fusion; RVAD, rib vertebral angle difference.

- Treatment with anterior-posterior spinal fusion indicated for myelomeningocele, congenital spinal deformity. Relative indications: NF, age < 10 years, > 75-degree curve, Marfan's syndrome

4. Kyphosis
   - Congenital
     a. Most commonly from failure of formation of elements
     b. Poor prognosis with high incidence of neurologic compromise
     c. Treatment of choice is posterior fusion if < 50 degrees; larger or stiffer curves may require anterior/posterior surgery or deformity resection
   - Scheuermann's
     a. Pathology: increased kyphosis with > 5 degrees of wedging in three consecutive vertebrae (differentiates from postural kyphosis)
     b. More common in males and overweight individuals
     c. Bracing if > 50 degrees, but poorly tolerated (Milwaukee brace)
     d. Surgery if progressive or continued pain, curve > 75 degrees; anterior surgery rarely needed if pedicle screws used
5. Cervical spine
   - Klippel-Feil syndrome
     a. Pathology: congenital fusion of cervical spine
     b. Presentation: low hair line, limited ROM, short neck
        - Associated with Sprengel's deformity (high scapula with limited abduction), renal abnormality.
        - Treatment: surgery only if neurologic deficit or intractable pain; otherwise, patient avoids contact sports/gymnastics
   - Instability (atlantoaxial)
     a. Associated with Down syndrome, Morquio syndrome, juvenile rheumatoid arthritis

Table 4.6 Clinical Manifestations and Treatment of Myelodysplasia in Children

Level	Muscles functioning	Limb position	Ambulatory status	Treatment
L1	Weak iliopsoas	Equinovarus foot	Nonambulatory	HKAFO
L2	Iliopsoas/adductor	Flexed hip, flexed knee, equinovarus foot	Nonambulatory	HKAFO
L3	Adductor/quad	Adducted/flexed hip, recurvatum of knee, equinovarus foot	Household ambulator	KAFO
L4	Quadriceps/tibialis anterior	Adducted/flexed hip, extended knee, cavovarus foot	Minimal community ambulator	KAFO
L5	Peroneals, hip abductors	Extended knee, calcaneovalgus foot	Community ambulator	AFO
S1	Gastroc/soleus	Foot deformity alone	Community ambulator	Normal shoe wear

Abbreviations: AFO, ankle–foot orthosis; HKAFO, hip–knee–ankle–foot orthosis; KAFO, knee–ankle–foot orthosis.

   b. No contact sports/gymnastics
   c. Surgery if neurologic defect (fusion)

6. Myelodysplasia
   - Caused by incomplete closure of spinal cord, early diagnosis with elevated α-fetoprotein in amniotic fluid (prevent with folate)
   - Spina bifida occulta: defect in posterior elements with no herniation
   - Meningocele: dural sac without neurologic elements
   - Myelomeningocele: dural sac with herniation of neural elements
   - Lowest functional level **(Table 4.6)**
   - L5 level generates calcaneus foot, treatment with transfer of anterior tibial tendon (avoid triple arthrodesis)
   - Bilateral dislocated hips of L3 or above should be left alone. Position of hips does not contribute to overall functional outcome at the thoracic level.
   - Soft tissue contractures should be treated to improve positioning and care.
   - Fracture may manifest as warmth/erythema only and is commonly missed, as only minimal energy is required to fracture.
   - Increased rate of latex sensitivity
   - Severe local kyphosis at level of defect may require excision of the deformity (kyphectomy)
   - **Rapid progression of scoliosis may be attributable to tethered cord in spina bifida occulta; order MRI.**
7. Pseudosubluxation
   - Can be normal finding before age 8 years
   - Most common at C2-C3, followed by C3-C4
   - Alignment of posterior elements remains anatomic
8. Atlantoaxial rotatory subluxation
   - May be due to retropharyngeal infection
   - Treatment:
     a. Presents < 1 week: collar, nonsteroidal anti-inflammatory drug (NSAIDs), physical therapy
     b. Presents > 1 week: traction ± halo traction
     c. Presents > 1 month: traction ± C1/C2 fusion if unstable or neurologic compromise present
9. Vertebral osteomyelitis
   - Enhancement of vertebral body (high on T2) on MRI
   - Treatment: obtain percutaneous biopsy and blood cultures
   - Appropriate antibiotics are first-line treatment

10. Diskitis
    - **Primary diskitis is a pediatric disease not seen in adults.**
    - Disk erosions on MRI
    - Bacterial infection of disk space and vertebral end plates
    - Treatment: empiric antibiotics to cover *Staphylococcus aureus*

XIII. Lower Extremity

1. DDH
    - Age: present at birth, manifestation variable
    - Increased risk in firstborn, positive family history, female sex, breech position
    - Exam: Ortolani (elevation/abduction of femur reduces hip), Barlow (posterior pressure and adduction dislocates). If age > 12 months, Ortolani/Barlow no longer useful. However, limited abduction will be present.
    - Pathology: deficiency in anterolateral acetabular coverage (index < 25 degrees)
    - Important imaging/classification
        a. Femoral head ossific nucleus should be present by 6 months of age.
        b. Use ultrasound to follow progress of treatment in Pavlik harness (see **Fig. 4.13**).
    - Treatment
        a. Pavlik harness if reducible hip and less than 6 months of age
        b. Reduction may be blocked by the pulvinar, transverse acetabular ligament, psoas tendon, inverted labrum, and limbus tissue.
        c. If does not reduce in Pavlik by 3 weeks, needs closed reduction ± adductor tenotomy and spica casting. Can consider abduction orthosis if child too young for closed reduction
        d. Presentation age 6–18 months: closed reduction/arthrogram, adductor tenotomy and spica with postreduction CT; if fails, then requires open reduction
        e. Age 18 months to 3 years: open reduction
        f. Age 3 to 8 years: osteotomy **(Table 4.7)**

Table 4.7 Pelvic Osteotomies for Treatment of Acetabular Dysplasia in Children

Osteotomy	Coverage	Triradiate	Orientation	Category	Volume	Surface	Fixation	Other
Dega	Posterolateral	Open/hinge	–	Reshaping	Reduced	Hyaline	None	Graft from ASIS; best for posterior coverage in CP
Pemberton	Anterior/lateral	Open/hinge	–	Reshaping	Reduced	Hyaline	None	Graft from ASIS
Salter	Anterolateral	Closed	Extend/ Adduct	Redirection	–	Hyaline	Pins	Mobility through symphysis, graft from ASIS
Triple	Anterolateral	Closed	Extend/ Adduct	Redirection	–	Hyaline	Pins or screws	Mobility through rami osteotomies, graft from ASIS
Ganz/peri-acetabular (PAO)		Closed	Free	Redirection	–	Hyaline	Screws	Leaves pelvic ring intact
Chiari	Subluxed/ incongruent hip	Closed	–	Salvage	–	fibrocartilage		Salvage osteotomy
Shelf	Incongruent hip	Closed		Salvage	–			Adds bone graft to acetabular edge

Abbreviations: CP, cerebral palsy; ASIS, anterior superior iliac spine.

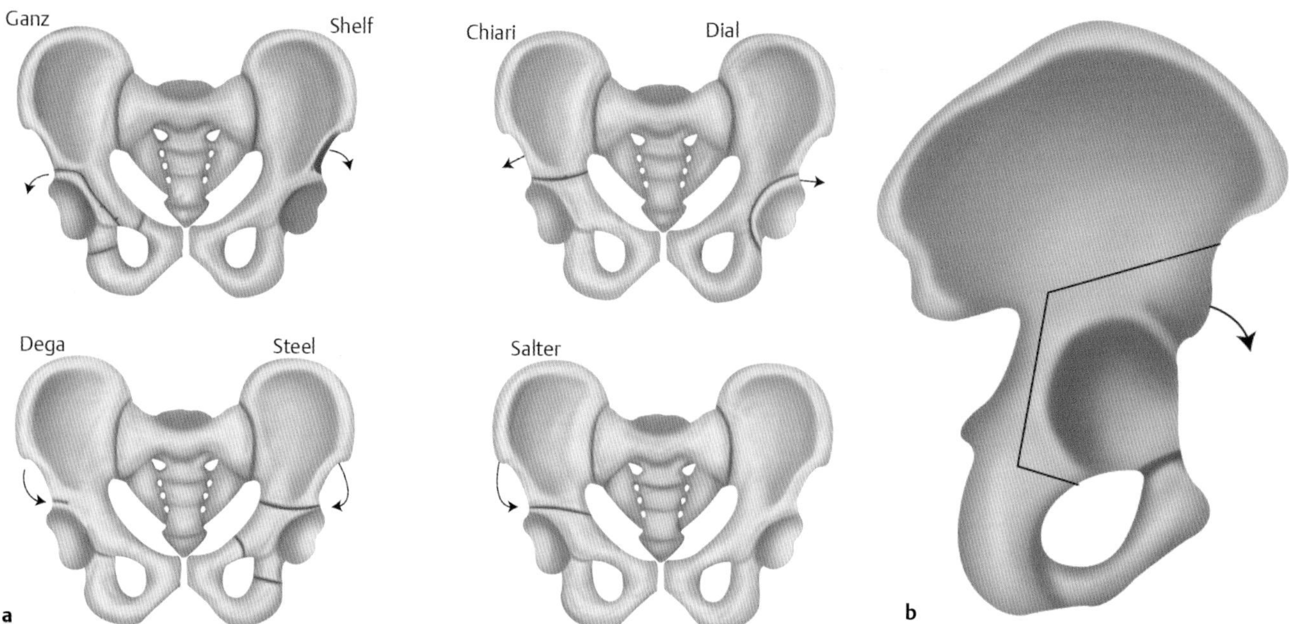

Fig. 4.16 **(a)** AP view of various pelvic osteotomies; **(b)** lateral view of ganz osteotomy. Note that dega osteotomy does not cross into the inner table. Extension of the dega osteotomy into inner table generates a pemberton osteotomy.

g. Periacetabular osteotomy (Ganz) for patients with closed triradiate cartilage

h. Teratologic dislocations (high riding, pseudoacetabulum in neonatal period) will not respond to bracing; surgery at 6–12 months

i. If Pavlik unsuccessful at 3–4 weeks, change to abduction orthoses **(Table 4.7** and **Fig. 4.16)**

2. Legg-Calvé-Perthes disease (LCPD)
   - Age: 4–8 years; predominantly males
   - Presentation: limp (with or without pain), effusion, decreased hip range of motion, Trendelenburg gait
   - Pathology: multiple theories exist; end result is vascular insult to femoral head with avascular necrosis
   - **Diseases that present similar to LCPD: Gaucher's, MED, SED, glycogen storage diseases**

   a. Phases of disease
      - Synovitic: 0–3 months
      - Fragmentation: 3–9 months
      - Reossification: 9–24 months
      - Remodeling: 2–4 years

   - Important imaging/classification:
   - **If bilateral and at same stage, consider MED**

   a. Lateral pillar classification (during fragmentation phase): head broken into thirds medial to lateral
      - Group A has no involvement of lateral pillar.
      - Group B has ≤ 50% involvement (superior outcome if age > 6 years)
      - Group C > 50% involvement (inferior outcomes)

   b. Catterall head at-risk signs: lateral calcification, Gage's sign (radiolucent defect between lateral epiphysis and metaphysis), lateral subluxation, metaphyseal cyst, horizontal growth plate

c. Worse outcome if < 50% lateral pillar height maintained (group C), lateral subluxation of the head, calcification lateral to epiphysis, V-shaped radiolucency in lateral epiphysis

- Treatment: may require "containment," with bracing or proximal femoral/acetabular osteotomy; this improves outcome for children > 8 years of age; first-line treatment is to reduce symptoms with NSAIDs, traction, limited weight bearing

3. SCFE

- **Slip occurs through hypertrophic zone of physis**

- Age: preteen/teen; most common in obese African Americans
- Presentation: males > females, left > right, hip or knee pain, check thyroid/renal laboratories if bilateral, age < 10, weight below 50th percentile; exam with obligate external rotation with hip flexion
- Pathology: weakness of perichondrial ring of Lacroix and "fracture" through hypertrophic zone of the physis; head displaces inferiorly and posteriorly relative to femoral metaphysis
- Important imaging/classification
  a. Frog lateral: most sensitive film
  b. Southwick angle (epiphyseal/shaft angle): measure of slip severity
  c. Stable/unstable determined by ability to bear weight
    - **Unstable slips where the patient is unable to bear weight have a higher rate of osteonecrosis (avascular necrosis).**
  d. Unstable slips more likely to have osteonecrosis (~ 50%)
- Treatment: no forceful reduction, single screw. Chronic deformity can be treated with flexion/internal rotation/valgus osteotomy of proximal femur.
- **Hypothyroidism and chronic renal failure are endocrine etiologies for SCFE; check thyroid-stimulating hormone (TSH) and bone morphogenic protein (BMP)**
  a. Check laboratories (TSH, BMP) to rule out endocrine etiology for slip.
  b. Contralateral pinning of patient who has endocrine disorder or of young patient is recommended.
- Outcome: limb shortening, loss of flexion and internal rotation, osteoarthritis. Anterior screws may impinge on acetabular labrum and produce tears/pain.
- Complication: avascular necrosis most common; risk higher with unstable slip

4. Coxa vara

- Age: may be present at birth, or develop from trauma or genetic predisposition (AD)
- Presentation: waddling gait, leg length discrepancy, positive Galeazzi sign, and abnormal gluteal fold
- Pathology: decreased neck shaft angle of proximal femur
- Important imaging/classification: lack of ossification at inferomedial neck on X-ray for developmental disease
- Treatment:
  a. Epiphyseal angle < 45 degrees: spontaneously corrects
  b. Epiphyseal angle 45–60 degrees: observe
  c. Epiphyseal angle > 60 degrees: valgus osteotomy
  d. Valgus osteotomy if neck shaft angle < 90 degrees, may include derotation; restoring abductor tension by distal/lateral transfer of greater trochanter may be helpful.

5. Proximal femur focal deficiency (PFFD)

- Age: congenital

- Presentation: short femur (varying severity) resulting in leg length discrepancy
- Pathology: defect in primary ossification center; associated with anterior cruciate ligament (ACL) deficiency and fibular hemimelia
- Important imaging/classification: stability of hip joint important in treatment decisions
  a. Aitken classification: class A/B have femoral head; class C/D do not have femoral heads
- Treatment: prosthetics, contralateral epiphysiodesis, lengthening, Van Ness rotationplasty, Steel procedure (fusion of femur to acetabulum, knee functions as hip); foot may be amputated to improve prosthetic fitting

6. Fibular hemimelia
   - Anteromedial bowing, associated with knee ligamentous instability and anatomic differences of the foot, which is typically in valgus position. Reconstruction vs. amputation depending on severity
7. Tibial hemimelia
   - Reconstruction vs. amputation depending on severity
8. Knee dislocation
   - Varying severity. Simplest form (hyperextension) generally responds to gentle manipulation and casting. All should undergo attempted serial splinting/casting for closed management.
   - Surgical procedure (open reduction, quadriceps plasty vs femoral shortening, ligamentous reconstruction) may be required.
   - More severe when associated with other syndromes.
9. Discoid lateral meniscus
   - Age: congenital lesion
   - Presentation: most common cause of clicking/clunking in pediatric knee
   - Imaging: continuous meniscal tissue on three sagittal MRI scans
   - **Look for three sequential MRI cuts that show the bow-tie shape of the anterior and posterior horns.**
   - Treatment: observation if asymptomatic; if painful or unstable at posterior horn (Watanabe type III), treat with saucerization ± stabilization
10. Osteochondritis dissecans (of knee)
    - **Osteochondritis dissecans of knee seen on the lateral surface of the medial femoral condyle; bone bruise from ACL rupture seen on the medial surface of the lateral femoral condyle**
    - Age: preteen/teen
    - Presentation: pain with use, local swelling; mechanical symptoms
    - Pathology: most commonly lesion is located on lateral surface of medial femoral condyle; may be associated with trauma
    - Imaging: can be seen best on a notch view with 30–50 degrees of knee flexion
      a. MRI classification system based on presence of fluid around the lesion (fluid surrounding lesion suggests poor prognosis, as does location on patella/lateral condyle)
    - Treatment: restricted weight bearing and immobilization initially, arthroscopic debridement if refractory to conservative efforts (retrograde drilling, excision)
11. Osgood-Schlatter disease
    - Age: teenage years
    - Presentation: anterior knee pain with exertion
    - Pathology: traction apophysitis of tibial tubercle

- Imaging: fragmentation of tibial tubercle or normal
- Treatment: symptomatic treatment predominates (ice/NSAIDs/quadriceps stretching); may require fragment excision persisting after maturity in severe cases.

12. Infantile Blount's disease
    - Age: up to 4 years
    - Presentation: overweight early walkers, bilateral
    - Pathology: abnormality in medial proximal tibial physis leading to genu varum with metaphyseal diaphyseal angle > 16 degrees
    - Important imaging/classification: Langenskiöld classification, based on degree of metaphyseal (early) and epiphyseal (late) deformity; progresses to complete bar formation
    - Treatment:
      a. Early (prior to epiphyseal changes) bracing if age < 3 years; if refractory in older patient (> 4 years), osteotomy to overcorrect deformity slightly to prevent recurrence
      b. Late: may require epiphysiolysis once bar has formed. Evolving indications for growth modulation as long as no bony bar present
13. Adolescent Blount's disease (age > 10 years): less severe and more often unilateral
    - Treatment: guided growth procedures (lateral epiphysiodesis)
14. Genu valgum
    - Age: normal from age 2–6, up to 15 degrees is within normal range
    - Pathology: persistent valgus in age > 6 years
    - Treatment: bracing usually ineffective; treatment with guided growth (medial growth modulation) if fails to resolve spontaneously
15. Posteromedial tibial bowing
    - Can be found normally or from oligohydramnios
      a. Associated with calcaneovalgus foot
    - Treatment: observe; spontaneous correction with resultant leg length discrepancy (~ 3 cm). May require either leg lengthening or contralateral epiphysiodesis in the future
16. Anteromedial tibial bowing/fibular hemimelia
    - Age: congenital
    - Pathology: anteromedial bowing, complete/partial absence of fibula, ball and socket ankle joint (secondary to subtalar coalition), equinovalgus foot, absence of lateral rays of the foot, ACL deficiency common, associated with PFFD
    - May require Syme amputation or below-knee amputation (BKA)
      a. BKA requires good quadriceps function and no knee flexion contracture. Reconstruction vs amputation depending on severity and patient preference
17. Anterolateral tibial bowing
    - **Anterolateral tibial bowing is seen in NF or fibrous dysplasia (FD), and conservative treatment for healing of a pseudoarthrosis is always attempted first. Pseudarthroses will not heal spontaneously; operative management needed. Preventative treatment includes clamshell orthosis to prevent fracture**
    - Age: congenital
    - Presentation: varies from bowing to complete pseudarthrosis
    - Pathology: most commonly congenital pseudarthrosis in setting of NF or FD
    - Treatment: total contact bracing initially, debridement/fixation with bone graft versus amputation if bracing fails

18. Clubfoot
   - Age: congenital
   - Presentation: foot positioned in cavus, adductus, varus, equinus
   - Pathology: deformed talar neck with plantar and varus orientation; shortening of surrounding soft tissue structures; equinovarus hindfoot, midfoot cavus, and forefoot supination and adductus; likely genetic contribution
   - Important imaging/classification: decreased talocalcaneal angle (< 35 degrees on lateral, < 20 degrees on AP), with talus and calcaneus becoming parallel. Imaging is less important. Clubfoot associated with spina bifida, arthrogryposis, etc., may not respond to ponseti. Presence of medial/posterior crease, muscle/neurologic abnormality portend worse treatment outcomes.
   - Treatment:
     a. **Treatment order can be remembered with the CAVE mnemonic: correct midfoot Cavus, hindfoot Adductus, hindfoot Varus, hindfoot Equinus.**
     b. Initial treatment is with casting (Ponseti casting), with first manipulation of supination to align first metatarsal with lateral rays; casting progresses to correct in the order CAVE; initial manipulation in cast is supination (elevation of first ray) to reduce cavus, lateral pressure on talar neck; requires weekly cast changes, and likely percutaneous tendon Achilles lengthening (TAL) prior to last cast
     c. Failed cast treatment may require posteromedial release. Complications: stiffness, recurrence, talonavicular subluxation
     d. If patient presents at age 3–10 years, treat with opening medial or lateral closing osteotomy.
     e. If patient presents at age 8–10 years with foot sensation, treat with triple arthrodesis.
   - Outcome
     a. Ponseti method: can have dynamic adduction/supination due to tibialis anterior overpull medially. Correct with split anterior tibial tendon transfer to lateral cuneiform.
        - Subtalar rigidity is a contraindication to transfer.
        - Outcome worse with extensive release. Surgical complications include dorsal bunion, osteonecrosis of talus, rigid pes planus, in-toeing gait.
        - Affected extremity usually smaller than contralateral normal extremity
        - Operative complication is dorsal bunion: strong toe flexors, weak peroneus longus, and weak gastroc/soleus complex with strong tibialis anterior results in flexion at first tarsometatarsal joint.
          - Treat with flexor hallucis longus (FHL) lengthening, dorsal capsulotomy, and flexor hallucis brevis (FHB) to extensor apparatus transfer
19. Calcaneovalgus foot
   - Age: Congenital
   - Presentation: foot hyperdorsiflexed, "stuck" on the front of the tibia; associated with posteromedial bowing and leg length discrepancy
   - Treatment: stretching/observation. Requires follow up for leg length discrepancy
20. Metatarsus adductus
   - **Associated with DDH**
   - Age: congenital
   - Presentation: apparent in-toeing
   - Pathology: associated with DDH
   - Treatment: depends on flexibility of foot
     a. If corrects to neutral with peroneal activation, usually responds to stretching

b. Passively correctable deformity treated with casting/bracing
c. Rigid deformity may require osteotomies (lateral shortening, medial lengthening), and usually are associated with a medial skin crease.

21. Skewfoot
  - Age: Congenital
  - Presentation: metatarsus adductus, lateral subluxation of navicular on the talus, valgus deformity of hindfoot
  - Important imaging/classification: AP X-ray of the foot will demonstrate multidirectional deformity
  - Treatment: nonoperative treatment is not indicated; each aspect of deformity is corrected with osteotomy in the affected segment
22. Congenital vertical talus
  - **Flexible flat foot is normal and can be seen due to ligamentous laxity; rigid flat foot is pathological and should be worked up.**
  - Age: Congenital
  - Presentation: rigid flat foot; associated with neural tube defects, arthrogryposis, rocker bottom deformity; need to rule out spinal abnormality
  - Pathology: dorsal dislocation of talonavicular joint
  - Important imaging/classification: oblique talus if talus lines up with metatarsal and navicular on plantarflexion lateral; vertical talus if anatomic axis of talus remains plantar to navicular and metatarsal on lateral X-ray with forced plantarflexion
  - Treatment: initially, stretching of dorsolateral tissue in preparation for surgery at age 6–12 months (always needed if vertical talus is present)
23. Tarsal coalition
  - Age: congenital lesion, but becomes symptomatic as coalition ossifies
  - Presentation: recurrent ankle sprains, pain/stiffness, rigid flatfoot, limited subtalar motion.
  - Pathology: abnormal connection between bones (most commonly calcaneonavicular followed by talocalcaneal)
  - Important imaging/classification: talar beaking may indicate presence of coalition, may require CT or MRI (most sensitive) to definitively assess
  - Treatment casting initially for all coalitions
    a. Calcaneonavicular: excision and interposed extensor digitorum brevis (EDB) or fat graft
    b. Subtalar (talocalcaneal): resection if < 50% middle facet, fusion if greater than or equal to 50% of the facet.
24. Flexible flatfoot
  - Generally bilateral, most often does not require treatment
  - University of California Biomechanics Laboratory (UCBL) orthosis is first line for painful flatfoot.
  - Lateral column lengthening and medial tightening may be used if refractory to other efforts.
25. Flatfoot in toddlers (ages 1–3 years)
  - Normal variant: as long as there is no pain or dysfunction, observation only
26. Accessory navicular
  - Age: congenital
  - Presentation: present in ~ 10% of population; if symptomatic, medial arch pain
  - Pathology: may be fused (cornuate) or separate bone within the posterior tibial tendon
  - Treatment: initially, immobilization/casting; recalcitrant cases, excision
  - Outcome: removal of accessory bone improves pain, but any associated deformity remains (flatfoot).

27. Cavus
    - Age: variable
    - Presentation: often progressive "high arched" foot
    - Pathology: may be due to neurologic pathology (tethered cord, CMT disease, etc.).
    - **Cavus foot can be secondary to neurologic abnormality; order spine MRI.**
    - Important imaging/classification: Coleman block test to evaluate rigidity of hindfoot deformity. If hindfoot varus corrects with the heel on block and first ray on the floor, only the forefoot needs to be addressed.
    - **Coleman block test evaluates if the hindfoot deformity is driven by the forefoot. If hindfoot varus corrects (supple deformity), then you only have to address the forefoot (see Fig. 10.46).**
    - Treatment
        a. Flexible hindfoot: plantar release, posterior tibial tendon transfer, dorsiflexion metatarsal osteotomy
        b. Rigid hindfoot: requires addition of lateralizing calcaneal osteotomy
        c. Severe rigid deformity: triple arthrodesis if all growth plates closed
28. Pediatric bunion (also see Chapter 10)
    - Age: usually present in preteen/teen years, bilateral common
    - Presentation: difficulty with shoe wear, pain
    - Pathology: associated with ligamentous laxity, familial inheritance; most pediatric bunions also have metatarsus primus varus
    - Treatment: accommodative shoe wear is primary; surgery for refractory cases
    - Outcome: recurrence is most common complication
29. Curly toes
    - May require release of toe flexors if symptomatic and fail conservative management
30. Polydactyly
    - Postaxial: AD inheritance
    - Normal motor milestones, not associated with syndromes
31. Limb length discrepancy
    - Normal expected growth in mm/year: proximal femur, 3; distal femur, 9; proximal tibia, 6; distal tibia, 3
    - Expected physis closure: females, ~ age 14 years; males, ~ age 16 years
    - Genu varum normal to age 2; after age 2 becomes genu valgum and becomes normal at age 4
    - Important imaging/classification: long leg films with ruler needed to determine source/severity of deformity. CT scanogram may be helpful if joint contractures are present.
    - Treatment: difference of 1 cm well tolerated and considered within normal limits
        a. If > 2 cm and < 5 cm, contralateral epiphysiodesis is planned depending on how much growth remains.
        b. If > 5 cm, lengthening is preferred. If > or equal to 5 cm, it should be lengthened
    - Outcome
        a. Lengthening procedures carry high complication rates (infection, nerve injury, nonunion). With intramedullary techniques, minor complications are reduced, but major complications (joint subluxation, nerve injury) persist.

Table 4.8 Common Limb Malalignments and Their Treatment

Age Group	In-Toeing	Treatment	Out-Toeing	Treatment
Infants	Metatarsus adductus	Observation, casting if refractory	Hip contracture (external rotation)	Observation
Toddlers	Internal tibial torsion	Observation unless severe (supramalleolar osteotomy age 7–10)	External tibial torsion	Observation unless severe (supramalleolar osteotomy age 7–10)
Children < 10 years	Femoral anteversion (W-sitters)	Observation	External femoral torsion	Observation

32. In-toeing/out-toeing (cite image from beginning of chapter)
    - Evaluate source with thigh–foot angle (15 degrees), foot progression angle, range of internal/external rotation (75/90 degrees in newborn, 55/45 degrees in 4-year-old) at the hip **(Table 4.8)**

XIV. Arthritis

1. Juvenile rheumatoid arthritis (JRA)
   - Age: most commonly 7–12 years, but can occur up to age 16
   - Presentation
     a. Oligoarticular
        - Four joints or fewer, usually larger joints
        - Can have eye involvement
     b. Polyarticular
        - Five or more joints, can involve cervical spine
        - Can have eye involvement
     c. Systemic
        - Small and large joints
        - Organ involvement
   - Pathology: autoimmune process of unclear etiology
   - Important imaging/classification: associated with iridocyclitis [most if antinuclear antibody (ANA) positive], needs ophthalmologic evaluation; serological evaluation not consistent for clinical diagnosis
   - Treatment: NSAIDs once septic arthritis has been ruled out
   - **Children with JRA require ophthalmology care.**
2. Transient synovitis
   - Most common cause of hip pain in childhood
   - Age: throughout childhood
   - Presentation: hip pain with movement; often follows viral illness
   - Pathology: unknown etiology; effusion causes pain
   - Important imaging/classification: the Kocher criteria are used to differentiate septic arthritis from transient synovitis: if three of the following criteria are positive, then 90% specific for septic arthritis; if only one, then likely to be transient synovitis:
     a. White blood cell count (WBC) > 12,000/mL
     b. Erythrocyte sedimentation rate (ESR) > 40
     c. Unable to bear weight
     d. Fever > 101.5
   - Treatment: NSAIDs once septic arthritis has been ruled out
   - Outcome: spontaneous resolution

3. Lyme disease
   - Age: any
   - Presentation: may have bull's-eye rash initially, but only present 80% of the time; migrating polyarthralgias
   - Pathology: caused by spirochete *Borrelia burgdorferi*
   - Treatment: doxycycline
   - Outcome: if caught early, can be eliminated; chronic lyme disease progresses to involve central nervous system
4. Septic arthritis
   - Age: the most likely bacterial infection varies with age **(Table 4.9)**
   - Presentation: pain, pseudoparalysis, fever
   - Pathology:
     a. Bacterial enzymes are toxic to chondrocytes, destroying articular surface rapidly
     b. Can spread from metaphyseal osteomyelitis in shoulder, elbow, ankle, hip (intra-articular metaphysis)
   - Important imaging/classification: if aspiration is negative with high clinical suspicion of septic joint, consider MRI to evaluate for synovitis.
   - Treatment: emergent irrigation and debridement indicated, followed by antibiotics
     a. Empiric antibiotics should include methicillin-resistant *Staphylococcus aureus* (MRSA) coverage (vancomycin)
   - Outcome: worse outcome predicted by delayed diagnosis, age < 6 months, associated osteomyelitis, or hip joint involvement
     a. Chronic septic arthritis results in destruction of the joint.
5. Osteomyelitis
   - Age: infectious organism varies with age **(Table 4.9)**
   - Presentation: variable acuity depending on causative organism, common result is pain
     a. Can be incited by local trauma with resultant hematogenous seeding
   - Pathology
     a. Involucrum: reactive bone
     b. Sequestrum: necrotic bone
     c. Most common bacteria is *S. aureus;* consider *Salmonella* if sickle cell patient
   - Treatment: intravenous (IV) antibiotics only if no abscess or necrotic bone (± percutaneous biopsy)
     a. Associated with deep venous thrombosis (DVT) if MRSA, surgery, C-reactive protein (CRP) > 6, age > 8 years
     b. Surgery indicated if no response to IV antibiotics alone; follow CRP to determine clinical effect

Table 4.9 Most Common Pediatric Infectious Agents

	Neonatal	Infantile	Toddler	Child	Adolescent
Community acquired	*Staphylococcus aureus,* group B streptococcus, *Escherichia coli, Klebsiella*	*S aureas, Kingella, Streptococcus pneumoniae, Neisseria meningitidis*	*S. Aureas, Kingella kingae, S. pneumoniae, N. meningitidis, Haemophilus influenzae*	*S. aureus,* group A streptococcus (GAS)	*S. aureus,* GAS, *Neisseria gonorrhoeae*
Nosocomial	*S. aureus, Streptococcus, Enterobacter, Candida*				

XV. Trauma

1. General
   - In polytrauma setting, patients with spine fractures have the highest mortality rate.
   - 75–80 mL average total blood volume per kg body weight
   - Those with head injury have the worst long-term prognosis.
   - Cast burns: increased risk with more layers of cast material, use of higher water temperature in prepration of cast, placement of a limb on a pillow while cast setting, higher with fiberglass overwrapped.
   - Consider intraosseous access if peripheral IV access unobtainable
2. Pediatric-specific fractures
   - Children's bones are more flexible than adults' and have a thicker periosteum, allowing incomplete fracture.
   - Torus/greenstick fractures
   - Physeal fractures
     a. Salter-Harris classification, types I–VI; increased risk of growth disturbance with increasing type
     b. Use mnemonic SALTR for Salter-Harris types I–V:
       - **S: type I, slipped (fracture through physis)**
       - **A: type II, above (fracture into metaphysis)**
       - **L: type III, lower (fracture into epiphysis)**
       - **T: type IV, through (fracture through metaphysis into physis and then exiting into epiphysis)**
       - **R: type V, rammed (crush injury to physis, diagnosed retroactively due to growth disturbance)**
       - **Type VI involves injury to perichondrial ring, can cause angular deformity**
   - Treatment
     a. MRI/CT scans can define location and extent of physeal involvement.
     b. Angular deformities treated by resection of physeal bar in those with > 2 cm of growth remaining and < 50% of physis involved
     c. Best success with young patients in peripheral physeal bars
     d. Growth arrest of > 50% of physis treated with ipsilateral growth arrest as well as contralateral epiphysiodesis/limb lengthening
3. Abuse
   - Presentation: scrapes/cuts most commonly, fractures second most
   - Risk factors
     a. Age < 3 years, multiple healing injuries/bruises, skin marks, burns, inconsistent history, neglect, delay in seeking care
   - Worrisome fractures
     a. Corner fractures; femur in nonambulatory patients; posterior rib; fractures in various stages of healing
   - Most common locations in order of frequency:
     a. Humerus, tibia, femur, diaphyseal, metaphyseal; diaphyseal is four times as common as metaphyseal; most common pattern is a single transverse fracture of a long bone
   - Greater than one third chance of further abuse if abuse is missed at initial presentation; 5–10% chance of mortality
4. Upper extremity
   - Birth injuries
     a. Occur at rate of 2:1,000 live births

b. Risk factors: large babies, shoulder dystocia, forceps delivery, breech position, prolonged labor

c. Categories
   - Erb-Duchenne syndrome: C5–C6, waiter's tip deformity (best prognosis)
   - Klumpke palsy: C8-T1 (poor prognosis)
   - Total plexus palsy: C5-T1, both sensory and motor (worst prognosis)
   - Treatment
     - ♦ Maintain passive ROM while motor returns (can take up to 18 months)
     - ♦ Release of subscapularis by age 2 can improve external rotation
     - ♦ Other options:
       - ▪ Contracture release
       - ▪ Latissimus/teres major transfers to external rotators
       - ▪ Tendon transfers to aid elbow flexion
       - ▪ Rotational humerus osteotomy
       - ▪ Microsurgical nerve grafting
   - Outcomes
     - ♦ Lack of biceps function at 6 months and Horner's syndrome are poor prognosticators.
     - ♦ Watch for fixed posterior shoulder dislocation because of muscle imbalance.

- Clavicle

a. Most frequent fracture in children, accounting for 8–15% of all pediatric fractures; most common obstetric fracture (accounting for 90% of fractures in delivery)

b. Mechanism: either direct, such as a blow to the clavicle, or indirect, such as a fall onto an outstretched hand; direct is more common and carries a higher risk of neurovascular/pulmonary injuries

c. Classified based on location: middle/medial/lateral thirds
   - 80% of fractures are middle third
   - 15% are lateral third
   - 5% are medial third
     - ♦ Medial fractures are normally Salter-Harris type I or II.
     - ♦ Lateral fractures are nondisplaced (type I) or displaced (type II).
     - ♦ Type II is further subdivided into IIA when fractured medial to coracoclavicular (CC) ligaments, and IIB when CC ligaments are torn.

d. Most clavicle fractures can be treated nonoperatively.

e. Treatment: based on location of fracture and age of patient
   - Absolute indications for operative treatment include open fractures, neurovascular compromise, and threatened skin not improved with closed reduction.
   - Medial fractures can be treated with a sling.
   - Midshaft fractures normally treated with sling for 4–6 weeks in patients age 2 or older, can treat supportively in patients younger than age 2
     - ♦ ORIF indicated if floating shoulder or potentially in polytraumatized patients; avoid treating with pins due to potential for migration
   - Lateral fractures most commonly treated with sling for 4–6 weeks; rare to require ORIF because CC ligaments remain attached to periosteal sleeve, so most patients with open physes can be treated only with sling; type IIA may require ORIF
   - Outcomes: complications rare in children
     - ♦ Periosteum protects deep structures

- ♦ Malunion rare due to high remodeling potential, possibility of cosmetic deformity from bony prominence
- ♦ Nonunion in 1–3%; never occurs in patients younger than age 12

• Acromioclavicular (AC) joint injuries

a. Mechanism: most commonly from direct blow onto acromion

b. Classification and treatment re the same as for adults; however, unlike AC injuries in adults, the CC ligaments remain intact in the pediatric population, with injury occurring through a split in the periosteum, with the distal aspect of the clavicle displacing superiorly.

• Sternoclavicular (SC) joint injuries

a. Mechanism: usually high-energy direct trauma to SC joint

b. Can be Salter-Harris type I or II fractures

c. Classification based on anterior or posterior displacement

d. Treatment: same as for adults; anterior high likelihood for recurrent dislocations though patients are often asymptomatic

e. Posterior require closed reduction in operating room (OR) with a thoracic surgeon available, given the risk to mediastinal structures

• Scapula

a. Accounts for 1–5% of fractures in adults and even rarer in children

b. Mechanism: in children, most of these fractures are a result of avulsions from glenohumeral joint injuries, and the remainder are from high-energy direct blows. Isolated scapula fractures are uncommon; suspect child abuse.

- ∘ High rate of other injuries, including to torso, chest, lung, and spinal column, as well as neurovascular injuries and other extremity injuries from high-energy trauma

c. Classified based on location:

- ∘ Body/neck make up > 50% of fractures
- ∘ Coracoid
- ∘ Acromion
- ∘ Glenoid

d. Treatment: most scapula fractures can be treated nonoperatively in either casting or with a sling.

- ∘ Indications for operative intervention vary by area.
- ∘ Body fractures that fail to unite may require partial excision.
- ∘ Scapula neck fractures associated with either clavicle fracture or instability are an indication for ORIF of the clavicle and scapula through a separate incision if displaced.
- ∘ Coracoid fractures that displace are associated with AC joint injury or lateral clavicle fracture and are an indication for ORIF.
- ∘ Acromion fractures that cause impingement should be treated with ORIF.
- ∘ Indications for ORIF of the glenoid include:
  - ♦ > 25% of glenoid surface and resultant instability
  - ♦ > 5 mm step-off
  - ♦ Subluxation of the humeral head
- ∘ Outcomes: most of the long-term sequelae of pediatric scapula fractures are due to associated injuries
  - ♦ Malunion can occur but is generally well tolerated.
  - ♦ Nonunion is extremely rare, but may require delayed ORIF with bone grafting.
  - ♦ Decreased motion may occur as a result of subacromial impingement.
  - ♦ Suprascapular nerve injury may result from fractures through the suprascapular notch.

- ♦ Posttraumatic osteoarthritis is rare but can be due to articular incongruity.

- Proximal humerus
  a. Ossification of proximal humerus occurs in stages: head ossified at 6 months of age, greater tuberosity between ages 1 and 3 years, and the lesser tuberosity between ages 4 and 5 years
  b. Mechanism: either direct, from a blow to the shoulder, or indirect, from a fall on an outstretched hand
  c. 90% of humeral growth occurs through the proximal humerus, making these fractures very amenable to nonoperative management.
  d. Neer-Horowitz classification system helps designate treatment:
    - Type I: < 5 mm displacement
    - Type II: < ⅓ humeral diameter displacement
    - Type III: ⅓–⅔ diameter displacement
    - Type IV: > ⅔ diameter displacement
    - Treatment: acceptable alignment dependent on age
      - ♦ Young children (age 1–4) can accept up to 70 degrees angulation and any amount of displacement
      - ♦ Older children (age 5–12): 40 degrees and 50% cortical contact
      - ♦ Adolescent (age 12-maturity): 20 degrees and no less than 70% cortical contact
    - Treatment is most commonly accomplished with closed reduction and a sling or coaptation splint.
      - ♦ Indications for open treatment:
        - Open fracture or neurovascular injury
        - Displaced intra-articular fracture
        - Irreducible fractures, commonly from interposed periosteum or biceps tendon
    - Outcomes: Because of the tremendous remodeling potential, most patients recover very well. Complications, such as avascular necrosis, loss of motion, and growth arrest, can occur, but do so more commonly in those treated surgically.

- Glenohumeral dislocations
  a. Vast majority occur in patients > age 10; > 90% are anterior
  b. Mechanism: either direct trauma to the shoulder or more commonly indirectly with forces transmitted through the humerus
    - Anterior dislocations commonly occur with the shoulder abducted, externally rotated and extended
    - Posterior dislocations occur with the shoulder adducted, internally rotated, and flexed and is usually due to seizure or shock
    - **Posterior dislocations because internal rotators are stronger than external rotators during muscular co-contraction.**
    - Treatment: Most shoulder dislocations can be treated with closed reduction and a brief period of sling immobilization for 2–4 weeks.
    - Most common cause of operative intervention is recurrent instability, age being the best predictor of recurrent dislocation.
      - ♦ > 60% recurrence when first dislocation occurs before age 21
      - ♦ 100% recurrence when initial dislocation occurs before age 10

- Humerus
  a. Cause of injury varies with age from birth injury to direct and indirect trauma in older children
  b. Mechanism: from a direct blow to the humerus, but can also occur from indirect trauma via a fall onto an outstretched hand

c. Treatment: very similar to that for adult humeral shaft fracture; a small percentage (~ 5%) can have a radial nerve palsy, which is usually transient and due to a traction injury

d. Fractures with <30 degrees of varus angulation can be treated nonoperatively in either a fracture brace or a sling
   - Children under age 3 can be treated either by pinning their shirt sleeve to the front of their shirt or by applying a sling and swathe.
   - Children age 3 and older can be treated in a fracture brace.
   - The following require operative intervention:
     - Open fractures
     - Polytrauma
     - Ipsilateral forearm or shoulder injuries

e. Outcomes: As with most pediatric fractures, outcomes are generally good, and malunion is well tolerated because of extensive shoulder ROM. Limb length discrepancy can occur but is most commonly asymptomatic.

f. Use the mnemonic Captain Roy Makes Trouble On Leave (or CRMTOL) for the elbow ossification order: Capitellum, Radial head, Medial epicondyle, Trochlea, Olecranon, Lateral epicondyle. These entities ossify in different ranges, but 2-year intervals is probably the easiest to remember.

- Elbow

a. Supracondylar humerus
   - Most common pediatric elbow fracture, accounting for half to three quarters of all pediatric elbow fractures
   - Peak is in age group 4–8 years, after which dislocations are more common
   - Mechanism: most commonly indirectly through a fall onto an outstretched hand, but occasionally due to a fall directly onto an elbow. These fractures are classified into flexion or extension types.
     - Extension type is the most common, accounting for 98% of supracondylar fractures

5. Gartland classification system:
   - Type I: nondisplaced
   - Type II: angulated with an intact posterior hinge/cortex
   - Type III: completely displaced
   - Treatment: Acceptable nonoperative treatment requires that the anterior humeral line intersects the anterior third of the capitellum. This can be achieved in type I and some type IIs. All type IIIs are operative.

a. Reduction can be obtained first in the coronal plane and then in the sagittal plane. This is done with extension and traction, then varus/valgus stress to correct the coronal plane, followed by an anterior force directed onto the olecranon while flexing the elbow. Reduction should be obtained

   - Can present with diminished/absent pulses. If pulses are absent then immediate closed reduction in the emergency room (ER) should be performed. If after closed reduction the hand remains pulseless and cool, then immediate reduction/pinning should be performed. If the hand remains perfused (without pulses), then surgery can be delayed.
   - Crossed pins have higher biomechanical stability than using only lateral pins, but they entail the risk iatrogenic injury to the ulnar nerve (medial pin). Pins are removed at 3–4 weeks.
   - The most devastating complication of supracondylar fractures would be compartment syndrome with Volkmann's ischemic contracture or vascular injury; occurs in < 1% of fractures.

- More common is a neurologic injury that occurs in ~ 10% of type III fractures; these are usually traction injuries, which can be observed.
- Extension type presents with anterior interosseous nerve (AIN) palsy (most common), and flexion type with ulnar palsy.
- Outcomes: can result in cubitus varus, which is primarily a cosmetic deformity that can be corrected at an older age with osteotomy.
- Lateral condyle
  a. Peak age is 6 years; these account for 15–20% of pediatric elbow fractures.
  b. Worse outcomes than with supracondylar fractures
     - Loss of motion
     - Missed/delayed diagnosis
     - Growth disturbance
     - Avascular necrosis
  c. Two classifications systems: Milch and Jakob
     - Milch I: Salter-Harris type IV
     - Milch II: Salter-Harris type II
  d. Jakob system better at guiding treatment
     - Jakob I: < 2 mm displacement, usually with intact articular surface (accounts for 40% of fractures)
     - Jakob II: 2–4 mm displaced
     - Jakob III: > 4 mm displaced
  e. Treatment: Jakob II and III are operative fractures. Jakob I is treated conservatively.
  f. Displacement/alignment best seen on internal oblique views
  g. Care must be taken to preserve posterior blood supply during ORIF
  h. Outcomes: can result in nonunion or late cubitus valgus, which can cause tardy ulnar nerve palsy
- Medial condyle
  a. Rare fractures, < 1% of all distal humerus fractures
  b. Occurs at ages 8–14 years
  c. Classifications and treatment are the same as those for lateral condyle fractures.
  d. Treatment: displaced fractures require ORIF
  e. Outcomes: complications can include nonunion, cubitus varus, osteonecrosis, or ulnar neuropathy
- Medial epicondyle
  a. Relatively common fracture; occurs at ages 10–12 years
  b. Can also occur chronically, known as Little League elbow, from flexor/pronator mass traction
  c. Treatment: up to 5–10 mm displacement can be treated with immobilization
     - Common to have fibrous union (up to 60%); however, > 90% have good/excellent function
  d. Rare indications for operative treatment
     - Incarcerated fragment in joint associated with dislocation
     - Displacement more than 1 cm
     - Associated ulnar nerve dysfunction
- Radial neck
  a. Peak incidence between ages 9 and 10 years
  b. Mechanism: commonly from a fall onto an outstretched hand, rarely due to direct trauma because of overlying muscular cushion

c. Associated with olecranon, medial epicondyle, and coronoid fractures
d. Most commonly a Salter-Harris type I or II fracture because of thick cartilage cap on radial head
e. O'Brien classification based on extent of angulation:
    - Type I: < 30 degrees
    - Type II: 30–60 degrees
    - Type III: > 60 degrees
f. Treatment
    - If angulation < 30 degrees, treat with splinting for 7–10 days, and then begin ROM exercises.
    - Require reduction if angulation > 30 degrees
        - ♦ Best accomplished with traction and varus stress with elbow supinated and extended
    - Require open reduction in pinning if:
        - ♦ Unstable postreduction
        - ♦ > 60 degrees angulation
        - ♦ > 4 mm displacement
    - After pinning, the arm should be casted in pronation and flexion
g. Outcomes: 15–25% of these fractures have a poor outcome, most commonly loss of ROM
    - Age < 10 years, < 30 degrees angulation: early and closed treatment have better prognoses
    - Late complications include radial head overgrowth in 20–40%, early physeal closure, posterior interosseous nerve (PIN) injury, synostosis, and osteonecrosis of the radial head
h. Elbow dislocation
    - Peak incidence at ages 13–14 years; occurs most often after physes are closed
    - Mechanism: fall onto a hyperextended arm with valgus stress; can also occur when a posterior force strikes a flexed elbow
    - Associated with multiple fractures, including medial epicondyle, radial head/neck, coronoid
    - Classified based on direction of displacement
        - ♦ Posterolateral account for > 90%
        - ♦ Anterior and divergent are rare
    - Treatment: closed reduction is the treatment of choice, followed by splinting, and then early active ROM beginning a week after injury.
    - Operative intervention may be necessary in these cases:
        - ♦ Postreduction incongruency that may be due to interposed medial epicondyle
        - ♦ Large associated coronoid fractures; may require ORIF
    - Outcomes: full recovery of motion and strength may take up to 6 months.
    - The most common complication is loss of terminal extension.
        - ♦ Neurologic injury occurs in up to 10%; if no improvement seen after 3 months, EMG and exploration warranted
        - ♦ Recurrent instability in < 1%
        - ♦ Heterotopic ossification occurs in 3–20%; greater risk with associated fractures
        - ♦ Vascular injury and compartment syndrome are rare, but have been reported
    - Distal humerus physeal separation

- ♦ Most common in infants
- ♦ Mechanism: due to birth injury, child abuse, or falls with hyperextension of the elbow
- ♦ In children younger than 3 years, it is a Salter-Harris type I fracture; in older children it is a Salter-Harris type II fracture.
- ♦ Most commonly displaces posteromedially
- ♦ Treatment: closed reduction and percutaneous pinning
- ♦ Outcomes: late complications include avascular necrosis of the medial condyle and cubitus varus

- ◦ Nursemaid's elbow
  - ♦ Mechanism: pulling on extended arm
    - ▪ Male-to-female ratio = 1:2
    - ▪ Left elbow ¾ of the time
    - ▪ Peak ages 2–3 years
  - ♦ Patient refuses to supinate/pronate, flex/extend elbow
  - ♦ Treatment: reduce by flexion and supination
  - ♦ Outcomes: recurrence in 5–30% of patients
- ◦ Olecranon
  - ♦ Peak age 5–10 years
  - ♦ One in five associated with other fractures, radial head/neck most commonly
  - ♦ **Commonly seen in OI**
  - ♦ Classified based on mechanism/pattern of injury
    - ▪ Flexion
    - ▪ Extension
      - • Varus
      - • Valgus
    - ▪ Shear
  - ♦ Treatment: based on pattern
    - ▪ Flexion: splinted in 5–10 degrees of flexion
    - ▪ Extension: correction of varus/valgus, splinting/casting
    - ▪ Splint/cast in hyperflexed position, posterior periosteum is intact and functions essentially as a tension band
  - ♦ Operative intervention required if there is displacement > 3 mm or comminution.

- Forearm

  a. Majority occur in children age > 5 years; most common during peak growth

  b. Mechanism: an indirect mechanism due to fall onto outstretched hand
  - ◦ Pronated hand = dorsal angulation
  - ◦ Supinated hand = volar angulation

  c. Treatment: most are treated with closed reduction and casting
  - ◦ Angulation corrects at ~1 degree/month or 10 degrees/year.
  - ◦ Up to 1cm of bayonet apposition is acceptable under age 10 years.
  - ◦ Rotation does not correct with growth.

  d. Acceptable nonoperative alignment varies by age/gender/fracture location
  - ◦ Females < 8 years and males < 10 years can accept 20 degrees in distal third, 15 degrees middle third, and 10 degrees proximal third.
  - ◦ Proximal fractures should be casted in supination, distal in pronation, middle in neutral rotation. This is especially important with greenstick injuries.

- Ratio of cast depth on AP to width (radioulnar) > 0.85 is associated with fracture displacement in cast.
- Radial styloid and biceps tuberosity should be 180 degrees apart.
- When treating operatively, intramedullary constructs and plating are associated with similar correction of radial bow.

- Monteggia fractures account for < 1% of forearm fractures in children.
  a. Most common in ages 4–9 years
  b. Classification is the Bado system, based on direction of radial head dislocation
    - Type I: anterior dislocation (most common in children)
    - Type II: posterior dislocation (most common in adults)
    - Type III: lateral dislocation
    - Type IV: radial head dislocation with radial shaft fracture
  c. Radial head dislocations are a variant of Monteggia injuries that occur with a plastic ulnar deformity.
  d. Treatment: nonoperative treatment can be accomplished in children age < 10 years, with < 10 degrees angulation and a located radial head postreduction.
    - Cast in up to 110 degrees flexion with full supination; this relaxes the biceps and tightens the interosseous membrane.
  e. Operative intervention required in these cases:
    - Ulnar comminution
    - Bado type IV injuries
    - Loss of, or unacceptable, reduction
  f. Outcomes: most common complications are nerve injury, commonly PIN (15–20% incidence) and heterotopic ossification (<10% incidence)
- Distal radius
  a. Very common physeal fracture in children
  b. Treatment: Salter-Harris types I and II can be treated with closed reduction and casting.
    - Acceptable alignment requires > 50% apposition, and no angular/rotational deformity can be accepted.
  c. Salter-Harris types III, IV, and V require ORIF; increasing type number correlates with increasing likelihood of growth disturbance
  d. Can lead to radial growth arrest, which is associated with:
    - Reduction > 7 days after injury
    - Multiple reduction attempts
- Galeazzi: radial shaft fracture with distal radioulnar joint (DRUJ) dislocation
  a. Peak incidence at age 9–12 years; rare injury, occurring in only 3% of children
  b. Classified based on position of radius in DRUJ dislocation
    - Dorsal displacement is associated with a supination force.
    - Volar is caused by a pronation force.
    - Treatment: reduction is obtained by using an oppositely directed force:
      - Pronation for dorsal injuries, supination for volar injuries
      - Acceptable alignment is based on age/angulation/displacement of radius fracture.
      - Treated by closed reduction and casting most commonly
      - Outcomes: persistent ulnar subluxation is the most common cause of malunion in these injuries.

6. Lower extremity
   - Pelvis

a. Mechanism: occurs from either high-energy mechanism causing disruption of ring or from avulsions
    - Hamstrings/adductors avulse from ischium
    - Sartorius avulses from anterior superior iliac spine (ASIS)
    - Rectus femoris avulses from anterior inferior iliac spine (AIIS)
    - Abdominals avulse from iliac crest
    - Iliopsoas avulse from lesser trochanter
b. Classified by Torode and Zieg and by Tile
    - Torode and Zieg:
        - ♦ Type I: avulsions
        - ♦ Type II: iliac wing
        - ♦ Type III: simple ring without instability
        - ♦ Type IV: ring with instability
    - Tile:
        - ♦ Type A: stable
        - ♦ Type B: rotationally unstable
        - ♦ Type C: rotationally and vertically unstable
c. Treatment: most can be treated nonoperatively with bedrest for 2–6 weeks, followed by progressive weight bearing
    - Operative intervention for unstable patterns with open-book injuries
    - Skeletal traction may be necessary for an unstable hip fracture dislocation.
    - Outcomes: malunion/nonunion is rare, though leg length discrepancy can occur with fractures that are vertically unstable.

- Hip

a. Mechanism: high-energy direct trauma responsible for the majority of cases
b. Major concern is disruption of blood supply to the femoral head
c. Delbet Classification system:
    - Type IA: nondisplaced transepiphyseal
    - Type IB: displaced transepiphyseal
    - Type II: transcervical
    - Type III: cervicotrochanteric
    - Type IV: intertrochanteric
d. Risk of avascular necrosis decreases with increasing type: nearly 100% in type IB, 50% in type II, 20–30% in type III, and less common in type IV.
e. Treatment: most pediatric hip fractures are operative, and treatment is based on type of fracture:
    - Type I: closed/open reduction and smooth/threaded pins based on patient age (smooth pins for younger children)
    - Type II: spica cast for nondisplaced versus closed reduction and pinning for displaced fractures, avoiding transphyseal pins
    - Type III: nondisplaced treated initially with traction, then spica cast in abduction; open/closed reduction with pinning if displaced, avoiding transphyseal pins
    - Type IV: nondisplaced treated with spica; displaced or unable to hold reduction in spica require ORIF
f. Outcomes: about 40% of pediatric hip fractures go on to develop avascular necrosis; growth arrest may occur in over half, especially if pins cross the physis; varus deformity or nonunion occur in 10–20% due to inadequate reduction or fixation; may require late valgus osteotomy with bone grafting. Choose good fixation over physis preservation

- Hip dislocations
   a. Mechanism: occurs at ages 2–5 years due to ligamentous laxity and softer cartilage, with another peak at ages 11–15 years due to sports and high-energy trauma.
   b. Classified based on anterior/posterior dislocation; posterior is more common
   c. Treatment: closed reduction, open if unable to achieve congruent reduction
   d. Outcomes: complications include avascular necrosis (10%), fractures either at time of injury or reduction, nerve injury in 2–10%, damage to cartilage in 5–10%
- Femur
   a. Most common at ages 2–4 years and in adolescents
   b. Mechanism: in young children who are nonambulatory, most are caused by abuse; ambulatory patients are less likely to experience abuse. Most adolescent femur fractures are due to high-energy trauma.
   c. Acceptable alignment is based on age:
      - Age < 2: 30 degrees varus/valgus, 30 degrees anterior/posterior, up to 1.5 cm shortening
      - Ages 2–5: 15 degrees varus/valgus, 20 degrees anterior/posterior, and 2 cm shortening
      - Ages 6–10: 10 degrees varus/valgus, 15 degrees anterior/posterior, 1.5 cm shortening
      - Age 11 to adulthood: 5 degrees varus/valgus, 10 degrees anterior/posterior, 1 cm shortening
   d. Treatment is based on age:
      - Younger than 6 months: Pavlik harness. Add relative contraindication to flexible nails if weight >110 lb or comminution
      - 6 months to 5–6 years: spica cast, may require traction if > 2.3 cm shortened, can also consider flexible nails/external fixator if shortened
      - 6–11 years: flexible nails if stable, ORIF/external fixation if unstable or proximal/distal fracture
      - Older than 11 years: possible flexible nails, but more commonly antegrade nail/lateral trochanteric entry nail if unstable
   e. Outcomes: malunion/nonunion in children is rare; piriformis nail associated with femoral head osteonecrosis; up to 2 cm of overgrowth can occur with spica casting, and most of the overgrowth occurs in the first 2 years after fracture; pulling traction through spica increases risk of compartment syndrome
- Distal femoral physis
   a. Majority are Salter-Harris type II fractures and occur in adolescents
   b. Mechanism: due to either high-energy trauma or varus/valgus or hyperflexion/extension injury
   c. Treatment: nonoperative treatment can be used for nondisplaced fractures; consists of long leg casting for 4–8 weeks
   d. Displaced or intra-articular fractures require open reduction and fixation most commonly with partially threaded cannulated screws. Salter-Harris type II fractures can be treated with percutaneous fixation after adequate closed reduction.
   e. Outcomes: complications include vascular injury, peroneal injury, instability, late deformity, stiffness, and premature physeal closure.
   f. Risk factors:
      - Displaced fracture (50–60% of growth arrest)
      - Fixation across physis
      - Surgical treatment

- Inadequate reduction

- Patella
  a. Very rare fracture, less than < 1% of fractures in children under age 16
  b. Mechanism: either from direct trauma to the patella (most commonly) or from sudden acceleration to the quadriceps
     - Patella sleeve fracture is an avulsion of cartilage by patellar tendon resulting in patella alta; requires surgical repair
  c. Treatment: fractures with < 3 mm of intra-articular displacement or 3 mm of diastasis can be treated in a long leg cast in extension if the extensor mechanism is intact.
  d. Displaced fractures require ORIF with sutures, screws, or tension band.
  e. Outcomes: can result in posttraumatic arthritis because of cartilage damage at time of injury or persistent articular step-off. Late complications include patella alta and quadriceps weakness.
- Knee dislocation
  a. Mechanism: high-energy injury
  b. High risk of vascular injury; check ankle-brachial index (ABI); risk of vascular injury low if ABI > 0.9
  c. Must be treated with emergent closed reduction, followed by monitoring for neurovascular compromise and compartment syndrome
- Proximal tibia
  a. Average age of occurrence: 14 years
  b. Mechanism: can occur due to high-energy direct trauma or from low-energy plant and twist mechanisms
     - Knee dislocation equivalent (check ABI)
  c. Treatment: nondisplaced fractures can be treated in a long leg cast.
  d. Displaced fractures or those with intra-articular extension require ORIF with pins or screws followed by casting.
  e. Late complications include angular deformity or growth disturbance due to premature closure of the physis.
     - In toddlers, proximal tibia fractures (Cozen fractures) are prone to valgus deformity due to medial overgrowth. This commonly corrects with growth and does not require intervention.
- Tibial spine
  a. ACL tear equivalent
  b. Mechanism: common after falls, indirect plant/twisting mechanisms
  c. Meyers and McKeever classification:
     - Type I: minimal/no displacement
     - Type II: anterior spine elevated, posterior not fractured
     - Type III: completely displaced spine
     - Type IV: comminuted
     - 80% are type I and II
  d. Essential to test medial collateral ligament (MCL)/lateral collateral ligament (LCL) for associated injury
  e. Treatment: types I and II can be casted in extension for 4–6 weeks; hemarthrosis can be aspirated under sterile conditions to aid in reduction of type II fractures.
     - Types III and IV require operative fixation with arthroscopy and ACL guide with the use of suture/pins/screws.
  f. Outcomes: more than half have some degree of loss of extension, either from stiffness or from malunion of type III fractures. Instability can occur if collateral ligament injury unrecognized.
- Tibial tubercle

a. Most common in males ages 14–16 years
b. Mechanism: due to sudden acceleration of quadriceps tendon. Risk factors are tight hamstrings, patella baja, Osgood-Schlatter disease, and physeal anomaly.
c. Watson-Jones classification:
  ◦ Type I: small fragment through secondary ossification center
  ◦ Type II: secondary ossification center fused with proximal epiphysis; fracture at level of proximal physis
  ◦ Type III: fracture through tibial epiphysis
  ◦ Treatment: majority of these fractures are operative. Nondisplaced type I fractures can be treated in a long leg cast in extension for 4–6 weeks.
    ♦ Remainder of fractures require ORIF with pins/screws/tension band construct; long leg cast in extension for 4–6 weeks
  ◦ **Outcomes: risk of compartment syndrome due to tearing of the recurrent anterior tibial artery**
d. Late complications: genu recurvatum from anterior physeal closure, patella alta from loss of reduction, knee stiffness and osteonecrosis of the fracture fragment

• Tibia
a. Average age of occurrence is 8 years; second most common fracture in child abuse
b. Mechanism: spiral tibia fractures with intact fibula are commonly due to low-energy twisting mechanism, whereas injuries with ipsilateral tibia and fibula fractures are more commonly due to high-energy mechanisms.
c. Toddler's fractures occur in young children and should be suspected in a child with normal X-rays who refuses to bear weight and has tibial tenderness.
d. Treatment: 95% can be treated with closed reduction and casting, given the thigh periosteum as well as the more common low-energy mechanisms.
  ◦ Up to age 12 years can correct 50% of angular deformity; age > 13 can correct less than 25% of angular deformity
e. Operative indications:
  ◦ Ipsilateral femur fracture
  ◦ Open injury
  ◦ Compartment syndrome
  ◦ Vascular injury
  ◦ Unable to maintain reduction in cast
f. Outcome:
  ◦ Time to union can be up to 12 weeks in adolescents, but malunion and nonunion are rare in children.

• Ankle
a. Most common in ages 8–15 years
b. Mechanism: due to twisting or less commonly from axial loading
c. Lauge-Hansen classification similar to that in adults, but these are physeal injuries:
  ◦ Supination–external rotation
  ◦ Supination–plantar flexion
  ◦ Supination–inversion (most common)
  ◦ Pronation–eversion–external rotation
d. Pediatric-specific ankle fractures are Tillaux and triplane
  ◦ Triplane occurs in ages 12–14 females, 13–15 males
    ♦ Triplane due to external rotation of the ankle through the physis in all three planes (axial/sagittal/coronal) (Saler Harris IV)

- Tillaux occurs in ages 13–16 years (usually older than triplane children)
  - Tillaux fractures due to avulsion of the anteroinferior tibiofibular ligament from anterolateral tibia (Saler Harris III)
- Treatment:
  - Nondisplaced fractures can be treated in a cast.
  - Operative indications:
    - Tillaux: > 2 mm vertical displacement or > 3 mm horizontal displacement
    - Triplane: > 2 mm articular step-off
    - Other fractures with intra-articular step-off > 2 mm: treatment is with open or closed reduction and fixation followed by casting
- Outcomes: complications include angular deformity from physeal arrest, leg length discrepancy, and posttraumatic arthritis from intra-articular step-off. Angular deformity/physeal arrest can sometimes be treated with epiphysiodesis, but in more mature patients may require osteotomy.

- Foot
  a. Tarsal fractures are rare in children.
  b. Talus fractures usually occur through the talar neck.
     - Operative indications include > 5-degree angulation or 5 mm displacement; most common complication is avascular necrosis.
  c. Calcaneus fractures are most commonly extra-articular and involve the apophysis; associated with lumbar spine and ipsilateral leg injuries
     - Operative indications include displaced intra-articular fractures as well as displaced anterior process fractures (high risk of nonunion).
  d. Lisfranc injury is extremely rare in children.
     - Operative indications include displacement more than 2 mm, angular deformity, dislocation that cannot be maintained in a cast
  e. Base of the fifth metatarsal fractures are different in children due to the apophysis; present beginning at age 8 and fuses at age 12 in females, age 15 in males
     - Treatment is the same as in adults.
  f. Phalanx fractures are as common in children as in adults; proximal first metatarsal most common foot fracture before age 5 years
     - Most are treated with closed reduction and buddy taping.
  g. Seymour fractures are Salter Harris fractures of the distal phalanx that involve the nail bed. They require irrigation and debridement along with pinning.
     - **These are frequently missed injuries that present late**

7. Spine (see Chapter 5)
   - Majority of spinal cord injuries occur under age 8 years
   - Due to elasticity of pediatric spine
   - Can have multiple causes:
     a. Transverse atlantal ligament injury
     b. Interspinous ligament injury
     c. Fracture through vertebral endplates
   - MRI can be helpful to diagnose
     a. Spinal cord injury without radiographic abnormality (SCIWORA) (defined before advent of MRI)
   - Treatment: based on location and severity of injury, generally external immobilization for up to 12 weeks

5

Spine

Matthew McDonnell, Alan H. Daniels, and Mark A. Palumbo

I. Anatomy of the Spine

1. Bony anatomy
   - **Because there are seven cervical vertebrae and eight cervical nerve roots, roots exit above their respective vertebrae until C8 exits below the C7 vertebrae. After this, thoracic and lumbar nerve roots exit below their respective vertebrae. This is important to understand when evaluating potential root impingement.**
   - Thirty-three vertebrae (seven cervical, 12 thoracic, five lumbar, five sacral, four fused coccygeal) comprise the osseous components of the spinal column **(Fig. 5.1)**.
2. Alignment
   - Cervical lordosis
   - Thoracic kyphosis (normal 20–40 degrees; average 35 degrees)
   - Lumbar lordosis (normal 40–70 degrees; average 55–60 degrees)
   - Sacral kyphosis
3. Topographic anatomy **(Table 5.1)**
   - **Topographic anatomy is important in planning your incision for surgical approaches.**
4. Cervical spine **(Fig. 5.2)**
   - C1 (atlas) consists of anterior arch, posterior arch, two lateral masses; has no vertebral body or spinous process
     a. C1 articulates with occipital condyles of skull via two superior-oriented facets.
     b. Occiput–C1 (atlanto-occipital) articulation responsible for ~ 50% of the neck flexion/extension arc
     c. Structures at risk during surgery: internal carotid artery from penetration of anterior cortex of C1 lateral mass; vertebral artery from lateral dissection on the posterior arch
   - C2 (axis) consists of a vertebral body and the dens (odontoid process), which articulates with the anterior arch of C1 via a diarthrodial joint.
     a. Synchondrosis between dens and body fuses around age 7
     b. Atlantoaxial C1-C2 articulation provides for ~ 50% of neck axial rotation

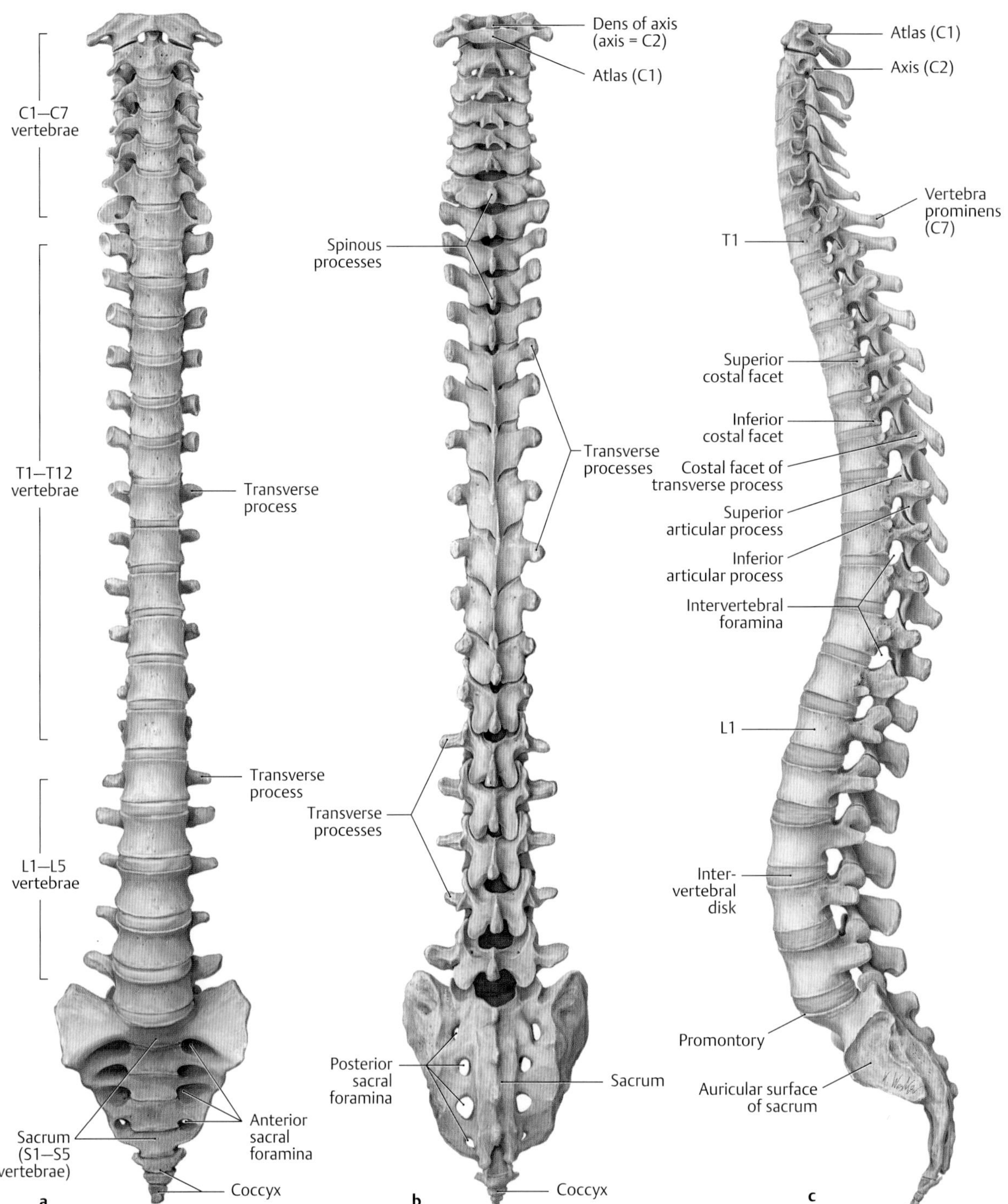

Fig. 5.1 The bony spinal column **(a)** Anterior view, **(b)** posterior view, **(c)** left lateral view. Note that, phylogenetically, the transverse processes of the lumbar vertebrae are rudimentary ribs. They are often known as costal processes therefore. (From Schuenke M, Schulte E. General Anatomy and the Musculoskeletal System: Thieme Atlas of Anatomy. New York: Thieme; 2005. Illustration by Karl Wesker.)

- Atlantoaxial joint complex
  a. Alar and transverse ligaments impart stability **(Fig. 5.3)**.
- **Know the plane in which these ligaments resist translation.**
  a. Transverse ligament attaches the posterior odontoid to each lateral mass of the atlas; major stabilizer of C1-C2; resists sagittal plan translation

b. Alar ligaments run obliquely from tip of dens to occiput; resists lateral translation of odontoid **(Fig. 5.4)**.

c. Vertebral artery travels in transverse foramina of C6 through C2, then travels through the transverse process and along the top of arch of C1

d. Carotid tubercle is anterior tubercle of transverse process of C6

5. Thoracic spine
   - T1 spinous process is long and prominent.
   - Spinous processes are angled and overlap the subadjacent level.
   - Costal facets allow articulation with ribs (present on thoracic vertebrae 1–12 and thoracic transverse processes of T1 through T9).
   - Articulations with rib cage make thoracic spine a stable region of vertebral column.
6. Lumbar spine
   - Large bodies are taller anteriorly than posteriorly, contributing to lumbar lordosis.
   - Laminae increasingly overlap the disk space level, moving from caudal to cranial; relevant when performing laminotomy for herniated nucleus pulposus (HNP) in mid/upper lumbar region
   - Sacralization of L5: transverse process of fifth vertebra fused to sacrum unilaterally or bilaterally
   - Lumbarization of S1: first sacral segment with rudimentary disk leading to additional motion segment (i.e., six lumbar vertebra)
   - **Recognizing sacralization or lumbarization is important when localizing the operative level in lumbar surgery and when placing iliosacral screws.**
   - Large-diameter pedicles; however, L1 and L2 pedicles have smaller diameter than T11 and T12

     a. Smallest pedicle isthmic width: L1
   - Pars interarticularis: osseous segment between superior and inferior articular processes; defect results in spondylolysis

     a. Posterior elements bear 20% of biomechanical load in upright position.
   - Iliolumbar ligament

     a. Stout ligament attaching transverse process of L5 to ilium

     b. Provides stability to lumbopelvic articulation; may be disrupted or avulsed from L5 transverse process in unstable vertical shear pelvic injuries
   - L5 nerve root is relatively fixed and is draped over the sacral ala; at risk from displaced sacral fractures and misplaced iliosacral screws (anterior)
7. Sacrum
   - Structure formed by fusion of five embryological sacral vertebrae
   - Four pairs of sacral foramina allow passage of ventral and dorsal branches of first four sacral nerve roots
   - Sacral canal opens caudally to sacral hiatus; contains fifth sacral root

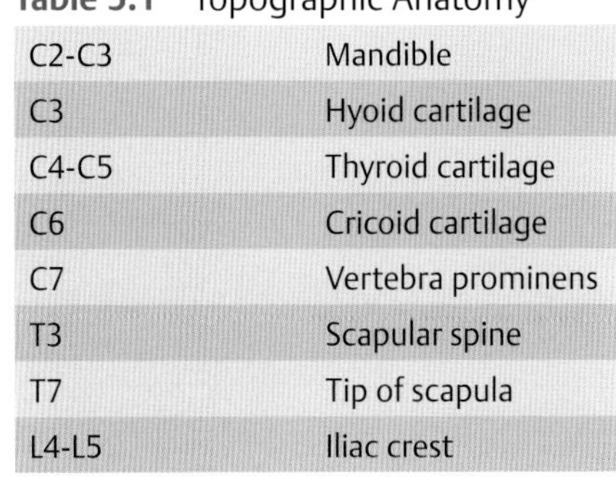

Table 5.1 Topographic Anatomy

Level	Landmark
C2-C3	Mandible
C3	Hyoid cartilage
C4-C5	Thyroid cartilage
C6	Cricoid cartilage
C7	Vertebra prominens
T3	Scapular spine
T7	Tip of scapula
L4-L5	Iliac crest

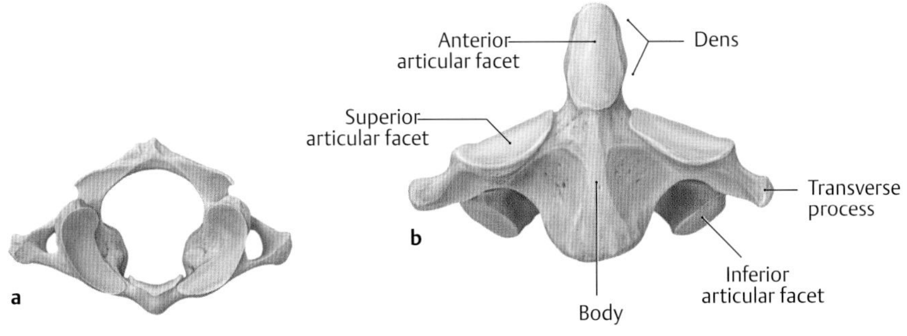

Fig. 5.2 **(a)** First cervical vertebra (atlas). **(b)** Second cervical vertebra (axis) (From Schuenke M, Schulte E. General Anatomy and the Musculoskeletal System: Thieme Atlas of Anatomy. New York: Thieme; 2005. Illustration by Karl Wesker.)

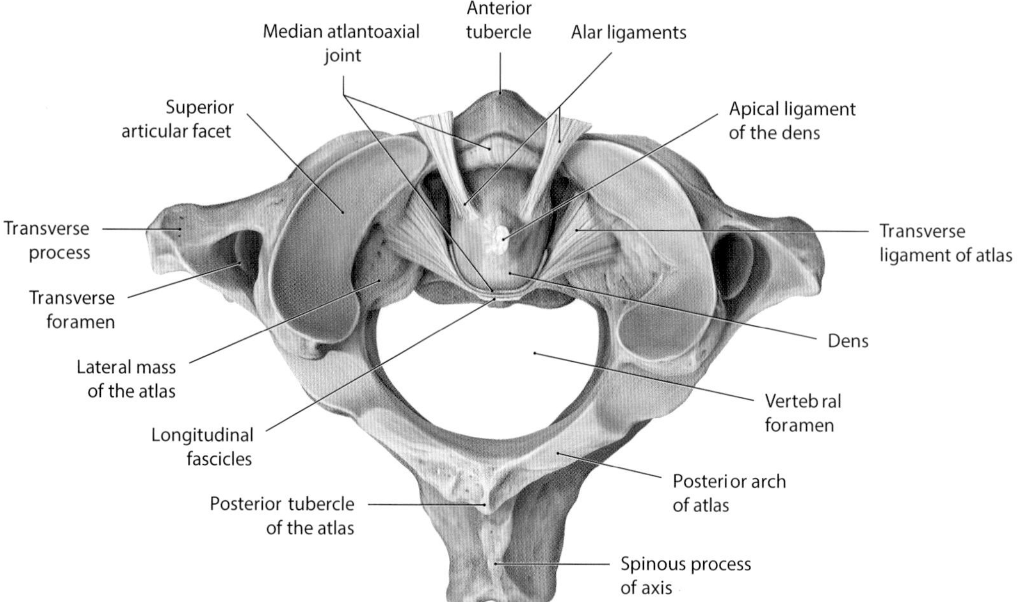

Fig. 5.3 The ligaments of the median atlantoaxial joint. Atlas and axis,superior view.(The fovea, while part of the median atlantoaxial joint, is hidden by the joint capsule.) (From Schuenke M, Schulte E. General Anatomy and the Musculoskeletal System: Thieme Atlas of Anatomy. New York: Thieme; 2005. Illustration by Karl Wesker.)

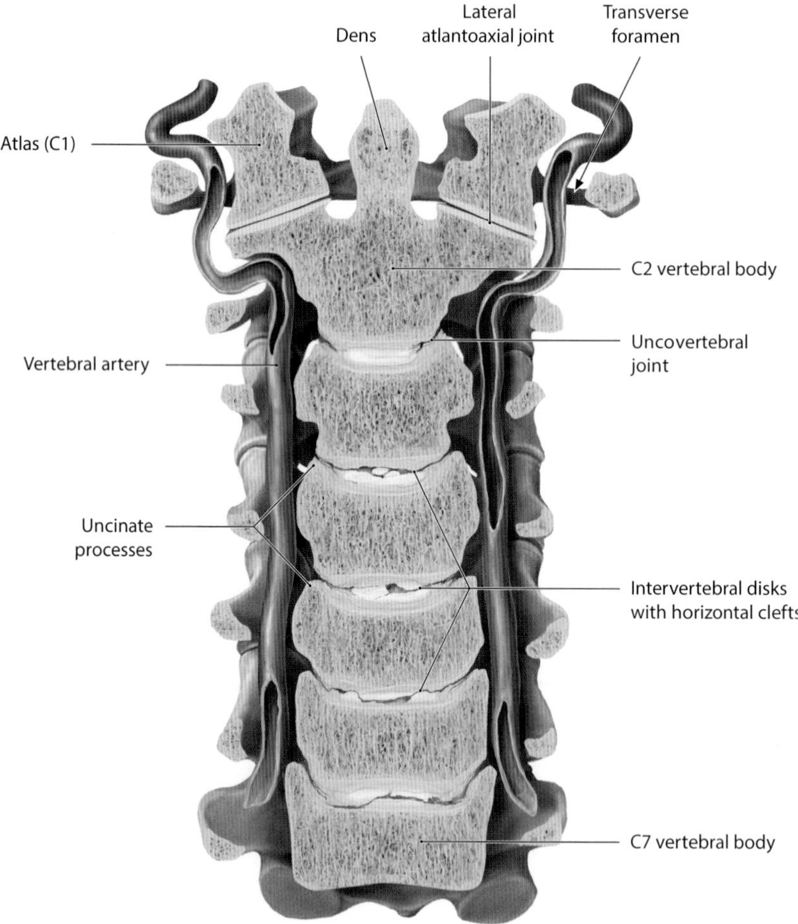

Fig. 5.4 Degenerative changes in the cervical spine (uncovertebral arthrosis). Coronal section through the cervical spine of a 35-year-old man, anterior view. Note the course of the vertebral arteries on both sides of the vertebral bodies. The development of the uncovertebral joints at approximately 10 years of age initiates a process of cleft formation in the intervertebral disks. This process spreads toward the center of the disk with aging, eventually resulting in the formation of complete transverse clefts that subdivide the intervertebral disks into two slabs of roughly equal thickness. The result is a progressive degenerative process marked by flattening of the disks and consequent instability of the motion segments (drawing based on specimens from the Anatomical Collection at Kiel University). (From Schuenke M, Schulte E. General Anatomy and the Musculoskeletal System: Thieme Atlas of Anatomy. New York: Thieme; 2005. Illustration by Karl Wesker.)

8. Spinal ligaments: contribute to spinal stability **(Fig. 5.5)**
   - Anterior longitudinal ligament (ALL)
     a. Thicker centrally than peripherally
     b. Generally thicker than posterior longitudinal ligament
     c. Strong and resists extension
   - Posterior longitudinal ligament (PLL)
     a. Thicker over vertebral body, thinner yet wider over disks
   - **Annular tears (and disk herniation) typically occur lateral to PLL expansion where it is weakest**

     b. Resists hyperflexion of vertebral column
   - Ligamentum flavum (LF)
     a. Strongest spinal ligament, elastic
     b. Runs from anterior surface of superior lamina to cranial surface of inferior lamina
     c. Functions to maintain extension of adjacent vertebrae
     d. Hypertrophy of LF contributes to neural element compression in degenerative spinal disorders
   - Interspinous ligaments **(Fig. 5.6)**
   - Supraspinous ligament: above C7 is continuous with ligamentum nuchae; limits flexion of vertebral column
9. Intervertebral disk (IVD) complex
   - IVD along with vertebrae above and below and along with associated facet joints at each level form the functional spinal unit (FSU)
   - Annulus fibrosis: outer, obliquely oriented, composed of type I collagen; highest tensile modulus to resist torsional, axial, and tensile loads
   - Nucleus pulposus: inner, type II collagen, predominantly water (decreases with aging, converted to fibrocartilage)
   - Lumbar spine intradiscal pressure highest in the sitting/flexed position with weights in hands; lowest in supine position
10. Facet joints
    - Orientation varies by spinal level and dictates plane of motion.
      a. Cervical: superior articular facets of the subaxial cervical spine (C3-C7) are oriented in a posteromedial direction at C3 and posterolateral direction at C7; variable transition between C3 and C7
      b. Thoracic: coronal plane orientation; resists translation and axial rotation but allows for sagittal plane motion
      c. Lumbar: superior articular facets oriented in posteromedial direction. Orientation is more vertical in sagittal plane in upper lumbar spine and becomes more coronal as you move in a caudal direction; coronal orientation resists anterior translation, vertical orientation resists axial rotation **(Fig. 5.7)**
    - Position of superior articular facet in relation to inferior articular process:
      a. Cervical spine: anterior and inferior
      b. Lumbar spine: anterior and lateral
    - Superior margin of superior articular process often contributes to nerve root compression in lumbar foraminal stenosis
11. Spinal cord anatomy
    - Structural anatomy
      a. Spinal cord extends from brainstem to L1-L2, terminating as the conus medullaris.

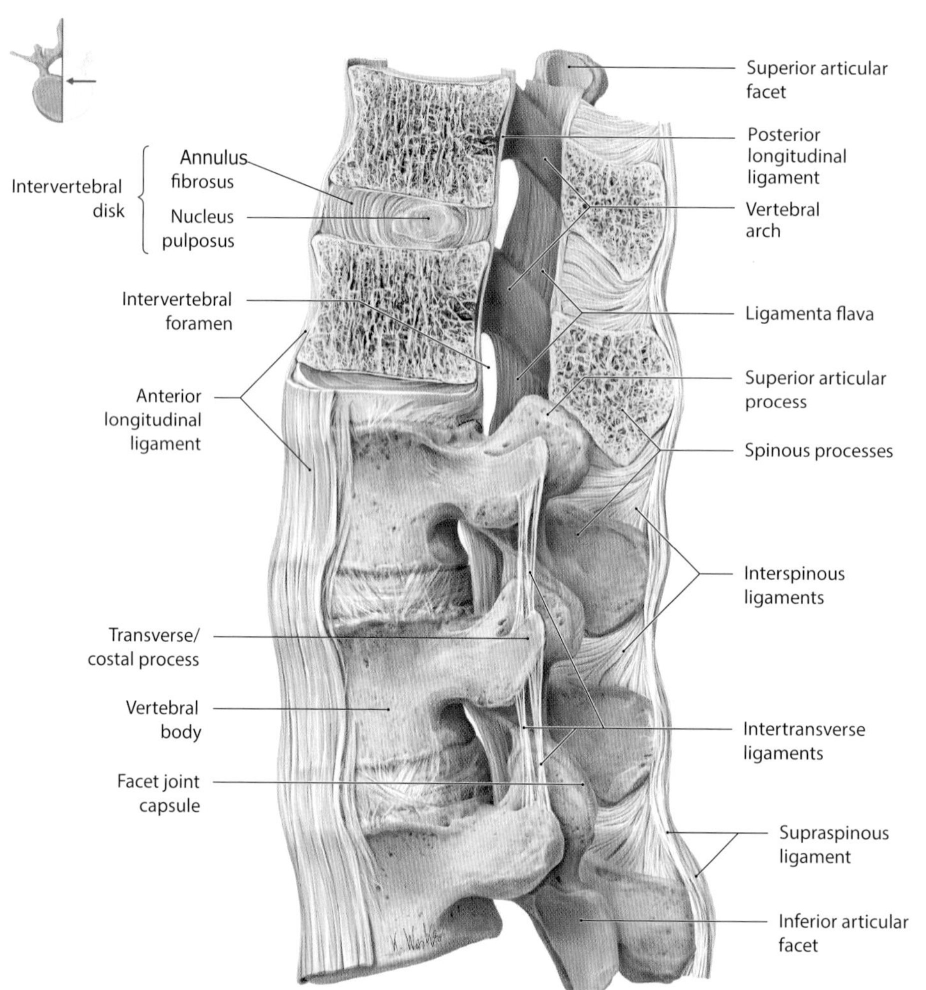

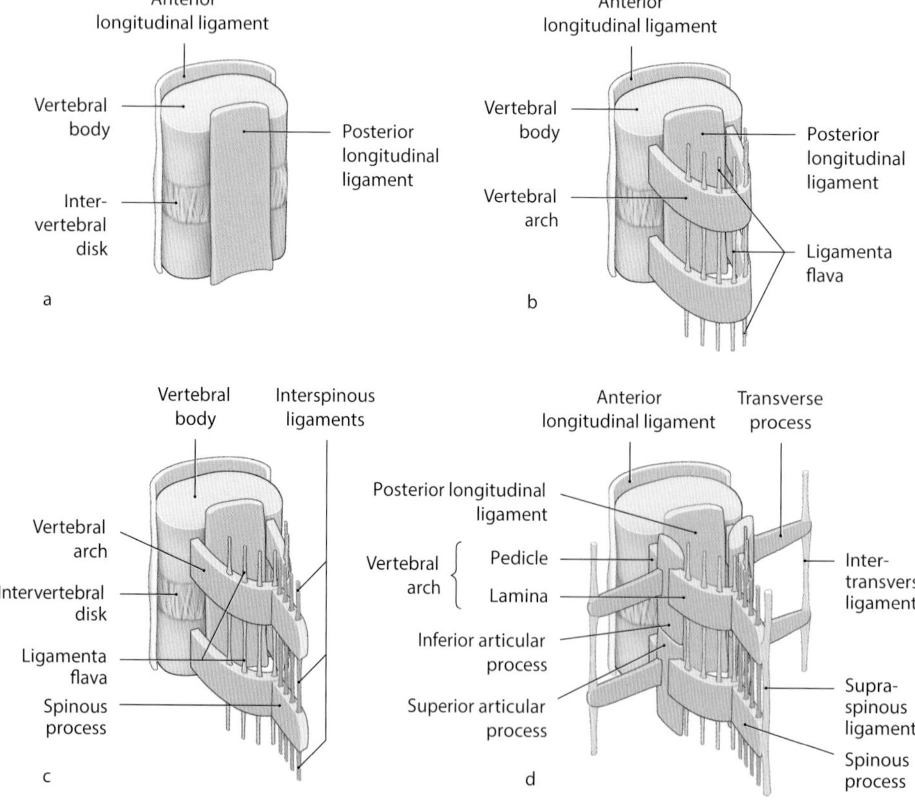

Fig. 5.5 **(a)** The ligaments of the spinal column. The ligaments of the spinal column bind the vertebrae securely to one another and enable the spine to withstand high mechanical loads and shearing stresses. The ligaments are sub-divided into vertebral body ligaments and vertebral arch ligaments. **(b)** Schematic representation of the vertebral body and vertebral arch ligaments. Viewed obliquely from the left posterior view. a. Vertebral body ligaments. b–d Vertebral arch ligaments (From Schuenke M, Schulte E. General Anatomy and the Musculoskeletal System: Thieme Atlas of Anatomy. New York: Thieme; 2005. Illustration by Karl Wesker.)

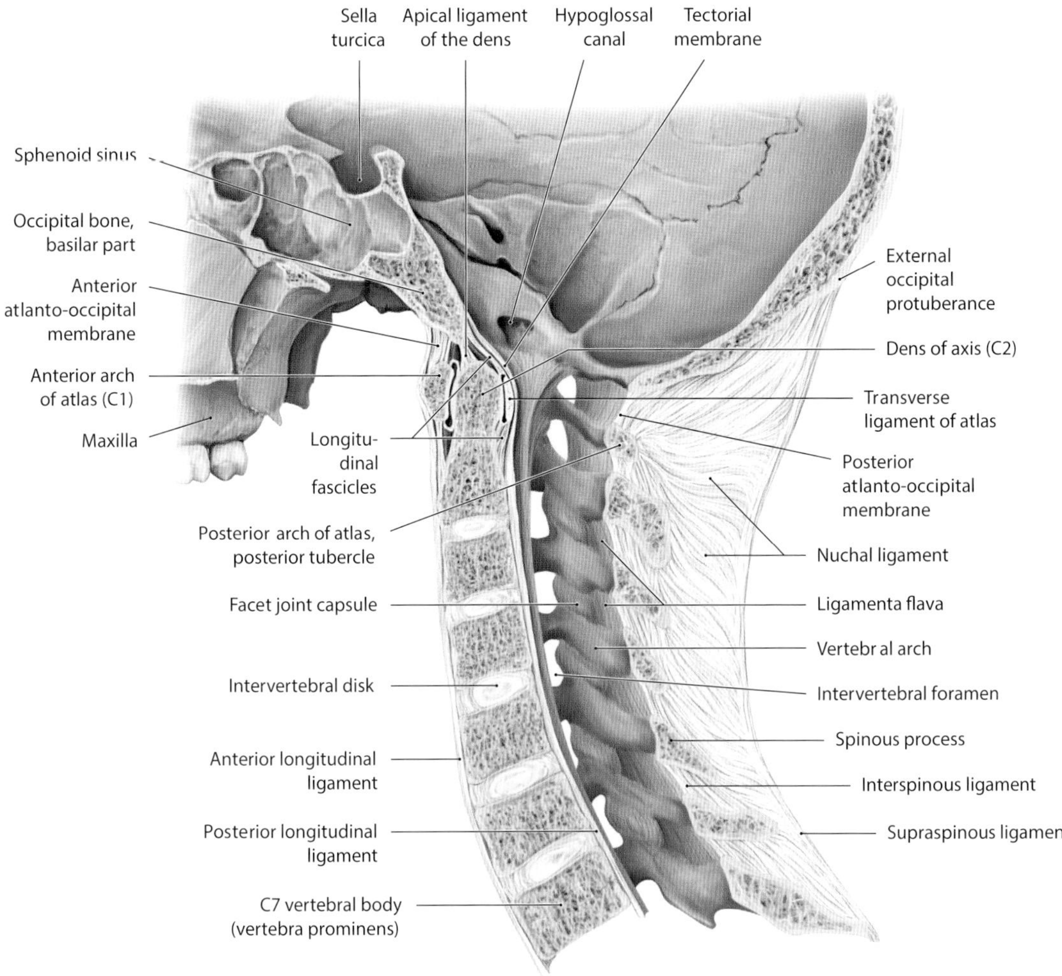

Fig. 5.6 The ligaments of the cervical spine:nuchal ligament. Midsagittal section,left lateral view. The nuchal ligament is the broadened, sagittally oriented part of the supraspinous ligament that extends from the vertebra prominens (C1) to the external occipital protuberance (see A; see also p.98 for the ligaments of the atlantooccipital and atlantoaxial joints). (From Schuenke M, Schulte E. General Anatomy and the Musculoskeletal System: Thieme Atlas of Anatomy. New York: Thieme; 2005. Illustration by Karl Wesker.)

b. Distal to conus medullaris the dural sac contains the cauda equine (a bundle of lumbar and sacral spinal nerves originating in the conus medullaris).
c. Dominant blood supply: anterior spinal artery
d. Vascular watershed area of thoracic cord located at T4-T9

- Functional anatomy
  a. Ascending (sensory) and descending (motor) tracts can be visualized in cross-section **(Fig. 5.8)**

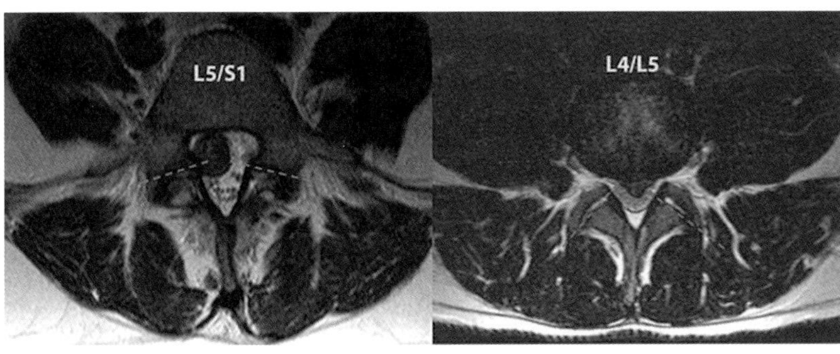

Fig. 5.7 Lumbar facet orientation: superior articular facets oriented in posteromedial direction. Orientation is more vertical in sagittal plane in upper lumbar spine and becomes more coronal moving in the caudal direction.

b. Know the spatial relationships of these tracts (Fig. 5.8).

- Dorsal columns: posterior, ascending fibers transmit proprioceptive, vibratory, and deep touch sensations
- Lateral spinothalamic: lateral, ascending fibers transmit pain and temperature sensations.
- Ventral spinothalamic: anterior, ascending fibers transmit light touch sensation.
- Lateral corticospinal: lateral, descending fibers transmit voluntary motor function.
  - Upper extremities: deep/central
  - Lower extremities: superficial/peripheral
  - Injured in central cord syndrome

- Central cord syndrome affects the upper extremity more than the lower due to the central location of the upper extremity fibers.
  a. Upper extremity motor deficits greater than lower extremity motor deficits due to deep/central location of upper extremity fibers of corticospinal tract
     - Anterior corticospinal: anterior, descending, voluntary motor
  b. Nerve roots **(Fig. 5.9)**
     - Thirty-one paired spinal nerves: eight cervical, 12 thoracic, five lumbar, five sacral, one coccygeal

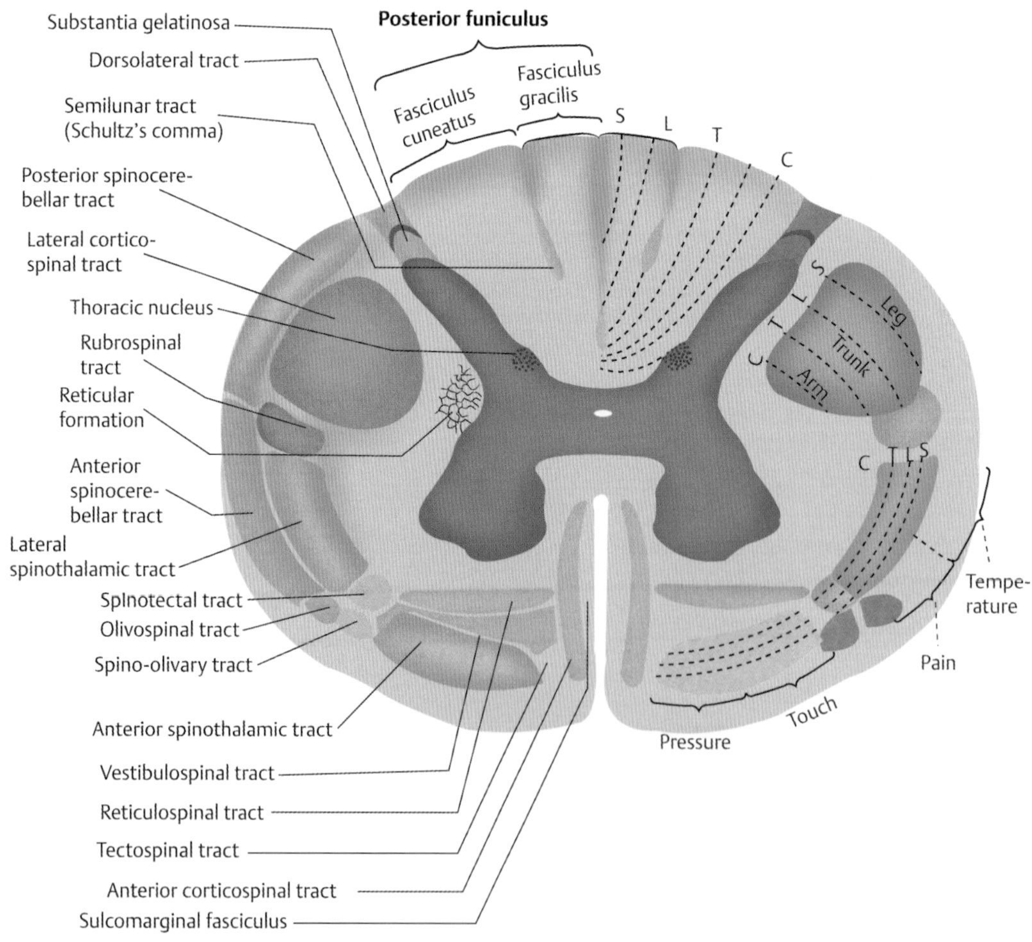

Fig. 5.8 Long tracts of the spinal cord. C, cervical; L, lumbar; and S, sacral; T, thoracic. (From Duus P. Topical Diagnosis in Neurology. New York: Thieme; 1998. Reprinted with permission.)

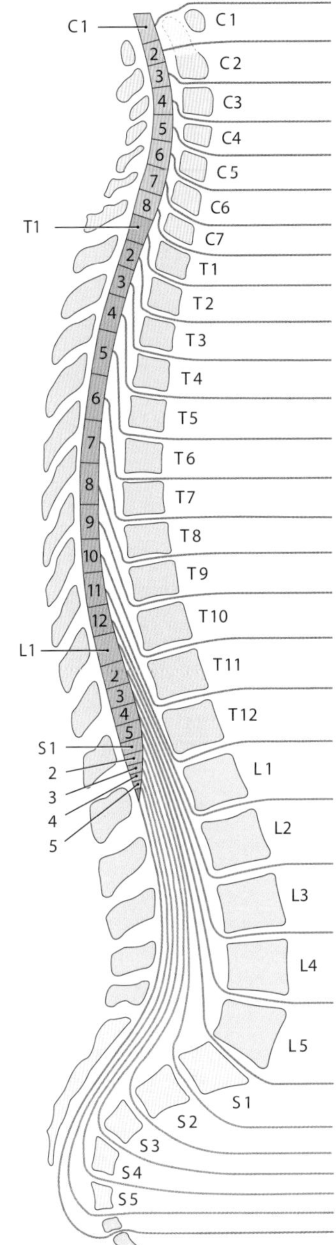

Fig. 5.9 Location and designation of spinal cord segments in relation to the spinal canal: right lateral view. The longitudinal growth of the spinal cord lags behind that of the spinal column, with the result that the cord extends only about to the level of the first lumbar vertebra (L1). Note that there are seven cervical vertebrae (C1–C7) but eight pairs of cervical nerves (C1–C8). The highest pair of cervical nerves exit the spinal canal superior to the first cervical vertebra. The remaining pairs of cervical nerves, like all the other spinal nerve pairs, exit inferior to the cervical vertebral body. The pair of coccygeal nerves *(gray)* has no clinical importance. (From Schuenke M, Schulte E. General Anatomy and the Musculoskeletal System: Thieme Atlas of Anatomy. New York: Thieme; 2005. Illustration by Karl Wesker.)

- In the cervical spine, the nerve root exits above its corresponding vertebral level (e.g., C5 root exits the C4–C5 foramen); in the thoracic and lumbar spine, the nerve root exits the foramen of its respective vertebral level (e.g., fourth lumbar root exits the L4–L5 foramen).
- Dorsal root/ganglia and ventral root converge to form the spinal nerve; once the nerve exits the foramen it gives off dorsal primary rami supplying muscles and skin of the neck and back, and a ventral ramus supplying the anterior trunk and all extremities.
- Sinuvertebral nerve: reenters the intervertebral foramen and innervates facet joints, annulus fibrosis, and IVD
  - Mediates/transmits pain signal in degenerative disk disease

c. Autonomic nervous system

- Sympathetic ganglia: three cervical, 11 thoracic, four lumbar, four sacral
- In cervical spine, ganglia lie posterior to carotid sheath and anterior to longus capitis muscle
- Horner's syndrome: disruption of inferior cervical ganglia (ptosis, miosis, anhidrosis)
- **Seen with preganglionic lower trunk brachial plexus lesions**
- Parasympathetic fibers from sacral levels for the pelvic splanchnic nerves combine with sympathetic fibers to form the hypogastric plexus; at risk with anterior lower lumbar dissection and can result in retrograde ejaculation
  - Neurologic levels **(Table 5.2)** and physical exam **(Fig. 5.10)**
    - Reflexes:
      - Generally, hyperreflexia, clonus and positive Babinski sign, are indicative of cervical myelopathy
      - Pathological reflexes:
        - ◊ Hoffman's sign: elicited by quickly flicking the middle finger into flexion; a positive sign is noted when thumb and index fingers flex in response; may indicate myelopathy
        - ◊ Inverted radial reflex: noted when thumb and fingers flex during brachioradialis reflex testing; may also indicate myelopathy
    - Special tests and provocative maneuvers:
      - Lhermitte's sign: shocklike sensation in trunk or extremities associated with axial load combined with flexion or extension of neck
      - Spurling maneuver: progressive rotation, lateral bending and extension of neck to affected side exacerbates symptoms of radiculopathy
      - Femoral nerve stretch test (L2-L4): flexing knee and hyperextending hip while patient is in a lateral decubitus position can reproduce symptoms of radiculopathy
      - Straight-leg raise (L4-S1): can be performed supine or sitting, a positive test reproduces symptoms of radiculopathy

Table 5.2 Neurologic Levels and Physical Exam

Root	Primary Motion	Tested Muscles	Sensory	Reflex
C5	Shoulder abduction Elbow flexion (palm up)	Deltoid Biceps	Lateral arm below deltoid	Biceps
C6	Elbow flexion (thumb up) Wrist extension	Brachioradialis ECRL	Thumb and radial hand	Brachioradialis
C7	Elbow extension Wrist flexion	Triceps FCR	Fingers 2, 3, 4	Triceps
C8	Finger flexion	FDS	Finger 5	–
T1	Finger abduction	Interossei (ulnar n.)	Medial elbow	–
Root	**Primary Motion**	**Primary Muscles**	**Sensory**	**Reflex**
L2,3	Hip flexion Hip adduction	Iliopsoas (*lumbar plexus, femoral n.*) Hip adductors (*obturator n.*)	Anterior and inner thigh	None
L3	Knee extension *(also L4)*	Quadriceps (*femoral n.*)	Lateral thigh, anterior knee, and medial leg	Patellar
L4	Ankle dorsiflexion *(also L5)*	Tibialis anterior (*deep peroneal n.*)	Lateral leg and dorsal foot	None
L5	Foot inversion Toe dorsiflexion Hip extension Hip abduction	Tibialis posterior (*tibial n.*) EHL (*DPN*), EDL (*DPN*) Hamstrings (tibial) and gluteus maximus (*inf. gluteal n.*) Gluteus medius (*sup. gluteal n.*)		
S1	Foot plantar flexion Foot eversion	Gastrocsoleus (*tibial n.*) Peroneals (*SPN*)	Posterior leg	Achilles
S2	Toe plantar flexion	FHL (*tibial n.*), FDL (*tibial*)	Plantar foot	None
S3,4	Bowel and bladder function	Bladder	Perianal	Cremaster

Abbreviations: DPN, deep peroneal nerve; ECRL, extensor carpi radialis longus; EHL, extensor hallucis longus; EDL, extensor digitorum longus; FCR, flexor carpi radialis; FDL, flexor digitorum longus; FDS, flexor digitorum superficialis; FHL, flexor hallucis longus; SPN, superficial peroneal nerve.

- **Reproduction of pain with a contralateral straight leg raise enhances specificity.**
  - ◊ Lasegue's sign: pain aggravated by dorsiflexion of ankle
  - ◊ Kernig's sign: pain aggravated by flexion of the neck

12. Surgical approaches
  - Anterior cervical (**Fig. 5.11**)
    a. Interval: between midline viscera (i.e., trachea and esophagus) and the carotid sheath
  - **Omohyoid muscle crosses surgical field in ventral approach**
    b. Complications
      - ∘ Dysphagia and dysphonia common; usually resolve
        - ♦ Equally likely after right/left sided approach
        - ♦ May require hospital admission if swallowing dysfunction severe in early postoperative course or if swelling is concerning
        - ♦ Work up for persistent problems: laryngoscopy/ear, nose, and throat (ENT) referral
        - ♦ Unilateral vocal cord dysfunction is contraindication to contralateral approach
      - ∘ Vocal cord paralysis and hoarse voice
        - ♦ Due to recurrent laryngeal nerve injury
        - ♦ Recurrent laryngeal nerve arises from vagus nerve at level of subclavian artery on right side (arises from aortic arch on left); injury results in unilateral vocal cord paralysis and hoarse voice

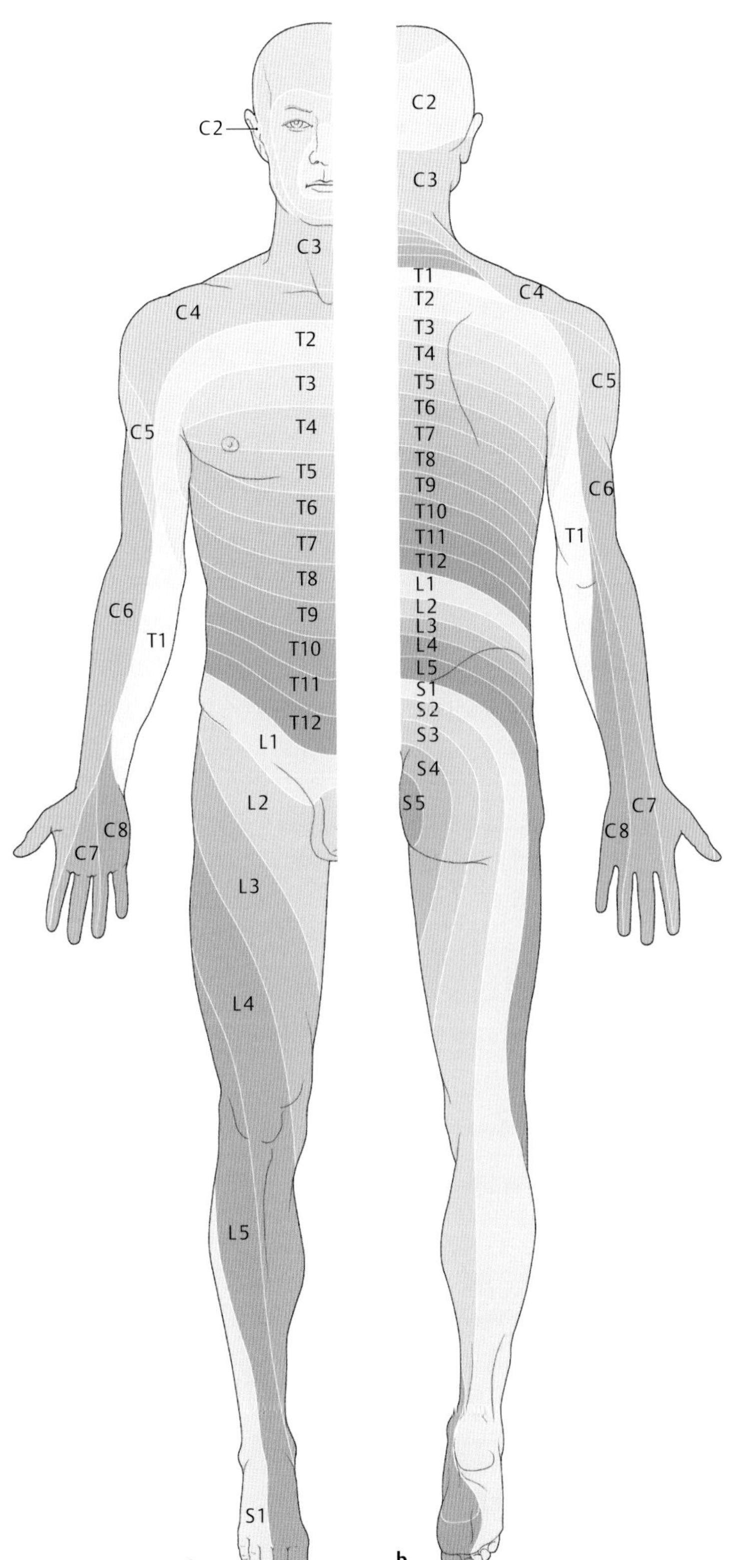

Fig. 5.10 The pattern of radicular (segmental) sensory innervation. The skin area supplied by a dorsal spinal nerve root is called a dermatome. Because the C1 segment consists entirely of motor fibers, it lacks a corresponding sensory field. Knowledge of radicular innervation is very important clinically. For example, when a herniated intervertebral disk is impinging on a sensory root, it will cause sensory losses in the affected dermatome. The area of sensory loss can then be used to locate the level of the lesion. Which intervertebral disk is affected? In a patient with shingles (herpes zoster inflammation of a spinal ganglion), the dermatome supplied by that ganglion will be affected (after Mumenthaler). (From Schuenke M, Schulte E. General Anatomy and the Musculoskeletal System: Thieme Atlas of Anatomy. New York: Thieme; 2005. Illustration by Karl Wesker.)

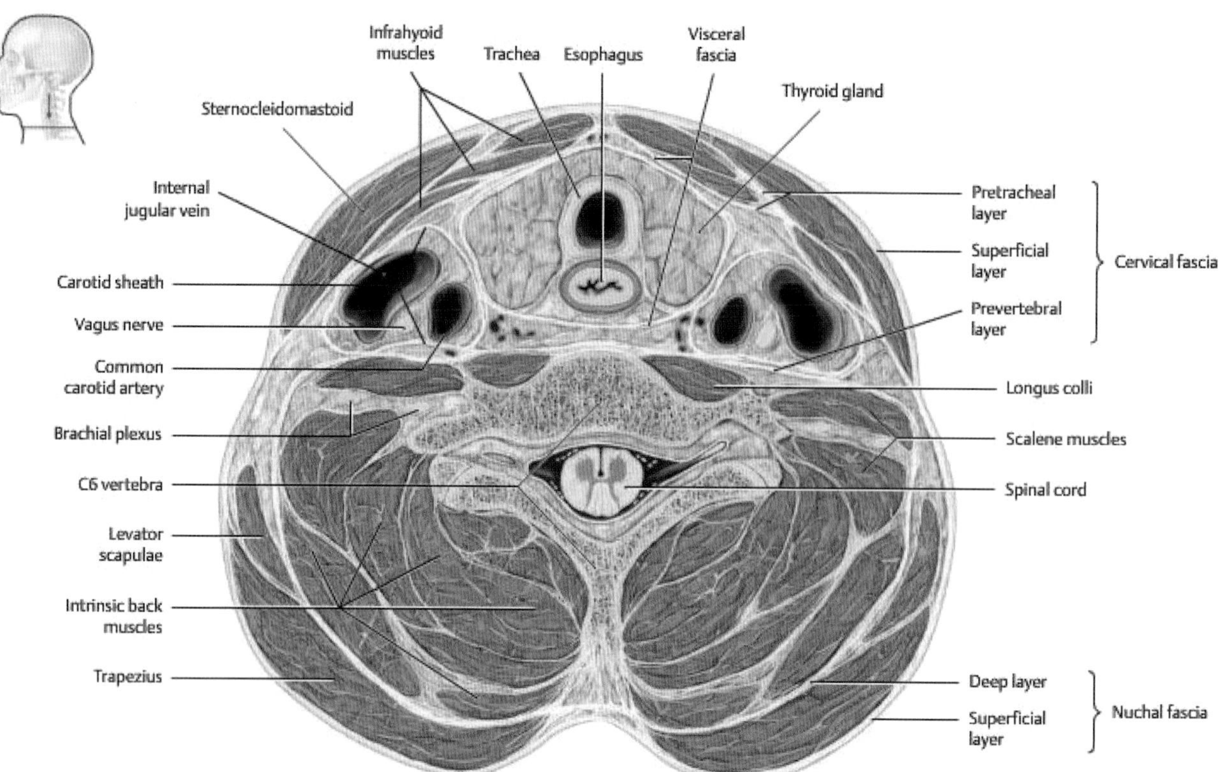

Fig. 5.11 Transverse section through the neck at the level of the C6 vertebra, superior view. (From Schuenke M, Schulte E. General Anatomy and the Musculoskeletal System: Thieme Atlas of Anatomy. New York: Thieme; 2005. Illustration by Karl Wesker.)

- Horner's syndrome: due to injury to sympathetic ganglion; injury to inferior stellate ganglion results in ptosis and constriction of the pupil
- Intraoperative nerve injury
  - C2–C3: hypoglossal nerve
    - Leads to tongue deviation *toward* side of injury
    - At risk with posterior C1-C2 transarticular screw placement
  - C4–C5: superior laryngeal nerve; injury leads to fatigue of voice, hoarseness
- Airway compromise
- **Acute dyspnea within the first 6–12 hours after surgery after cervical spine surgery may indicate an enlarging hematoma, and the incision should be emergently reopened.**
  - < 24 hours: hematoma; may warrant urgent decompression
  - 24–72 hours: laryngopharyngeal edema; may require definitive airway control
  - Late (> 72 hours): abscess, cerebrospinal fluid (CSF) accumulation, construct failure
  - Airway complication prevention
    - Consider maintaining intubation for 24–48 hrs postop for complex/prolonged procedures with extensive dissection, and for surgical time > 5 hours, with > 300 mL blood loss, focused above C3–C4
  - Risk factors: exposure of more than three vertebral bodies, exposures involving the C2-C4 levels, blood loss > 300 mL, surgical time > 5 hours, and patients undergoing combined anterior/posterior procedures
- Vertebral artery injury: dissection lateral to the uncinate process can lead to injury to the vertebral artery as it ascends in the transverse foramen of the cervical vertebrae.

- ♦ Most asymptomatic due to collateral flow
- ♦ Injury to dominant artery may result in vertebral artery insufficiency (dizziness, dysarthria, dysphagia, diplopia, blurred vision, and tinnitus) or hindbrain infarct.

c. Revision surgery
   - Revision anterior approach safest within 2 weeks of initial surgery before adhesion formation
   - > 2 weeks postop, posterior approach may be advised
   - Revision for pseudarthrosis
     - ♦ Posterior fusion has higher fusion rate, lower reoperation rate, higher blood loss, longer hospitalization, increased complication rate compared with anterior revision

- Posterior cervical
  a. Interval: midline paracervical muscles
  b. Risks:
     - Vertebral artery: vulnerable with lateral dissection at level of C1; exits transverse foramen, travels medially and superiorly, and enters atlanto-occipital membrane
     - C5 palsy postoperatively: most common nerve palsy after posterior approach, motor dominant
- Transthoracic
  a. Interval: through rib bed usually one to two levels above site of anterior column pathology
  b. Leads to reduced pulmonary function postoperatively that often remains long-term
  c. Risks:
     - Intercostal neurovascular bundle
     - Aorta, segmental arteries, artery of Adamkiewicz, thoracic duct (use right sided approach to avoid)
     - Lung pleura
     - Esophagus
- Posterior thoracolumbar
  a. Interval: midline approach
  b. Risk:
     - Segmental vessels
- Anterior lumbar
  a. Transperitoneal or retroperitoneal
  b. Structures at risk:
     - **injury to hypogastric plexus can lead to retrograde ejaculation.**
     - Transperitoneal: bladder, bowel, great vessels (bifurcation at L4-L5 disk), median sacral artery, lumbar superior hypogastric plexus (retrograde ejaculation), sympathetic chain descends along anterolateral aspect of spine into the pelvis
     - Retroperitoneal: great vessels, hypogastric plexus (retrograde ejaculation), ureters

13. Halo placement
   - Appropriate pin placement: 1 cm above lateral third of orbit at or below equator of skull
   - Adults/adolescents: usually four pins at 8 inch-pounds of torque
   - Children: require more pins (8–10) at 2–4 inch-pounds of torque
   - **Adults get four pins at 8 inch-pounds, and children get the opposite, eight pins at 4 inch-pounds.**
   - Contraindications: skull fracture, skin defect over pin site

- Structures at risk:
  a. Sinus in too medial-frontal a position; supraorbital nerve
  b. Temporalis fossa/muscle in too lateral a position
  c. Too much traction: cranial nerve VI (abducens) palsy

II. Spinal Trauma

1. Spinal cord injury
   - Background
     a. Most common in young males
     b. Most common causes: motor vehicle accidents, falls, gunshot wounds, and recreational/sports injuries
     c. Cervical spine clearance: computed tomography (CT) or magnetic resonance imaging (MRI) required in obtunded patient
     d. Spinal shock
        - Characterized by flaccid areflexic paralysis and sensory loss
        - Absent bulbocavernosus reflex
        - Some neurologic recovery may occur when spinal shock resolves
        - Typically resolves within 48 hours and is marked by return of bulbocavernosus reflex
        - **The level of injury cannot be determined until spinal shock has resolved.**
        - Following spinal shock, hyperreflexia, spasticity, and clonus develop.
     e. Neurogenic shock
        - **Know the difference in clinical presentation between neurogenic and spinal shock.**
        - Systemic hypotension caused by interruption of sympathetic output to heart and peripheral vasculature; relative bradycardia (differentiates from hypovolemic shock)
        - Treatment: vasopressor support
   - Classification:
     a. Complete/incomplete
        - Complete injury: no preservation of sensorimotor function caudal to the injured spinal segment
        - Incomplete injury: partial preservation of sensorimotor function caudal to the injured spinal segment
        - Neurologic level: most caudal segment of spinal cord with intact sensory function and at least grade 3/5 motor function
        - Thorough neurologic examination establishes the level of spinal cord injury following the return of the bulbocavernosus reflex.
        - Complete and incomplete injuries can be distinguished by the absence or presence of sacral sensation or distal sparing.
     b. American Spinal Injury Association (ASIA) classification
        - **ASIA classification goes from worst (A) to best (E).**
        - ASIA A: complete loss of sensory and motor function below level of injury
        - ASIA B: sensory function but no motor function below level of injury
        - ASIA C: sensory function and partial preservation of motor function, but key muscle groups less than grade 3/5 strength
        - ASIA D: sensory function and useful motor (at least half the muscles have a grade of at least 3/5) below level of injury

- ASIA E: normal
  - Function following spinal cord injury (according to level):
    - C1, C2, C3: ventilator dependent with limited talking; electric wheelchair with head or chin control
    - C4: possibly ventilator independent; electric wheelchair with head or chin control
    - C5: ventilator independent likely; electric wheelchair with hand control; unable to live independently
    - C6: manual wheelchair; able to live independently
    - C7: improved use of a manual wheelchair; independent transfers
    - **Patient can independently transfer only if C7/triceps function is maintained.**

- Medical management of spinal cord injury
  a. Hemodynamic, respiratory, and cardiac support/monitoring; maintenance of mean arterial pressure (MAP) > 85–90 mm Hg
  b. High-dose methylprednisolone: controversial due to question of efficacy and associated risks; use is based on hospital policy
    - Proposed mechanism of action: reduced tumor necrosis factor-α (TNF-α) expression
    - National Acute Spinal Cord Injury Study (NASCIS III) protocol:
      - Indicated for patients with acute, nonpenetrating spinal cord injuries when treatment initiated within 8 hours of injury
      - Less than 3 hours from injury: 30 mg/kg bolus, followed by 5.4 mg/kg/h for 24 hours
      - 3 hours to less than 8 hours from injury: 30 mg/kg bolus, followed by 5.4 mg/kg/h for 48 hours
- Incomplete spinal cord injury syndromes
  a. Brown-Séquard syndrome
    - Penetrating trauma
    - Ipsilateral loss of motor function and contralateral loss of pain and temperature sensation
    - Best prognosis
  b. Central cord syndrome
    - Hyperextension injury (often in setting of preexisting cervical spondylosis/stenosis)
    - Patients with cervical stenosis
    - Bilateral upper > lower extremity weakness and sensory loss
    - 35–45% chance of ambulation in ASIA C injuries in patients aged > 50 years
    - Fair prognosis
    - Most common incomplete spinal cord injury syndrome
  c. Anterior cord syndrome
    - **Anterior cord has worst prognosis; Brown-Séquard has best prognosis**
    - Incomplete motor deficit below the level of injury
    - Sensory deficit caused by injury to spinothalamic tract; posterior columns preserved (proprioception and vibration)
    - Worst prognosis
- Surgical management
  a. Decompression prior to 24 hours after spinal cord injury is associated with improved neurologic outcome, defined as an improvement of at

least 2 grades on the ASIA C impairment scale at 6 months' follow-up (Surgical Timing In Acute Spinal Cord Injury Study)

- Cervical spine fractures

- Occipital condyle fractures
  a. Type I: impacted/comminuted condyle fracture resulting from axial load
    - Mechanism: compression
    - Alar ligaments and tectorial membrane intact
    - Treatment: cervical collar

  b. Type II: occipital condyle fracture with extension to or involvement of basilar skull
    - Mechanism: compression
    - Alar ligaments and tectorial membrane usually intact
    - Treatment: cervical collar

  c. Type III: avulsion fracture of occipital condyle
    - Mechanism: distraction
    - Results from avulsion of alar ligament
    - Concern for underlying occipitocervical dissociation
    - Treatment: immobilization in collar or halo versus surgery (occipitocervical fusion) depending on amount of displacement

- Occipitocervical dissociation
  a. Background
    - Commonly fatal
    - Radiographically often challenging to diagnose **(Fig. 5.12)**
      - ♦ Radiographic measurements:
        - Powers ratio: distance from basion to posterior arch divided by distance from anterior arch to opisthion
          - Value > 1.0 indicates atlantoaxial instability, possibly secondary to occipitocervical dissociation (anterior dislocation) **(Fig. 5.13)**

  b. Harris method
    - Basion–axial interval: distance from basion to line drawn tangential to posterior border of C2
      - ♦ Less than 4 mm or greater than 12 mm is abnormal
    - Basion–dens interval: distance from basion to tip of odontoid
      - ♦ Greater than 12 mm is abnormal

  c. Traynelis Classification
    - Type I: anterior displacement of occiput on the atlas
    - Type II: longitudinal distraction; any traction applied to type II injury can result in progression of existing deficit
    - Type III: posterior subluxation or dislocation

  d. Treatment
    - Light traction may help reduce type I and III injures
    - Immediate application of halo vest followed by occipital-cervical fusion with instrumentation for unstable injuries

- C1 (atlas) fractures
  a. Isolated anterior or posterior arch fracture: nonsurgical treatment with immobilization

  b. Lateral mass fracture: nonsurgical treatment with immobilization

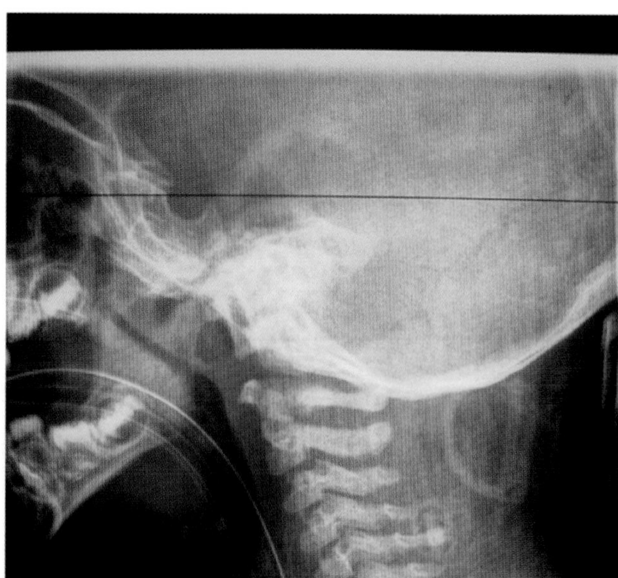

Fig. 5.12 Lateral radiograph of young child involved in high-speed motor vehicle accident demonstrating occipitocervical dissociation. The patient succumbed to the injury.

c. Jefferson burst fracture
  - Mechanism: axial load causing bilateral fractures of the anterior and posterior arches
  - Greater than 7 mm lateral mass displacement indicative of transverse ligament rupture
  - Atlantodens interval (ADI)
    - Greater than 3 mm: transverse ligament disruption
    - Greater than 5 mm: transverse and alar ligament disruption
  - Treatment
    - Intact transverse ligament (< 7 mm lateral mass displacement or ADI < 3 mm): halo vest immobilization or hard collar
    - Transverse ligament disruption (> 7 mm lateral mass displacement or ADI > 3 mm): C1-C2 fusion or occipitocervical fusion

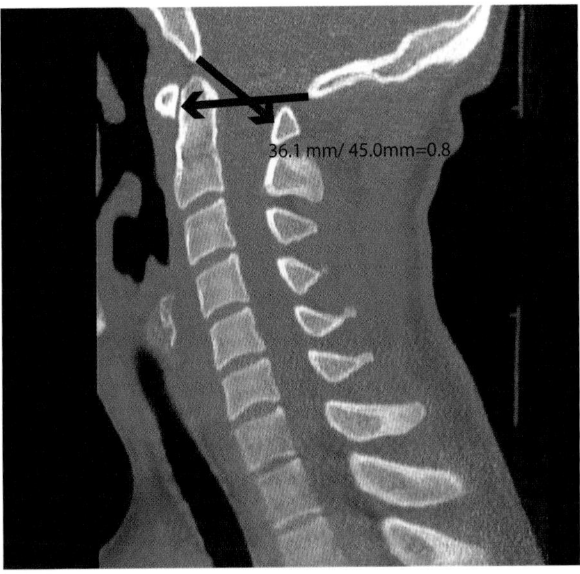

Fig. 5.13 Midsagittal computed tomography (CT) of the upper cervical spine demonstrating the Powers ratio. This is determined by dividing the distance between the tip of the basion to the spinolaminar line by the distance from the tip of the opisthion to the midpoint of the posterior aspect of the of C1 anterior arch. A value > 1 indicates possible instability.

- C2 (axis) fractures

a. Odontoid fracture
  - Type I: avulsion fracture of tip of odontoid
    - Treatment: collar
  - Type II: fracture through waist of odontoid process at the junction with the body
    - Treatment dependent on patient and fracture characteristics; options include anterior odontoid screw, posterior C1–C2 fusion, halo or collar
    - Elderly patient
      - Poor tolerance of halo immobilization
      - Early posterior C1-C2 fusion if patient able to tolerate surgery
      - If patient unable to tolerate surgery, consider collar and progression to fibrous union
    - Young patient
      - Nondisplaced fracture: consider halo (or collar) immobilization
      - Displaced fracture or risk for nonunion: anterior screw placement versus posterior C1-C2 fusion
    - Risks of nonunion: greater displacement, increased angulation, posterior displacement
    - Contraindications to anterior screw fixation: barrel chest, osteoporosis, subacute or chronic fractures, extensive comminution
  - Type III: fracture through body
    - Treatment: collar/halo

a. Hangman fracture
  - Bilateral fractures of par interarticularis with spondylolisthesis
  - Classification
    - Type I: hyperextension and axial load injury with minimal (< 3 mm) displacement and no angulation
    - Type II: hyperextension and axial load usually followed by rebound flexion; fracture displacement > 3 mm with angulation of fracture
    - Type IIa: flexion-distraction injury with significant angulation but minimal translation/displacement; involves injury through disk space; critical to recognize and thus avoid traction, which can further displace the fracture
    - **Avoid traction with type IIa fractures.**

- Type III: flexion-distraction injury followed by extension; fracture involves bilateral pars and bilateral C2-C3 facet dislocations
- Treatment
  - Type I: cervical collar or halo
  - Type II: initial traction in extension followed by immobilization in halo vest
  - Type IIa: avoid traction, which can cause severe overdistraction; immobilization in halo vest
  - Type III: surgical reduction and posterior C2-C3 fusion
  - Surgical treatment options for nonunion of type II injuries include C1-C3 posterior fusion and C2-C3 anterior interbody fusion.

- Subaxial cervical spine fractures (C3-C7)
  a. Allen-Ferguson classification based on mechanism
    - Compressive flexion
    - Distractive flexion
    - Compressive extension
    - Lateral compression
    - Distractive extension
    - Lateral flexion

  b. Treatment based on injury severity: Subaxial Cervical Injury Classification System (SLIC) assigns points based on fracture morphology, status of the discoligamentous complex, and neurologic status of the patient.
  c. Cervical burst fractures and "teardrop" (compressive flexion) fractures are associated with high rate of neurologic injury and are often unstable.
  d. Facet fracture-dislocations
    - Injury mechanism: flexion-distraction
    - Obtunded patient: neurology intact, order MRI; if no disk herniation, then perform closed reduction with traction
    - Awake/cooperative patient: closed reduction safe with frequent neurologic exams prior to MRI
    - Closed reduction with Gardner-Wells tongs or halo and progressive application of traction: may require > 100 lb
    - Treatment
      - Unilateral facet dislocations without significant displacement/posterior ligamentous injury can be treated nonoperatively; close clinical and radiological follow-up necessary
      - Bilateral facet dislocations or posterior ligamentous injury generally require surgical stabilization.

- SCIWORA: spinal cord injury without radiographic abnormality (prior to advent of MRI)
  a. Pediatric patients
  b. Best predictor of neurologic outcome: severity of initial injury
- Pediatric C2–C3 pseudosubluxation: seen in half the children < 8 years of age
- Halo vest immobilization
  a. Indications: Jefferson C1 fractures, type II or III odontoid fractures, type II hangman fracture, selected subaxial injuries

- **Halo vest treatment used for Jefferson C1 fractures, Type II or III odontoid fractures, Type II Hangman fracture, and select subaxial injuries**

  b. Complications
    - Abducens nerve (CNVI) palsy: decreased ability to laterally deviate eyes due to traction on nerve
    - Pin loosening or infection

- Supraorbital nerve injury
- Dural penetration

2. Vertebral compression fractures
   - Background
     a. Mechanism: associated with osteoporosis and low energy trauma
     b. Spine is the most common site for an osteoporotic fracture.
     c. Prior compression fracture and reduced bone mineral density are the biggest risk factors for a new compression fracture.
     d. Associated with 20% risk of future fracture
   - Rule out pathological origin in patient with atypical radiograph findings, history of cancer, or constitutional symptoms
   - Neurologic injury rare
   - MRI useful for differentiating acute from chronic compression fractures
   - Treatment
     a. Medical management of osteoporosis (see Chapter 1)
        - Bisphosphonates for T score less than –1
        - American Academy of Orthopaedic Surgeons (AAOS) clinical practice guideline: acute spinal compression fracture (neurologically intact) should be treated with calcitonin for 4 weeks (moderate evidence).
     b. Analgesics for pain
     c. Activity modification and early mobilization with physical therapy
     d. Percutaneous vertebral augmentation (vertebroplasty, kyphoplasty)
        - Controversial
        - May consider for patients with intractable pain
        - May provide pain relief; efficacy lacks support from prospective, randomized, controlled study
        - AAOS clinical practice guideline recommends against vertebroplasty (strong evidence)
3. Thoracolumbar Fractures
   - Background
     a. Mechanism: traumatic injuries to thoracolumbar spine usually result of high-energy blunt trauma
     b. Thoracolumbar junction: biomechanical transition zone between rigid thoracic spine (rib cage) and more flexible lumbar spine
     c. Transitional anatomy of the TL junction. This region is prone to fractures and dislocation due to anatomic and biomechanical factors. Anatomic factors: facet orientation is changing, ribs 11–12 do not articulate with the rib cage. Biomechanical factors: transition between rigid T-spine and more mobile L-spine. Line of gravity passes through T12-L1 bodies.
   - Magerl classification
     a. Type A: compression fractures caused by axial loading
     b. Type B1: distraction injury with ligamentous injury posteriorly
     c. Type B2: distraction injury with osseoligamentous injury posteriorly
     d. Type C: multidirectional, unstable fracture dislocation with high incidence of neurologic injury
   - Denis classification
     a. Divides spine into three columns
        - Anterior column: anterior longitudinal ligament, annulus, and anterior half of vertebral body
        - Middle column: posterior half of vertebral body and annulus, and the posterior longitudinal ligament

5 Spine

- Posterior column: pedicle, facets, lamina, spinous process, transverse process, ligamentum flavum, interspinous ligament, supraspinous ligament **(Fig. 5.14)**

b. Compression fractures involve anterior column only with intact middle column

c. Burst fractures involve anterior and middle columns with widening of interpedicular distance and retropulsion of vertebral body into canal; posterior column involvement also possible (usually a sagittal plane fracture through lamina)

- o Occur due to axial load

d. Flexion-distraction injuries result in failure of posterior and middle columns in tension; anterior column fails in compression.

- Highest association with abdominal visceral injuries
- Ligamentous injuries in the adult nearly always require surgery

e. Fracture-dislocations result from failure of all three columns.

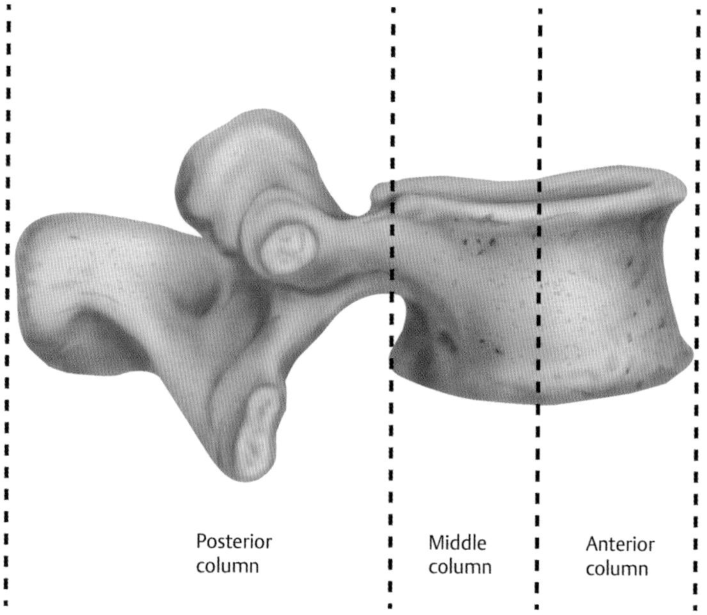

Fig. 5.14 Three-column Denis division of vertebral column.

- Thoracolumbar Injury Classification and Severity Score (TLICS)
  a. Highly reliable system; helps predict need for operative intervention
  b. Based on injury morphology, neurologic status, and integrity of posterior ligamentous complex
  c. Score 0–3: nonoperative treatment
  d. Score 4: either operative or nonoperative treatment
  e. Score > 4: operative treatment
  f. TLICS grading system **(Table 5.3)**
- Associated injuries
  a. High association with noncontiguous spinal injury
  b. High incidence of intra-abdominal or bowel injury
- Treatment
  a. Nonsurgical
    - Indication: stable spinal column injury without neurologic deficit
      - ♦ Compression fractures
      - ♦ Burst fractures with < 50% loss of height, < 50% canal compromise, < 30 degrees kyphosis
      - ♦ Type B2 (bony) flexion distraction injuries
    - Method: thoracolumbar orthosis
  b. Surgical
    - Neurologically intact patients: surgery associated with higher incidence of complications at 5 years compared with nonsurgical treatment; no difference in patient outcome compared with thoracolumbosacral orthosis (TLSO) treatment
    - Indication: neurologic deficit associated with compressive lesion or biomechanical instability
      - ♦ Burst fractures with > 50% loss of height, > 50% canal compromise, > 30 degrees kyphosis: unilateral symptoms may indicate entrapment of caudal root(s) in lamina fracture. Treatment: decompression and posterior instrumented spine fusion
      - ♦ B1 (ligamentous) flexion-distraction injury
      - ♦ Fracture-dislocation

- ♦ Multiply injured patient: allows for early mobilization
- ◦ Sacral fractures (see Chapter 3)

- Background
  a. Result of high-energy trauma
  b. Commonly associated with pelvic and spine fractures
  c. May be associated with sacral root deficits
- Classification
  a. Zone 1: fractures within region extending from sacral ala to lateral border or neuroforamina
     - ◦ Most common sacral fracture
     - ◦ Lowest incidence of neurologic deficit
  b. Zone 2: fractures involving the neuroforamina
     - ◦ Incidence of neurologic deficit ~ 30%
     - ◦ If unilateral, patient may still have normal bowel and bladder function.
  c. Zone 3: fractures involving sacral bodies and canal
     - ◦ Least common
     - ◦ May be horizontal or vertical
     - ◦ Highest association with neurologic deficit (~60%) and involvement of bilateral sacral roots
- Treatment
  a. Generally dictated by pelvic injury and stability of pelvic ring
  b. Sacral decompression warranted in setting of neurologic deficit
  c. H- or U-shaped zone 3 sacral fractures (spinopelvic dissociation) require spinopelvic instrumentation/fusion.

4. Special considerations
- Gunshot wounds
  a. Steroids are not indicated as treatment in gunshot wounds to the spine.
  b. Surgical treatment
     - ◦ Spine unstable (rare scenario)
     - ◦ Dural leak
     - ◦ Incomplete deficit with retained bullet
  c. Otherwise, nonoperative treatment preferred
  d. Broad-spectrum IV antibiotics if bowel transected
- Ankylosing spondylitis/diffuse idiopathic skeletal hyperostosis (DISH):
  a. Fused spine with high potential for instability
  b. Epidural hematoma common
  c. Treatment: decompression (if deficit) and long segment instrumented fusion
  d. Must fuse long segment above and below injury due to long lever arm created by bony fusion of spine

Table 5.3 Thoracolumbar Injury Classification and Severity Score (TLICS) Grading System

TLICS System	
Parameter	**Points**
Morphology	
Compression	1
Burst	2
Rotation/translation	3
Distraction	4
Posterior ligamentous complex (PLC) disruption	
Intact	0
Suspected	2
Disrupted	3
Neurologic status	
Intact	0
Nerve root	2
Cord, conus medullaris: complete	2
Cord, conus medullaris: incomplete	3
Cauda equina	3
Operative Management Decision Protocol	
Management	
Nonoperative treatment	0–3
Nonoperative or operative treatment	4
Operative treatment	> 4

Source: Adapted from Vaccaro AR, Lehman RA Jr, Hurlbert RJ, et al. A new classification of thoracolumbar injuries: the importance of injury morphology, the integrity of the posterior ligamentous complex, and neurologic status. Spine (Phila Pa 1976) 2005;30(20):2325–2333.

III. Degenerative Conditions of the Cervical Spine

1. Background
- Pathoanatomy: a cascade of degenerative events leads to cervical spondylosis

a. Ratio of keratin sulfate to chondroitin sulfate increases; water content within disk decreases

b. Degeneration leads to loss of disk height, herniation/calcification, end-plate osteophytes, buckling of ligamentum flavum, arthrosis of facet and uncovertebral joints (of Luschka)

c. Alteration in sagittal plane alignment (loss of normal lordosis)

d. Increased segmental motion

e. Neural impingement

- Clinical presentations: axial neck pain, radiculopathy and myelopathy

2. Axial neck pain
   - Overview

     a. Insidious onset, episodic

     b. Exacerbated by neck motion, particularly extension

     c. Occipital headaches common
   - Imaging

     a. Indications
       - History of traumatic event
       - Prolonged duration of symptoms
       - Coexistent radiculopathy or myelopathy
       - Constitutional symptoms or known history of cancer or inflammatory arthritis

     b. Plain radiographs
       - Anteroposterior (AP): uncovertebral degenerative changes, vertebral body fractures
       - Lateral: altered sagittal alignment, disk-space narrowing, end-plate osteophytes, listhesis, fractures
       - Oblique: neuroforaminal stenosis, facet arthrosis
         - ♦ **Oblique views enable visualizing the foramen and identifying stenosis caused by osteophyte formation.**
       - Flexion-extension views: instability, listhesis
       - Odontoid view (open mouth): odontoid fractures, atlantoaxial arthrosis

     c. CT scan: used to delineate bony anatomy

     d. MRI or CT myelogram: used to diagnosis neural compression, infections, neoplasms
   - Treatment

     a. Nonsurgical management is mainstay of treatment

     b. Nonsteroidal anti-inflammatory drugs (NSAIDs)

     c. Physical therapy

     d. Short-term immobilization (soft collar)

     e. Surgical fusion after failure of prolonged conservative management; controversial; unproven efficacy

3. Cervical radiculopathy
   - Pathoanatomy: compression of exiting nerve root secondary to:

     a. Soft disk herniation: nucleus pulposus compresses nerve root exiting from cord or within foramen.

     b. Hard disk: root compression from end-plate osteophyte/calcified annulus (± uncovertebral osteophytes)

     c. Other contributing factors: loss of disk space height, facet joint hypertrophy, malalignment (listhesis)

     d. Chemical pain mediators and inflammatory cytokines [interleukin-1 (IL-1), IL-6, TNF-α, prostaglandins, substance P, bradykinin]

- Overview
  a. Symptoms: neck pain, unilateral shoulder pain, arm pain (or sensory alteration) in distribution of affected root
  b. Typically one root (but can involve multiple roots)
  c. C6 root (C5-C6 level) and C7 root (C6-C7 level) most commonly affected
  d. Cervical roots exit above their corresponding pedicle; posterolateral disk herniation or foraminal stenosis produce radiculopathy of the exiting nerve (e.g., pathology at C5-C6 leads to C6 radiculopathy)
     - Example: C5–6 posterolateral disk herniation leads to C6 nerve impingement, which leads to decreased sensation thumb/index finger, diminished brachioradialis reflex, weak biceps/brachialis, and wrist extensors.
     - **Know the expected neurologic deficit based on a posterolateral disk herniation at a given cervical level.**
  e. Provocative tests elicit (Spurling's maneuver) or diminish (shoulder abduction relief sign) radicular symptoms; must differentiate radiculopathy from upper limb peripheral nerve entrapment disorders
- Imaging: see Axial neck pain, above
- Treatment
  a. Nonsurgical: initial treatment
     - Short-term immobilization in soft collar
     - NSAIDs, corticosteroids, narcotics
     - Physical therapy
     - Cervical epidural steroid injections
  b. Surgical treatment
     - Anterior cervical decompression and fusion (ACDF)
     - Anterior decompression and disk arthroplasty: results comparable to ACDF
     - Posterior decompression (laminoforaminotomy)

4. Cervical myelopathy
- Overview
  a. Clinical syndrome due to compression and dysfunction of spinal cord (in relation to cervical spondylosis) **(Fig. 5.15)**
  b. Natural history: stepwise progression separated by periods of neurologic stability
  c. Osseoligamentous pathology produces cord dysfunction by direct mechanical compression or ischemia related to anterior spinal artery compromise.
  d. Presentation
     - Upper extremity clumsiness; inability to manipulate fine objects
     - Gait instability; loss of balance
     - Lhermitte sign: neck flexion eliciting electric shock like sensations radiating down spine or extremities
     - Weakness and sensory symptoms (numbness/paresthesias) in upper limbs
     - Bowel and bladder symptoms: late in disease progression
     - Hyperreflexia, Hoffman sign, inverted radial reflex, clonus, extensor plantar response (Babinski)
     - Patients may have concomitant radiculopathy or peripheral nerve disease; lack of neck pain common
- Classification
  a. Nurick classification: determined based on lower extremity function/ambulatory status

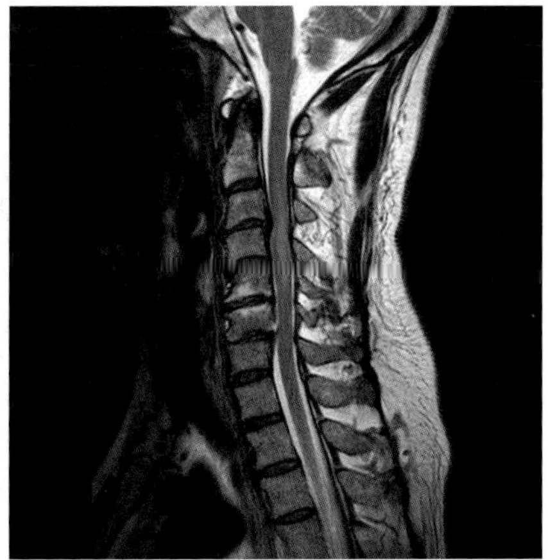

Fig. 5.15 Midsagittal MRI of the cervical spine demonstrating cervical stenosis secondary to congenital narrowing, disk herniation, and spondylosis.

b. Ranawat classification: takes into account symptoms of upper extremity and lower extremity

- Imaging: refer to axial neck pain
- Treatment: generally surgical

a. Early intervention improves prognosis.

b. Selection of surgical technique depends on multiple variables, including primary direction of compressive pathology, overall sagittal alignment, number of levels involved, surgeon training/experience, and patient factors.

c. Anterior procedures

  - Cervical diskectomy and fusion (one or more levels)
  - Single or multilevel corpectomy and fusion
  - Hybrid anterior decompression and reconstruction (corpectomy plus diskectomy)

d. Posterior laminectomy with or without fusion

  - Postlaminectomy kyphosis may lead to recurrent myelopathy: cord draped over kyphotic segment
  - **Contraindicated in kyphotic cervical spine**

e. Laminoplasty

  - **Beware of C5 nerve root palsy after laminoplasty; treat with observation.**
  - Motion preserving: no fusion performed
  - Postoperative segmental (usually C5) nerve root palsy is known complication
    - ♦ Motor dominant palsy most common
    - ♦ Recovery common; may take weeks to months
  - May not be effective in patient with significant kyphosis (decompression relies on dorsal translation of cord)
  - Postoperative neck pain and stiffness common: preoperative neck pain is relative contraindication
  - Contraindication: fixed cervical kyphosis

5. Cervical stenosis

- Reduction in space available for the spinal cord and nerve roots
- Classification:

a. Congenital/developmental

b. Acquired

  - Traumatic
  - Degenerative

- Absolute stenosis: canal diameter < 10 mm on lateral imaging
- Relative stenosis: canal diameter 10–13 mm
- Pavlov/Torg ratio (canal width/vertebral body diameter)

a. Should be 1.0 or greater

b. Less than 0.8 is risk factor for neurologic impairment following trauma

- Hyperextension injury and minor trauma can lead to spinal cord injury/central cord syndrome with or without fracture

6. Ossification of the posterior longitudinal ligament (OPLL)

- Overview

a. Common in Asian population

b. Cause unclear and likely multifactorial

c. Potential cause of cervical myelopathy

- Presentation: patients may be asymptomatic or present with frank cervical myelopathy
- Imaging: refer to axial neck pain
- Treatment
  a. Treatment generally surgical if myelopathy present
  b. Treatment principles the same as for cervical myelopathy
  c. Note the potential for dural defect/erosion with anterior approach.
    - Laminoplasty generally a very effective posterior decompressive procedure for OPLL

IV. Thoracic Disk Herniation

1. Presentation
   - Often asymptomatic; occurs in up to 40% of individuals
   - Posterolateral or foraminal herniations may lead to chest wall pain and numbness.
   - Large, central herniations can produce myelopathy.
2. Treatment
   - Anterior decompression for central herniations; associated with spinal cord dysfunction
   - Posterolateral decompression: safe and effective for paracentral and foraminal herniations

V. Low Back Pain and Degenerative Conditions of the Lumbar Spine

1. Low back pain (LBP)
   - Epidemiology
     a. Major cause of morbidity and disability in the United States
     b. 15% annual incidence; 80% of individuals will experience LBP at some point in their lives.
   - Causes
     a. Myofascial strains
     b. Discogenic pain
     c. Facet joint arthropathy
     d. Spondylolisthesis
     e. Lumbar spinal stenosis
     f. Sacroiliac joint dysfunction
   - Evaluation
     a. History and physical examination with careful neurologic assessment to differentiate spinal from nonspinal causes of back pain
        - Atraumatic back pain without neurologic findings: reassurance, limited analgesics, early return to functional activities as tolerated
        - Exception: "red flag" symptoms that may indicate worrisome etiology of LBP (e.g., infection or neoplasm)
          - "Red flags": history of cancer; extremes of age; unexplained weight loss, night pain, or pain with rest; persistent fevers; history of IV drug abuse; immunocompromised state; recent bacterial infection
     b. Radiographs
        - Radiography is best initial diagnostic test for evaluating diskogenic LBP.

- Obtain X-rays if concern raised about tumor, fracture, or infection.
- If primary complaint is back pain, generally defer X-rays for 4–6 weeks in absence of "red flags."
- AP/lateral X-rays: disk degeneration, other osseous or soft tissue abnormalities, malalignment
- Oblique views: defect of pars interarticularis (spondylolysis)
- Flexion/extension views: instability/spondylolisthesis

c. MRI
- Obtained in setting of back pain unresponsive to 3 months of nonoperative management
- Obtain immediately for LBP in case of suspected malignancy or infection (or major neurologic deficit, e.g., cauda equina syndrome)
- Also generally indicated for LBP associated with a clinically significant motor deficit (monoradiculopathy)
- MRI with gadolinium is the best study for assessing recurrent disk herniation/stenosis in patients with prior surgery.

d. CT myelography
- Largely replaced by MRI but useful in assessing spinal fusion and when MRI contraindicated (e.g., pacemaker/defibrillator), and in traumatic brachial plexus injuries for signs of nerve root avulsion

e. Waddell signs: inappropriate signs and symptoms that may indicate nonorganic component of back pain or malingering
- Superficial, diffuse, nonanatomic tenderness
- Simulation tests (axial loading, spinopelvic rotation)
- Distraction tests (straight leg raise when patient distracted or seated)
- Regional nonanatomic disturbances
- Overreaction

2. Disk herniations **(Fig. 5.16)**
- Disk degeneration characterized by loss of hydration of nucleus pulposus and decrease in number of viable cells
- **Most common level L5-S1, followed by L4-L5**
- May occur centrally, posterolateral/paracentral (most common), foraminal or extraforaminal/far lateral
- **Posterolateral/paracentral disk herniation affects the traversing nerve root (L4-L5 herniation affects L5).**
- **Far lateral (intra/extraforaminal) disk herniation affects the exiting nerve root (L4-L5 herniation affects L4); know the location of disk herniation and the associated deficit**
- Morphology
  a. Protrusion: eccentric bulge with intact annulus
  b. Extrusion: disk material has extruded through annulus but remains contiguous with disk space
  c. Sequestration: herniated nucleus that is no longer contiguous with disk space (free fragment)
- Presentation
  a. Varying degrees of low back pain and radicular leg pain
  b. Radicular pain in dermatomal pattern of affected nerve root
  c. Positive nerve root tension signs (straight-leg raise or femoral nerve stretch test)
  d. Positive contralateral straight-leg raise test is most specific.
- Diagnostic testing

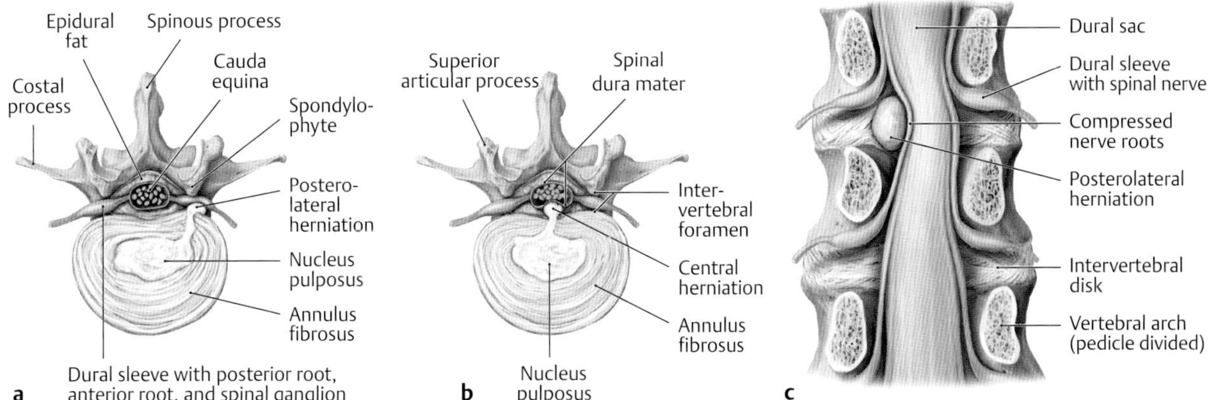

Fig. 5.16 Lumbar disk herniation. **(a)** Posterolateral herniation, superior view. **(b)** Posterior herniation, superior view. **(c)** Posterolateral herniation, posterior view (the vertebral arches have been removed to demonstrate the lumbar dural sac and corresponding nerve roots). (From Schuenke M, Schulte E. General Anatomy and the Musculoskeletal System: Thieme Atlas of Anatomy. New York: Thieme; 2005. Illustration by Karl Wesker.)

a. X-rays
b. MRI
c. Electromyogram (EMG) rarely required; can help rule out alternative causes of lower extremity symptomatology (e.g., peripheral neuropathy, tarsal tunnel syndrome, piriformis syndrome)

- Cauda equina syndrome
  a. Usually secondary to large central disk herniation
  b. Characterized by pain (back of buttocks/thighs), numbness (saddle anesthesia), varying degrees of motor weakness in lower extremities, bowel or bladder dysfunction (urinary retention, check post-void residual)
  c. Surgical emergency
  d. Immediate MRI and decompression warranted
    - CT myelogram in patients with contraindication to MRI (pacemaker)
  e. Best results of decompression within first 24–48 hours; timing of surgery most predictive of outcome
- Treatment of lumbar radiculopathy
  a. Nonoperative: initial treatment is nearly always nonoperative
    - Vast majority of patients recover by 3 months
    - NSAIDs
    - Physical therapy
      - ♦ Activity modification
      - ♦ Progressive early mobilization/ambulation
    - Other modalities
      - ♦ Muscle relaxants
      - ♦ Epidural steroid injections
      - ♦ Oral steroids
  b. Surgery
    - Rarely indicated before 6 weeks (early intervention for progressive and functionally significant motor deficit (or cauda equina syndrome)
      - ♦ Outcomes worse in workers' compensation cases
    - Indications: intractable radicular pain, clinically significant neurologic deficit, failure of nonsurgical management
    - Optimal candidate: patient with predominance of radicular pain and neurologic exam findings that correlate with MRI lesion

- Procedure of choice: laminotomy with excision of displaced nucleus pulposus and decompression of affected nerve root
- Spine Patient Outcomes Research Trial (SPORT):
  - At 2-year follow-up, no significant differences in primary outcome measures for operative group compared with nonoperative group
  - Surgical treatment of disk herniation leads to early and sustained pain relief.
  - Results of diskectomy are generally better when surgery performed within 6 months of symptom onset.
- Operative complications
  - Dural tear: suture repair with watertight closure
    - Pia/arachnoid seal within 2–3 days. Dural edges heal with fibroblastic proliferation.
    - Leads to postural headaches and nausea if leak persistent
  - Postoperative chronic back pain; progressive IVD degeneration
  - Recurrent disk herniation: treatment outcome same as for primary herniation
  - Postoperative disk space infection: treat with needle biopsy and culture-specific antimicrobial therapy (unless there is frank epidural abscess)
  - Nerve root injury/dysfunction
  - Vascular injury due to anterior disk perforation: flip patient to supine position, emergent laparotomy, and vessel repair
    - Common iliac vein: most often injured

3. Facet cysts (synovial cysts)
   - May lead to spinal stenosis and radiculopathy
   - Treatment: laminotomy/laminectomy with cyst excision
4. Degenerative disk disease (DDD)
   - MRI findings often do not correlate with presence or severity of symptoms.
   - Symptoms not directly correlated with MRI: treatment is cognitive intervention, physical therapy, exercise
   - In selected patients, advanced DDD with associated severe back pain may benefit from lumbar fusion.
   - Intradiscal electrothermal therapy (IDET) has demonstrated no significant benefit over placebo in controlled trials.
5. Lumbar stenosis **(Fig. 5.17)**
   - May cause back pain and neurogenic claudication
     a. Consider vascular claudication in differential diagnosis.
     b. Neurogenic versus vascular claudication **(Table 5.4)**
   - Conservative treatment: physical therapy, Williams flexion exercises, NSAIDs, bracing, epidural steroid injection (ESI)
     a. Most patients experience some pain relief within the first 3 months.
   - Surgical intervention: decompression (laminectomy- foraminotomies, medial facetectomies)
     a. Can consider interspinous decompression with the X-STOP, the interspinous process decompression system, although contraindicated in cauda equina syndrome, osteoporosis
     b. Patients treated surgically have better pain and function scores at 4 years compared with nonsurgical patients (SPORT)
   - Reasonable to consider arthrodesis in setting of degenerative scoliosis, degenerative spondylolisthesis/instability, pars interarticularis fracture, or recurrent disk herniation

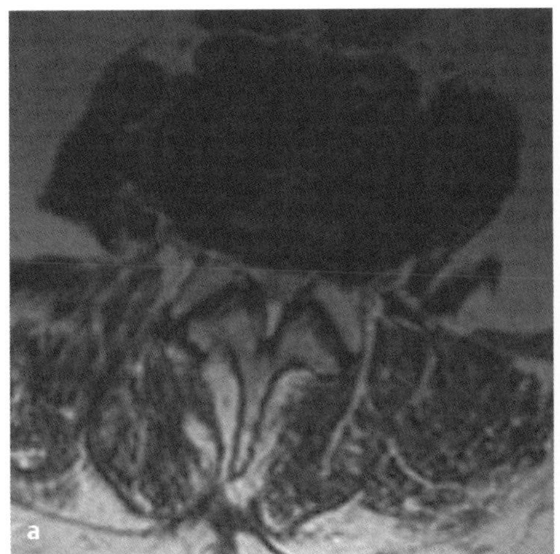
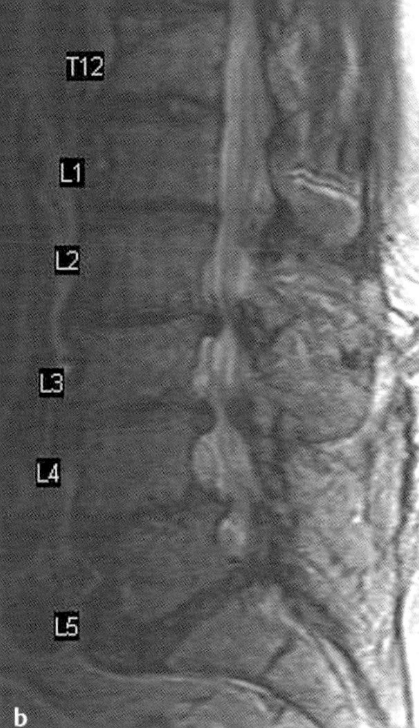

Fig. 5.17 Lumbar stenosis. **(a)** Axial and **(b)** sagittal MRI deonstrating lumbar spondylosis and spinal stenosis.

- Surgical complications:
  a. Residual foraminal stenosis due to inadequate decompression most common explanation for persistent symptoms of leg pain following decompressive laminectomy
  b. Increased risk of surgical site complications with epidural morphine and steroid paste
  c. New-onset neurologic dysfunction:
     - Postoperative spinal epidural hematoma
     - Screw malposition
       - ♦ Treatment: immediate surgical exploration decompression
  d. Adjacent segment disease: 25% have symptomatic adjacent segment degeneration at 5- to 10-year follow-up
  e. Smoking leads to increased rate of pseudarthrosis. Smoking cessation for 6 months leads to improved fusion rates.
     - **Decreased fusion rate in smokers due to diminished revascularization of cancellous bone graft**

Table 5.4 Neurogenic Versus Vascular Claudication

	Vascular Claudication	Spinal Stenosis
Quality of pain/symptoms	Cramping, tightness, or tiredness	Same symptoms as with claudication or tingling, weakness, or clumsiness
Location of symptoms	Buttock, hip, thigh, calf, foot	Buttock, hip, thigh
Low back pain	No	Frequently present
Relieving factors	Rapid relief with rest	Relief with sitting or otherwise changing position
Associated conditions	Atherosclerosis and decreased pulses	History of lower back problems

6. Lumbar spondylolisthesis
   - Etiology: degenerative, isthmic (associated with pars defect), congenital/dysplastic, pathological, postsurgical, or traumatic
   - Isthmic spondylolisthesis: common in athletes (rowers, gymnasts)
     a. Pars defect (spondylolysis) in athlete treatment: activity restriction and bracing
     b. If conservative treatment fails: pars repair or fusion
   - High-grade spondylolisthesis of L5/S1 most often associated with L5 root symptoms/signs
   - Meyerding classification: based on lateral X-ray
     a. Grade 1: 0–25%
     b. Grade II: 26–50%
     c. Grade III: 51–75%
     d. Grade IV: 76–100%
     e. Spondyloptosis: > 100%
   - Risk factors for progression:
     a. Young age at presentation
     b. Female gender with slip angle > 10 degrees
     c. High-grade slip
     d. Dome-shaped/inclined sacrum
     e. Pelvic incidence (PI)
        - PI is the angle subtended by a line perpendicular from the cephalad end plate of S1 and a line connecting the center of the femoral head to the center of the cephalad end plate of S1
        - Increased angle of pelvic incidence believed to increase risk of progression of slippage
   - Treatment after failed conservative management: posterior decompression and instrumented fusion.
     a. Isolated stand-alone interbody fusion generally not indicated when instability evident
     b. In high-grade L5-S1 slips, L4-S1 fusion may be required.
   - Operative slip reduction risks L5 nerve root injury.
   - Posterior instrumentation with or without interbody support [posterior lumbar interbody fusion (PLIF), transforaminal lumbar interbody fusion (TLIF), anterior lumbar interbody fusion (ALIF), axial lumbar interbody fusion (AxialLIF)] or transvertebral support (fibular strut, transvertebral pedicle screw) commonly used for high-grade listhesis
     a. Pedicle screws decrease pseudarthrosis rate
7. Sacroiliac joint pain
   - Pain over posterior sacroiliac (SI) joint or posterior sacroiliac spine (PSIS) that often radiates to groin or buttocks
   - Diagnosis
     a. FABER test: *f*lexion, *ab*duction, *e*xternal *r*otation of involved extremity
     b. Gaenslen test: patient experiences pain when lying on the affected side without support
     c. Manual compression test
   - Treatment
     a. NSAIDs
     b. Physical therapy
     c. SI injections for refractory cases (also play diagnostic role)
     d. Fusion rarely indicated

8. Coccygodynia
    - Pain with activities that put pressure on the coccyx
    - More common in women after pregnancy or trauma
    - May be idiopathic
    - Sometimes associated with fracture
    - Often self-limiting
    - Diagnosis
        a. Pain and point tenderness over coccyx
        b. Radiographs or MRI to rule out traumatic etiology
    - Treatment
        a. NSAIDs
        b. Physical therapy
        c. Sitting donut pillow
        d. Local injections
        e. Surgery: high failure rate, rarely indicated

VI. Inflammatory Disorders of the Spine

1. Overview
    - Disorders characterized by inflammatory changes in the bone, connective tissue, and synovium of the spine
    - Initial laboratory workup: complete blood count (CBC), erythrocyte sedimentation rate (ESR), C-reactive protein (CRP)
2. Rheumatoid arthritis
    - Chronic, systemic autoimmune disorder
    - Positive rheumatoid factor in 85% of individuals
    - Destructive synovitis is seen in synovium-lined joints due to autoimmune response.
    - Spine involvement occurs in ~ 60% of individuals and is usually restricted to the cervical spine.
    - Clinical presentation varies
        a. Asymptomatic
        b. Neck pain; occipital headaches (C2 root/greater occipital nerve irritation)
        c. Deformity (kyphosis, torticollis)
        d. Neurologic compromise: radiculopathy ± myelopathy
    - Characterization of spinal involvement:
        a. Atlantoaxial instability
            - Results from erosion of synovial joints and destruction of transverse, alar and apical ligaments, leading to atlantoaxial subluxation and instability
            - Pannus develops posterior to dens and may result in cord compression
            - Potential instability necessitates cervical spine dynamic radiographs for surgical clearance in patients with rheumatoid arthritis (RA) undergoing general anesthesia.
            - Anterior ADI of greater than 7–10 mm or posterior space available for the cord of less than 13 mm is relative contraindication to elective nonspinal surgery without prior C1–C2 stabilization
            - Radiographic parameter that predicts outcome: posterior ADI > 13 mm
        b. Superior migration of the dens and basilar invagination
            - Occurs after erosion and destruction of occipitoatlantal joints, atlantoaxial joints, and lateral masses

    - May result in brainstem compression and vertebrobasilar vascular insufficiency
  c. Subaxial subluxation
    - Occurs due to progressive erosion of facet joints and posterior ligamentous structures
    - Multilevel subluxation is common and can lead to kyphotic deformity ("stepladder" appearance)
- Diagnostic workup
  a. Lateral radiographs required to assess posterior ADI, anterior ADI, migration of dens, subaxial subluxation
  b. Flexion-extension radiographs required to evaluate dynamic instability
    - Posterior ADI < 14 mm or anterior ADI > 9 mm associated with increased risk of progressive myelopathy
  c. Methods of evaluating basilar invagination **(Fig. 5.18)**
    - Chamberlain's line:
      - ♦ Line from dorsal margin of hard palate to posterior edge of foramen magnum
      - ♦ Dens > 6 mm above Chamberlain's line: basilar invagination
    - McCrae's line:
      - ♦ Defines the opening of the foramen magnum
      - ♦ Impaction present if odontoid tip above this line
    - McGregor's line:
      - ♦ Line drawn from the posterior edge of the hard palate to the caudal posterior occiput
      - ♦ Cranial settling is present when the tip of dens > 8 mm above McGregor's line in men and > 9.7 mm in women
    - Disadvantage: hard palate position may vary with facial anomalies
    - Ranawat's line:
      - ♦ Center of C2 pedicle to a line connecting anterior and posterior C1 arches
      - ♦ Normal measurement in men is 17 mm, whereas in women it is 15 mm

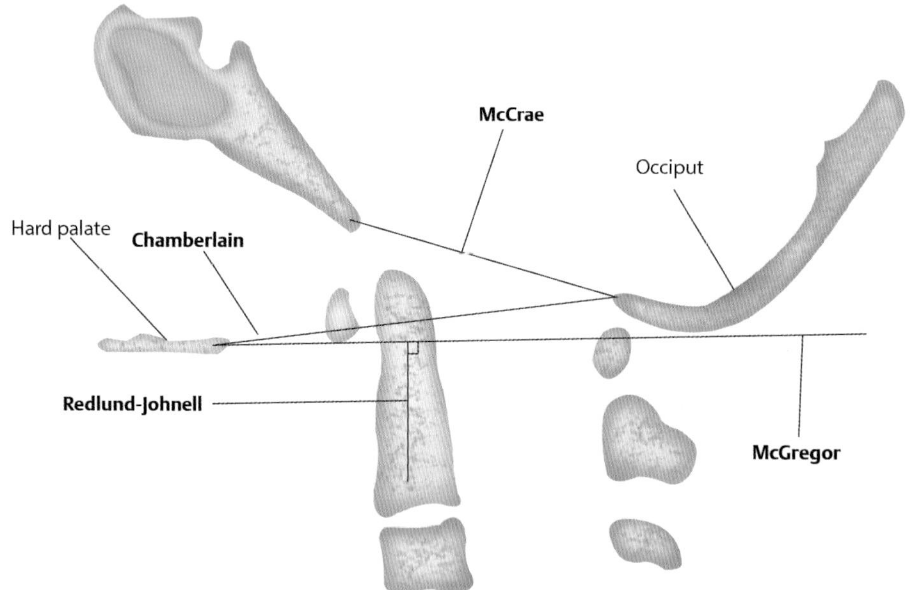

Fig. 5.18 Methods of evaluating basilar invagination. Disadvantage: hard palate position may vary with facial anomalies.

- ♦ < 13 mm: impaction
  - ♦ < 7 mm: associated with medullary compression
- ◦ Wackenheim line
  - ♦ Used to determine anterior/posterior subluxation
  - ♦ Drawn down the posterior surface of the clivus; its inferior extension should barely touch the posterior aspect of the odontoid tip
  - ♦ Relationship does not change in flexion and extension.
- ◦ Clark stations
  - ♦ Divide odontoid process into thirds in the sagittal plane
  - ♦ Normally, anterior ring of atlas is adjacent to the top (cephalad) third of the axis (station I)
  - ♦ Mild cranial settling if adjacent to middle third (station II)
  - ♦ Severe cranial settling if ring of atlas adjacent to base of axis (station III) **(Fig. 5.19)**

- Ranawat classification of myelopathy
  a. Class I: no neurologic deficit
  b. Class II: subjective weakness, paresthesia, hyperreflexia
  c. Class III: objective weakness and upper motor neuron signs
    - ◦ Class IIIa: patient is ambulatory
    - ◦ Class IIIb: patient is nonambulatory
  d. Treatment
    - ◦ Nonsurgical treatment
      - ♦ Disease modifying antirheumatic drugs (methotrexate, sulfasalazine, hydroxychloroquine sulfate), and agents targeting TNF-α (etanercept, infliximab) and IL-1 (Anakinra)
      - ♦ Oral steroids
      - ♦ Goal is to alleviate pain and prevent neurologic compromise
    - ◦ Surgical treatment
      - ♦ Considered for intractable pain or neurologic deficit/myelopathy
      - ♦ Prognosis for improvement guarded in patients with Ranawat class III myelopathy

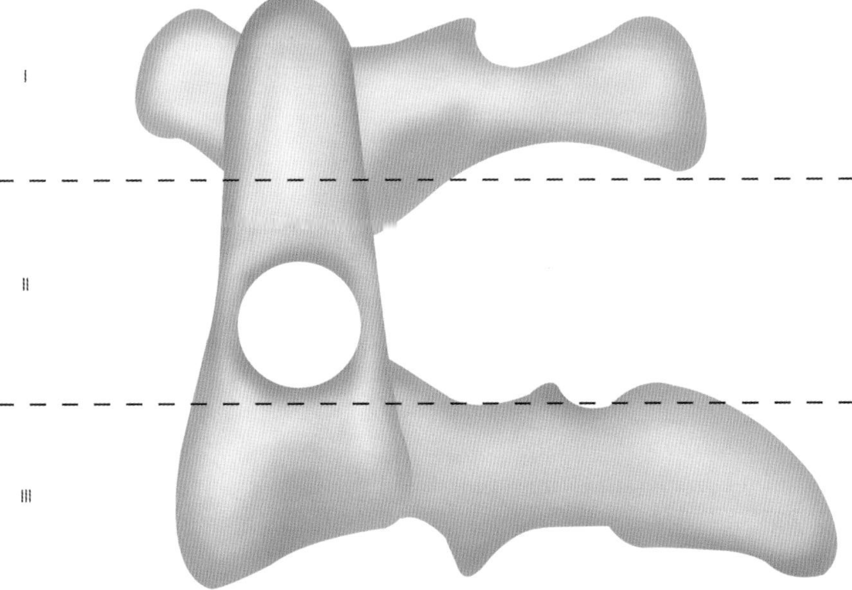

Fig. 5.19 Severe cranial settling in ring of atlas adjacent to the base of the axis (station III).

- ♦ C1-C2 fusion for atlantoaxial instability (posterior ADI < 14)
  - ♦ Occiput–C2 fusion in setting of basilar invagination; C1 arch removal may be required if decompression necessary
  - ♦ Posterior fusion usually required for subaxial subluxation

3. Seronegative spondyloarthropathies
   - Background
     a. Predominantly affects the entheses (bony insertions of ligaments and tendons)
     b. Associated with human leukocyte antigen (HLA)-B27
     c. Negative rheumatoid factor (RF)
     d. Sacroiliitis/spondylitis
     e. Associated conditions
        - Arthritis of large joints of appendicular skeleton
        - Anterior uveitis
        - Aortic stenosis and regurgitation
        - Restrictive lung disease
        - Ileitis/colitis
   - Ankylosing spondylitis
     a. Predominantly effects males in third decade of life
     b. HLA-B27 positive
     c. Associated with bilateral uveitis and sacroiliitis
     d. Inflammation of entheses leads to bony erosions followed by formation of new bone and eventual ankylosis
     e. Bridging syndesmophytes form along inflamed annulus fibrosis
        - Radiographs demonstrate bridging marginal syndesmophytes (characteristic bamboo spine).
     f. Sacroiliitis common
        - Pain often localized to low back and SI joint regions (most common presentation)
        - Obliteration of SI joint (erosion of iliac side seen first) visible on radiographs and helps differentiate from DISH
     g. Ankylosing spondylitis and fracture **(Fig. 5.20)**
        - Patients with ankylosing spondylitis and new onset back or neck pain should be carefully evaluated for fracture.
        - Fracture occurs between two rigid spinal segments; usually involves all three columns and is inherently unstable
        - High incidence of neurologic injury secondary to resultant instability or epidural hematoma formation
        - May require corrective osteotomy surgery for fixed kyphotic deformity (of cervicothoracic or lumbar spine) and sagittal imbalance
        - Treatment requires long segment instrumentation above and below the fracture due to the long lever arm created by the disease.
   - Diffuse idiopathic skeletal hyperostosis (DISH)
     a. Affects middle-aged or older individuals
     b. More common in patients with diabetes and gout
     c. Associated with extraspinal ossification of peripheral joints and with increased risk of heterotopic ossification after total hip arthroplasty
     d. Characterized by nonmarginal syndesmophytes (in contrast to ankylosing spondylitis)
        - **No SI joint involvement in DISH**
     e. Seen most commonly in the thoracic spine

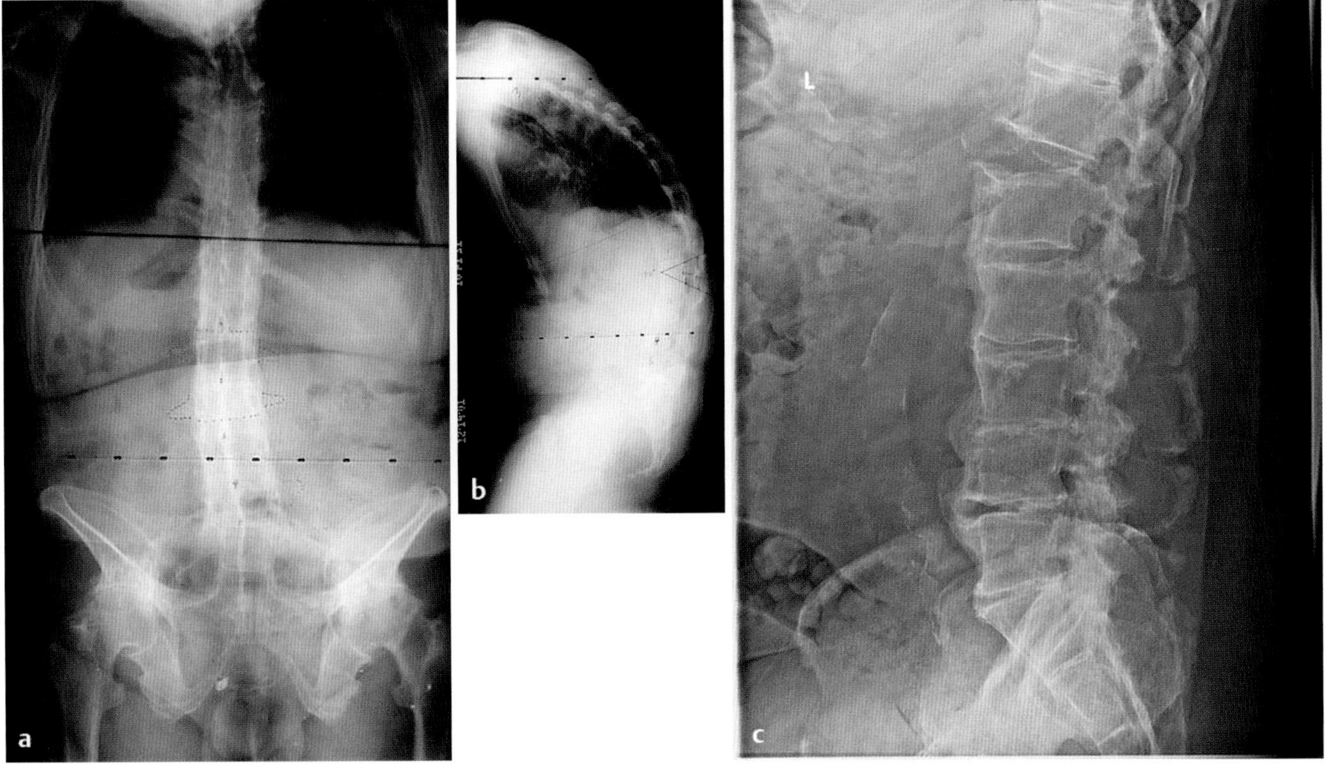

Fig. 5.20 Ankylosing spondylitis versus diffuse idiopathic skeletal hyperostosis (DISH). **(a)** Anteroposterior (AP) and **(b)** lateral radiograph showing ankylosing spondylitis with bridging marginal syndesmophytes. **(c)** Lateral lumbar radiograph with T12-L1 fracture/dislocation through DISH segment with nonmarginal syndesmophytes.

- Large anterior syndesmophytes of the cervical spine may cause stridor or dysphagia.

f. DISH and fracture
- Rigid spine that is susceptible to fracture; similar to patients with ankylosing spondylitis
- Low threshold to obtain imaging for appropriate fracture workup
- Fractures are generally unstable, necessitating surgical stabilization.

- Psoriatic arthritis
  a. HLA-B27 association
  b. Patients with psoriatic spondylitis develop noncontiguous ankylosis with the presence of both marginal and nonmarginal syndesmophytes as well as diskovertebral erosions.
  c. Cervical spine involvement with presentation similar to rheumatoid arthritis
  d. Treatment is predominantly medical (as with RA) in the form of disease-modifying antirheumatic drugs (DMARDs) and TNF-α blocking agents.
  e. Surgery sometimes indicated if severe kyphotic deformity or for severe cervical involvement and myelopathy
- Enteropathic arthritis
  a. HLA-B27 association
  b. Similar in presentation and treatment to ankylosing spondylitis
- Reiter syndrome
  a. Mnemonic: "Can't see, can't pee, can't climb a tree."
  - Conjunctivitis/uveitis
  - Urethritis

- Reactive arthritis thought to occur following infection
- Large joint arthritis (usually knees, ankles, spine)
- Sacroiliitis and nonmarginal syndesmophytes seen in patients with spinal involvement

VII. Adult Spinal Deformity

1. Evaluation: standing, long-cassette AP and lateral scoliosis X-rays from femoral heads to external auditory meatus
2. **Most significant predictor of disability: sagittal plane imbalance**
3. Canal and neuroforaminal stenosis most often occur in the concavity of a scoliotic curve.
4. Spine curves < 30 degrees rarely progress, whereas curves > 50 degrees often progress.
5. Untreated adolescent idiopathic scoliosis (AIS) with curve > 60 degrees leads to higher rates of acute and chronic back pain.
6. Spinopelvic parameters **(Fig. 5.21)**
7. Pelvic incidence: measured on lateral standing radiograph; angle formed by drawing perpendicular line from midpoint of sacral end plate and line connecting that point with the center of the femoral head
   - Pelvic incidence = Sacral slope + Pelvic tilt
   - Pelvic tilt refers to the vertical position of the sacrum. A line is drawn from the center of the S1 end plate to the center of the femoral head. A second vertical line (parallel with the side margin of the radiograph or perpendicular to the floor) is drawn intersecting the center of the femoral head. The angle between these two lines is the pelvic tilt.
   - Sacral slope is determined by the angle formed between a line parallel to the superior end plate of S1 and a line parallel to the floor.
   - A low pelvic incidence implies a low pelvic tilt and lower lumbar lordosis. Patients with greater lumbar lordosis (high pelvic incidence) have increased shear forces at the lumbosacral junction.
   - Normal mean pelvic incidence: children, 47 degrees; adults, 57 degrees
   - Mean pelvic incidence in low-grade spondylolisthesis, 65 degrees; in high-grade spondylolisthesis, 80 degrees
   - Adult spinal deformity surgery should attempt to match the lumbar lordosis to the pelvic incidence, or risk over- or under-correction
8. C7 plumb line
   - Vertical line drawn from center of C7 body to the ground, measured in relation to posterosuperior corner of body of S1; line anterior to S1 corner equates with positive sagittal balance, whereas posterior line equates with negative sagittal balance; positive sagittal balance, especially > 10 cm, poorly tolerated and correlates with outcome in adult spinal deformity patients **(Fig. 5.21)**
   - Assesses sagittal balance
9. Scoliosis (adult) (see Chapter 4 for pediatric scoliosis)
   - Surgical indications
     a. Rapid curve progression
     b. Symptomatic canal/neuroforaminal stenosis unresponsive to nonoperative measures
     c. Cosmesis
     d. Severe back pain associated with curve (and/or associated stenosis)
   - Surgery
     a. Decompression: central decompression plus lateral recess decompression often necessary

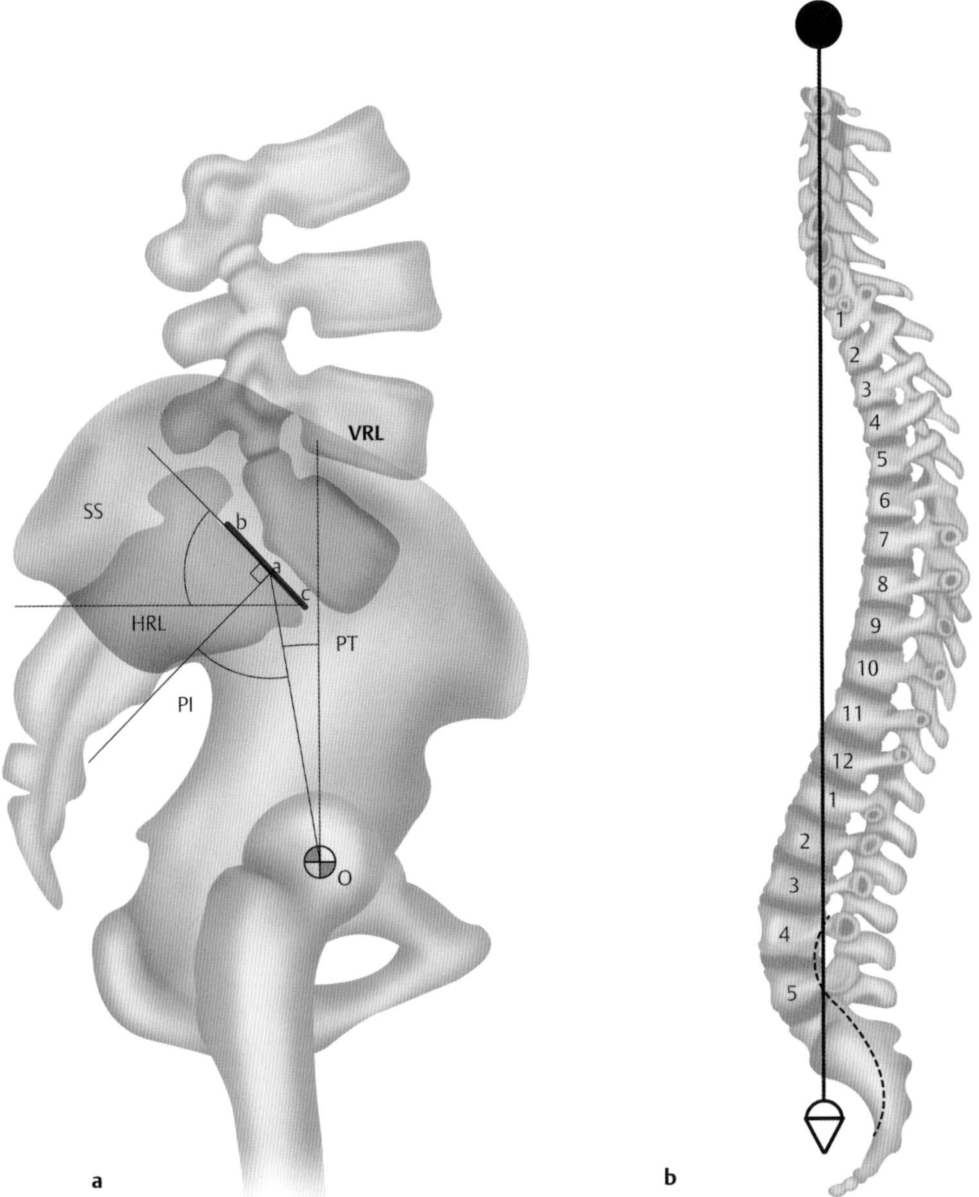

Fig. 5.21 Spinopelvic parameters. **(a,b)** C7 plumb line. HRL; horizontal reference line; O, femoral head center; PI, pelvic incidence; PT, pelvic tilt; SS, sacracl slope; VRL, vertical reference line.

b. Instrumented fusion indicated in curve progression, back pain, listhesis
c. Higher pseudarthrosis rates with isolated thoracoabdominal approach
d. High failure rates if long construct ends at L5
   - Surgery can stop at L5 if L5/S1 is healthy (facet joints and disk)
e. Instrument/fuse to sacrum and ilium; higher fusion rates and fewer sacral insufficiency fractures
f. Also better correction of sagittal balance

10. Kyphosis (also see Chapter 4)
    - May occur due to Scheuermann's disease (> 5-degree wedging of three or more consecutive levels), trauma, or proximal junctional kyphosis (PJK)
    - Osteoporotic compression fractures: increased risk of future compression fractures as sagittal alignment moves anterior and load transferred to superior adjacent vertebra
    - Surgery: instrumentation must extend to first lordotic segment caudally to avoid junctional kyphosis.

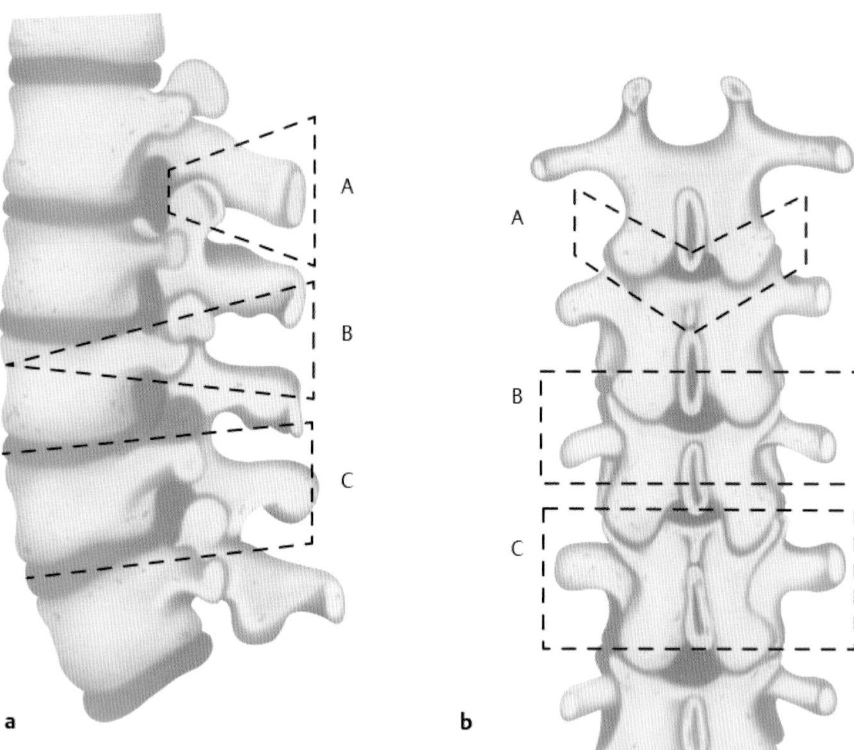

Fig. 5.22 **(a,b)** Posterior spinal osteotomies: A, Smith-Petersen osteotomy; B, pedicle subtraction osteotomy; C, vertebral column resection.

- Osteotomy may be necessary to correct fixed positive sagittal imbalance.
  a. Smith-Petersen osteotomy
    - For correction of mild sagittal imbalance, or for more severe imbalance if multiple osteotomies are performed
    - Allows for 10 degrees of correction per osteotomy
  b. Pedicle subtraction osteotomy (PSO): a closing wedge procedure that provides correction without having to resect intervertebral disk
    - Useful for more severe sagittal imbalance
    - Allows correction of 30–35 degrees of sagittal deformity
  c. Vertebral column resection (VCR)
    - Indicated for most severe deformities
    - Allows correction of up to 45 degrees, and may allow for greater coronal realignment

11. Posterior spinal osteotomies **(Fig. 5.22)**

VIII. Infections of the Spine

1. Disk space infections and vertebral osteomyelitis
   - Disk space infections
     a. A pediatric disease unless it starts in the end plate in an adult and spreads to the disk space
     b. Almost exclusively in children, due to preserved vascularity of the disk
     c. *Staphylococcus aureus* most common organism; gram-negative organisms also common
     d. Infections of the spine unrelated to a surgical procedure frequently develop secondary to hematogenous seeding
   - Vertebral osteomyelitis
     a. Incidence rising

b. Clinical presentation remains nonspecific and is associated with delay in diagnosis.
c. More common in older, debilitated patients
d. IV drug users and immunocompromised at risk
e. *S. aureus* most common organism
f. Hematogenous seeding
g. Secondary disk space infection
   - Infection usually begins in vascular end plates with subsequent penetration and spread into the avascular disk space.

- Diagnosis: signs and symptoms often nonspecific, resulting in delay in diagnosis
  a. Back pain/tenderness
  b. Pain with spinal motion, walking, standing, sitting
  c. Fever
  d. Laboratory studies
     - Elevated ESR
     - CRP
     - White blood cell (WBC) count (high normal or mildly elevated; nonspecific)
     - Blood cultures positive in approximately one third of patients
     - CT-guided biopsy may be required to identify organism.
  e. Radiographic studies
     - Loss of lumbar lordosis (diskitis): earliest finding
     - Osteopenia (vertebral osteomyelitis)
     - Disk space narrowing/destruction: later in disease process
     - End-plate erosion
     - MRI with gadolinium enhancement is diagnostic test of choice.
     - Bone scan can also be used to make the diagnosis.
- Treatment
  a. Six to 12 weeks of culture-specific IV antibiotics
  b. Brace, supportive care
  c. Surgical intervention indicated in patients who have failed medical management or patients with neurologic deficit, progressive deformity, or if needed to establish diagnosis
     - Irrigation/debridement, corpectomy, instrumentation, fusion may be necessary
- **In general, spinal infections involve the end plates and disk space, whereas most metastatic neoplasms primarily involve the vertebral body.**

2. Epidural abscesses
   - Bacterial infections that results in the accumulation of pus in the epidural space of the spinal canal
   - Lesions most commonly extend from an adjacent focus of vertebral osteomyelitis/diskitis
   - Usually located in the posterior epidural space in the thoracic or lumbar spine
   - Less commonly occur in cervical spine, where they tend to be located in the anterior epidural space
   - Most common organism is *S. aureus*; gram-negative rods account for minority of infections
   - Variable clinical presentation, often misdiagnosed or diagnosed in delayed manner

- Diagnosis
  a. Back or neck pain
  b. More commonly present with constitutional symptoms than patients with osteomyelitis or diskitis
  c. High risk of neurologic deficits from direct compression of neural elements and ischemic injury resulting from thrombosis/vasculitis
  d. Laboratory studies
     - Elevated ESR, CRP, WBC
     - Blood cultures positive in more than half of cases
     - Ultimate diagnosis confirmed with cultures from the abscess
  e. Imaging studies
     - Plain radiographs often normal unless evidence of adjacent osteomyelitis/diskitis
     - MRI with gadolinium is test of choice
- Treatment
  a. Surgical decompression with abscess evacuation (and spinal stabilization if necessary) is the treatment of choice.
  b. IV antibiotics following surgical decompression
  c. Nonsurgical treatment generally reserved for neurologically intact patients who are poor surgical candidates (or with small epidural collections in the mid/lower lumbar spine)

3. Tuberculosis (TB) involving the spine
   - Most common granulomatous infection of the spine
   - Relatively rare; however, incidence has increased with growing number of immunocompromised hosts.
   - The spine is the most common location of extrapulmonary TB.
     a. Most common in lower thoracic/upper lumbar spine
   - **Unlike pyogenic infections, the nidus originates in the metaphysis of vertebral bodies, sparing the disk space; often confused with tumors.**
   - Spreads under the anterior longitudinal ligament to contiguous levels or may even result in skip lesions
   - Destruction of vertebral body may lead to instability and kyphotic deformity.
     a. Disk space preserved
   - Diagnosis
     a. Pain or discomfort in thoracic back region (most common location)
     b. Focal kyphosis (typically with delayed presentation after vertebral collapse)
     c. Constitutional findings are common, such as fever and weight loss.
     d. Laboratory studies
        - ESR, CRP, WBC may be normal or elevated
        - Positive purified protein derivative (PPD) test
        - Sputum cultures in patients with pulmonary disease may show acid-fast bacilli.
        - Biopsy of spinal lesion should include testing for acid-fast bacilli.
     e. Imaging studies
        - Plain radiographs may be normal or may demonstrate peri-diskal erosions, scalloping of anterior vertebral bodies, or extensive bony destruction and focal kyphosis in later stages of disease.
        - Preservation of disk space on plain radiographs and MRI
        - Chest radiographs may be abnormal if pulmonary disease present.
        - MRI with gadolinium is test of choice.

- Treatment
  a. Pharmacological therapy often required for at least 6–12 months (isoniazid, rifampin, pyrazinamide, and either streptomycin or ethambutol)
  b. Surgical treatment required for patients with neurologic deficit, abscess, failure of conservative management, spinal instability or progressive kyphosis.

4. Postoperative infections
   - Treatment of postoperative lumbar disk space infection following diskectomy:
     a. No neurologic deficit, no fluid collection: IV antibiotics
     b. No neurologic deficit, with fluid collection: irrigation/debridement/IV antibiotics
     c. Neurologic deficit: irrigation/debridement + IV antibiotics
     d. Hardware can often be retained; do not remove hardware if instability present

IX. Miscellaneous Facts

1. The use of continuous fluoroscopy increases the radiation exposure.
2. The most common sentinel event in spine surgery is wrong-level surgery.
3. The most common nonanesthetic cause of reversible change to intraoperative neuromonitoring is patient positioning.
4. The Oswestry Disability Index is a highly specific spine outcome instrument.
5. In Jehovah's Witness patients, if high blood loss surgery is anticipated, use a cell saver with continuity maintained through a closed circuit.
6. Fasciculations occur in lower motor neuron disorders. Spasticity and exaggerated deep tendon reflexes occur in upper motor neuron disorders.
7. Intraoperative monitoring changes in anterior cervical spine surgery may occur due to retractor placement compressing the carotid artery.
8. Transcranial motor evoked potential (tcMEP) monitoring is the most effective means of detecting intraoperative evolving motor tract injury.

6

Adult Hip and Knee Reconstruction

Scott Ritterman, John Froehlich, and Matthew Miller

I. Total Hip Replacement

1. Anatomy
   - Ball-and-socket joint
     a. Socket deepened by thick flexible labrum
     b. Cotyloid fossa: floor of acetabulum, no cartilage, ligamentum teres
        ◦ Radiographic marker "teardrop" is formed by:
          ♦ Quadrilateral plate from inside pelvis
          ♦ Cotyloid fossa from floor of acetabulum
     c. Adult's main blood supply to femoral head from medial femoral circumflex artery
   - Surgical approaches
     a. Anterior (Smith-Petersen approach)
        ◦ Internervous plane
          ♦ Sartorius (femoral nerve) and tensor fascia lata (superior gluteal nerve) superficially
          ♦ Gluteus medius (superior gluteal nerve) and rectus femoris (femoral nerve) deep
        ◦ Ascending braches of the lateral circumflex artery must be cauterized or ligated.
        ◦ Lateral femoral cutaneous nerve typically exits the pelvis laterally just inferior to the inguinal ligament, but there are several anatomic variants.
     b. Anterolateral (Watson Jones)
        ◦ Intermuscular plane
          ♦ Tensor fascia lata and gluteus medius (superior gluteal nerve)
          ♦ Traditionally requires trochanteric osteotomy for adequate exposure of the hip joint
     c. Direct lateral
        ◦ No intermuscular plane
          ♦ Splits anterior third of gluteus medius and minimus, and anterior portion of vastus lateralis
        ◦ Dislocate hip anteriorly
        ◦ Can lead to Trendelenburg gait postoperatively due weakness of gluteus medius and possible damage to superior gluteal nerve
          ♦ Superior gluteal nerve lies 3–5 cm proximal to greater trochanter on the underside of the gluteus medius muscle
          ♦ Prone to injury by stretching or transection

d. Posterior approach
   - No intramuscular plane
     - Split gluteus maximus muscle (inferior gluteal nerve)
     - Tag and divide piriformis tendon; alternatively, can spare tendon and retract
     - Short external rotators are detached and reflected with posterior capsular flap used to protect the sciatic nerve during dissection
     - Hip extension and knee flexion will protect the sciatic nerve from excess stretch intraoperatively.
   - Increased dislocation risk if capsule is not repaired with the posterior approach
   - **Most common reason for sciatic nerve injury is errant retractor placement. Hematoma can form postoperatively as a result of postop anticoagulation, which can cause sciatic palsy as well. Treatment is evacuation of hematoma. Females, revision surgery, and patients with severe hip dysplasia (congenital dislocation) have highest risks of nerve injury.**

2. Physical examination
   - Normal range of motion (ROM)
     a. Flexion: 135 degrees
     b. Extension: 10–15 degrees
     c. Abduction: 45 degrees
     d. Adduction: 30 degrees
     e. Internal rotation: 35 degrees
     f. External rotation: 45 degrees
   - **Hip rotation can be checked in both flexion and extension. Excessive femoral anteversion results in increased internal rotation in extension, which may not be obvious or present in flexion.**
   - Motor function
     a. Hip flexion against resistance from a seated position
        - Test for iliopsoas impingement (snapping hip) with the patient seated, pain with resisted flexion
     b. Adduction
     c. Abductors: lay patient on contralateral side and keep leg abducted against resistance
     d. Knee extension against resistance (quad strength)
   - Gait examination
     a. Antalgic: shortened stance phase, unloading painful limb
     b. Abductor lurch (Trendelenburg gait)
        - When the abductors are deficient, the pelvis tilts down toward the contralateral side during single-limb stance. In compensation, the trunk leans toward the deficient side to maintain the center of gravity over the weight-bearing limb. See Trendelenburg test, below.
   - Leg length discrepancy (LLD)
     a. Always should be evaluated preoperatively and intraoperatively
        - Common cause of litigation
     b. Some people have small LLD at baseline and most can tolerate up to 1 cm difference
     c. True LLD
        - Actual lengthening measured with anteroposterior (AP) pelvis, comparing distance between lesser trochanter and transischiac line, teardrop line, or some other fixed point **(Fig. 6.1)**

d. Apparent LLD: perceived leg length difference
   - Hip flexion/adduction contracture
   - Scoliosis, pelvis obliquity
   - Lengthening after long-term shortened limb (chronic femoral neck fracture, acetabular protrusio)

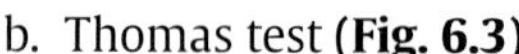

e. Measurements
   - Anterior superior iliac spine (ASIS) to medial malleolus
   - Umbilicus to medial malleolus

- Special tests

a. Trendelenburg test **(Fig. 6.2)**
   - To test the left abductors, ask the patient to stand on the left leg. If the patient's pelvis tilts to the right, then the test is positive, indicating weak/deficient abductors of the left hip.

b. Thomas test **(Fig. 6.3)**
   - To test for a hip flexion contracture, ask the patient to lie in the supine position, and, placing one hand under the patient's lower back to prevent excessive lumbar lordosis, flex the unaffected hip as much as possible. Lift the patient's affected limb and release. The leg should return to the examination table with the lower back in contact with the examiner's hand.

c. Impingement test
   - Flex hip to 90 degrees
   - Pain with internal rotation and adduction

d. Labral shear test
   - Pain with circumduction of the hip (like McMurray maneuver for the hip)

- Differential diagnosis of hip joint pain

a. Trochanteric bursitis/tight iliotibial band (ITB)
   - Tenderness centered over greater trochanter; check Ober test

Fig. 6.1 Actual lengthening measured with anteroposterior (AP) X-ray of the pelvis, comparing the distance between the lesser trochanter and the ipsilateral ischial spine.

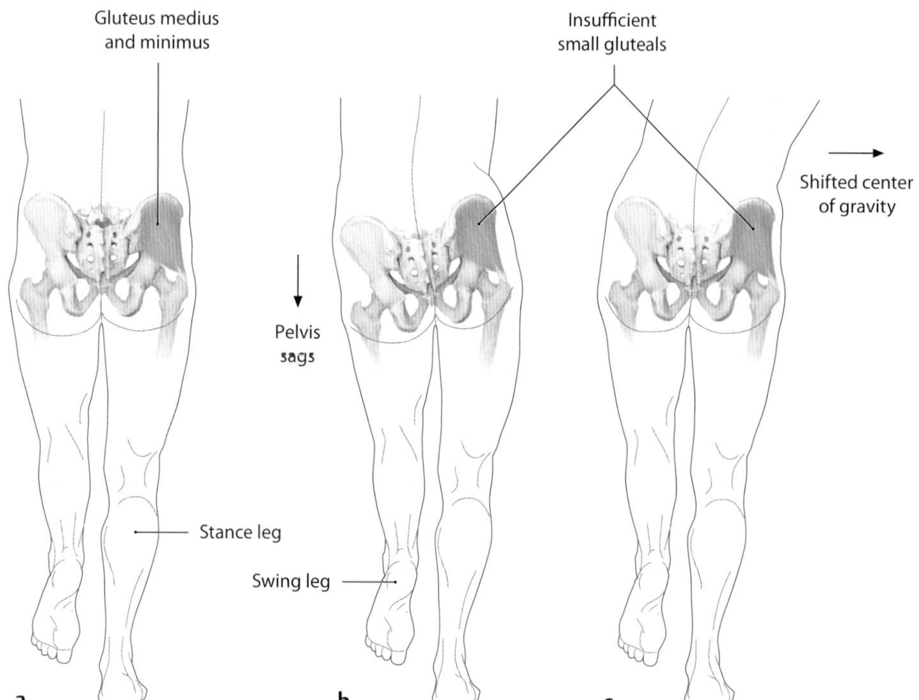

Fig. 6.2 **(a–c)** Trendelenburg test. (From Schuenke M, Schulte E. General Anatomy and the Musculoskeletal System: Thieme Atlas of Anatomy. New York: Thieme; 2005. Illustration by Karl Wesker.)

b. Sacroiliac (SI) joint inflammation

c. FABER (*f*lexion, *ab*duction, and *e*xternal *r*otation) test: pain with flexion, abduction, external rotation in the SI joint region

d. Lumbar radiculopathy (see Chapter 5)

- Radicular symptoms extending beyond the knee
- Evaluate with lumbosacral spine X-ray and possibly magnetic resonance imaging (MRI)

e. Intrapelvic pain

- Hernia
- Pelvic inflammatory disease (PID)
- Diverticular disease

f. Diagnostic hip injection with local anesthetic can help differentiate between intracapsular and extracapsular causes of pain.

3. Hip disease

- Dysplasia

a. Developmental malalignment of the hip joint

b. Typically presents in fourth to seventh decades with arthritis of the hip joint

c. May be subtle or pronounced

- Abnormal biomechanics lead to degenerative changes within the hip joint.
- Time of presentation depends on the degree of dysplasia.

d. Acetabular dysplasia

- Coverage
  - ♦ Under-coverage of femoral head: typically anterior and laterally
    - Lateral center-edge angle **(Fig. 6.4)**
    - Normally 25–40 degrees; < 20 degrees is typical in developmental dysplasia of the hip (DDH)
  - ♦ Over-coverage of femoral head
    - Center-edge angle > 40 degrees can lead to pincer type impingement as the hip flexes and abducts.
- Version
  - ♦ Acetabular retroversion (normally anteverted)
  - ♦ Crossover sign
    - Radiographic cardinal lines/landmarks **(Fig. 6.5)**
    - When anterior wall crosses posterior wall medial to the weight-bearing lateral rim
    - May be present in those with pincer-type femoroacetabular impingement (FAI)

e. Femoral dysplasia

- Head–neck dysplasia (also see Chapter 8)
  - ♦ Cam lesion reduces the native head/neck ratio, leading to early femoral neck impingement during normal ROM
  - ♦ Pistol grip deformity seen on radiograph
  - ♦ Alpha angle: formed by a line drawn from the center of the femoral head through the center of the femoral neck and a line drawn from the center of the femoral head to the head/neck junction; alpha angle > 50–55 degrees indicates a likely cam lesion
  - ♦ Demonstration of alpha angle **(Fig. 6.6)**

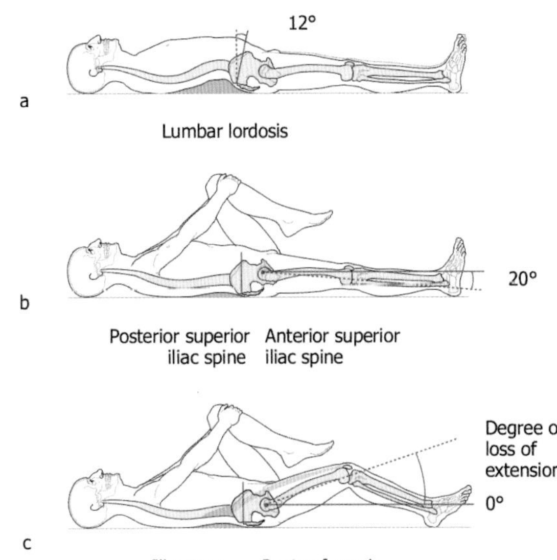

Fig. 6.3 **(a–c)** Thomas test. (From Schuenke M, Schulte E. General Anatomy and the Musculoskeletal System: Thieme Atlas of Anatomy. New York: Thieme; 2005. Illustration by Karl Wesker.)

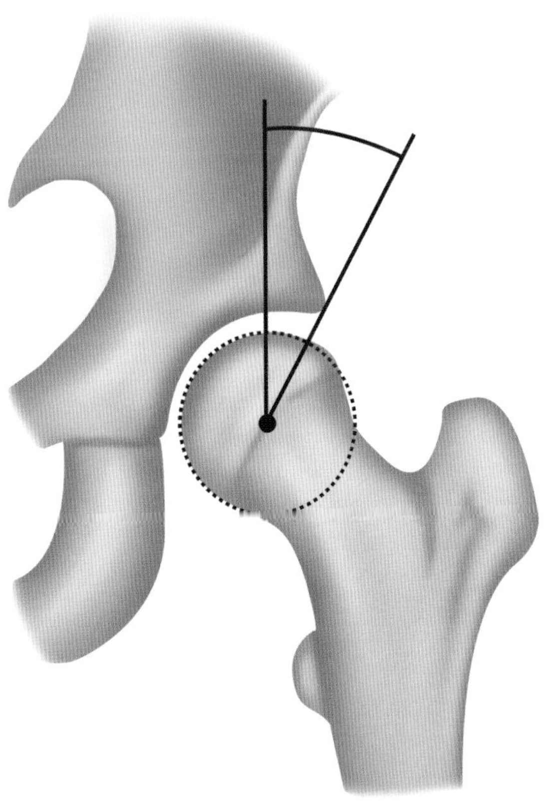

Fig. 6.4 Lateral center-edge angle.

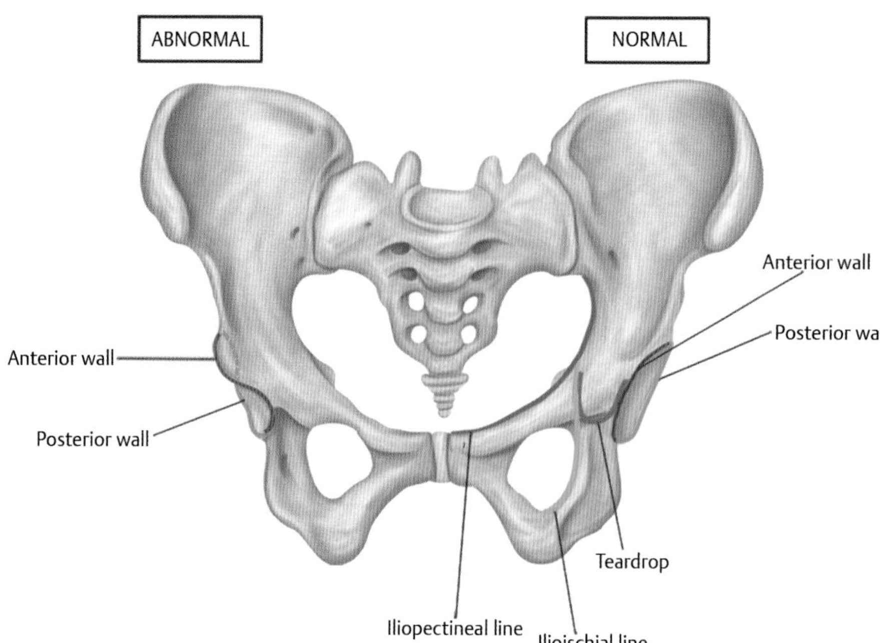

Fig. 6.5 Radiographic cardinal lines/landmarks.

f. FAI (also see Chapter 8)

- **Abnormal impingement can be from the acetabulum or from the femur; evaluate the radiograph to delineate the etiology of the impingement.**
- Abnormal contact between anterior rim of acetabulum and femoral neck, leading to block in motion and pain, decreased internal rotation
- Pincer type: labrum caught between bony surfaces
  - Occurs with acetabular retroversion or over-coverage
    - Crossover sign seen on X-ray
  - Labrum is damaged
- Cam type: raised area of proximal femur impinges on anterior acetabulum during hip flexion
- Combined: features of both cam and pincer type
  - Damage to chondral surface of acetabulum
- Presentation
  - Pain with hip flexion and internal rotation
  - Decreased internal rotation or obligate external rotation with flexion

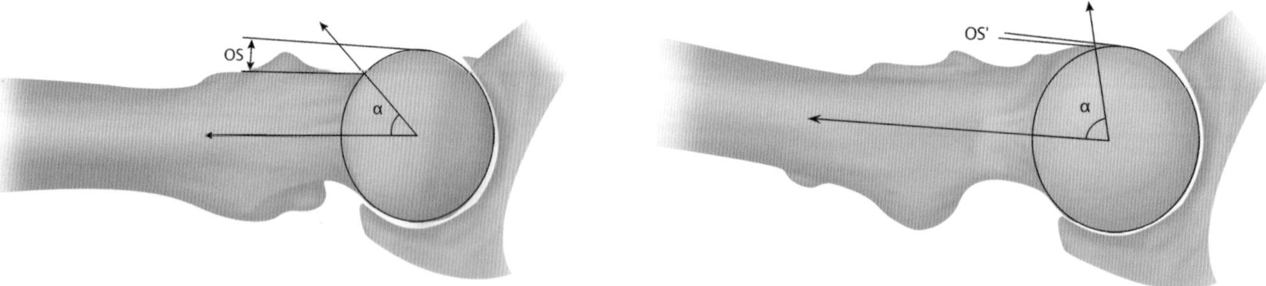

Fig. 6.6 Alpha angle: formed by a line drawn from the center of the femoral head through the center of the femoral neck and a line drawn from the center of the femoral head to the head/neck junction. (Alpha angles > 50–55 degrees indicates a likely cam lesion.) OS, offset (femoral head-neck offset).

- Treatment: aimed at cause of dysplasia
  - Ganz periacetabular osteotomy (PAO); used to correct acetabular dysplasia
    - Osteotomize around the acetabulum while leaving the posterior column intact to redirect the native acetabulum.
    - Goal is to medialize the joint and gain lateral/anterior coverage of the femoral head.
      - Joint medialization decreases joint reactive forces.
      - Correction of acetabular version, lateral center-edge angle
  - Anterior hip decompression
    - Arthroscopic versus open
    - **Nerve injury is the most common complication of hip arthroscopy. The pudendal nerve is at risk due to traction needed to access the hip. Traction should not be applied for longer than 2 hours. The pudendal nerve exits the pelvis through the greater sciatic notch, and reenters through the lesser sciatic notch. It provides sensation to external genitalia**
    - Debridement of cam lesion
    - Debridement of anterior acetabulum (rim trim)
    - Repair/debride torn labrum
  - Proximal femoral osteotomy
    - Varus producing osteotomy
      - Typically done after PAO with insufficient lateral coverage (insufficient center-edge angle)
    - Valgus producing osteotomy
      - Typically for femoral neck nonunion in adults
  - Total hip considerations with hip dysplasia
    - Acetabulum is shallow, deficient superiorly and anteriorly.
    - Femoral neck may be short with excessive anteversion.
    - Proximal migration of femoral head may exist (chronic shortening of leg and neurovascular structures).
      - Insufficient abductors may need to be transferred distally with trochanteric osteotomy.
      - Shortened hamstrings and adductors may need to be lengthened.
      - Shortened sciatic nerve
      - **Sciatic nerve palsy may occur after excessive lengthening during total hip arthroplasty (THA).**
        - ◊ Susceptible to injury if leg lengthened > 2–3 cm, although can occur with less
        - ◊ May require femoral shortening osteotomy (subtrochanteric)

- Osteonecrosis
- **The medial femoral circumflex artery is the dominant blood supply to the femoral head in adults.**

a. Loss of blood supply to femoral head

b. Posttraumatic
   - Femoral head necrosis after femoral head or neck fracture, or traumatic or iatrogenic hip dislocation

c. Idiopathic: avascular necrosis (AVN)
   - Demographics: third and fourth decades of life
   - Presentation: acute or progressive groin pain, decreased/painful internal rotation and flexion

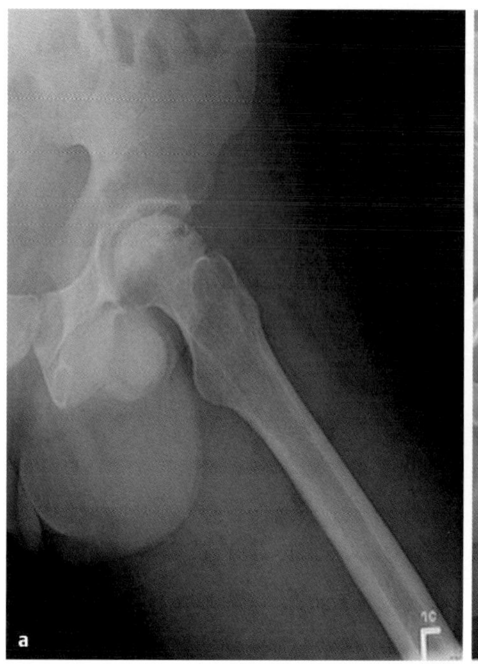

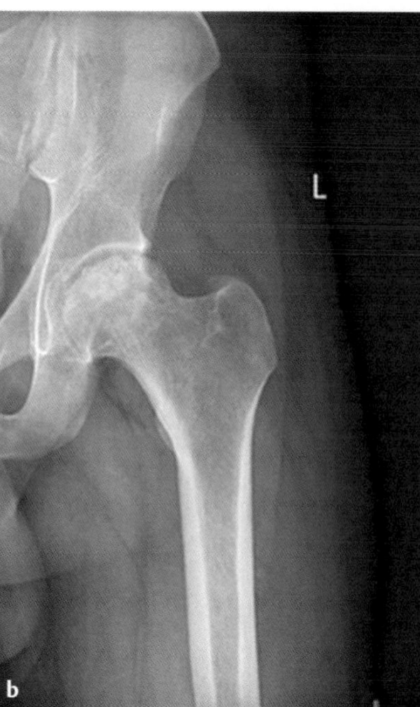

Fig. 6.7 **(a)** A crescent sign can be seen, with slight lucency in the subchondral bone of the femur with flattening of the head. **(b)** The femoral head eventually collapsed about 18 months later.

- Risk factors:
  - Alcoholism
  - Corticosteroids
  - Hypercoagulability
    - Sickle cell anemia
      - 75% of asymptomatic patients with osteonecrosis develop symptoms/collapse if untreated
- Imaging
  - Radiographs: AP pelvis, AP lateral hip
    - Look for sclerosis or cystic changes in femoral head
    - Crescent sign **(Fig. 6.7)**
    - Collapse of femoral head
    - Ficat classification **(Table 6.1)**
  - MRI
    - Edema within the femoral head/neck
    - Always check contralateral hip for asymptomatic disease.
- Treatment
  - Nonsurgical
    - Activity modification: limited weight bearing
    - Weight loss

Table 6.1 Ficat Classification

Grade	Findings
0	Pain without radiographic or MRI findings
I	Normal radiograph with edema within femoral head on MRI
II	Radiograph with sclerotic changes to femoral head
III	Femoral head flattening with crescent sign on radiograph
IV	Femoral head collapse, loss of joint space, osteoarthritis

- Nonsteroidal anti-inflammatory drugs (NSAIDs)
- Bisphosphonates: can prevent/delay collapse if given in the early stages

- Surgical
  - Core decompression
    - Tunnel(s) drilled up the femoral neck into the head to allow decompression and revascularization; often combined with bone grafting
    - May be effective early in disease before crescent sign and collapse occur (Ficat grades I and II)
  - Vascularized fibular graft
    - Free tissue transfer to place vascularized autograft into the femoral head
    - Pain at donor site/leg following vascularized fibula transfer may indicate a tibial stress fracture; evaluate with MRI.
  - Total hip replacement
    - Most reliable treatment for AVN with collapse
  - **Can also consider hip fusion in young laborer**
    - Young patient with Ficat grade III or IV (collapse present)

- Osteoarthritis

a. Progressive cartilage loss leads to weight bearing on subchondral bone
   - Demographics: fourth to eighth decades of life; females > males
   - Presentation: progressive groin pain with weight-bearing activities; decreased rotation; external rotation and flexion contractures due to long-standing joint inflammation
   - Imaging
     - Weight-bearing AP pelvis, AP hip, cross-table lateral of hip
   - Treatment
     - Nonsurgical
       - Activity modification with continued low-impact exercise
       - Weight loss
       - NSAIDs
       - Crutch/cane: placed in contralateral hand will off-load weight during stance phase
       - Intra-articular corticosteroid injection (fluoro or ultrasound guided)
     - Surgical
       - Hip fusion
         - **Ideal position is 0–5 degrees external rotation, 0–5 degrees adduction, 20–35 degrees flexion**
         - Typical candidate is a young male laborer with debilitating arthritis who needs to continue working
         - Unilateral disease
         - One-third increase in energy needed to ambulate
         - As with any fused joints, increased stresses are translated to adjacent joints, which become arthritic (spine, knee)
       - Fusion to THA
         - **Must have hip abductors present to convert a hip fusion to an arthroplasty for stability; otherwise, will require a constrained liner for stability**
         - Often done for adjacent joint disease (lumbosacral spine most commonly, knee)

    - Function directly related to integrity of abductor complex
    - Preoperative electromyogram (EMG) required to test abductors
    - Deficient abductors require constrained hip liner or tripolar articulation
  - Hip resurfacing arthroplasty
    - Intended for active young male patients
    - Larger head should confer greater static stability
    - Metal-on-metal resurfacing of femoral head and acetabulum
    - Advantages include preservation of bone stock, lower wear without polyethylene liner, retain large femoral head size and therefore lower dislocation risk
    - Contraindications
      - ◊ Osteoporosis, coxa vara, femoral neck cyst
      - ◊ Abnormal acetabular anatomy
      - ◊ Significant leg length discrepancy
      - ◊ Smaller anatomy
      - ◊ Renal disease
      - ◊ Metal allergy
    - Complications
      - ◊ Periprosthetic femoral neck fracture up to 4% and is the most common reason for revision before 20 weeks
      - ◊ Metal-on-metal debris is generated, leading to T-cell immune response; see Metal-on-metal wear, below.
- Hemiarthroplasty
  a. Typically used for femoral neck fractures in low demand, elderly patients
  b. Unipolar hemiarthroplasty refers to a one-piece head that is attached to the neck of the implanted femoral component. A bipolar hemiarthroplasty refers to an articulating head within the larger head component. In theory, this more equally distributes shear forces, leading to less wear of the native acetabulum as well as a greater range of motion. However, motion within the inner bearing decreases over time. There is no difference in outcomes.
  c. Low demand, infirm patient without antecedent hip/groin pain
  d. Advantage is large head size, allowing for more stability and lower dislocation rate
    - Preserve the labrum, repair hip capsule for greatest postoperative stability
  e. Active patients develop groin pain due to chondrolysis and have superior outcome with total hip replacement
- Total hip arthroplasty
  a. Use THA for active patients with arthritis and displaced femoral neck fracture.
  b. Higher dislocation rate with femoral neck fracture than elective THA for osteoarthritis (OA)

4. Basics of total hip replacement
- Bearing surfaces
  a. Soft: ceramic on polyethylene (PE), metal on PE
  b. PE: hydrocarbon molecule
    - Ultra-high molecular weight polyethylene (UHMWPE) has been in use for > 40 years
      - ♦ Mechanical properties depend on percentage of PE in
        - Amorphous phase
        - Crystalline phase

- Highly cross-linked UHMWPE
  - Better wear characteristics
- Significantly reduces wear compared with conventional UHMWPE
  - Less mechanical strength
- Need to find compromise between the two

- **Steps in PE liner production: 1, manufacture; 2, sterilize; 3, cross-link; 4, melt/anneal; 5, package**
- Manufacturing
  - Direct compression molding from powder has the best wear characteristics.
  - **During manufacturing via ram-bar extrusion, calcium stearate was once added to PE to prevent sticking to equipment; results in increased wear, and reduced mechanical properties; no longer used but still tested**
- Sterilization
  - Low-dose irradiation (2.5–4 Mrd) is best mode
  - Irradiation (at higher dose) also allows cross-linking to occur
- Cross-linking of hydrocarbon chains between molecules of PE provides greater wear resistance.
  - **Why cross-link? More wear resistant, more resistant to adhesive and abrasive wear; smaller wear particles**
- Irradiation of PE creates free radicals that can bind either:
  - Oxygen: oxidized PE, chain scission, and no cross-linking occurs; greatly increased wear
  - Other PE molecules: in an oxygen-free environment (typically in the presence of inert gases such as argon), free radicals bind other PE molecules and form cross-links (which is good)
- Therefore, irradiation must be done in an oxygen-free environment!
- **Sterilization of polyethylene and packaging in air lead to premature polyethylene wear and osteolysis, and is a commonly tested concept.**
- Irradiation in larger amounts of radiation (5–20 Mrad) creates highly cross-linked polyethylene
  - Better wear resistance than cross-linking with lower dose of irradiation
  - Decreased mechanical strength compared with regular cross-linked PE, more brittle
  - Smaller wear particles
- Heating of PE after cross-linking is required to remove excess free radicals. Melting removes all free radicals; annealing removes some.
  - Affects the structure of PE
    - Crystalline: ideally 45–65% of PE
      - Greater percentage of crystallinity leads to greater mechanical strength
    - Amorphous
      - Where cross-linking occurs
  - Melting
    - Less free radicals, better resistance to oxidation in vivo
    - Reduces mechanical properties; lowers crystallinity
  - Annealing: heating PE to less than melting point
    - Better mechanical properties than melting (decreased wear) due to higher crystallinity

- Higher risk of free radicals and resulting oxidation in vivo

- Vitamin E can be added to reduce free radicals by blending or infusion.
- Shelf life: vacuum-sealed package
  - Remaining free radicals have the potential to oxidize while PE sits on the shelf awaiting use.
  - Concern about odd-sized components that may sit on shelf for extended time
  - **Two reasons for irradiating: (1) sterilization (2.5–4 Mrad); (2) creation of free radicals for cross-linking to form highly cross-linked PE (5–20 Mrad)**
- All PE components regardless of means of sterilization will begin to oxidize once implanted and exposed to environment.
- PE wear products lead to osteolysis (see below)

c. Hard bearing surfaces
- Metal
  - Alloys consisting of cobalt, chrome, molybdenum, nickel, and other substances are used for bearing surfaces due to their resistance to corrosion.
  - Titanium is too soft to use as a bearing surface but has a stiffness similar to bone and is therefore ideal for use in both femoral implant and acetabular shell.
    - Titanium has a Young modulus of 115 GPa.
    - **Relative Young's modulus of common materials from highest (stiffest) to lowest:**
      - **Ceramic**
      - **Cobalt-chromium (CoCr)**
      - **Steel**
      - **Titanium**
      - **Cortical bone**
      - **Tantalum**
      - **Cement**
      - **Polyethylene**
      - **Cancellous bone**
      - **Cartilage**
  - Scratches too easily, leading to increased wear if used for bearing surface (head)
- Theoretically, metal-on-metal (MOM) bearings have a lower wear rate, generate smaller wear particles compared with PE bearings, and allow the use of a large head, conferring greater joint stability.
- Imprecise placement of components, especially an over-abducted or anteverted cup, can lead to edge loading and generation of a large number of wear particles, increasing serum cobalt and chromium ion concentrations, and stimulating a T-cell response (see Metal-on-metal wear, below).
- Ceramic: alumina ceramic and zirconia ceramic
  - Ceramic on ceramic (COC)
    - Low wear
    - Fewer particles than in MOM
    - Bio-inert debris
    - Limited head size, less optimal fluid film mechanics (see below)
    - Can entail squeaking, possibly due to component malposition

- Risk of fracture
  - First-generation ceramic implants susceptible to fracture, due to manufacturing imperfections and brittle materials
  - Current-generation ceramic implants have significantly lower fracture rates
  - Low toughness (limited plastic deformation) (see Chapter 12)
  - After fracture, must revise with COC bearing
  - **When a ceramic component fractures, revision must always be with COC. Small fragments always remain and would cause rapid PE wear.**
  - **When exchanging prosthetic heads for any reason and retaining femoral components, a jacket should be placed on the retained trunnion. A new ceramic head cannot be placed directly on an old trunnion, as it will lead to fracture of the new femoral head.**

- Advantages of hard-on-hard bearings
  - Potential to decrease osteolytic wear, which was a main issue with conventional PE
  - Much smaller wear particles generated for MOM or ceramic components
    - 0.015–0.12 μm compared with 0.2–7 μm for hard on soft (polyethylene)
    - Smaller particles are not recognized by macrophages.
    - Immune response is mediated by lymphocytes.
- MOM hips have very low wear rate but generate many more particles (see below)

d. Lubrication
- Boundary
  - Occurs while at rest and slow walking
  - Two bearing surfaces in contact
- Hydrodynamic
  - Two bearing surfaces are completely separated by fluid.
  - **Lambda ratio**
    - **Takes into account roughness, head size, viscosity, angular velocity**
    - **Greater than 3 indicates fluid film mechanics**
  - More smooth bearing surfaces leads to hydrodynamic lubrication
  - Larger head size
    - ≥ 38 mm is most likely to achieve hydrodynamic lubrication
  - Requires angular motion to achieve hydrodynamic lubrication; must be walking
    - Surface roughness
  - Bearing surfaces must be very smooth
    - Ceramic > metal > PE
      - Ceramic Ra < 0.01 μm
      - Metal Ra 0.01 μm
      - PE Ra several μm

e. Sphericity
- Variation leads to small high points and localized stress points, which negatively affects lubrication.
- Measured as "out of roundness" in μm

- 9- to 10-µm heads have more PE wear than 0.5-µm heads.

f. Radial clearance
  - Difference in radius of curvature of the head and the cup
    - ♦ Equatorial contact
      - Head is larger than the cup.
      - High friction
        - No space for fluid to enter or exit
    - ♦ Polar contact
      - Head is smaller than the cup.
      - One point of contact
      - High stress at point of contact and poor lubrication
    - ♦ Midpolar contact (ideal)
      - Radius of curvature of head is slightly smaller than that of cup.
      - Fluid is able to enter the joint and lubricate the bearing surfaces.
      - Cannot have complete congruence or fluid cannot enter to lubricate joint

g. Wear
  - Any process that leads to breakdown of bearing surfaces, resulting in particulate debris, increased friction, and altered biomechanics
  - Volumetric wear
    - ♦ Calculated, though exact equation is debated
    - ♦ Directly related to size of prosthetic head
    - ♦ Larger heads lead to greater volumetric wear
  - Linear wear
    - ♦ Wear rates above 0.1 mm per year are at high risk of osteolysis.
      - Any new polyethylene with wear rates < 0.1 mm/year should have minimal osteolysis (> 10 billion particles/gram of tissue)
    - ♦ Measured on radiograph
    - ♦ Penetration of femoral head into the liner
    - ♦ **Smaller heads have greater linear wear, less volumetric wear**
  - Adhesive wear
    - ♦ PE particles pulled off form liner during gait cycle
    - ♦ Most important in generation of PE debris in hips
    - ♦ **Cross-linking of PE has led to decreased adhesive and abrasive wear and has significantly decreased the risk of osteolysis.**
  - Abrasive wear
    - ♦ Rough femoral head scratches and mechanically damages PE liner
  - Third body wear
    - ♦ Any material between the two bearing surfaces; cement, metal shavings, bone, etc.
    - ♦ Debris between two bearing surfaces wears/scratches the weaker one
  - Run-in wear
    - ♦ Higher wear rate within the first 1 million cycles of THA use (bedding in period)
    - ♦ Decreases thereafter as it goes into steady-state phase
    - ♦ High stress points on surfaces polished out
  - Stripe wear
    - ♦ Seen with ceramic prosthetic heads
    - ♦ Occurs with lift-off separation when the femoral head contacts the rim of the shell as it separates from the socket

- ♦ Crescent-shaped line on femoral head and corresponding on cup, near edge
  - ♦ Surface wear 1–60 μm deep
  - ♦ Seen more commonly in those cups that are vertically oriented
- ◦ Hip edge loading: radiograph shows an over-abducted cup
  - ♦ Stresses concentrate on edge of acetabular shell
    - ▪ To prevent, need to make sure that midpolar contact occurs, and the cup should not be abducted past 45 degrees **(Fig. 6.8)**

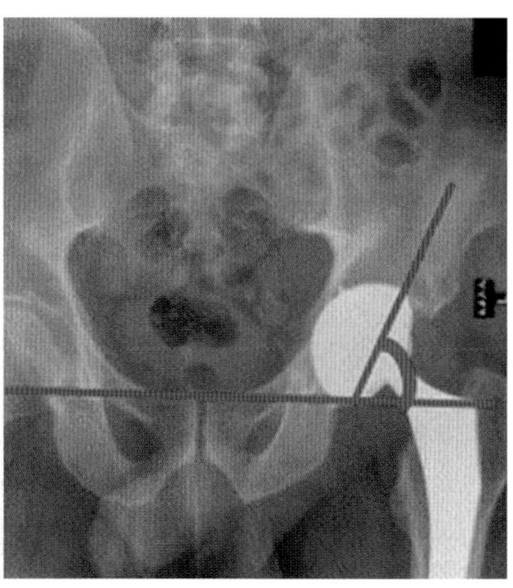

Fig. 6.8 Hip radiograph showing an over-abducted cup. To prevent excessive bearing surface wear in MOM reconstruction, cup abduction angle must be optimized. Cup abduction angle target should be 40 degrees.

- Implant fixation

a. Biological

- ◦ Biological fixation: dynamic relationship between bone and prosthesis with ability to remodel over time
- ◦ Prosthesis must be coated to allow bone ingrowth or ongrowth.
- ◦ Beware of devascularized bone.
  - ♦ Patients who have been irradiated may not be able to support bony ingrowth (requiring tantalum cup and multiple screw fixation or cement for fixation).
- ◦ Press fit versus line-to-line technique
  - ♦ Press fit refers to preparing bone (either femur or acetabulum) to a certain size and then inserting an implant that is slightly larger (1–2 mm). Compressive hoop stresses provide the initial fixation while bone ongrowth/ingrowth occurs.
  - ♦ Line-to-line technique refers to preparing the femur or cup to a certain size and inserting the same-size implant. Acetabular shell requires screws if placed in this fashion; femoral stem is fully porous coated for initial rigid fixation.
    - ▪ For both, the long-term fixation is biological.
- ◦ Porous coating: allows for bone ingrowth
  - ♦ Porosity
    - ▪ Too little porosity will not leave enough room for ingrowth.
    - ▪ Too much porosity will lead to failure due to shear forces.
    - ▪ 40–50% porosity is ideal
      - • Pore depth
        - ◊ Deeper is better to some extent.
      - • Pore size
        - ◊ 50–400 μm is ideal pore size
      - • Micromotion
        - ◊ < 30 μm for bone ingrowth
        - ◊ > 150 μm leads to fibrous fixation
      - • Proximal or metaphyseal loading
        - ◊ Stems that are coated proximally will lead to proximal ingrowth and loading of proximal bone (preventing stress shielding).
- ◦ Grit blasting: allows for bone ongrowth
  - ♦ Surface roughness
    - ▪ Difference in height between peaks a valleys
    - ▪ Rougher the surface, greater the fixation
  - ♦ Typically diaphyseal fitting with more stress shielding proximally because of diaphyseal loading/stress
    - ▪ Fully coated stems will gain fixation distally into the diaphysis.
    - ▪ Stress shielding may occur, which leads to decreased bone density and remodeling proximally.

- **Distally fixed implants can lead to stress shielding of the proximal femur/greater trochanter.**

♦ More function of stem stiffness
  - Thicker stems
  - Cobalt is stiffer than Titanium, and Titanium is stiffer than cortical bone

♦ Hydroxylapatite-coated stems have shorter time frame to achieve biological fixation.
  - $Ca_{10}(PO_4)_6(OH)_2$

♦ **Rule of 50's for bony ingrowth:**
  - **Less the 50 μm between bone and prosthesis**
  - **Less than 50 μm of motion for good ingrowth**
  - **Pore size of prosthesis between 50 and 150 μm**
  - **Porosity no greater than 50%**

b. Cemented
  - Static fixation, diaphyseal loading
  - Relies on interdigitation between cement and trabecular bone
  - Long-term failure in young active patients
    ♦ Will fatigue at stress points in mantle; does not remodel
    ♦ Cemented cups fail earlier than femur
      - Too much shear and tensile forces
      - Cement stronger in compression, fails in tension/shear
  - The femur must be appropriately broached and cleared of any marrow or fat debris.
  - A canal restrictor is placed within the femoral canal 1.5–2 cm distal to the eventual tip of the prosthesis.
  - The canal is back-filled with cement from distal to proximal.
    ♦ The cement is pressurized.
    ♦ Component is centralized in the cement mantle and held in position until cement hardening.
    ♦ Cement mantle should be at least 2 mm on every side and cement should occupy two thirds of the canal and the prosthesis the remaining one third.
    ♦ A mantle defect is a point where the prosthesis touches the bone and is a high stress point, susceptible to fracture.
    ♦ **Precoating of the femoral component with cement adds an additional interface where fixation failure can occur.**
    ♦ Osteopenic bone has improved fixation with cemented components. Porous bone allows increased interdigitation of cement.

- Acetabular component screw placement
  a. Required for line-to-line acetabular component placement
  b. Line between ASIS and center of fovea splits acetabulum into halves
  c. Line two is perpendicular at the center of the acetabulum, dividing into four quadrants
  d. Structures at risk **(Fig. 6.9)**:
    - **Posterior superior is safe zone for screws**
    - Posterior superior (safe zone for screw placement): sciatic nerve and superior gluteal nerve and artery

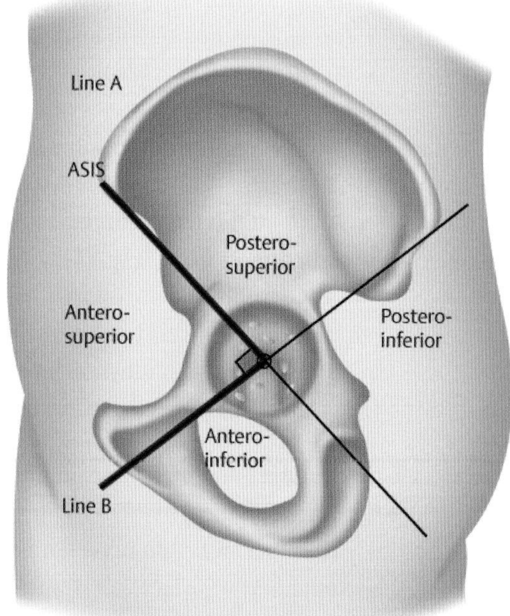

Fig. 6.9 Acetabular component screw placement. Required for line-to-line acetabular component placement. Antero-superior zone marked by red is the "zone of death." ASIS, anterior superior iliac spine.

        - Posterior inferior: sciatic nerve, inferior gluteal nerve and artery, internal pudendal nerve and artery
        - Anterior inferior: obturator nerve and artery
        - Anterior superior: external iliac artery (death zone)
- Stability
  a. Static stability
    - Acetabular/head component congruency
    - Component positioning
      - Alignment shell
        - 15–30 degrees' anteversion
      - Check the cross-table lateral hip X-ray to look for cup version
      - Excessive version in either direction will increase dislocation in that direction
        - 35–45 degrees' abduction
      - Femur
        - 10–15 degrees' anteversion
        - Excessive femoral anteversion or retroversion can cause early impingement as well as dislocation.
    - Combined version of components
      - Goal: a total of 40–45 degrees' combined femoral and acetabular anteversion
      - Check for impingement of the neck on the cup as well as bony impingement.
  b. Dynamic stability
    - Muscles, tendons, ligaments, capsule
      - Abductor tension and offset
        - Soft tissues
          - Tension of abductors (gluteus medius and gluteus minimums)
          - Correct soft tissue tension requires preoperative templating to re-create normal offset, leg length, and hip biomechanics
        - Offset: distance from the center of the femoral head to the greater trochanter
          - If offset is too large: tissues are too tight, leading to trochanteric pain
          - If offset is too small: incompetent abductors, impingement (greater trochanter can impinge on superior acetabulum during abduction, rotation}, dislocation **(Fig. 6.10)**
          - Medializing the acetabular cup (shortening **B**) to the radiographic "teardrop" with decrease the joint reactive forces.
          - Abductor force counteracts the body weight force. Decreasing the abductor force by poor soft tissue tensioning or shortened neck length will increase the joint reactive force.
          - Joint reactive forces are minimized by placing the acetabular shell in an inferior and medial position and increasing the femoral component offset.

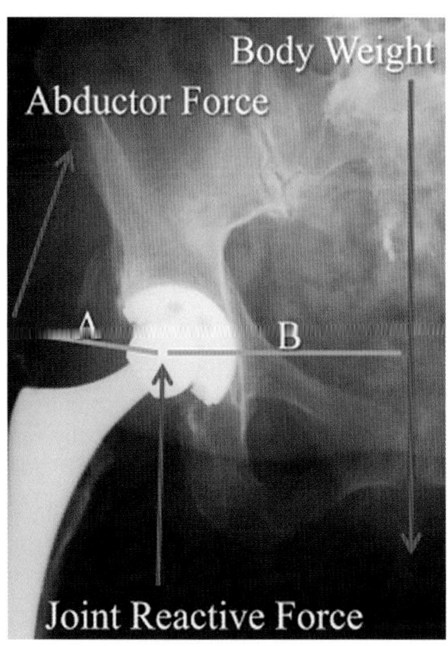

Fig. 6.10 Mechanical forces about the hip.

- Dislocation
  a. Incidence 1–2% of primary THA, up to 25% in revisions
  b. Major complication following hip replacement, and most common complication after any revision hip arthroplasty
  c. Primary arc of motion is motion of the artificial hip within the socket before any neck/liner or bony impingement occurs.
    - Larger heads have larger primary arcs of motion, imparting greater stability.

- ♦ At extremes of motion, the femoral neck impinges on the acetabular component or liner.
- ◦ Excursion distance: distance from the start of impingement to complete dislocation
  - ♦ Larger heads have larger excursion distances (more stability).
- ◦ Factors to note in the history:
  - ♦ Time since replacement or revision
  - ♦ Symptoms of infection
  - ♦ Normal activity or extreme of motion
  - ♦ Trauma
  - ♦ Number of dislocations
  - ♦ Neuromuscular issues
    - ▪ Parkinson's disease
    - ▪ Neuropathy

d. Risk factors: female (largest risk factor), osteonecrosis, obesity, age > 70 years, inflammatory arthritis, neuromuscular conditions

e. Reduction: anesthesia and closed reduction in the emergency room or operating room; move hip through ROM afterward
- ◦ Evaluate with AP radiographs of the pelvis and AP and lateral hip radiographs.
- ◦ Check for previous radiographs and compare component positioning.
- ◦ Check erythrocyte sedimentation rate (ESR), C-reactive protein (CRP) to rule out infection
- ◦ Anterior hip dislocation
- ◦ **Position of affected leg often indicates direction of dislocation**

f. Hip is extended, externally rotated

g. Reduce by extending the hip with traction and external rotation and then gentle internal rotation.
- ◦ Posterior hip dislocation

h. Hip is flexed, internally rotated

i. Reduce by flexing knee and hip, applying traction while internally and externally rotating hip with patient under full sedation
- ◦ If there is obvious impingement within normal ROM: high likelihood of recurrent dislocation
- ◦ More than two dislocations: likely will be recurrent and need revision
- ◦ Closed treatment
  - ♦ Posterior dislocation: placing the patient in a knee immobilizer will limit hip flexion as well.
  - ♦ Anterior dislocation: abduction brace, if needed, prevents hip extension, external rotation, and adduction.
  - ♦ Assist devices for ambulation
  - ♦ Strict adherence to restricted motion

j. Operative management
- ◦ Dislocations that occur in routine daily activities or without a readily apparent cause typically result from problems with either component alignment or soft tissue functioning.
- ◦ Component alignment
  - ♦ THA with a retroverted cup will continue to dislocate posteriorly, and the cup position should be revised.
  - ♦ A neck with a large skirt can impinge on the liner/cup, and the femoral component should be revised if it leads to impingement.

- Head exchange
    - Larger head/neck ratio confers greater ROM and stability,
    - No skirt around neck: skirt decreases head/neck ratio, causing impingement against cup
- Polyethylene wear: polyethylene exchange, ± component change if loose
- Trochanteric advancement for incompetent abductors
    - Only works if abductors are still functioning
    - Surgeon must be confident in performing fixation and in the patient's ability to heal
    - Restores abductor tension
- Trochanteric escape occurs when the trochanter and attached muscles are no longer competent and have actually displaced superiorly and laterally.
    - Usually after repaired osteotomy that fails to heal or trochanteric fracture
    - Weak abductor strength, increased joint reactive force
    - Lack of compression results in increased dislocation risk.
    - May require conversion to constrained liner
- Revision to constrained liner
    - **Can only use if the component positioning is correct**
    - Prosthetic femoral head is contained within the liner, which confers greater static stability.
    - Useful when the abductors are incompetent or have been debrided (infection, metallosis, etc.)
    - Forces are transmitted to the cup/bone interface; therefore, catastrophic failure of the cup can occur instead of dislocation.
    - Patient must be able to follow the instruction to limit the ROM, as excess motion will lever the cup loose.
    - Perform only if components are already in the correct position and dislocation continues.
    - Ring failure in a constrained prosthesis can lead to dislocation of a constrained femoral head.
- Resection arthroplasty (Girdlestone procedure)
    - Resection of femoral head and neck leads to pseudarthrosis of the hip joint.
    - Weight bearing is allowed.
    - Typically reserved for those patients with persistent infection or those who are minimally ambulatory

- Osteolysis: resorption of bone due to physiological response to wear debris
  a. PE wear generated by:
    - Cyclic loading of the femoral head in PE liner
    - Wear on the back side
        - Between liner and cup
        - Failed or inadequate locking mechanism leads to motion.

  b. Mechanism
    - Submicron-sized particles are phagocytosed by macrophages.
    - **Activated macrophages release cytokines:**
        - **Tumor necrosis factor-α**
        - **Interleukin-1**
        - **Interleukin-6**

- ♦ **Transforming growth factor-β**
- ♦ **Receptor activator of nuclear factor kappa B (RANK) ligand (RANKL)**
- ♦ **Vascular endothelial growth factor (VEGF)**

- ◦ RANK–RANKL system
  - ♦ Cytokine release by macrophages leads to osteoblast production of RANKL.
  - ♦ RANKL binds to RANK receptor on osteoclast.
  - ♦ Osteoclast activation leads to bone resorption.
  - ♦ **Osteoprotegerin (OPG) intercepts RANKL. OPG binds RANKL and prevents it from binding to RANK receptor. This blocks osteoclast differentiation/activation and bone resorption.**

c. Osteolysis can occur anywhere in the effective joint space.

d. Effective joint space extends to the proximal and distal aspect of the prosthesis.
  - ◦ Often occurs around acetabular screws
  - ◦ Osteointegration of components can prevent PE debris from reaching the bone.

e. Circumferentially coated porous implant may prevent PE debris from traveling down the canal, thereby preventing osteolysis distally by decreasing the effective joint space.
  - ◦ **Effective joint space refers to the joint itself as well as any part contacted by the prosthesis, including acetabular screws and the entire femoral component. Pressure within the joint causes fluid (and debris) to be pushed along the pressure gradient. In the case of a PE bearing, any area within the effective joint space is susceptible to osteolysis.**
  - ◦ Osteolysis around a well-fixed acetabular cup can be treated with PE liner exchange and bone grafting through screw holes with or without an iliac trapdoor; must be an implant with a reasonable track record, in good alignment

f. X-ray findings
  - ◦ Bony resorption around the femoral component
  - ◦ Large lytic lesions of the acetabulum or femur
  - ◦ Periprosthetic fracture

g. Radiostereometric analysis (RSA)
  - ◦ Most accurate way to measure polyethylene wear

h. Can be used to test two materials to see which has lower wear rates
  - ◦ Three or more radiopaque tantalum beads are placed in the bone around the implant.
  - ◦ Compare immediate postoperative X-ray to future follow-up X-ray.
  - ◦ Must place at index procedure

- Metal-on-metal wear

a. Very small (nanometer-sized) particles
  - ◦ Lymphocytes are main inflammatory cells mediating the response to MOM wear.

b. Cobalt (Co) and chromium (Cr) ions generated
  - ◦ Serum and urine levels (> 10 parts per billion) correlate with wear debris.
  - ◦ Higher ion levels correlate with abnormal wear, though the exact cutoff values for concern are undetermined.
    - ♦ Edge loading of MOM components generates a very large number of particles.

- ♦ Activity levels do not correlate with metal ion levels.
- ♦ No increased cancer risk has been demonstrated.

c. Biological response to MOM debris
- ∘ Hypersensitivity reaction
  - ♦ Rare
  - ♦ Occurs right after implantation
    - ▪ Nickel (Ni) allergy
    - ▪ Ni present in small amounts in Co-Cr alloy.
- ∘ MOM debris wear
  - ♦ Occurs with both MOM bearings as well as "trunnionosis."
  - ♦ **Trunnionosis refers to debris generated by fretting and crevice corrosion of metal head on metal trunnion; more common in large diameter femoral heads**
  - ♦ Production of many wear particles leads to generation of metal ion debris, which activates a T-cell response.
  - ♦ Proinflammatory cytokines released, including RANKL
  - ♦ Presentation
    - ▪ Pain and dull ache about hip/groin
    - ▪ Late dislocation
    - ▪ May have palpable mass
    - ▪ Pseudotumor
      - • Aseptic inflammatory tissue, which forms around hip joint
      - • Mixed fluid collection and solid mass common on metal-suppression MRI [metal artifact reduction sequences (MARS)]
      - • Effusion can be diagnosed with ultrasound.
      - • Aspiration of joint fluid yields milky white fluid and can be confused with infection.
  - ♦ Histology
    - ▪ Look for a slide with many lymphocytes
    - ▪ Atypical lymphocytic and vasculitis-associated lesion (ALVAL)
      - • Treatment
    - ▪ Asymptomatic
      - • Should check metal ion levels once.
        - ◊ If normal, reevaluate in 6–12 months.
        - ◊ If elevated, follow with advanced imaging and closely monitor for symptoms.
    - ▪ Symptomatic
      - • Remove source of metal ion wear.
      - • Decompression of pseudotumor
        - ◊ High risk of subsequent dislocation
      - • Use ceramic head with titanium sleeve on PE or COC components for revision

5. Periprosthetic joint infection (PJI)
- • Up to 1–2% of primary THA, 3% after revision THA
- • Most commonly *Staphylococcus aureus* or *Staphylococcus epidermidis*
- • Acute infections within 2–4 weeks after implantation

  a. Typically *S. aureus, Streptococcus* species, or gram-negative rods

  b. Acute hematologic infections may occur many years after a joint replacement in the setting of recent invasive procedures, including dental, gastrointestinal, or urologic procedures

- Chronic infection include those present for > 4 weeks
  a. Typically coagulase-negative *Staphylococcus* or gram-negative rods
  b. Bacteria create a biofilm around the prosthetic components as soon as 48 hours after the start of the infection, making eradication of infection without component removal very difficult.
- Presentation can vary from subtle pain to frank sepsis:
  a. Pain
  b. Fever
  c. Severely limited ROM secondary to pain and joint effusion
- Volume of hip capsule is greatest in flexion and external rotation, which is the position the hip will assume when a large joint effusion is present.
  a. Inability to bear weight
  b. Draining sinus is pathognomonic of PJI
  c. Dehisced wound
  d. Dislocation
     - **Always order ESR/CRP when working up THA dislocation**
- Risk factors
  a. Obese
  b. Diabetic
  c. Smokers
  d. Intravenous (IV) drug abusers
  e. Immunosuppressive drugs
  f. Steroids
- Laboratory
  a. ESR
     - More sensitive than specific
     - Elevation occurs slower than with CRP and remains elevated longer.
     - Remains elevated for up to 90 days following surgery
  b. CRP
     - Very sensitive
     - Elevation occurs quickly and should normalize by 6 weeks post-operative.
- Imaging
  a. Radiography
     - Loosening or osteolysis
       - ♦ Early osteolysis may indicate infection.
     - Periosteal bone formation and scalloping resorption are commonly seen.
  b. Bone scan
     - Technetium (Tc)-99m detects increased blood flow to reactive areas in bone.
     - May be useful in cases of indolent infections, no bacterial growth from aspiration cultures
     - Sensitive, but not very specific (cannot differentiate from aseptic loosening)
     - Can show increased uptake for up to 12–18 months following a joint replacement
  c. Positron emission tomography (PET) scan
     - Fluorinated glucose tracked to areas of high metabolic activity, which can indicate infection
     - Highly sensitive and specific

- **Threshold for PJI: acute PJI (≤ 6 weeks): CRP > 10 mg/L, > 20,000 nucleated cells/μL, > 90% polymorphonuclear (PMN) cells on cytology; chronic PJI (> 6 weeks): ESR > 30, CRP > 10 mg/L, > 80% PMN cells on cytology, > 3,000 nucleated cells/μL**

- Aspiration: thresholds for acute PJI and chronic PJI are listed in the margin box.
  a. Crystal analysis
  b. Gram stain and culture
  c. Repeat aspiration can be very useful when initial aspirations are equivocal.
  d. Polymerase chain reaction (PCR) can be used to amplify bacterial DNA to aid in detection if infection is highly suspected but no bacteria can be cultured.
- Treatment
  a. Less than 4 weeks from implantation or symptom onset
    - Debridement of soft tissues about joint
    - Multiple cultures from different sites, each with clean instruments to avoid sample contamination
    - Removal of all modular components (PE liner, metal head)
    - Copious irrigation
    - Check component stability
    - Antibiotics tailored to isolated bacteria
      - ♦ Low success rate with *Staphylococcus* infections
  b. Chronic infection > 4 weeks
  c. Two-stage revision is gold standard
    - Debridement, cultures
    - Removal of components
    - Placement of articulating spacer
      - ♦ Preservation of joint space
      - ♦ Preservation of motion
  d. Heat-stable antibiotics, including vancomycin, gentamicin, and tobramycin, should be mixed with cement.
    - Typically 6–8 weeks of parenteral antibiotics based on isolated bacteria and normalization of inflammatory markers
    - Re-aspiration with negative cultures and low nucleated cell count as well as normalization or trend toward normalization of CRP/ESR prior to any reimplantation (aspiration no sooner than 2 weeks after antibiotics end)
  e. Hip resection arthroplasty/implant removal
    - Salvage for chronic infection
    - Inadequate remaining bone stock
    Poor health of patient
    - Forms pseudarthrosis
    - Weight bearing allowed
    - Limited mobility but high chance of infection eradication with removal of all foreign material
      - ♦ Antibiotic prophylaxis after total joint replacement
    - No clear evidence or guidelines to follow for antibiotics after joint replacement
- International consensus meeting on PJI
  a. Dental antibiotic prophylaxis use should be individualized based on patient risk factors.

b. High-risk patients, including those with the following risks, should receive prophylaxis:
   - Immunosuppression
   - Inflammatory arthropathies
   - Insulin-dependent diabetes
   - Hemophilia
   - Poor dental hygiene as determined by a dentist

c. Consensus regarding the importance of good dental hygiene despite the lack of evidence to support it

6. Aseptic loosening
   - Presentation
     a. Thigh (loose femur) or groin (loose cup) pain while weight bearing
     b. Start-up pain: pain upon standing/ambulating after sitting for a prolonged period of time
   - Workup
     a. Imaging
        - Radiographs are typically sufficient
        - Subsidence
          - ♦ Subsidence of femoral component leads to decreased abductor tension and increased dislocation risk.
          - ♦ Compare postoperative films to the current films; measure the difference in height between the center of the femoral head and the greater trochanter.
        - Thick femoral cortices
          - ♦ "Pistoning" (loose prosthesis moving up and down with ambulation) of the prosthesis can lead to thickened-appearing cortices on AP X-ray
        - Pedestal sign
          - ♦ Bone formation distal to the stem within the canal in response to motion
        - Calcar hypertrophy or erosion in stems with collars; should see calcar wasting or remodeling with osteointegrated stems
     b. Laboratory
        - ESR/CRP should be normal
        - Bacterial/fungal culture
          - ♦ Hold for as long as 28 days for organisms that are difficult to culture
     c. Always aspirate, multiple times if equivocal
        - White blood cell (WBC) count $< 3,000$ cells/mm^3, $< 80\%$ PMNs
     d. Treatment
        - One-stage revision with press-fit components
        - Intraoperative cultures

7. Revision THA
   - Most common reason for a revision is instability/dislocation
   - Most common complication of revision THA is instability and dislocation (even if isolated liner exchange with stable components)
     a. More complications: infection, dislocation, nerve injury/palsy, fracture
     b. Remove and replace loose components.
     c. Preoperative planning essential; obtain previous operative reports.
        - Identify acetabular and femoral bone defects.
        - Identify adequate bone to be used for fixation.
     d. Revision implants

- Intact acetabulum: a porous coated shell with multiple acetabular screws
- Can cement a PE cup into a well-fixed porous cup
  - 1–2 mm cement mantle
  - Score with high-speed bur both the back of the PE liner and the cup for better fixation.
  - Can change version to limited degree
- Deficient acetabulum
  - Cavitary bone loss: loss of cancellous bone without loss of supportive acetabular rim
  - Segmental bone loss: loss of bony support to the implant; loss of medial wall, rim, or column
  - Treatment based on type of bone loss:
    - Cavitary loss: treat with particulate allograft to fill defect, and obtain rim fit with hemispherical cup.
    - Segmental defects: treat with hemispherical highly porous cup with multiple screws ± augments for significant boney defects.
    - Cage and allograft reconstructions have high failure rate by 10 years.
  - Custom implants: triflange
    - Three-dimensional (3D) computed tomography (CT) reconstruction preoperatively
    - Custom implant to fill acetabular defect with drill holes placed based on the CT reconstruction
    - Expensive
- Deficient femur
  - If there is at least 4 cm of intact diaphysis, then a cylindrical fully porous coated implant can be used and should extend 2–3 cm distal to previous stem or at least two cortical diameters distal to the cortical defect.
  - If there is less than 4 cm of intact diaphysis, then a tapered revision stem is indicated. Long-stem tapered implants allow stable fixation over much shorter lengths of isthmic diaphysis.
  - Impaction allograft can be used to reconstitute deficient proximal femoral bone.
  - Large amounts of cancellous allograft are impacted into the remaining femoral canal.
  - Component is then cemented into this bed of allograft bone.
  - Most common complication is subsidence of implant.

- Trochanteric osteotomies **(Fig. 6.11)**
  a. Standard trochanteric osteotomy **(A)**
    - Requires detachment of vastus lateralis fibers from vastus tubercle
    - Rarely used now for primary THA, may be useful for difficult exposures (protrusio, fused hip). Complication rate 18× higher than with posterior approach.
  b. Trochanteric slide **(B)**
    - More commonly used during revision hip surgery
    - Does not require vastus lateralis detachment
    - Greater surface area for healing
    - Osteotomy typically completed from posterior to anterior direction and allows mobilization of the bony block with both abductor and vastus lateralis tendons anteriorly

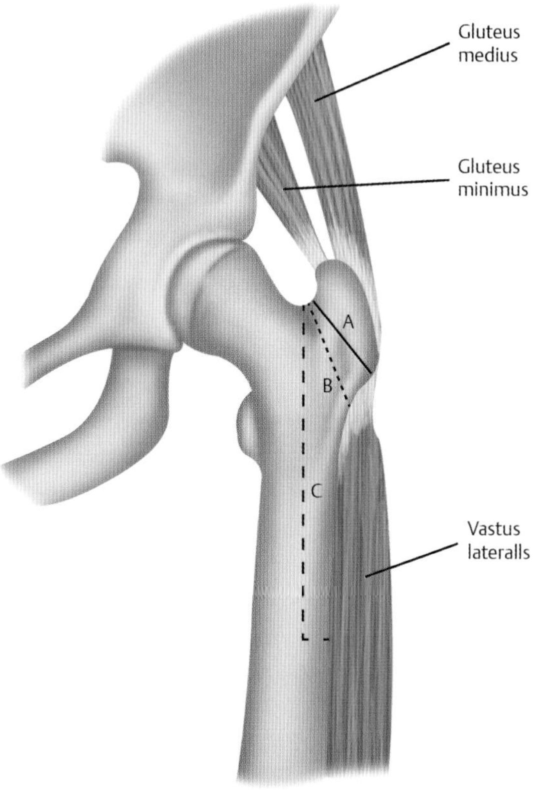

Fig. 6.11 Trochanteric osteotomies. **A,** standard trochanteric osteotomy; **B,** trochanteric slide osteotomy; **C,** extended trochanteric osteotomy. Lines indicate where cuts are made for the three different osteotomies.

c. Extended trochanteric osteotomy **(C)**
   - Greater exposure for revision surgery
   - Access to femoral canal to remove well-fixed implants or cement
   - Roughly 10–15 cm osteotomy measuring from tip of greater trochanter

d. Fixation techniques
   - Cables, cerclage wires, ± claw plate

- Periprosthetic fracture

a. Intraoperative
   - Femur
     - Proximal
       - May require cables/wires placed above and/or below the lesser trochanter
       - May require plate fixation if involves the greater trochanter
       - Typically occurs proximally due to wedge effect of implant/broach
       - Visualize the medal calcar to evaluate for fracture
     - Middle
       - Cables both above and below fracture
       - Bypass fracture by two cortical diameters with new stem
       - Structural allograft if needed for structural support
     - Distal
       - Fixation of fracture with plate, screws, cables if fracture cannot be bypassed with new stem
     - **When there is a change in resistance to broaching, suspect a fracture and check an X-ray if it is not visualized.**
   - Acetabulum
     - Assess stability
     - If stable, add screws for additional stability, may protect weight bearing for 8–12 weeks
     - If unstable, revision with screws, jumbo cup, or reduction and fixation of fracture and cup placement, bone grafting
     - **Under-reaming of acetabulum by 2 mm increases fracture risk.**

b. Pelvic discontinuity: treatment based on healing potential
   - Good healing potential: should be treated in compression with compression plating, structural or particular allograft
   - Poor healing potential: should be treated with distraction technique or custom triflange implant

c. Vancouver classification **(Table 6.2)**: radiographs determine classes A–C
   - A_G: Greater trochanter fracture
     - May require cable ± trochanteric plate if displaced
   - A_L: Lesser trochanter fracture
   - B1: Fracture about stem, well fixed
     - Open reduction and internal fixation (ORIF) plates and cables
     - Proximally coated stems only need to be well fixed in the metaphyseal area to be considered stable **(Fig. 6.12)**
   - B2: Fracture about stem, loose stem
     - Revision with cylindrical fully porous coated stem
   - B3: Fracture about stem, significant proximal bone loss
     - Treated with ORIF and tapered revision stems, fully porous coated stem, or tumor prosthesis
   - C: Fracture distal to stem

Table 6.2 Vancouver Classification

Type	Subtype	Description
A	A_G	Greater trochanter fracture: treated conservatively if non/minimally displaced with bracing and restriction of active abduction for 6–8 weeks; requires fixation if displaced
	A_L	Lesser trochanter fracture: treat conservatively
B	B1	Fracture about the implant with stable fixation of prosthesis; fracture can be fixed with plate, screw, cable construct.
	B2	Fracture about the implant with unstable prosthesis fixation; revision of femoral component indicated due to instability; need to place diaphyseal fitting, fully coated press-fit stem that bypasses fracture site by at least two cortical diameters
	B3	Fracture about the implant with inadequate bone stock remaining; requires diaphyseal fitting stem, ± impaction grafting, ± megaprosthesis
C		Fracture distal to stem of implant; must assess stability of implant; if stable, can fix with plate/cable construct; if unstable, must revise with diaphyseal fitting, fully coated press-fit stem that bypasses fracture site by at least two cortical diameters

- ♦ Typically can be reduced and internally fixed if implant is stable
- ◦ Cemented stems
  - ♦ If mantle compromised, requires revision to cementless stem and ORIF

- Iliopsoas impingement
  a. Pain with resisted hip flexion from a seated position
  b. Groin pain after THA without loosening or infection
  c. Uncovered cup rim at anterior wall (evaluate with cross table lateral)
  d. Anesthetic injection into the iliopsoas sheath is diagnostic.
  e. Cause determines treatment, which could include cup revision, liner and head revision, arthroscopic debridement, or iliopsoas release.
- Historic THA outcomes
  a. Charnley cemented PE cup failure
    - ◦ 10 years: 5%
    - ◦ 20 years: 15–20%
    - ◦ 35 years: 20–30%

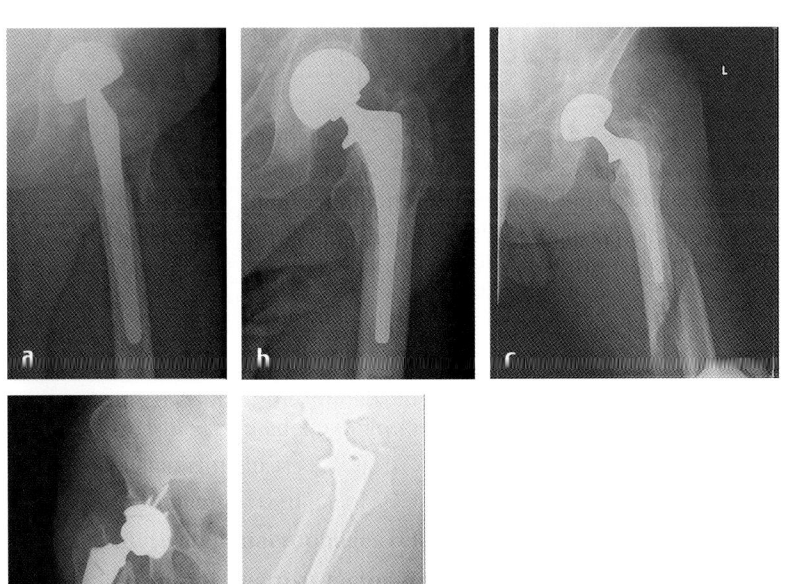

Fig. 6.12 **(a)** $A_{(g)}$; **(b)** $A_{(l)}$; **(c)** B1; **(d)** B2; **(e)** B3. Proximally coated stems only need to be well fixed in the metaphyseal area to be considered a B1 fracture.

II. Total Knee

1. Anatomy
   - Rotating hinge joint
     a. Femur
        - Medial condyle larger than lateral

     b. Tibia
        - Medial plateau is concave
        - Lateral plateau is convex
   - Both deepened by fibrocartilaginous meniscus
   - Mechanical axis of leg
     a. Center of femoral head to the center of talus
     b. Should bisect the knee joint
        - If line is medial to the center of the joint, identifies varus knee alignment
        - If line is lateral to the center of the joint, identifies valgus knee alignment
   - Anatomic axis
     a. The anatomic axis is used intraoperatively as a guide to re-create the physiological mechanical axis.
     b. Line drawn down the diaphyseal of the femur and the tibia
        - Distal femur is average of 9 degrees of valgus with respect to the longitudinal axis of the femur
        - Proximal tibia is average of 3 degrees of varus with respect to the longitudinal axis of the tibia
        - Combined result is average of 6 degrees of valgus anatomic axis
   - Extensor mechanism
     a. Q angle: angle formed between axis of quadriceps tendon (ASIS to center of patella) to the axis of the patellar tendon (center of patella to tibial tubercle)
        - Men 14 degree
        - Women 17 degrees
        - Must be maintained or even decreased during total knee replacement
   - Surgical exposure **(Fig. 6.13)**
     a. Medial parapatellar
        - Offers extensile exposure to the knee joint
        - Allows eversion or subluxation of patella
        - External rotation when the knee is flexed helps deliver the patellar tendon laterally with the subluxed/everted patella, which reduces tension on the extensor mechanism and can help prevent avulsion of the patellar tendon from the tubercle.

     b. Midvastus
        - Inferiorly similar to parapatellar but at superomedial corner of patella incision angles 45 degrees to split the vastus medialis oblique (VMO)
        - Splits muscle away from neurovascular supply
        - Easier eversion/subluxation of patella than subvastus approach

     c. Subvastus
        - Inferiorly similar to parapatellar but at the level of the patella turns medially to separate the vastus medialis from the intermuscular septum

     d. Lateral parapatellar
        - Sometimes used with fixed valgus deformity or lateral compartment partial knee replacement

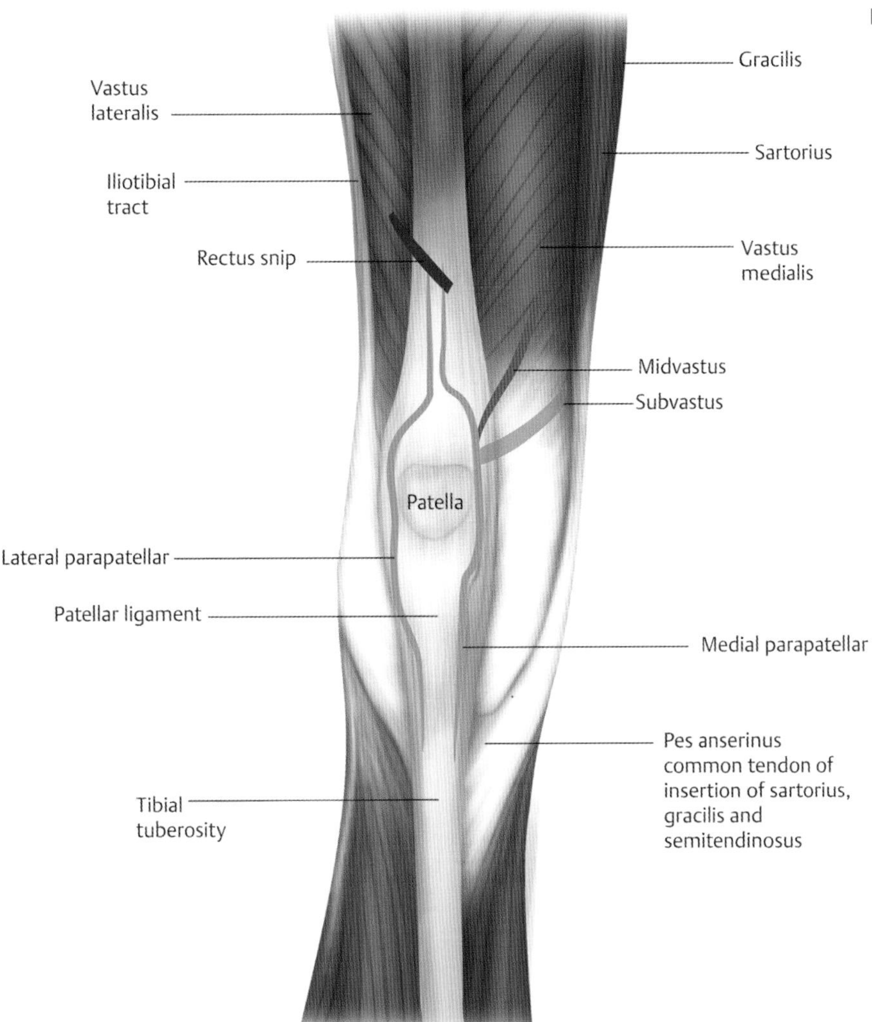

Fig. 6.13 Surgical exposures about the knee.

e. Quadriceps snip
   - Extension of medial parapatellar approach
   - Oblique incision in line with vastus lateralis fibers at 45 degrees to the original incision
   - Relieves tension on extensor mechanism, allowing eversion/subluxation of the patella.
   - No change in postoperative protocol/rehab

f. Quadriceps turndown
   - Extension of medial parapatellar approach down the lateral side of the patella
   - Patella and patellar tendon are turned down and the joint is exposed
   - Blood supply entering laterally from the lateral geniculate continues to supply the patella and quad tendon
   - Significantly compromised quadriceps function makes this exposure obsolete.

g. Tibial tubercle osteotomy
   - Useful for removing well-fixed stem extensions and incarcerated hardware; repair with wires through bone tunnels or screw fixation

- Physical Exam
  a. Inspection
     - Varus/valgus alignment

        - Correctable versus non correctable deformity
        - Previous incisions
        - Skin changes
    - Palpation
        - Tenderness
        - Bony landmarks
        - Effusion, ballotable patella
        - Quadriceps atrophy, VMO atrophy
        - Crepitus
        - Patellofemoral tracking
            - Increased femoral anteversion or external tibial torsion both effectively increase the Q angle and lateral patellar subluxing forces
    - Normal ROM
        - Flexion 0–140 degrees (some hyperextension may be seen; compare with other leg)
        - Internal rotation 0–10 degrees with knee flexed
        - External rotation up to 30 degrees with knee flexed

2. Gait examination
    - Varus/valgus thrust
        a. Pathological movement of knee joint during early stance phase due ligamentous laxity
        b. In a varus thrust gait the knee joint moves laterally during stance phase due to lax ligaments laterally.
    - Antalgic gait shortened stance phase on affected side
3. Flexion contracture
    - With patient supine, apply gentle pressure to the knee in a downward direction until resistance is met.
        a. 10-degree contracture if you can slide flat hand under knee
        b. 15- to 20-degree contracture if you can slide fist under knee
4. Stability
    - Varus/valgus stress may indicate ligament laxity.
        a. Assessed at both full extension and 30-degree flexion (to isolate collateral ligaments)
    - Anterior cruciate ligament (ACL)/posterior cruciate ligament (PCL) assessed with anterior and posterior drawer and Lachman maneuver (dictates potential reconstruction options)
5. Extensor mechanism
    - Extensor lag
        a. Lacking terminal extension
    - Motor strength
    - Palpate VMO, quad, and patellar tendons
6. Meniscal exam (see Chapter 8)
7. Common differential diagnosis of knee pain
    - **Beware of hip pathology that presents as knee pain.**
    - Arthritis
    - Patellofemoral pain
    - Meniscal pathology
    - Osteonecrosis
    - Pes anserine bursitis (tenderness and fullness at pes)
    - Lumbar radiculopathy
    - Hip pathology

8. Osteoarthritis
   - Demographics: between fifth and eighth decades of life, females > males
   - Presentation: progressive onset of pain with weight bearing, recurrent effusions, altered alignment and gait
   - Risk factors: family history, older age, female sex, obesity
   - Imaging: weight-bearing AP, 30-degree flexed posteroanterior (PA), sunrise, lateral radiographs
     a. 36-inch cassette useful for assessing overall limb alignment
     b. **Weight-bearing PA view in 30 degrees of flexion will pick up early arthritic changes on the posterior condyles of the femur.**
   - Treatment:
     a. Nonoperative
     b. American Academy of Orthopaedic Surgeons (AAOS) Clinical Practice Guidelines:
        - Strong evidence *for* recommending low-impact aerobic exercises, neuromuscular education, strengthening, and the use of NSAIDs (oral or topical) or tramadol
        - Moderate evidence *for* recommending weight loss for body mass index (BMI) > 25
        - Moderate evidence *against* recommending lateral wedge shoe orthotic for medial compartment disease
        - Strong evidence *against* recommending glucosamine, chondroitin, and injectable viscosupplementation
        - Strong evidence against arthroscopy with lavage/debridement for osteoarthritis
     c. Weight loss
     d. Off-load the joint
        - Cane/crutch on contralateral side
        - Moves center of gravity over the good side during stance phase on symptomatic side
     e. Activity modification
     f. NSAIDs
        - Provide good analgesia and anti-inflammatory effect
        - Contraindicated in those with history of peptic ulcer disease
        - Caution with strong family history or personal history of stroke or myocardial infarction (MI)
        - Must check renal function every 6 months
     g. Glucosamine/chondroitin sulfate
        - Natural, no side effects
        - No proven benefit
     h. Viscosupplementation
        - Given as either one or a series of intra-articular injections
        - Hyaluronic acid
          - Backbone of extracellular matrix of articular cartilage
        - Expensive
        - AAOS recommendation against use in osteoarthritis of the knee
     i. Intra-articular steroid injections
        - Therapeutic and diagnostic when combined with local anesthetic; do not use with epinephrine, as it results in chondrolysis
        - Decrease inflammation within joint and provide significant pain relief
        - Degrades cartilage over time

- Should only be given every 3–6 months
- Useful for nonsurgical candidates, those already planning a joint replacement (not within 6 weeks of surgery), and those with inflammatory arthritis

9. Operative intervention
   - Osteotomy
     a. For active patients typically of ages < 50 years
   - Extra-articular osteotomy
   - High tibial osteotomy (HTO) for varus malalignment and medial compartment arthritis most commonly
     a. Ideal candidate is young healthy laborer
     b. Can provide years of pain relief
     c. Medial opening wedge
        - Add slight posterior slope to tibia
     d. Lateral closing wedge
        - Must take down proximal tibiofibular joint
        - Injury to common peroneal nerve possible
     e. Both risk injury to popliteal vessels/tibial nerve
     f. Contraindications
        - Inflammatory arthritis, multicompartment arthritis, varus thrust, BMI > 35, flexion contracture > 15 degrees, < 90 degrees' flexion, > 20 degrees' varus
        - Patella baja is a low-riding patella, which may abut the proximal tibia and impede flexion. It is the most common complication of an HTO.
     g. Makes conversion to total knee replacement much more challenging
   - Distal femoral osteotomy
     a. Correct supramalleolar angular deformity
     b. Typically varus producing for valgus distal femur
        - Unicompartmental replacement [unicompartmental knee arthroplasty (UKA)]
        - **Know the contraindications for HTO and UKA.**
     c. Best for unicompartmental arthritis
        - Medal compartment
        - Most common
          - ♦ Patella-femoral
          - ♦ Lateral
          - ♦ Medial and lateral compartment UKA had no difference in survivorship
     d. Advantages:
        - Smaller surgical dissection than with total knee arthroplasty (TKA), less blood loss, less painful procedure
        - Retains ACL, resulting in a more normal feeling knee
        - Shorter hospitalization
        - Faster recovery than HTO/TKA
     e. Disadvantages
        - Worse long term survivorship than TKA
        - Technically more demanding than TKA
     f. Contraindications
        - Multicompartment arthritis
        - ACL deficiency
          - ♦ Increased shear stress on remaining cartilage and replacement components, leading to early failure

- Varus/valgus fixed deformity > 15 degrees
- Flexion contracture >10 degrees
- Inflammatory arthritis
- Morbid obesity
- Meniscectomy in other compartment of same knee

g. Complications
   - Tibial stress fracture

h. Evidence suggests that patients have better outcomes with high-volume surgeons

10. Total knee replacement (see below)
11. Osteonecrosis
    - Spontaneous osteonecrosis of the knee (SPONK)
      a. Demographics: typically females > 50 years
      b. Risk factors: same as for osteonecrosis of hip
      c. Presentation
         - Acute onset of pain without significant degenerative changes
         - Pain at medial femoral condyle (most common location)
      d. Imaging
         - Radiographs: AP and lateral, may not reveal pathology until late in disease
      e. MRI: edema within bone on T2-weighted scan early in disease
      f. Treatment
         - Nonoperative
           - ♦ Limited weight bearing, activity modification
           - ♦ NSAIDs
           - ♦ Weight loss
         - Operative
           - ♦ Percutaneous drilling and grafting/chondroplasty
           - ♦ UKA for small lesions
           - ♦ TKA for large lesions
           - ♦ Basics of total knee replacement
           - ♦ Goals
             - ▪ Maintain or restore mechanical alignment of the limb **(Fig. 6.14)**
             - ▪ Necessary to distribute forces equally along joint line
           - ♦ Excessive varus or valgus alignment will lead to asymmetric wear, pain, and early failure
12. Femoral anatomic/mechanical axis
    - Distal femoral cut should be perpendicular to mechanical axis of the leg and 4–7 degrees' valgus from the anatomic axis of the femur.
    - 36-inch long leg films necessary to template, especially when planning deformity correction
      a. Tibial anatomic/mechanical axis should be the same: 0 degree cut
         - Preserve or restore the joint line
13. Knee function (ligaments and extensor mechanism) work best with restored joint line
    - Remove and replace same amount of bone/prosthesis
    - Removing more distal femur will raise the joint line and contribute to patella baja (see below).
    - Do not raise joint line by more than 8 mm.
      a. Balance ligaments for stable knee

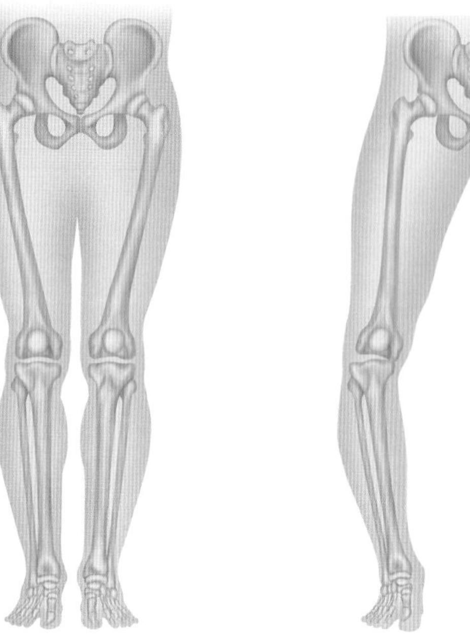
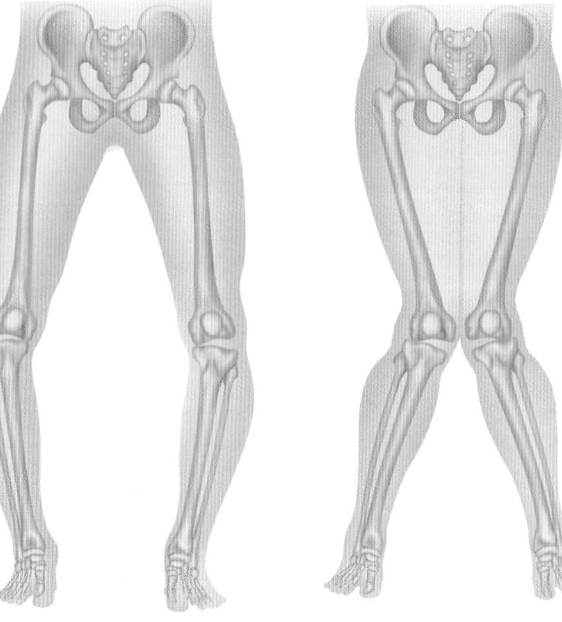

Fig. 6.14 Varus and valgus alignment.

- Must release on concave side of deformity; must be balanced in both flexion and extension, and should be confirmed with trial implants
- Two schools of thought regarding balancing a total knee:
  a. Gap balancing
     - Ligament releases are done prior to bony cuts.
     - Builds joint line based on soft tissue tensioning, which may lead to elevation of the joint line
     - Uses tensiometers or spacer blocks to balance gaps
  b. Measured Resection
     - Measured resection of the femur and tibia to preserve the native joint line with ligament releases as needed thereafter
- In reality, the line between the two schools of thought is blurred, with measured resection of both the femur and tibia with ligament balancing as needed (before or after bony cuts).
- **Releases to regain alignment should come from the contracted concave side.**
- **Osteophyte removal should be done prior to any soft tissue releases.**
- Varus: release medially (in order)
  a. Medial osteophytes
  b. Deep medial collateral ligament (MCL) on tibial side
  c. Posteromedial corner (semimembranosus insertion)
  d. Superficial MCL
- Valgus: release laterally (in order)
  a. Lateral osteophytes
  b. Tight in extension: posterior ITB
  c. Tight in flexion: release popliteus
  d. Lateral collateral ligament (LCL) should be released if the valgus knee is tight in both flexion and extension.

- Sagittal plane balancing (gap balancing)
  a. Goal is to have equal flexion and extension gaps, which enables stability through full ROM
  b. Generally, if the balancing issue is asymmetric, then the femur should be altered. If the issue is symmetric, the tibia should be altered **(Fig. 6.15)**
  c. Sagittal plane balancing **(Table 6.3)**
  d. Flexion instability
     - Posterior stabilized (PS) knee: causes effusion and pain, may lead to dislocation (jumping the post)
     - Rotating platform: can result in poly spin-out
  e. Flexion tightness
     - Treat with increasing tibial slope
       - As the knee flexes, the contact point between the femur and tibia moves posteriorly. Adding 3 degrees of posterior slip will open up the flexion space.
     - Downsize femur
     - Recess PCL in cruciate retaining (CR) knee
     - Shift tibial tray posteriorly (effectively de-tensions PCL)
  f. Flexion contracture: releases from femur with knee flexed to 90 degrees, which moves the neurovascular structures behind the knee posteriorly
     - Posterior osteophytes
     - Posterior capsule
     - Gastrocnemius origin
     - Femoral rollback **(Fig. 6.16)**
       - Contact point between the femur and tibia moves posteriorly as the knee flexes to allow for greater flexion than if the point were stationary.
       - Prevents femur from impinging on the tibia during flexion
       - Controlled by the function of the ACL and PCL in the native knee
       - In a PCL-retaining prosthesis, the PCL provides some rollback, although normal kinematics not restored.
       - In a PCL-substituting prosthesis, the action of the cam on the PE post moves the point of contact posteriorly.
       - Extensor mechanism alignment and function
         - Quadriceps (Q) angle (see below) **(Fig. 6.17)**
           - Men: 14 degrees
           - Women: 17 degrees

14. Primary TKA
- Surgical indications after failed medical management
  a. End-stage osteoarthritis
  b. Posttraumatic arthritis
  c. Inflammatory arthritis
  d. SPONK
  e. Acute/chronic symptomatic ACL tear with arthritic changes
  f. Patients not suitable for reconstruction
- Prosthesis design
  a. Least constrained to most constrained as follows:
     - Cruciate retaining (CR): PCL-retaining knee will allow more flexion. The PCL alone can re-create femoral rollback to a certain degree.
       - Allows more flexion and stops the femur from impinging on posterior tibial plateau, which would limit flexion

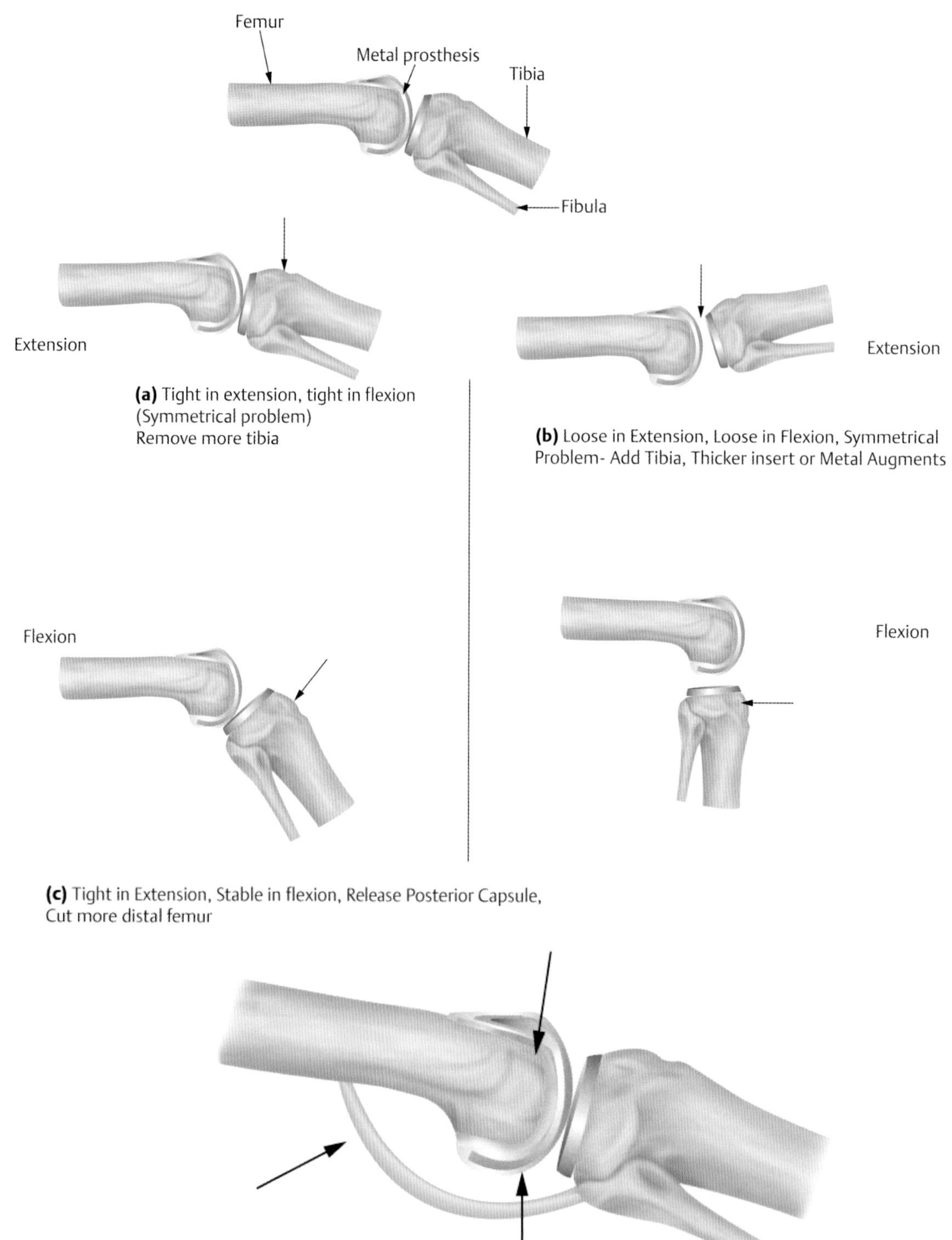

Fig. 6.15 Flexion and extension gap balancing in total knee replacement. Generally, if the balancing issue is asymmetric, then the femur should be altered. If the issue is symmetric, the tibia should be altered. **(a)** Tight in extension, tight in flexion (symmetrical problem). Remove more tibia. **(b)** Loose in extension, loose in flexion (symmetrical problem). Add tibia, thicker insert, or metal augments. **(c)** Tight in extension, stable in flexion. Release posterior capsule. Cut more distal femur.

(d) Stable in Extension, Tight in Flexion, cut more posterior femur and downsize femoral component, can also release the PCL and medial posterior tibial slope

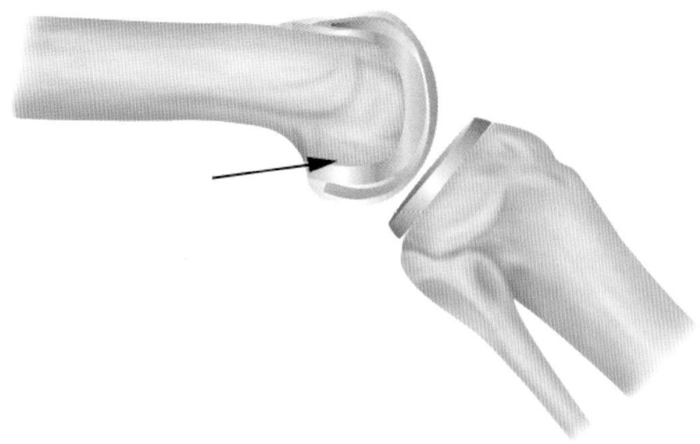

(e) Stable in Extension, Loose in Flexion, add posterior femoral augments or a larger femoral component. Can also fill posterior femur with cement approved to metal augment. Can also translate femoral component posteriorly

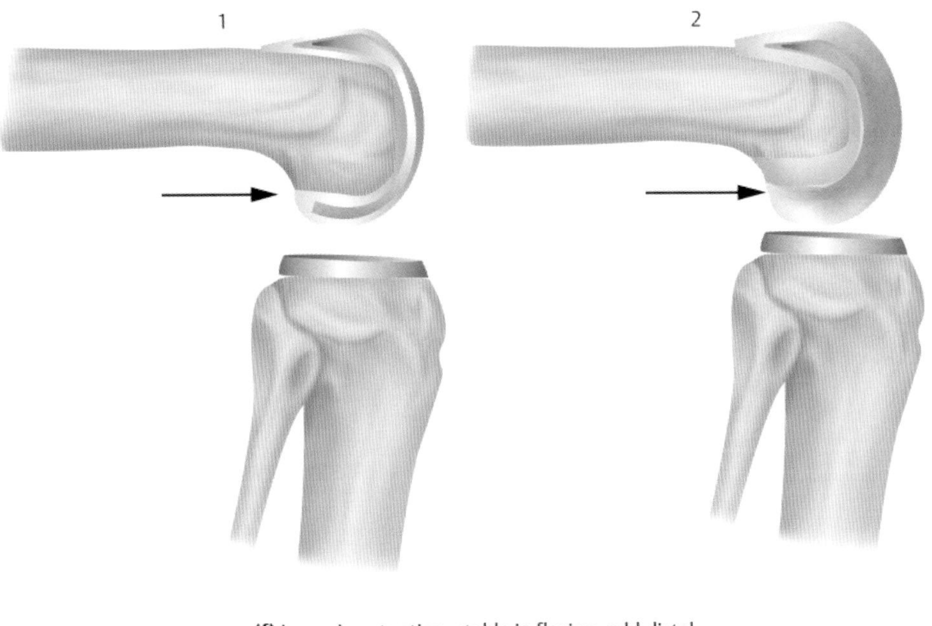

(f) Loose in extention, stable in flexion, add distal femoral augments to the femoral component.

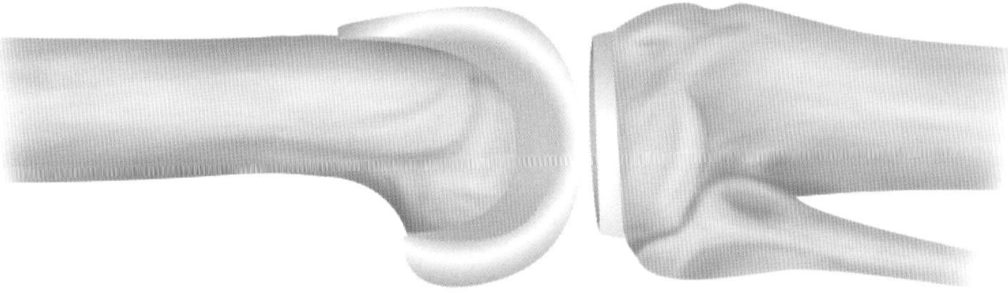

Fig. 6.15 (*continued*) **(d)** Stable in extension, tight in flexion. Cut more posterior femur and downsize the femoral component. May release PCL if intact, increase posterior tibial slope, or move tibial component posterior to increase flexion gap. **(e)** Stable in extension, loose in flexion. Add posterior femoral augments or a larger femoral component. Can also fill posterior femur with cement that is approved for the metal augment. Can also translate femoral component posteriorly. **(f)** Loose in extension, stable in flexion. Add distal femoral augments to the femoral component.

Table 6.3 Sagittal Plane Balancing (Gap Balancing)

		Flexion		
		Loose	**Stable**	**Tight**
Extension	**Loose**	Upsize PE liner until balanced (or add tibial augments)	Distal femoral augments	1. Downsize femoral component size and increase PE liner thickness (or add tibial augments) 2. Resect more tibia, add distal femoral augments
	Stable	Distal femoral augments/upsize femoral component size	Stable	1. Downsize femoral component size 2. Add tibial slope
	Tight	1. Resect more distal femur and upsize PE liner (or add tibial augments) 2. Resect more distal femur and upsize femoral component with posterior femoral augments	1. Resect more distal femur keeping the same size component 2. Posterior capsular release	Cut more tibial bone

Abbreviation: PE, polyethylene.

- Can lead to earlier PE wear due to less congruent PE, more roll/slide rollback, especially if PCL is tight
- PCL insufficiency following CR knee presents as pain, instability in flexion, recurrent effusions, a feeling of "giving out," weakness.

- Cruciate substituting
  - Anterior constrained (AC) or ultracongruent (UC)
  - Backup option for CR knee with incompetent PCL
  - Anterior lip on PE liner increases congruency
- Posterior stabilized (PS)
  - Tibial PE post in middle of knee with cam

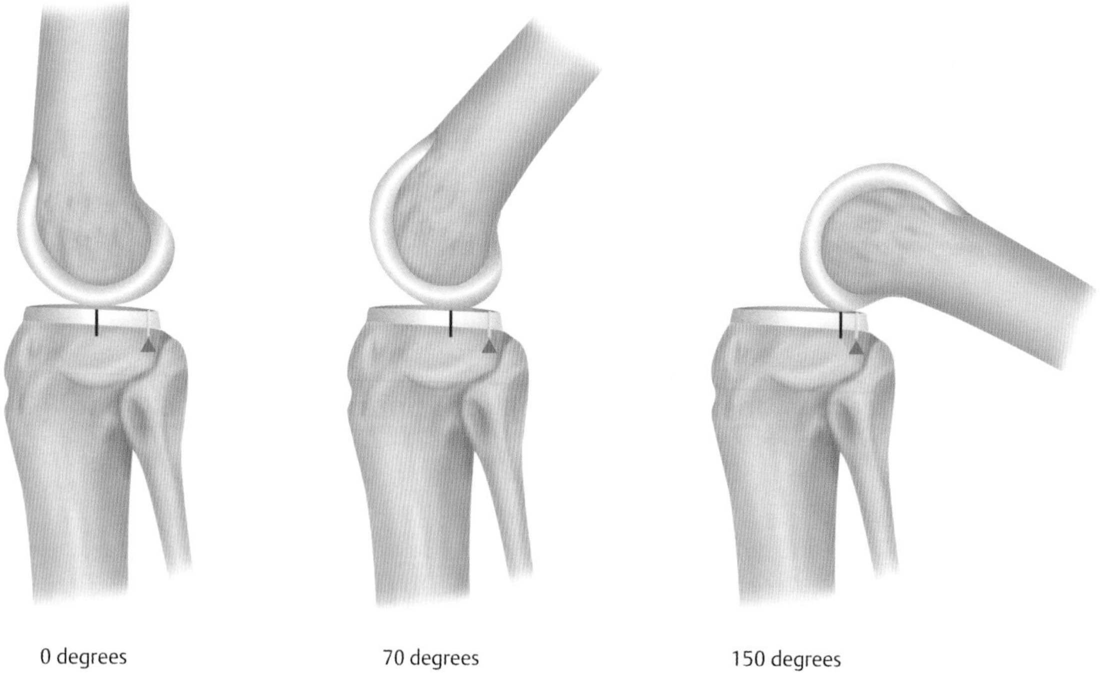

Fig. 6.16 Femoral rollback.

- ♦ During flexion, bar in femoral prosthesis contacts post, and further flexion pushes femur posterior on the tibia.
- ♦ **The post in the PS liner does NOT constrain movement in the varus/valgus plane.**
- ♦ More congruent PE liner, less stress to prosthesis–bone interface
- ♦ Easier to balance remaining ligaments without PCL
- ♦ Always use PS knee for:
  - ▪ TKA after patellectomy
  - ▪ Prior PCL trauma
- ♦ In hyperextension, the femoral cam contacts the anterior surface of the PE post, which can cause damage to the post.

A. Mobile Bearing (Rotating Platform)

1. PE component rotates on polished tibial surface
2. In theory, reduces stress on the bone prosthesis due to increased conformity with the femoral condyles in the anterior to posterior plane, which lowers overall shear forces and thus PE wear. Literature shows equivocal outcomes to fixed bearing PE liner.
3. Risk of spinout if loose flexion gap
   - Occurs when PE liner turns 90 degrees and gets stuck; may be reducible or may require open reduction ± revision for flexion instability
     a. Condylar constrained
        - ◦ Tall post that confers some varus/valgus stability for revision knees
        - ◦ Similar to PS knee but the post is both taller and wider
        - ◦ Will not compensate for complete collateral ligament loss
        - ◦ Higher stresses are transferred to the bone/prosthesis interface when a constrained system is used. Tibial and femoral stems are used to transmit stress evenly to a larger area of host bone.
        - ◦ **Constraint refers to the intrinsic stability of the prosthesis both in the varus/valgus and anterior posterior directions and is important in significant to severe ligamentous laxity or large bony defects.**
        - ◦ High post restricts varus/valgus motion:
          - ♦ Allows 2–3 degrees of varus-valgus and 2 degrees of internal rotation
          - ♦ Used for MCL/LCL laxity
          - ♦ Flexion gap laxity: better tolerated with tall post
          - ♦ Neuropathic joints in diabetics or those with syphilis typically require at least a constrained, nonhinged prosthesis with both tibial and femoral stems.

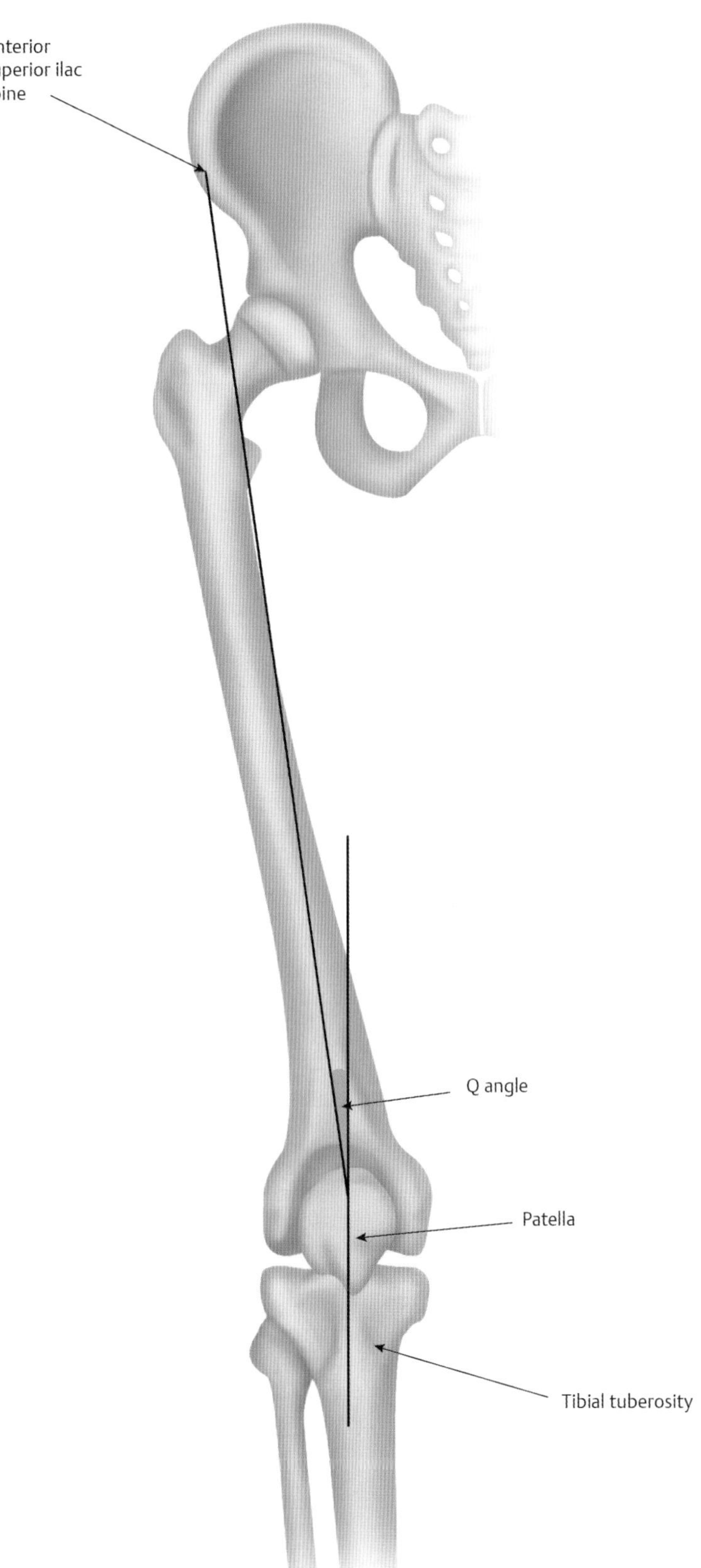

Fig. 6.17 Quadriceps (Q) angle.

b. Constrained-hinged
   - Femur and tibia linked with connecting bar and bearing.
   - Rotating PE liner on tibial plate allows some rotation.
     - Reduces rotational forces on bone–prosthesis interface
     - Uses
       - Global ligament instability, complete MCL or LCL loss
       - Hyperextension instability
         - Hyperextension deformity seen in post-polio syndrome
       - Resection of knee for tumor/infection
     - Always use both tibial/femoral stems
       - Share high torsional loads
         - Component positioning
       - Femoral component
         - Distal femoral cut is perpendicular to the mechanical axis of the limb
         - Placed centrally or cheated laterally on the distal femur; if medial, then Q angle is increased
         - Slight external rotation (3 degrees) is ideal
           - ◊ Internal rotation of femoral component leads to increased patellofemoral contact stress.
           - ◊ Internal rotation of the femoral component also leads to an increased flexion gap laterally and decreased medially. The native tibia has 3 degrees of varus inclination but commonly the cut is made perpendicular to the mechanical axis of the tibia.
           - ◊ External rotation delivers the patella laterally and makes the flexion gap equal medially and laterally.
         - Three important landmarks for femoral component rotation:
           - ◊ Anteroposterior axis (Whiteside's line): top of trochlear groove to the top of the intracondylar notch
           - ◊ Epicondylar axis: about neutral rotation, between medial/lateral epicondyles
           - ◊ Posterior condylar axis: flex knee to 90 degrees; beware of deficient lateral femoral condyles in chronically valgus knee
           - ◊ **Note that if the lateral condyle is deficient (valgus knee), then the posterior condylar axis is much more internally rotated, and if used for referencing may result in an internally rotated femoral component.**
       - Tibial component: must be slightly externally rotated
         - Internally rotating tibial component leads to increased Q angle (by effectively externally rotating the tibial tubercle).
         - Center of tibial component should be placed roughly between medial and central third of tibial tubercle.
       - Patellar component: ideally placed medial or central
         - Medializing the component allows the resurfaced patella to sit more naturally in the trochlea.

- Patellofemoral articulation

a. Most common complication: abnormal patellar tracking

b. Quadriceps (Q) angle: angle formed by the intersection of the extensor mechanism axis above the patella with the axis of the patellar tendon
   - Increased Q angle during TKA leads to greater lateral patella subluxation forces
   - Prosthetic knee has a less constrained patellofemoral joint than a native knee.

- Goal is to maintain or restore normal patellofemoral mechanics.

c. Fixation techniques
   - Cemented TKA is gold standard; > 90% success rate
   - Uncemented: no significant long-term data

d. Cementing technique
   - Mixed under vacuum suction
   - Clean with pulsatile saline lavage and dry all bone surfaces
   - Apply cement to tibial baseplate and femoral component, making sure to add to the posterior condyles and finger pack cement into cancellous bone surface.
   - Applied to patellar button
   - **Excessive antibiotics placed within the cement, with the goal of treating or preventing infection, can decrease its mechanical properties. Limit to 1 g per bag of cement in primary TKA. For treatment of periprosthetic joint infections, higher concentrations of antibiotics are desirable (up to 5 g per bag of cement)**

e. Complications
   - Patella baja: shortened patellar tendon (may present before or after a TKA)
   - Knee flexion is limited as the patella impinges on the tibia.
   - Pain, stiffness, and block to full flexion

f. Insall-Salvati ratio: 1:1 ratio of patella length to patellar tendon length as measured on lateral radiograph from inferior patella to tibial tubercle with knee flexed at 30 degrees; ratio of > 1.2 may be seen in patella baja.

g. Risk factors: HTO, tibial tubercle shift, prior trauma, elevation in joint line

h. Treatment
   - Lower joint line by using distal femoral augments and resecting more tibia.
   - Contour anterior PE liner to prevent impingement of patellar tendon.
   - Tibial tubercle osteotomy can be used in revision TKA with patella baja.
     - ♦ Move tubercle superiorly
     - ♦ Protect in hinged-knee brace postoperatively

4. Osteolysis
   - Similar to THA; wear particles generated by cyclic loading of PE liner
   - Phagocytosed by macrophages, which start a cascade leading to osteoclast activation and bone resorption around implants

   a. Seen as radiographic lucencies about the component, which may lead to component loosening and need for revision

5. Catastrophic wear of PE
   - Macroscopic failure of PE (versus long-term submicron wear)
   - More common in the knee

   a. PE thickness: UHMWPE needs to be at least 8 mm

   b. Take more tibial bone if needed to get at least an 8-mm PE insert.

   - Articular geometry: PE that is flat leads to higher stresses at the points of contact and can lead to early failure; modern PE liners are more congruent, share contact loads, less catastrophic failure
   - Artificial rollback: improperly balanced CR knees using flat PE components designed to facilitate rollback, may actually result in paradoxical anterior slide and lead to early polyethylene failure
   - PE needs to be irradiated in oxygen-free environment.
   - PE machining: direct compression molded PE from powder

6. Aseptic loosening
   - Loosening of components without evidence of infection
   - Startup pain is major driving factor in presentation
   - Workup
     a. Imaging: radiographs demonstrate complete 1-mm radiolucent lines around loose components or cement mantles.
     b. Bone scan is useful for confirming mechanical loosening.
     c. ESR, CRP, and WBC should all be within normal limits.
     d. Aspiration of knee:
        - Nucleated cell count should be < 1,500–3,000 cells/mm^3 and < 80% PMNs.
        - Hold cultures for 21–28 days to diagnose Propionibacterium acnes and other slow growers.
        - Send for fungal/acid-fast bacilli (AFB) cultures in at-risk populations.
   - Treatment
     a. Single-stage revision of loose components with standard technique
     b. Augments and stems may be needed after implant removal.
     c. Back-side wear
        - Wear that occurs between the PE liner and the tibial base plate, which can occur in both fixed and mobile bearing designs and can significantly contribute to osteolysis
        - Mobile bearing PE liner on tibial baseplate
        - Micromotion occurs when locking mechanism on stabilized PE liner is insufficient or fails.
        - All-polyethylene tibial components have no metal base plate and therefore no back-side wear.
7. Knee stiffness
   - Best predictor of postoperative motion is preoperative motion
   - Hamstring overpull: weak extensor mechanism after surgery leads to imbalanced hamstrings and flexion contracture,
     a. This will usually resolve in 6 months with physical therapy.
   - Poor ROM after TKA
     a. If ROM < 90 degrees at 6 weeks, consider recommending manipulation. After 12 weeks, risk of periprosthetic fracture increases due to maturation of scar tissue.
     b. Notching of the anterior cortex of the femur risks fracture during manipulation.
     c. Under sedation, the knee is progressively flexed and adhesions within the joint are broken up. Release of scar tissue bands can be felt and heard as the adhesions are released. Manipulation is less effective at treating flexion contractures.
     d. Aggressive physical therapy and pain control to maintain motion
     e. Use of continuous passive motion (CPM) after TKA has shown no improvement in clinical outcome or eventual ROM.
8. Peroneal nerve palsy
   - Presentation
     a. Inability to dorsiflex ankle and great toe
     b. Decreased sensation over the dorsum of the foot and the first web space
   - Risk factors
     a. Valgus knee > 20 degrees' correction and flexion contracture
     b. Correction of valgus and flexion deformities is most commonly associated with peroneal nerve palsies postoperatively.

c. Epidural anesthesia
   - Patients may not realize they have a deficit.
d. Preoperative neuropathy

- Treatment
  a. Remove compressive dressing and flex the knee.
  b. Ankle-foot orthosis to prevent foot drop
  c. Operative
     - Chronic peroneal nerve palsies status post-TKA (> 3 months): consider EMG/nerve conduction study (NCS) to identify level of damage.
     - Open exploration and release nerve if entrapped

9. Patellofemoral tracking issues
   - Most common complaint after TKA
   - Intraoperatively, let the tourniquet down and reassess if there is questionable patellar tracking at time of closure.
   - Anything that increases Q angle will increase forces on the patella.
     a. Internally rotated tibia component
     b. Internally rotated femoral component
     c. Medialized femoral component
   - Failure to release lateral patellar retinaculum when tight
   - Lateral placement of patellar button increases lateral subluxation forces.
   - Can assess patellofemoral articulation with Merchant or sunrise view radiograph
   - Component revision should only be undertaken with a clear task and objective in mind.
10. Patellar clunk: lump of fibrous tissue forms on posterior quad tendon
    - Gets stuck in box of PS knee as knee comes into extension, 30–45 degrees
    - Pops out with full extension
    - Treatment is arthroscopic or open debridement.
11. Infected TKA
    - Workup is similar to that for infected THA.
    - Basic imaging to assess for loose components; may include radiography, bone scan, or CT scan if there is significant bone loss
    - CRP, ESR, WBC may or may not be elevated depending on severity and acuity of infection.
    - Aspiration, more than once, as needed
    - **AAOS Clinical Practice Guidelines strongly recommend aspiration for abnormal ESR or CRP with concern about periprosthetic knee infection, and repeat aspiration if any discrepancy in results. Guidelines strongly recommend against intraoperative Gram stain to rule out infection.**
    - Gram stain/culture
    - Fungal cultures, acid-fast bacilli stains
    - Suspected infected joint should always be aspirated prior to initiation of antibiotics except in the systemically ill patient in extremis/sepsis.
    - Management
      a. Acute infections are those within 4 weeks of implantation or symptom onset. An attempt can be made to perform extensive debridement, irrigation, and modular component exchange.
         - Often unsuccessful for *Staphylococcus* infections
      b. Chronic or late infections typically require two-stage revision.
      c. Always know what organism you are treating. Re-aspirate the knee if needed.

d. PCR analysis of synovial fluid if cultures are negative and if high suspicion of infection
   - Component removal with placement of antibiotic spacer and treatment with 6–8 weeks of organism-specific parenteral antibiotics
   - Always aspirate the knee prior to reimplantation to assess eradication of infection.
   - Once inflammatory markers (CRP/ESR) return to normal or trend toward normal, discontinue antibiotics for 4–6 weeks. Reimplantation can be offered.
     - ♦ Will likely require the use of stemmed implants ± augments when bone defects are present
   - Biofilms form on chronically infected components.
     - ♦ Bacteria colonize components and create an extracellular matrix made of polysaccharides.
     - ♦ Difficult to treat; antibiotics cannot penetrate; requires removal of all foreign material

12. Revision TKA
- Goals
  a. Identify a problem preoperatively to be targeted.
     - Do not revise components without identifying the source of pain.
  b. Removal of prosthesis with bone preservation
  c. Restore bony defects.
  d. Restore joint line.
  e. Restore mechanical axis alignment.
  f. Balance ligaments in flexion and extension.
  g. Stable component fixation
- Implants
  a. Less constrained: typically not used for revision cases
     - PS: does not constrain any movement varus/valgus
     - PCL integrity difficult to predict/evaluate
  b. Constrained
     - Typically needed due to bone defects and ligamentous incompetence
     - Tibial and femoral stems should be used to better distribute stresses of a constrained component
- Metaphyseal bone damage
  a. Medullary stems help share torsional and weight-bearing load
  b. Cavitary defects
     - < 1 cm deep: cement
     - ≥ 1 cm deep: metal augments
  c. Very large defects
     - Strut allograph
     - Megaprosthesis
  d. Cement metaphyseal components
  e. Press-fit diaphyseal stems
     - Can also cement shorter stems
- Knee reconstruction after component removal
  a. Start with tibial side: establish joint line
     - 1.5–2 cm above the fibular head
       - ♦ Size femur to restore flexion gap
       - ♦ Balance ligaments
       - ♦ Watch out for patella baja

13. Periprosthetic fracture
    - Determine the stability of implants. Stable implants can be retained, and the fracture can be reduced and fixed. Loose implants need to be removed and revised.
    - Evaluation
        a. Radiographs
        b. Bone scan or metal-subtraction MRI if high suspicion of the findings with normal radiographs
    - Femur fracture
        a. Risk factors:
            - Female gender
            - Rheumatoid arthritis
            - Chronic steroid therapy
            - Osteopenia
            - Anterior femoral cortex notching during anterior distal femur cut
        b. Treatment
            - Nondisplaced fracture can be treated closed, with immobilization, as long as components are stable.
            - Patients who are not good candidates for surgery can be treated in a cast/brace.
            - Displaced
                - ♦ Loose components: revision with long stem implants to bypass defect
            - Stable
                - ♦ Plate fixation
                - ♦ Distal femoral locking plate is used when components appear stable.
                - ♦ Antegrade nail
                - ♦ Retrograde nail
                - ♦ Nail must fit through open box in femoral prosthesis. Usually only for CR implants. Ensure adequate sizing prior to procedure (no box present in PS for nail to be inserted retrograde).
                - ♦ Arthrotomy to visualize and protect PE liner during reaming/nail insertion
            - Revision with long stem
                - ♦ Especially with very distal fracture
            - Mega-prosthesis for non-reconstructable fractures
    - Tibial fracture
        a. Evaluation is same as for femur fractures.
        b. Treatment
            - Nondisplaced fractures can be casted.
            - Displaced fractures with stable components should be reduced and fixed.
            - Fractures with loose components should be revised.
                - ♦ Long press-fit stem that bypasses fracture is preferred.
    - Patella fracture
        a. Rate of fracture is up to 5% for resurfaced patellae, 0.05% for unresurfaced patellae
            - Risk factors include too much patellar resection (thinner than 12 mm), patellar button design, obesity, male gender
            - **Unresurfaced patellae have a lower risk of fracture but higher rate of revision.**
        b. Type I fractures are nondisplaced and can be immobilized in extension for 6 weeks.

c. Type II fractures are displaced and should be reduced and fixed with likely removal of loose prosthesis.
d. Type III fractures have an intact extensor mechanism with a loose patellar component that should be removed.
e. If unsalvageable:
   - Patellectomy, must have PS implant
   - Wound breakdown
     - Most blood supply enters medially (medial superior and inferior geniculate arteries).
     - Lateral superior geniculate artery is very important to maintain after medial parapatellar arthrotomy; can lead to AVN of the patella and fracture.
       - At risk with lateral release

- Anterior knee with multiple incisions
  a. Attempt to use or incorporate the lateralmost incision acceptable for exposure to preserve medially based blood supply to the skin overlying the anterior knee. If new incision necessary, try to maintain 7-cm skin bridge.
- Prior trauma with tissues loss
  b. When planning for TKA through scarred skin and tissue, subcutaneous soft tissue expanders can be used to mobilize excess skin in the preoperative period.
     - Saline is placed within the spacer each week to expand the skin about the knee. The spacer is removed at the time of TKA.
- Chronic infection with tissue loss or wound healing issues
  a. Medial gastrocnemius flap
     - Proximally based blood supply from medial sural artery
     - Good excursion, can be used all the way to the lateral side for coverage
  b. Lateral gastrocnemius flap
     - Can only be used for lateral defects
     - Proximally based blood supply from lateral sural artery
       - Pulled over peroneal nerve leading to frequent nerve palsy

14. Extensor mechanism disruption
   - Patellar tendon injury more common than quad tendon
     a. Marked extensor lag, patella alta
     b. Drop-lock knee brace for nonoperative candidates
     c. Primary suture repair typically fails
     d. Typically need repair of native tendon along with some form of augmentation, either allograft or Marlex mesh
        - Reconstruction with graft in bone tunnel at tibial tubercle. Postoperative cast for 6 weeks in extension. Rehab with active-assist ROM over 3 months. Patient will regain flexion, but will also likely regain extensor lag.

III. Blood Management During Total Joint Replacement

1. Transfusions are associated with increased risk of infection after joint replacement surgery.
   - Tranexamic acid
     a. Prevents activation of plasminogen to plasmin
     b. Derivative of lysine
     c. Prevents clot breakdown
     d. Given intravenously or topically
     e. Decreases perioperative blood loss and transfusion rates

2. Thromboembolic disease after TKA/THA
   - Virchow's triad
     a. Venous stasis
     b. Hypercoagulability
     c. Vessel wall injury
   - Those with a prior deep venous thrombosis (DVT) are at high risk for forming another.
   - 35–40% of patients undergoing THA/TKA without some form of prophylaxis develop a DVT.
   - Nonpharmacological management:
     a. Sequential compression devices: placed on lower leg or feet
     b. Compression of skeletal muscle leads to release of tissue plasminogen activator (TPA)-like substances, which help breakdown venous clots.
     c. Early ambulation: decreases risk of venous thromboembolism (VTE) disease and postoperative pulmonary complications
   - Common medications
     a. Warfarin: inhibits the vitamin K–mediated carboxylation of clotting factors II, VII, IX, X, protein C, protein S
     b. Rivaroxaban, fondaparinux: Xa inhibitor
     c. Dabigatran: direct IIa inhibitor
     d. Enoxaparin: binds and accelerates action of antithrombin III
     e. Aspirin: inhibits cyclooxygenase 1 and 2 (COX-1, -2)
   - Factor V Leiden
     a. Autosomal-dominant mutation of factor V protein
     b. Mutation that prevents activated protein C–mediated cleavage of factor V
     c. Increased risk of DVT formation
        - Prothrombin G20210A mutation (should be on same level as factor V Leiden)
          - Genetic mutation in prothrombin gene
          - Elevated serum prothrombin levels
          - Hypercoagulable state

7

Shoulder, Elbow, and Upper Extremity Sports

Stacey Elisa Gallacher and Andrew Green

I. Anatomy

1. Bony and articular anatomy **(Fig. 7.1)**
   - Clavicle
     a. First bone to ossify (at 5 weeks' gestation), last to fuse (medial clavicular physis at 25 years of age)
     b. Most common musculoskeletal injury at birth is clavicle fracture
   - Scapula **(Fig. 7.2)**
     a. Glenoid orientation: 7 degrees' retroversion to 10 degrees' anteversion
     b. Suprascapular notch: superior transverse scapular ligament (artery above, nerve below)
     c. Spinoglenoid notch: inferior transverse scapular ligament (artery and nerve both below)
     d. Coracoacromial ligament: forms anterior superior aspect of coracoacromial arch, restrains superoanterior displacement of humeral head; preserve when massive irreparable rotator cuff tear present
        - **Acromial branch of thoracoacromial artery on medial aspect: can be a cause of bleeding during acromioplasty. Thoracoacromial artery is a branch of the axillary artery. Acromial branch emerges between pectoralis major and deltoid; enters vessel network over the acromion**
   - Humerus **(Fig. 7.3)**
     a. Humeral head retroverted 20 degrees; average diameter 44–46 mm and is smaller in women than in men; head is mean 130-degree angle to shaft
     b. Anatomic neck: location of capsular attachment
     c. Surgical neck: juncture of shaft with tuberosities
     d. Greater tuberosity: attachment for rotator cuff muscles and tendons; supraspinatus, infraspinatus, teres minor
     e. Lesser tuberosity: attachment of subscapularis
     f. Bicipital groove: transverse humeral ligament restrains biceps long head tendon
     g. Posterior spiral groove: radial nerve, 13 cm superior to trochlea

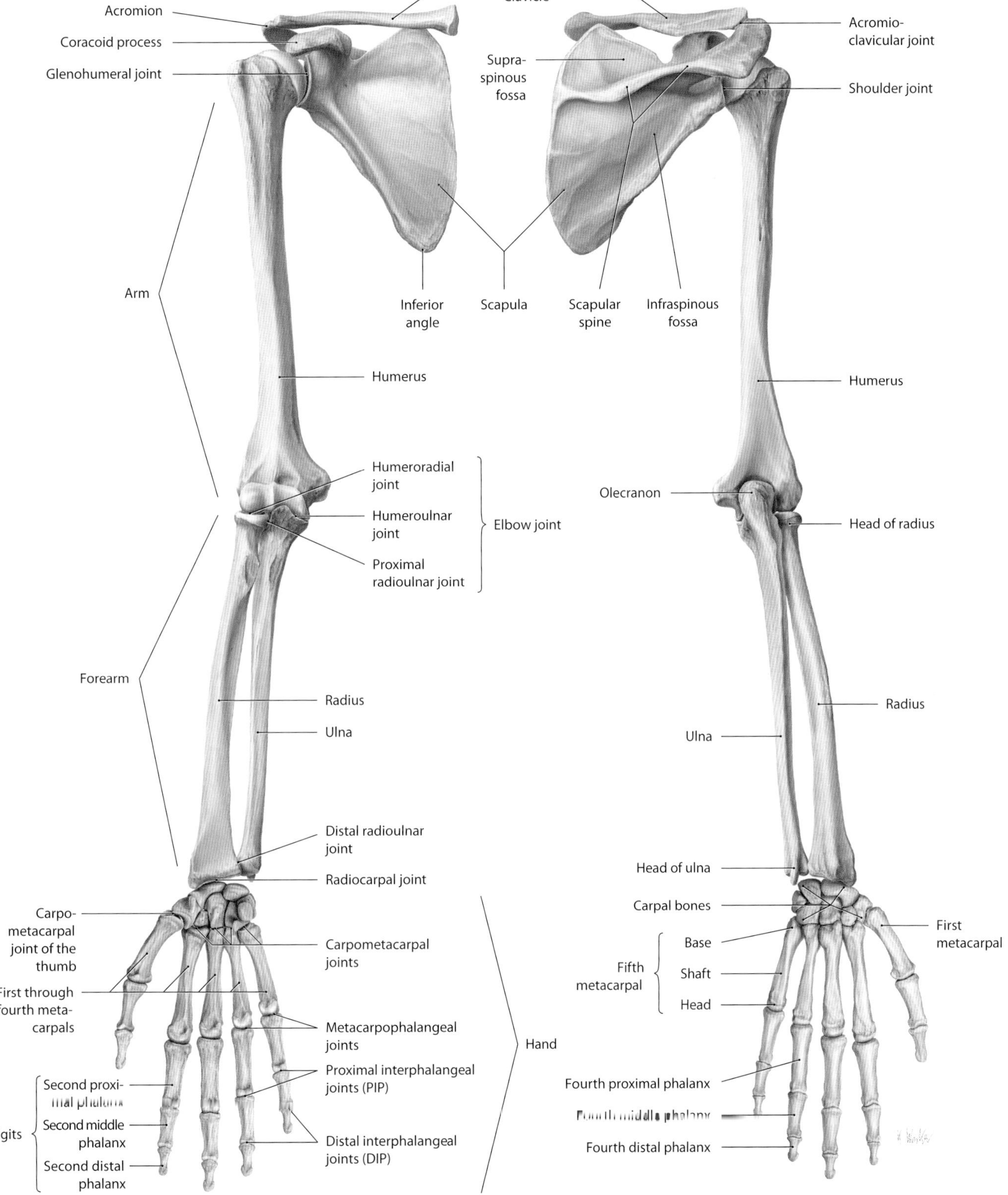

Fig. 7.1 Shoulder and elbow bony anatomy. (From Schuenke M, Schulte E. General Anatomy and the Musculoskeletal System: Thieme Atlas of Anatomy. New York: Thieme; 2005. Illustration by Karl Wesker.)

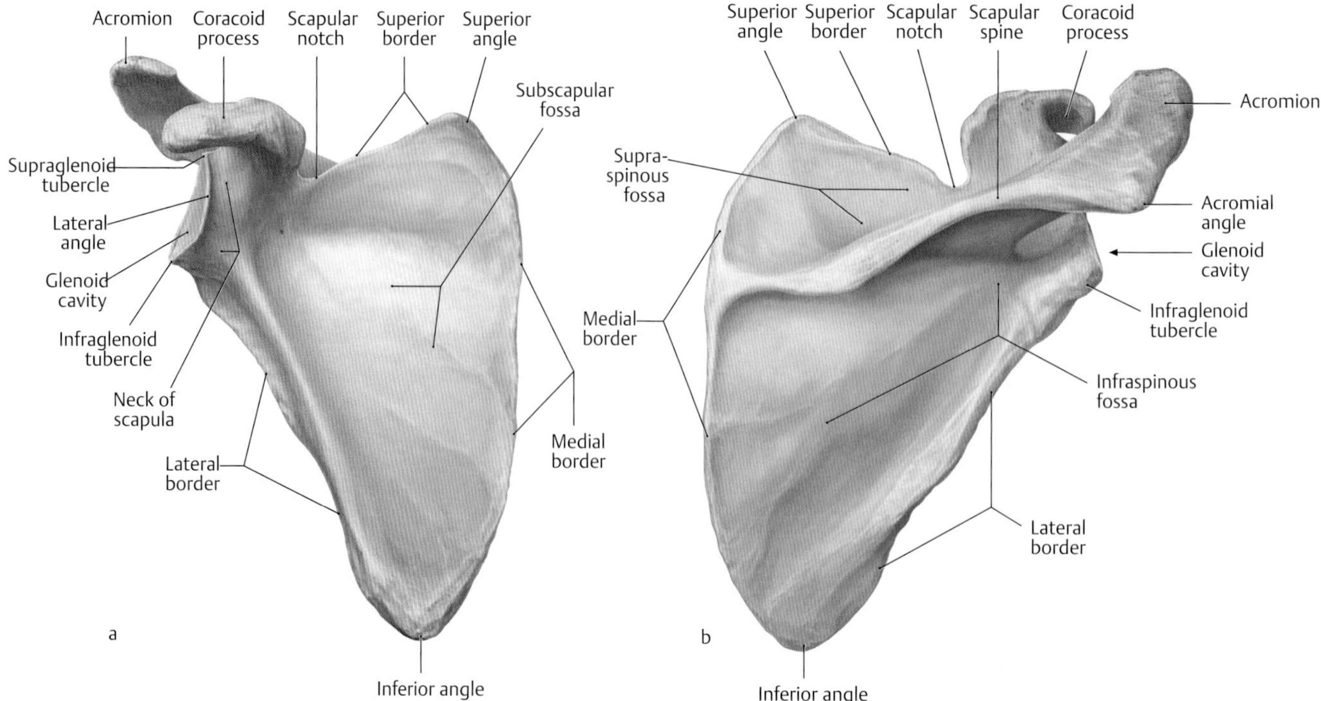

Fig. 7.2 The right scapula. **(a)** Lateral view. **(b)** Anterior view. (From Schuenke M, Schulte E. General Anatomy and the Musculoskeletal System: Thieme Atlas of Anatomy. New York: Thieme; 2005. Illustration by Karl Wesker.)

- Glenohumeral joint: ball and socket; large degree of motion; most frequently dislocated major joint **(Figs. 7.4** and **7.5)**
  a. Range of motion: 40 degrees of extension to 150–170 degrees of forward elevation; 20–40 degrees of adduction to 160–180 degrees of abduction
  b. Position of arthrodesis: 20–30 degrees of abduction, 20–30 degrees of forward flexion, 20–30 degrees of internal rotation
  c. Static restraints: labrum, capsule, ligaments, negative intra-articular joint pressure **(Figs. 7.6, 7.7, 7.8, 7.9)**
    - Static restraints **(Table 7.1)**
    - Anterior band of inferior glenohumeral ligament restricts anterior translation of arm in 90 degrees of abduction and maximal external rotation.
    - Middle glenohumeral ligament: limits anterior translation
    - Superior glenohumeral ligament: limits inferior translation
    - Coracohumeral ligament: primary restraint to inferior humeral translation; also important for posterior stability
    - Coracoacromial ligament: restrains anterior and inferior translation; resection increases glenohumeral joint translation
  d. Dynamic restraints: rotator cuff is main dynamic restraint; serves to compress humeral head against glenoid and contributes to concavity compression
    - Concavity compression is most important stabilizer in midrange of motion.
  e. Rotator cable: thickening of supraspinatus and infraspinatus tendons; borders the avascular zone of rotator cuff near insertion; decreases stress at avascular zone

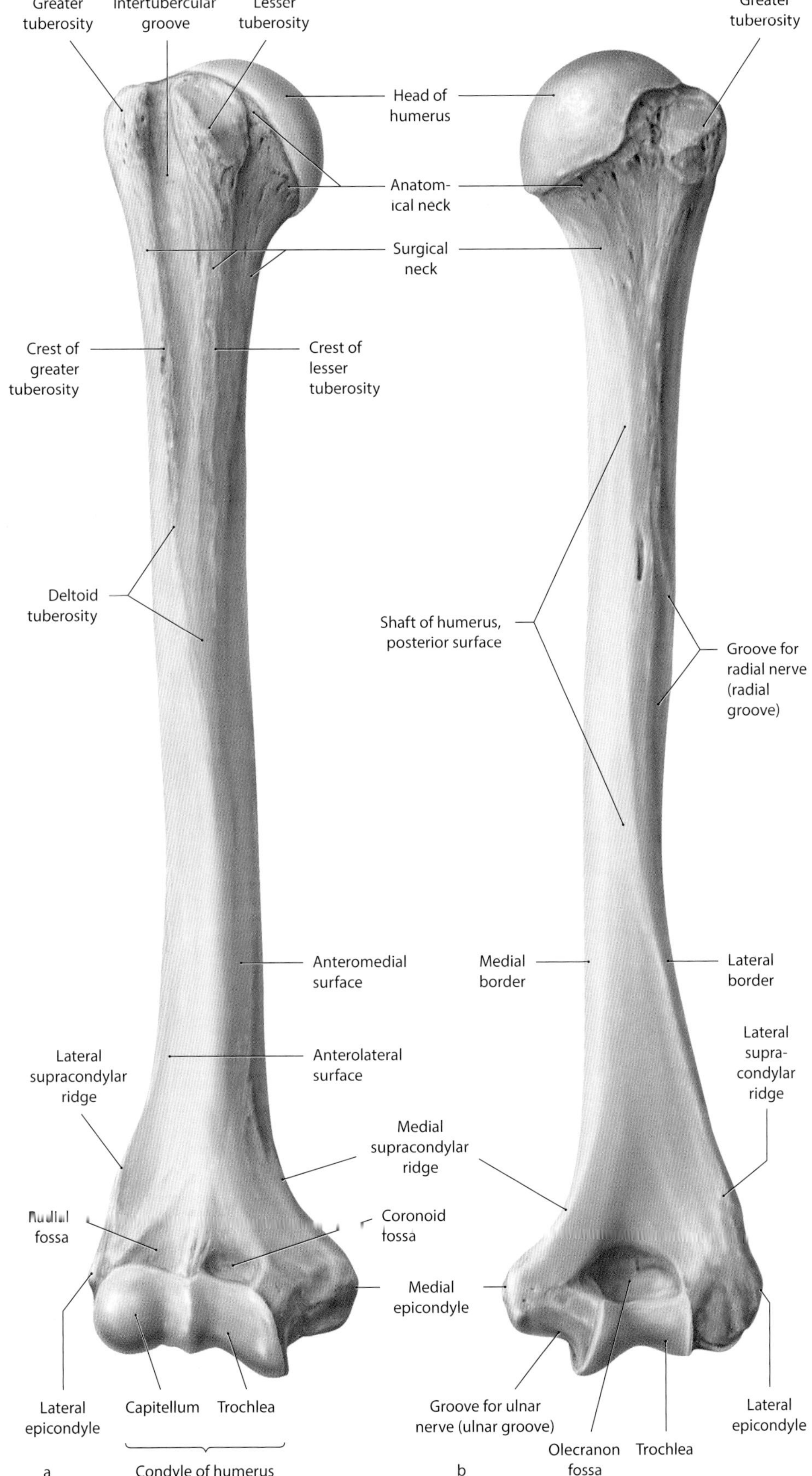

Fig. 7.3 The right humerus. **(a)** Anterior view. **(b)** Posterior view. (From Schuenke M, Schulte E. General Anatomy and the Musculoskeletal System: Thieme Atlas of Anatomy. New York: Thieme; 2005. Illustration by Karl Wesker.)

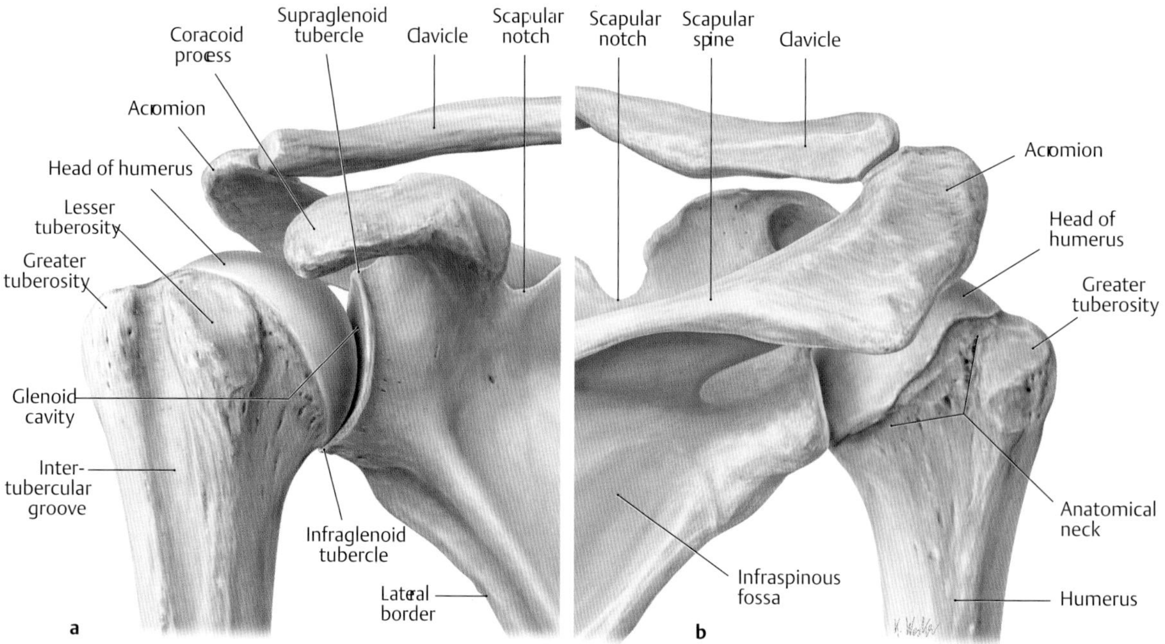

Fig. 7.4 Bony anatomy of glenohumeral joint. **(a)** Anterior view. **(b)** Posterior view. (From Schuenke M, Schulte E. General Anatomy and the Musculoskeletal System: Thieme Atlas of Anatomy. New York: Thieme; 2005. Illustration by Karl Wesker.)

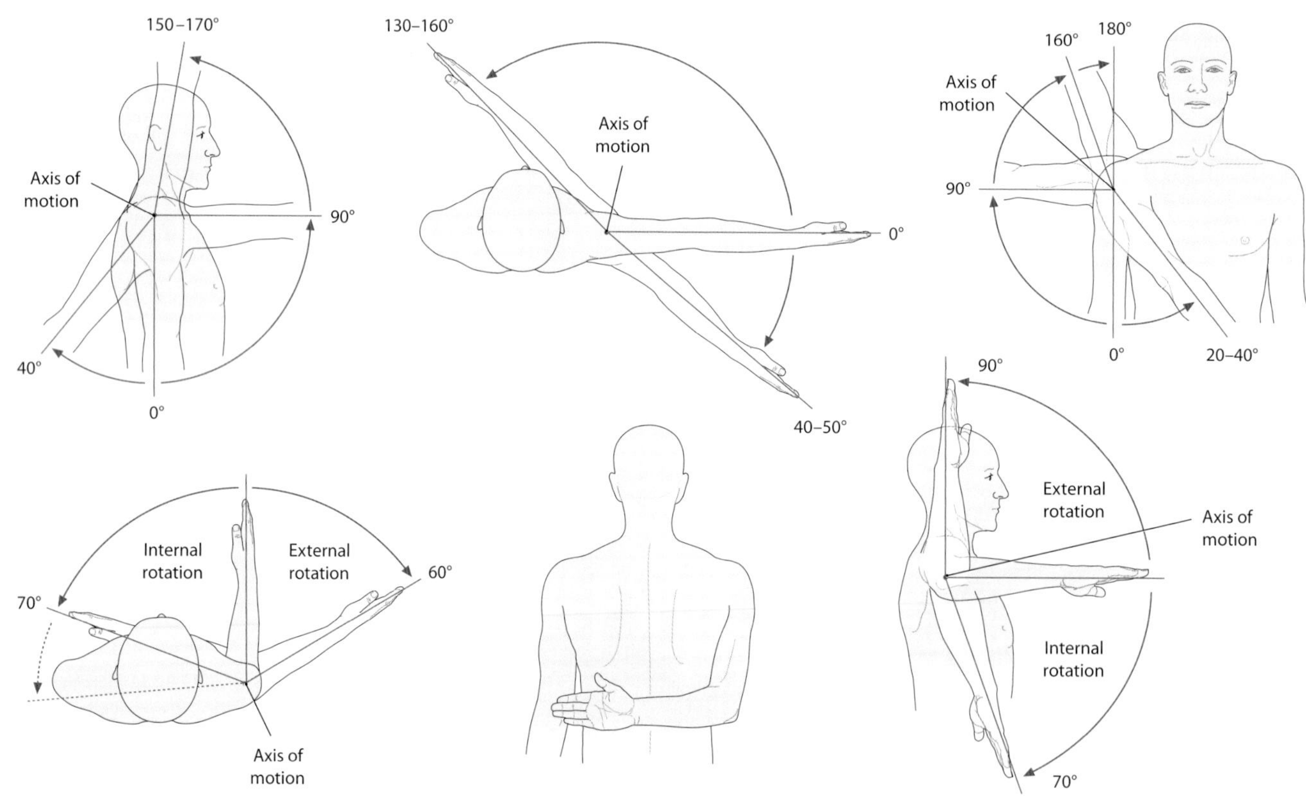

Fig. 7.5 Normal shoulder range of motion. (From Schuenke M, Schulte E. General Anatomy and the Musculoskeletal System: Thieme Atlas of Anatomy. New York: Thieme; 2005. Illustration by Karl Wesker.)

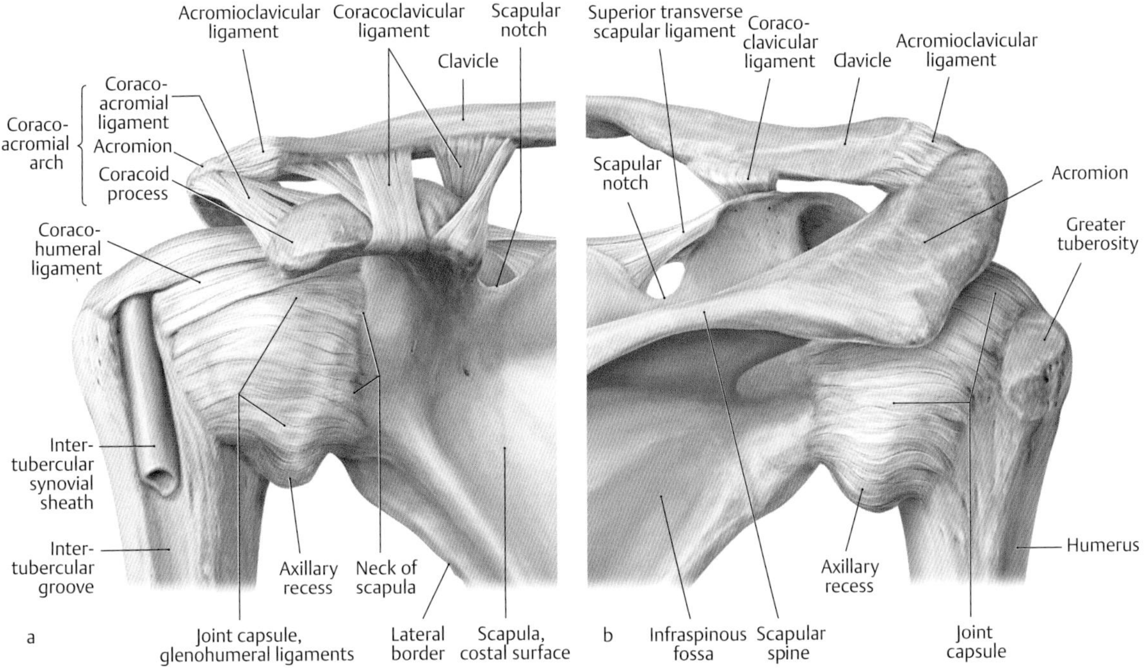

Fig. 7.6 Ligaments and capsule of the glenohumeral joint. **(a)** Anterior view. **(b)** Posterior view. (From Schuenke M, Schulte E. General Anatomy and the Musculoskeletal System: Thieme Atlas of Anatomy. New York: Thieme; 2005. Illustration by Karl Wesker.)

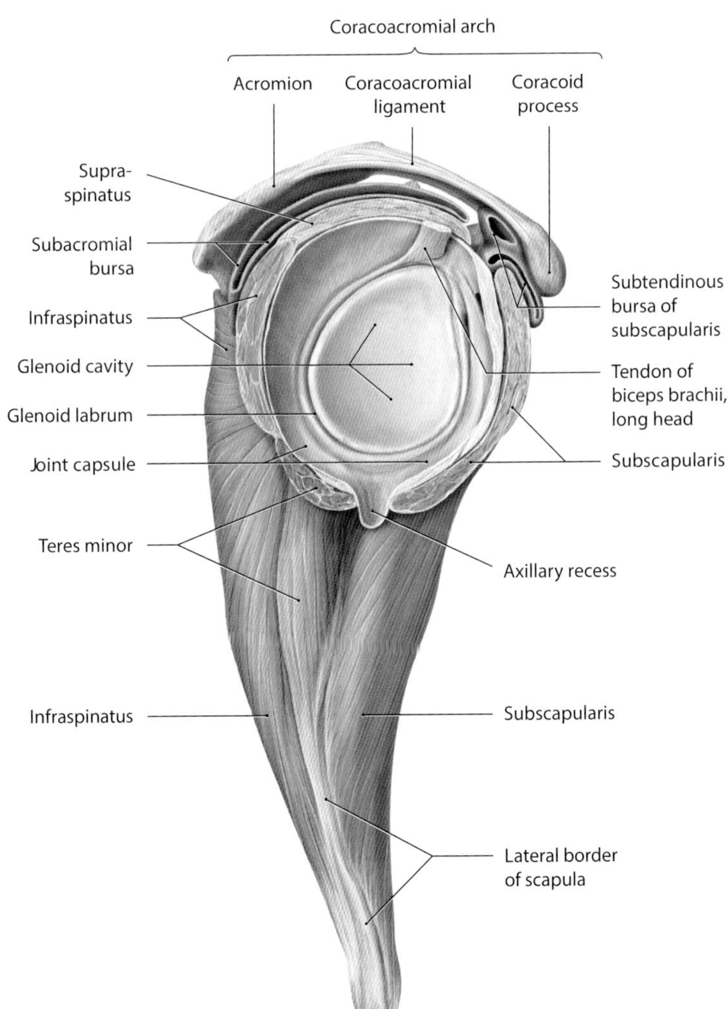

Fig. 7.7 Subacromial bursa and glenoid cavity of the right shoulder joint. (From Schuenke M, Schulte E. General Anatomy and the Musculoskeletal System: Thieme Atlas of Anatomy. New York: Thieme; 2005. Illustration by Karl Wesker.)

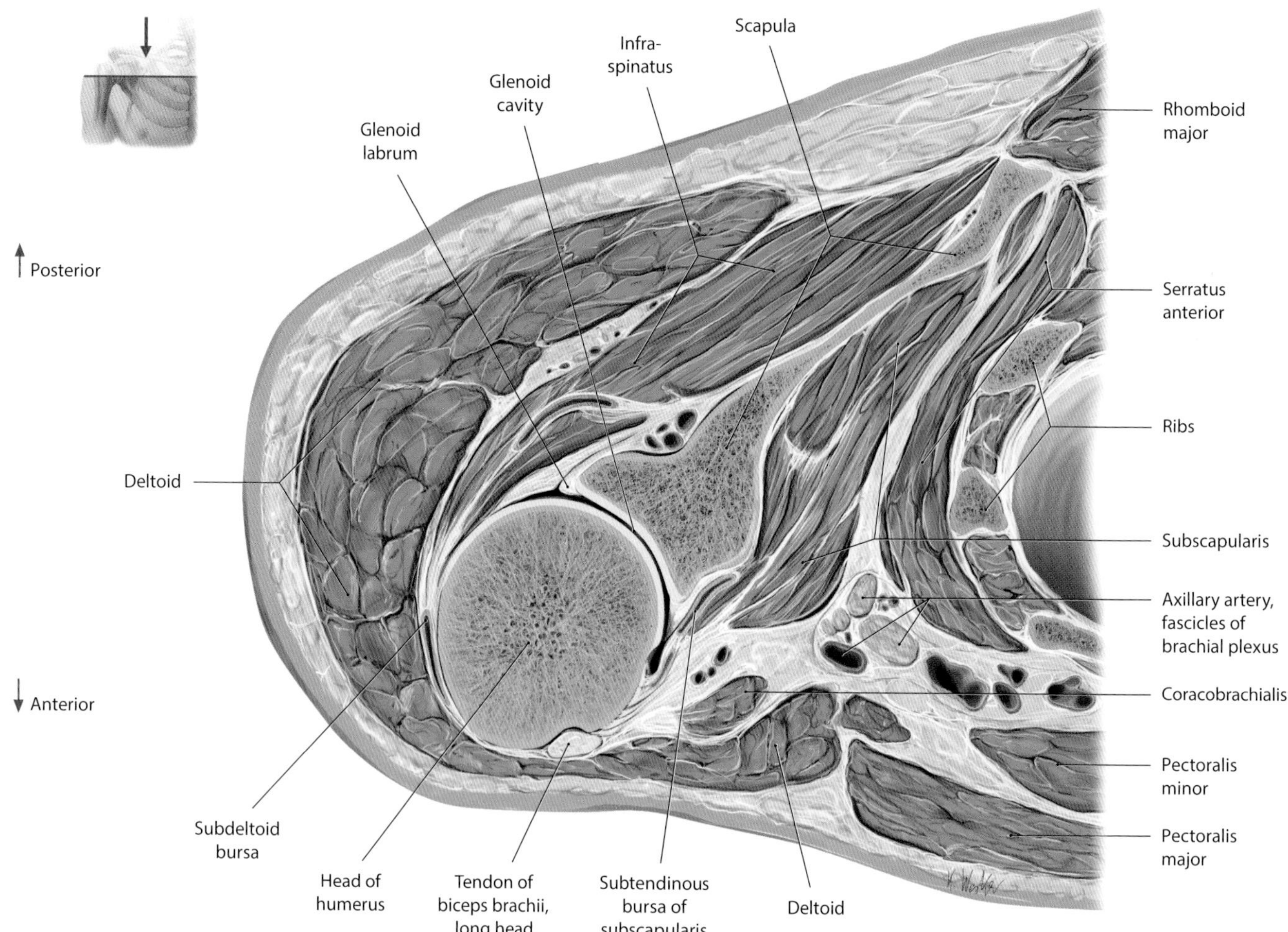

Fig. 7.8 Transverse section through the right shoulder joint. Superior view. (From Schuenke M, Schulte E. General Anatomy and the Musculoskeletal System: Thieme Atlas of Anatomy. New York: Thieme; 2005. Illustration by Karl Wesker.)

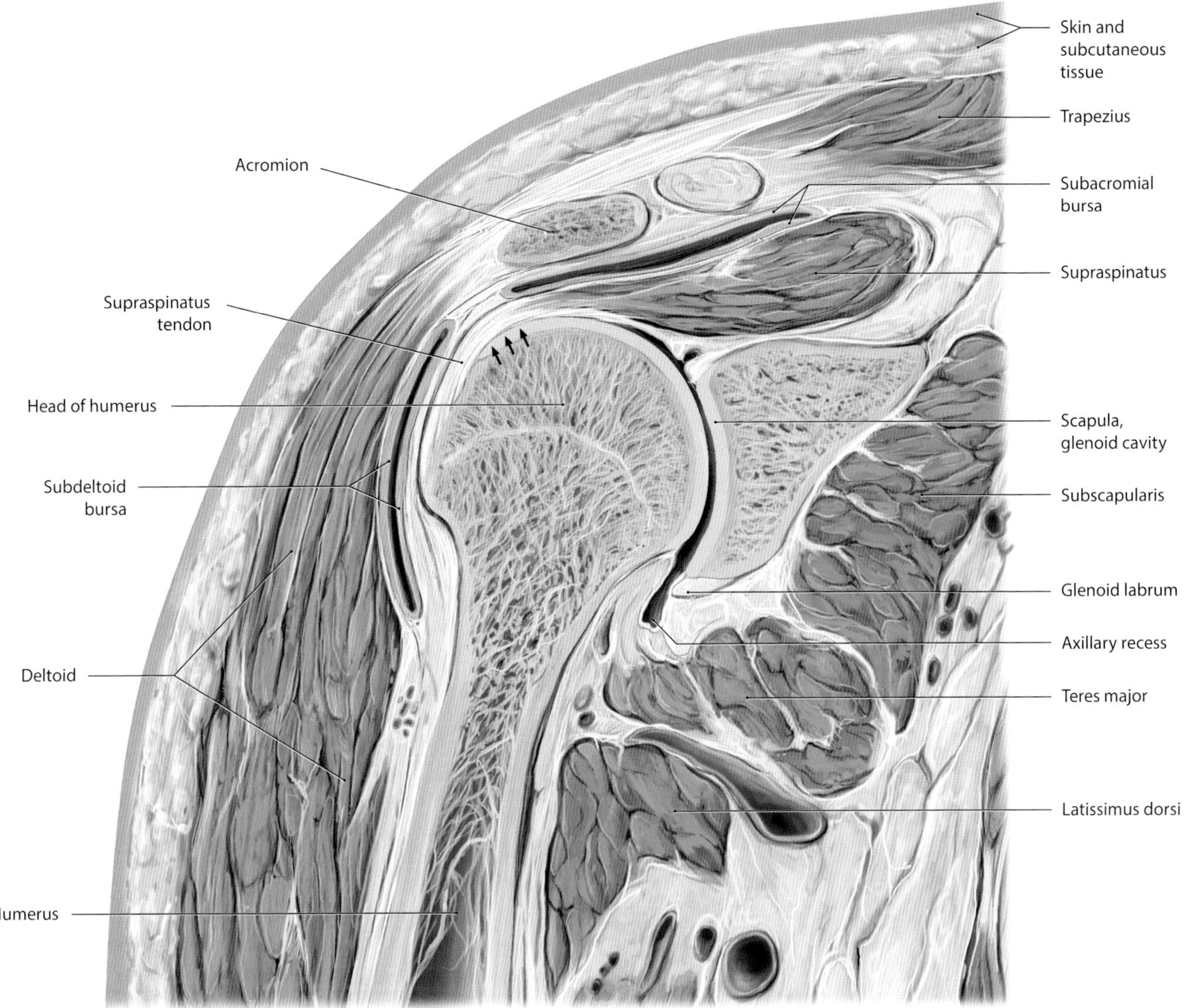

Fig. 7.9 Coronal section through the right shoulder joint. Anterior view. (From Schuenke M, Schulte E. General Anatomy and the Musculoskeletal System: Thieme Atlas of Anatomy. New York: Thieme; 2005. Illustration by Karl Wesker.)

Table 7.1 Glenohumeral Ligaments

Structure	Arm Position When Ligament Is Active	Function
Coracohumeral ligament	Adducted arm	Limits inferior translation, external rotation
Superior glenohumeral ligament	Adducted arm	Limits inferior translation, external rotation
Middle glenohumeral ligament	45 degrees of abduction	Limits anterior translation
Inferior glenohumeral ligament	Abduction external rotation	Limits anterior and inferior translation

f. Buford complex **(Fig. 7.10)**: anatomic variant not to be confused with an anterior labral tear; cord-like middle glenohumeral ligament, absent anterosuperior labral complex; normal variant if repaired results in lack of external rotation

- Sternoclavicular joint: medial clavicle articulates with manubrium
  a. 30 degrees of upward elevation with arm elevation from 30 to 90 degrees
  b. Posterior capsule/ligaments most important stabilizers
  c. Serendipity view to evaluate radiographically (40-degree cephalic tilt) versus computed tomography (CT) scan
- Acromioclavicular joint **(Fig. 7.11)**
  a. Acromioclavicular ligaments: prevent anteroposterior (AP) displacement
  b. Coracoclavicular ligaments: trapezoid is anterolateral, conoid posteromedial and strongest; prevent superior displacement of clavicle
  c. Zanca view for radiographic evaluation (10-degree cephalic tilt, one-half voltage)
- Scapulothoracic articulation **(Fig. 7.12)**
  a. Angled 30 degrees anterior and 3 degrees superior tilt
  b. Ratio of scapulothoracic to glenohumeral joint motion during abduction = 1:2
- Elbow **(Fig. 7.13)**
  a. Range of motion: 0 degrees' extension to 145 degrees' flexion; 70 degrees' pronation; 85 degrees' supination; function range of motion is 30–130 degrees of flexion-extension and 50/50 pronation/supination
  b. Position of arthrodesis: unilateral in 90 degrees of flexion and up to 7 degrees of valgus; if bilateral, fuse one in 110 degrees of flexion for feeding and the other at 65 degrees of flexion for perineal hygiene

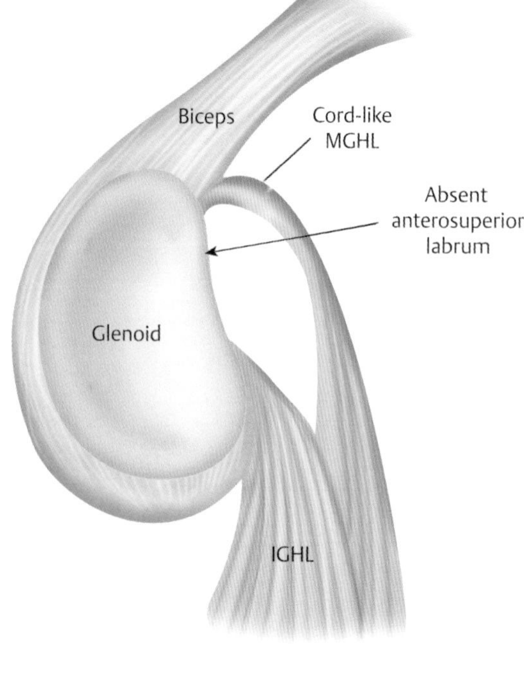

Fig. 7.10 Buford complex. IGHL, inferior glenohumeral ligament; MGHL, middle glenohumeral ligament.

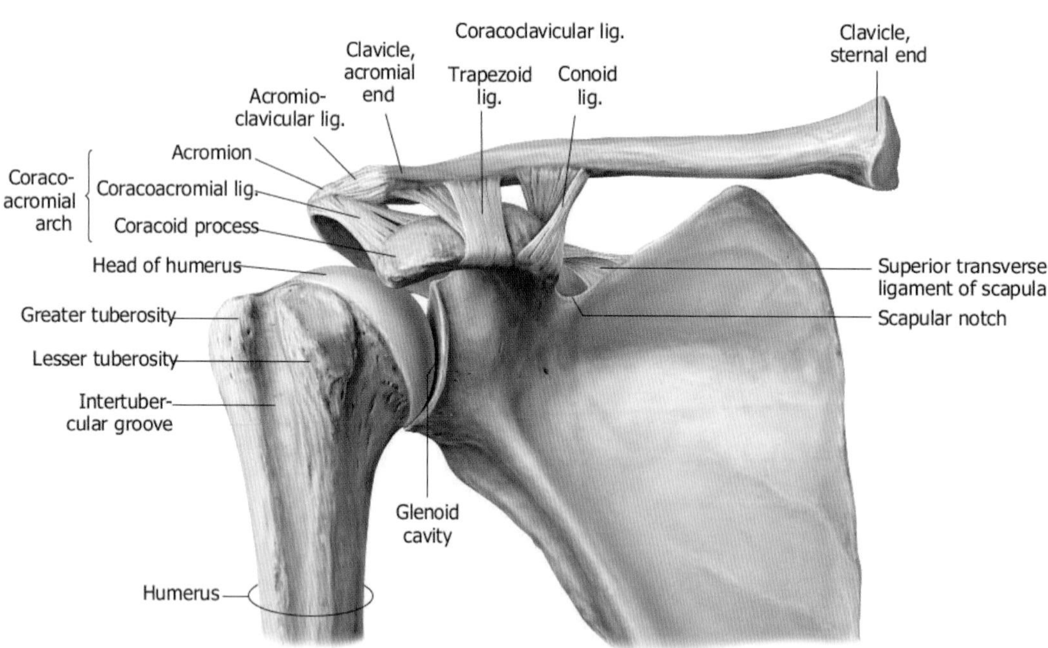

Fig. 7.11 The acromioclavicular joint and its ligaments. Anterior view. (Modified from Schuenke M, Schulte E. General Anatomy and the Musculoskeletal System: Thieme Atlas of Anatomy. New York: Thieme; 2005. Illustration by Karl Wesker.)

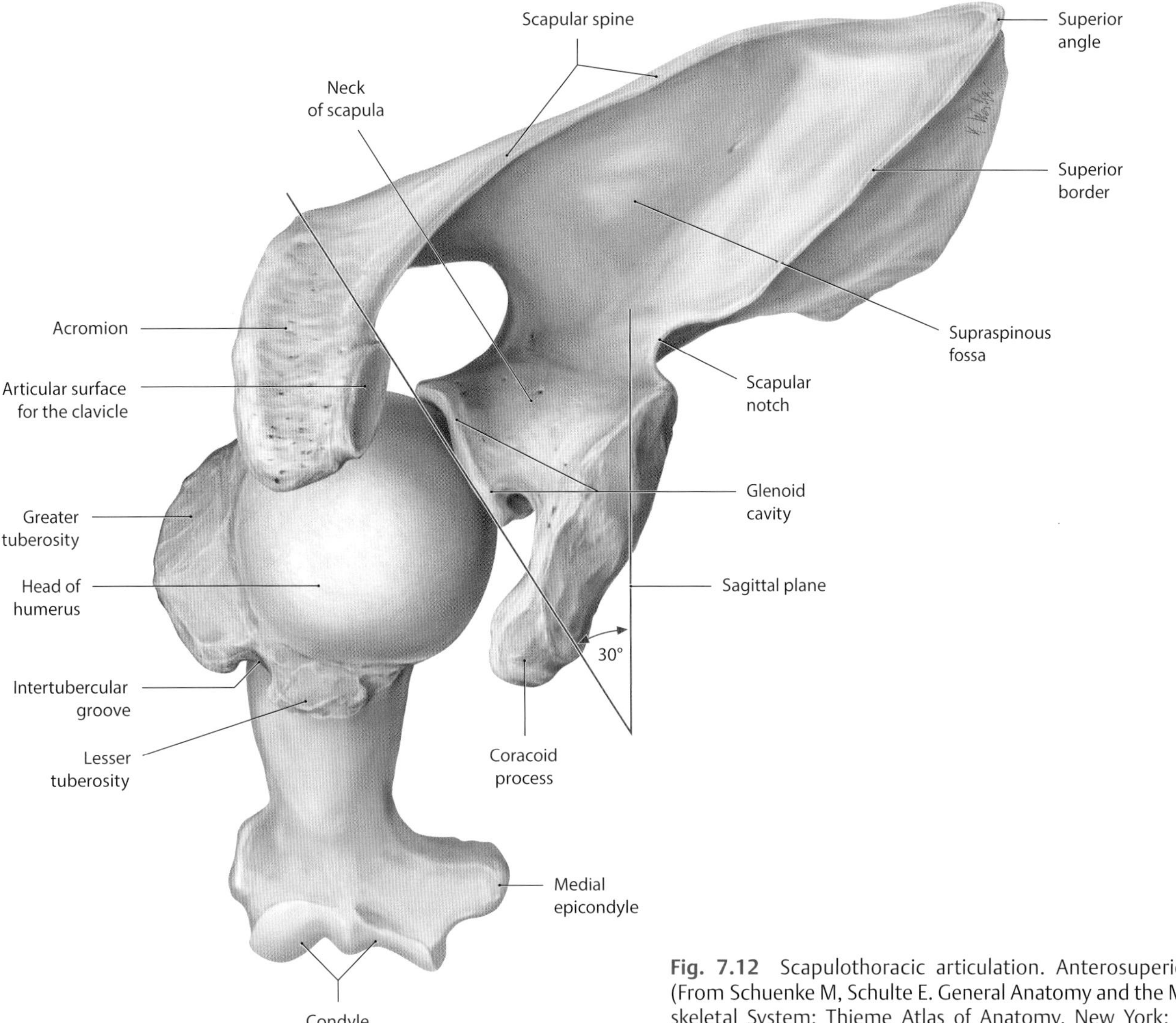

Fig. 7.12 Scapulothoracic articulation. Anterosuperior view. (From Schuenke M, Schulte E. General Anatomy and the Musculoskeletal System: Thieme Atlas of Anatomy. New York: Thieme; 2005. Illustration by Karl Wesker.)

c. Distal humeral joint surface has 7 degrees' valgus, 30 degrees' anterior tilt, 5 degrees' internal rotation
d. Maximal joint distention occurs at 70–80 degrees of flexion; effusion up to 20 cc of fluid results in flexed position of elbow
e. Distal anterior capsular attachment is located 6 mm distal to coronoid (tip of coronoid is intra-articular).
f. Ligaments (**Fig. 7.14**):
   - Medial collateral ligament: anterior, posterior, transverse bundles
     - Anterior bundle most important stabilizer against valgus stress; originates on medical epicondyle and attaches 18 mm distal to tip of coronoid on sublime tubercle (anteromedial facet of coronoid); primary stabilizer of elbow against valgus stress from 20–120 degrees of motion; Tommy John reconstruction
     - Posterior bundle: tight from 60–120 degrees, elongates with flexion and has larger change in tension during motion than anterior bundle

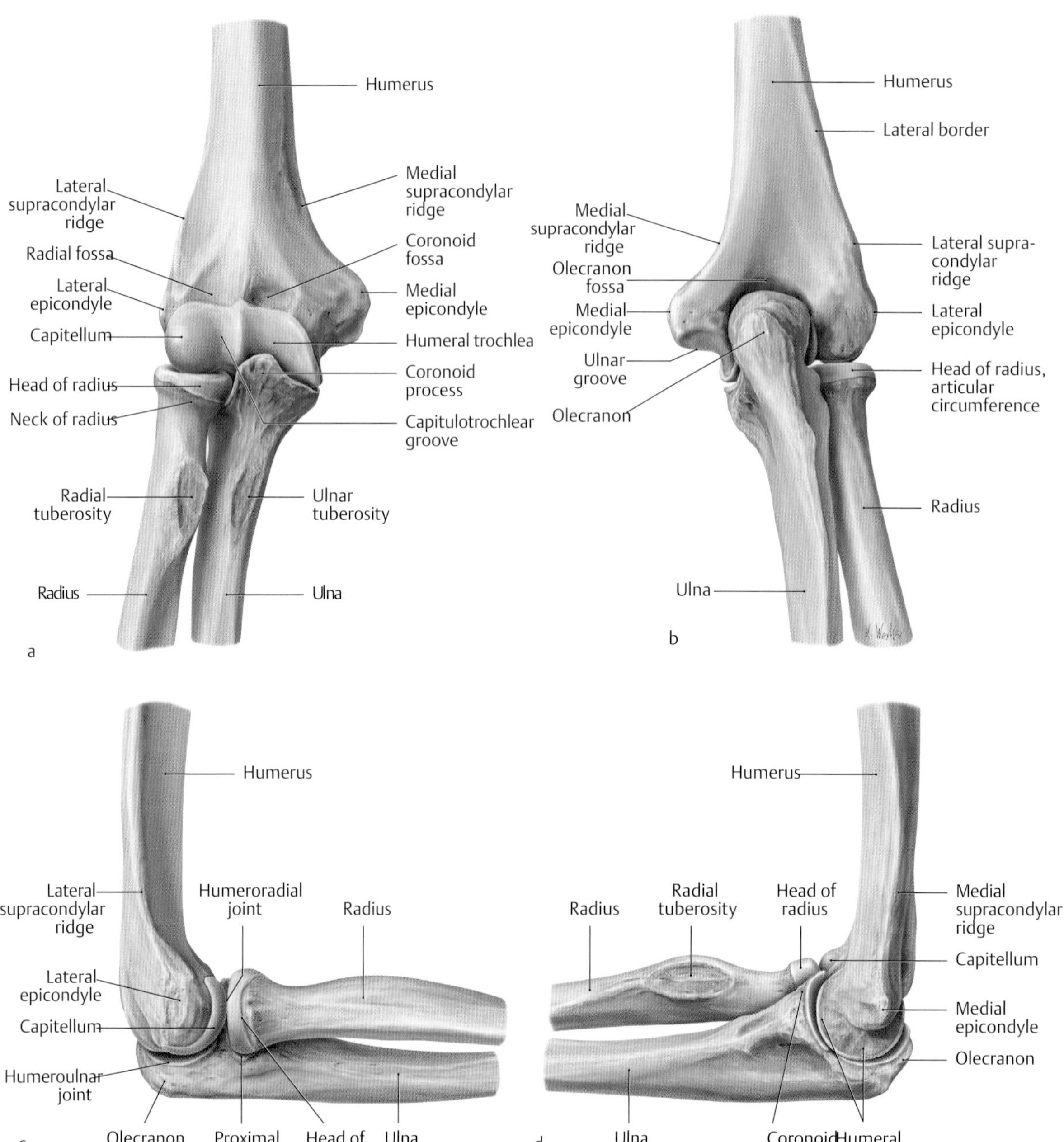

Fig. 7.13 Elbow joint bony and articular anatomy. **(a)** Anterior view. **(b)** Posterior view. **(c)** Lateral view. **(d)** Medial view. (From Schuenke M, Schulte E. General Anatomy and the Musculoskeletal System: Thieme Atlas of Anatomy. New York: Thieme; 2005. Illustration by Karl Wesker.)

- Lateral collateral ligament complex: composed of lateral ulnar collateral ligament; annular ligament, which attaches to radial neck; and the oblique cord
  - Lateral ulnar collateral ligament (LUCL): lateral epicondyle to ulna crista supinatoris; deficiency results in posterolateral rotatory instability
  - Most common elbow dislocation is posterolateral: all ligaments and capsule can be torn

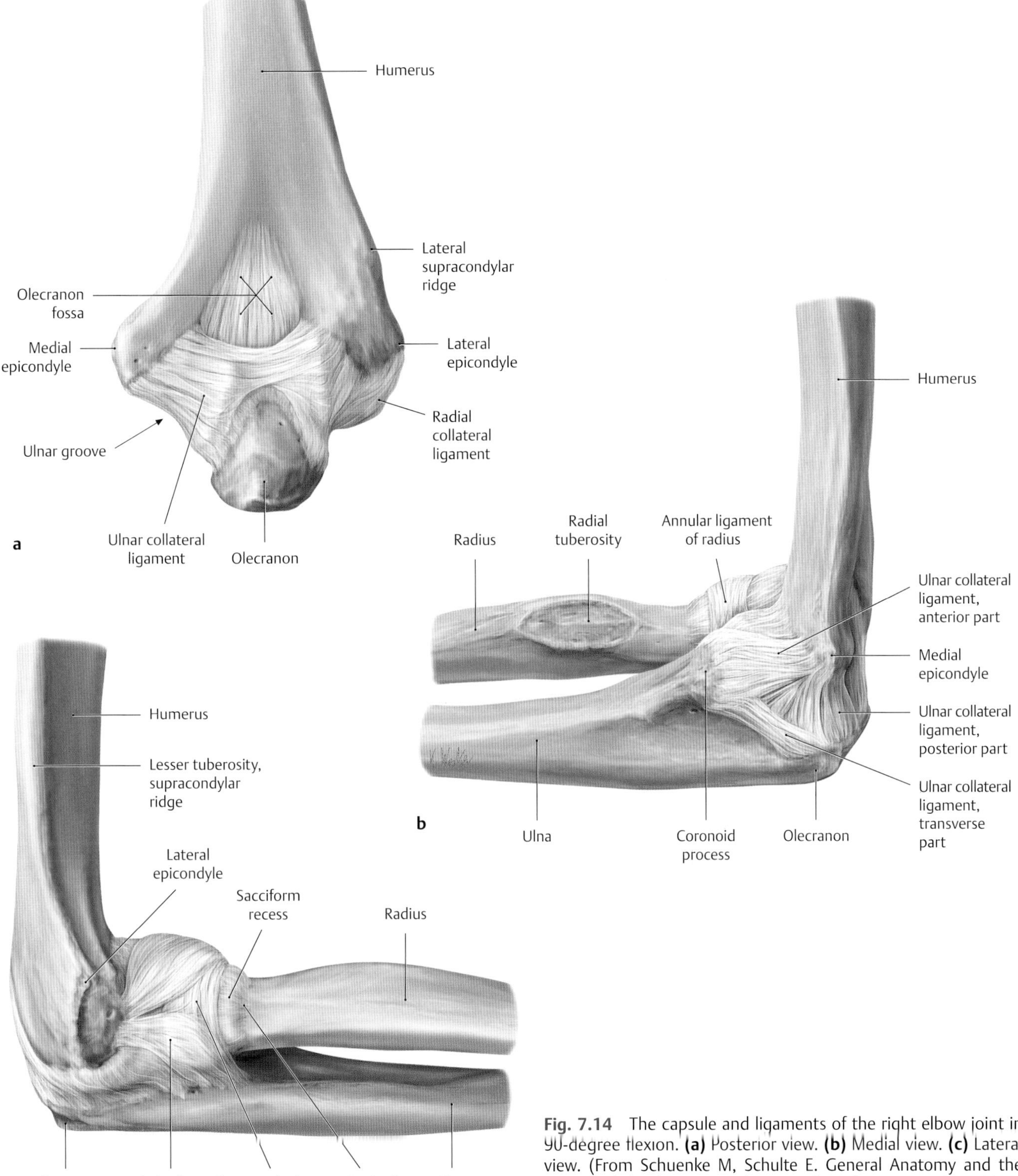

Fig. 7.14 The capsule and ligaments of the right elbow joint in 90-degree flexion. **(a)** Posterior view. **(b)** Medial view. **(c)** Lateral view. (From Schuenke M, Schulte E. General Anatomy and the Musculoskeletal System: Thieme Atlas of Anatomy. New York: Thieme; 2005. Illustration by Karl Wesker.)

2. Muscles (**Figs. 7.15, 7.16, 7.17, 7.18, 7.19, 7.20, 7.21, 7.22**)
   - Muscles including origin, insertion, innervations, action (**Table 7.2**)
   - Long head of biceps tendon has posterior or posterior dominant attachment to superior glenoid labrum in 70% of patients; collagen fibers of long head of biceps tendon and superior glenoid labrum overlap
   - Rotator cuff: supraspinatus, infraspinatus, and teres minor attaching to greater tuberosity; subscapularis attaching to lesser tuberosity; average supraspinatus insertion (footprint) from medial to lateral is 14–16 mm

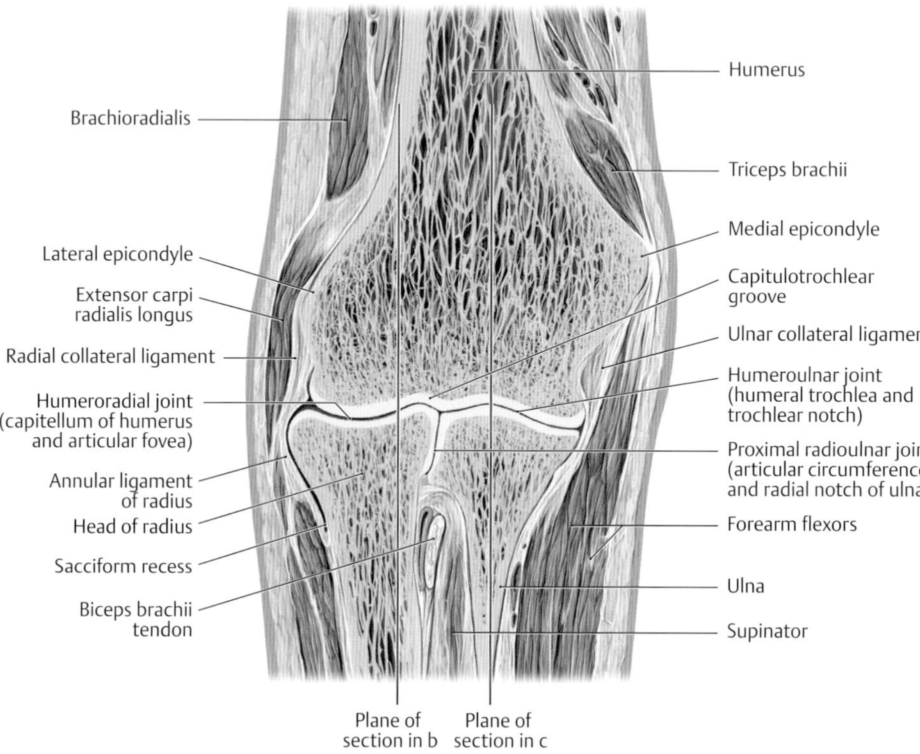

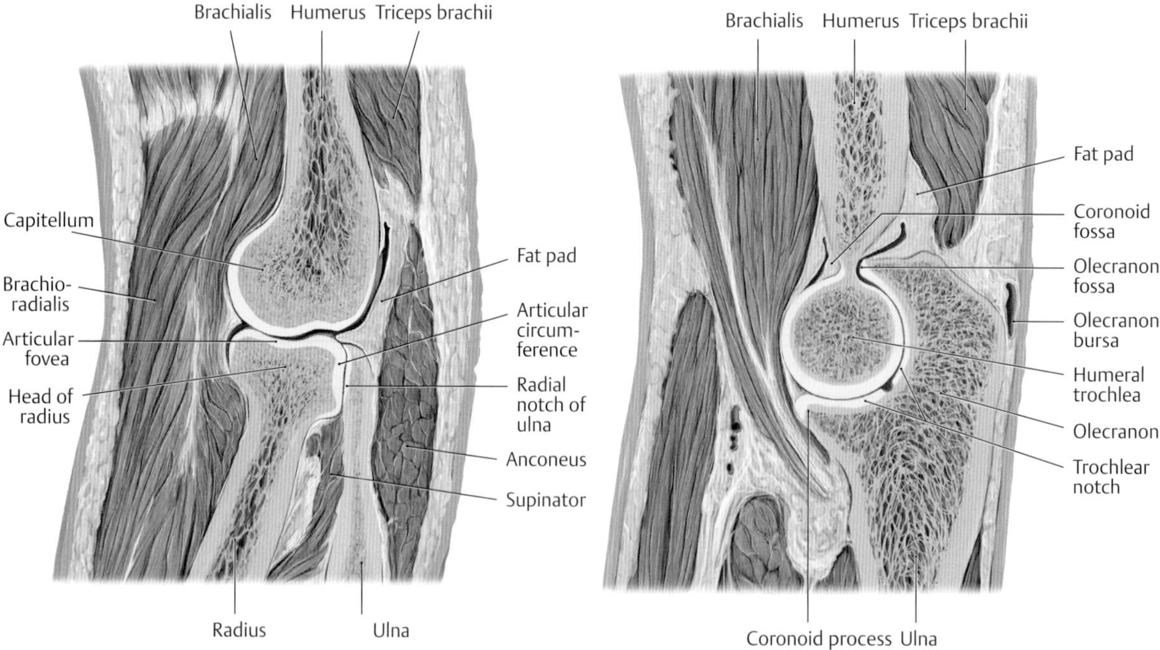

Fig. 7.15 Coronal and sagittal sections through ulnohumeral joint. (From Schuenke M, Schulte E. General Anatomy and the Musculoskeletal System: Thieme Atlas of Anatomy. New York: Thieme; 2005. Illustration by Karl Wesker.)

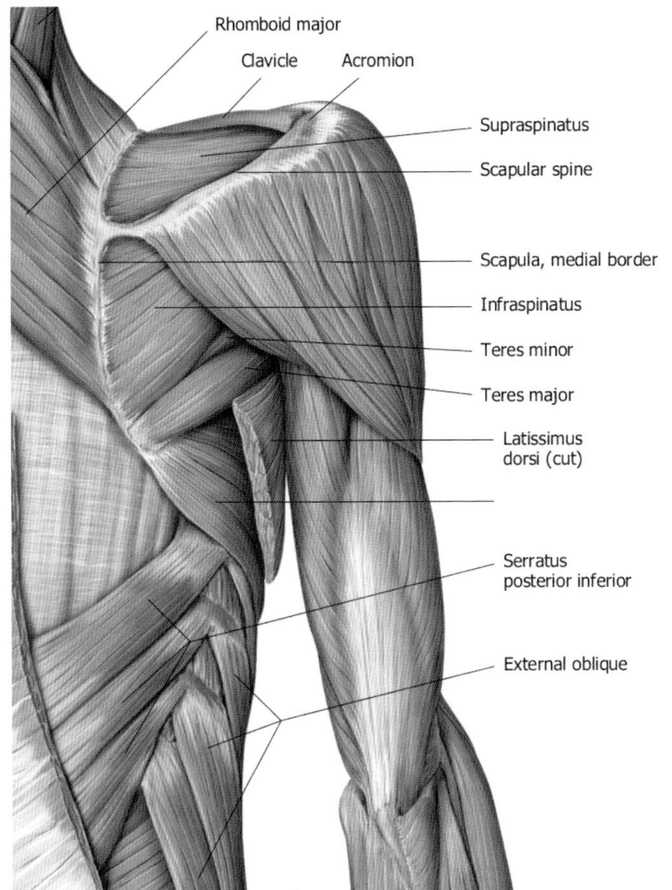

Fig. 7.16 Posterior muscles of the shoulder and arm. (From Schuenke M, Schulte E. General Anatomy and the Musculoskeletal System: Thieme Atlas of Anatomy. New York: Thieme; 2005. Illustration by Karl Wesker.)

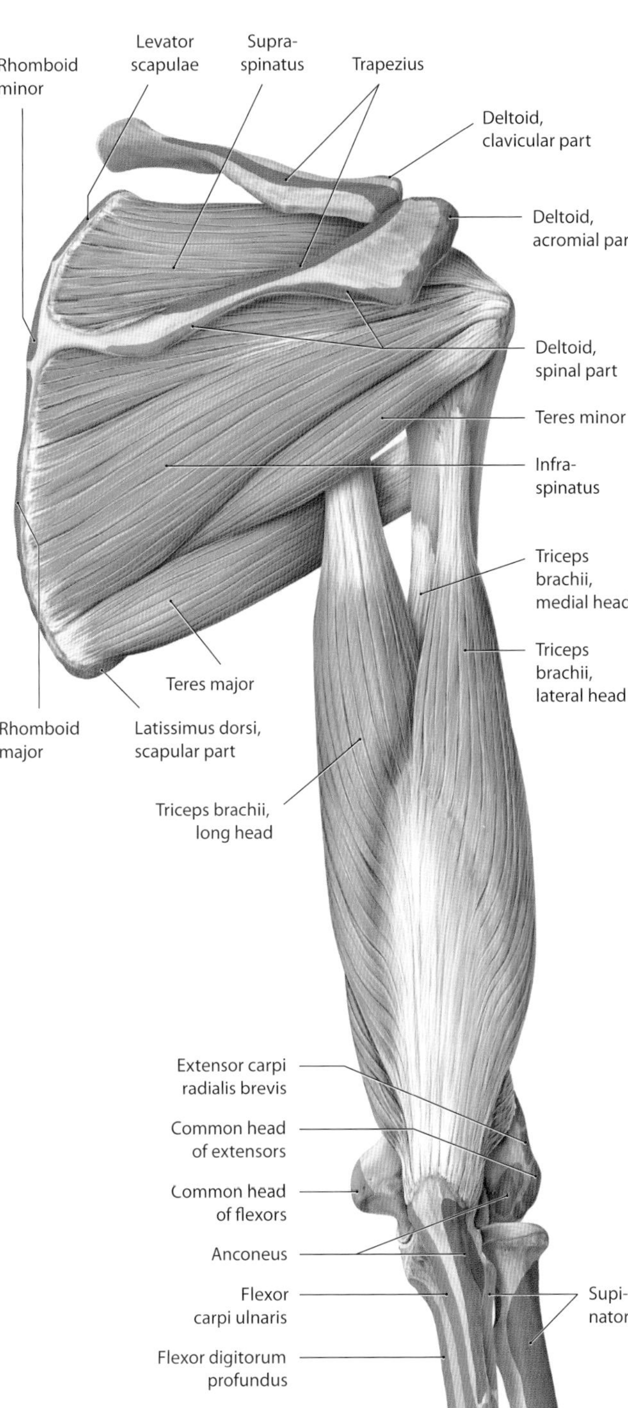

Fig. 7.17 Posterior muscles of the shoulder and arm. (From Schuenke M, Schulte E. General Anatomy and the Musculoskeletal System: Thieme Atlas of Anatomy. New York: Thieme; 2005. Illustration by Karl Wesker.)

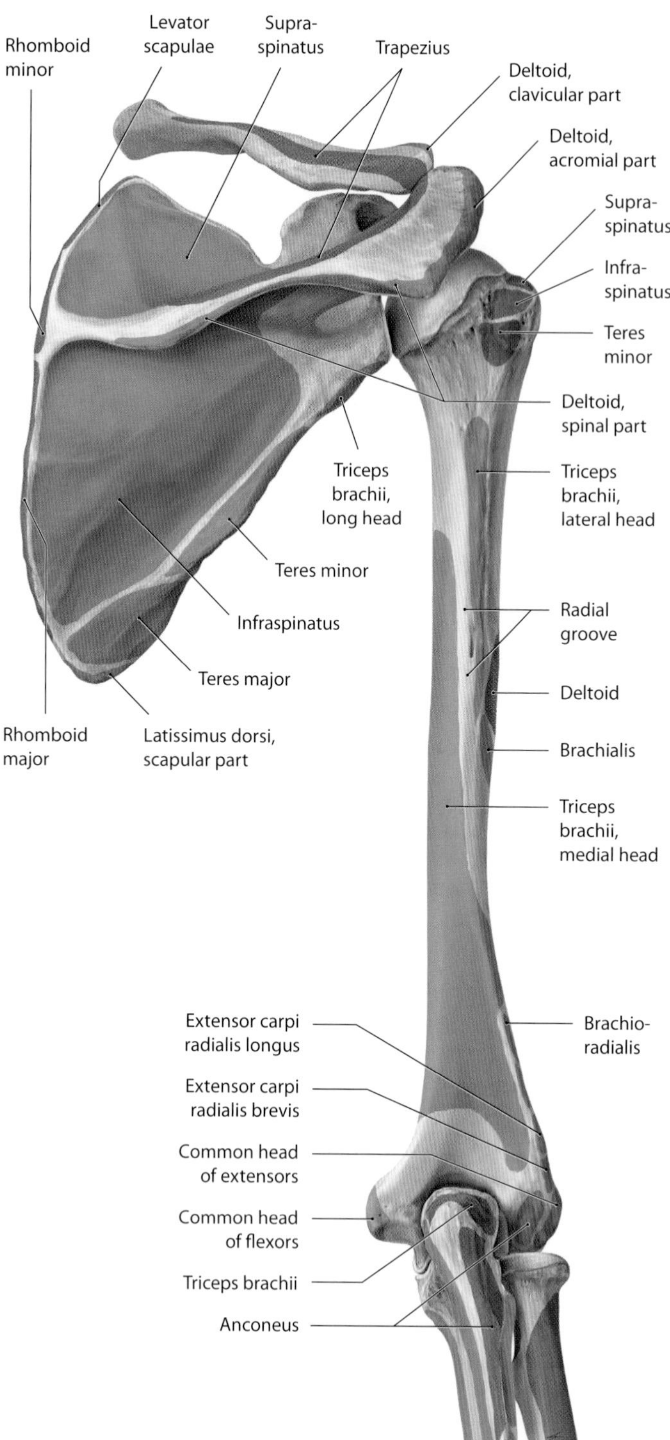

Fig. 7.18 Origin and insertion of muscles of shoulder and arm. (From Schuenke M, Schulte E. General Anatomy and the Musculoskeletal System: Thieme Atlas of Anatomy. New York: Thieme; 2005. Illustration by Karl Wesker.)

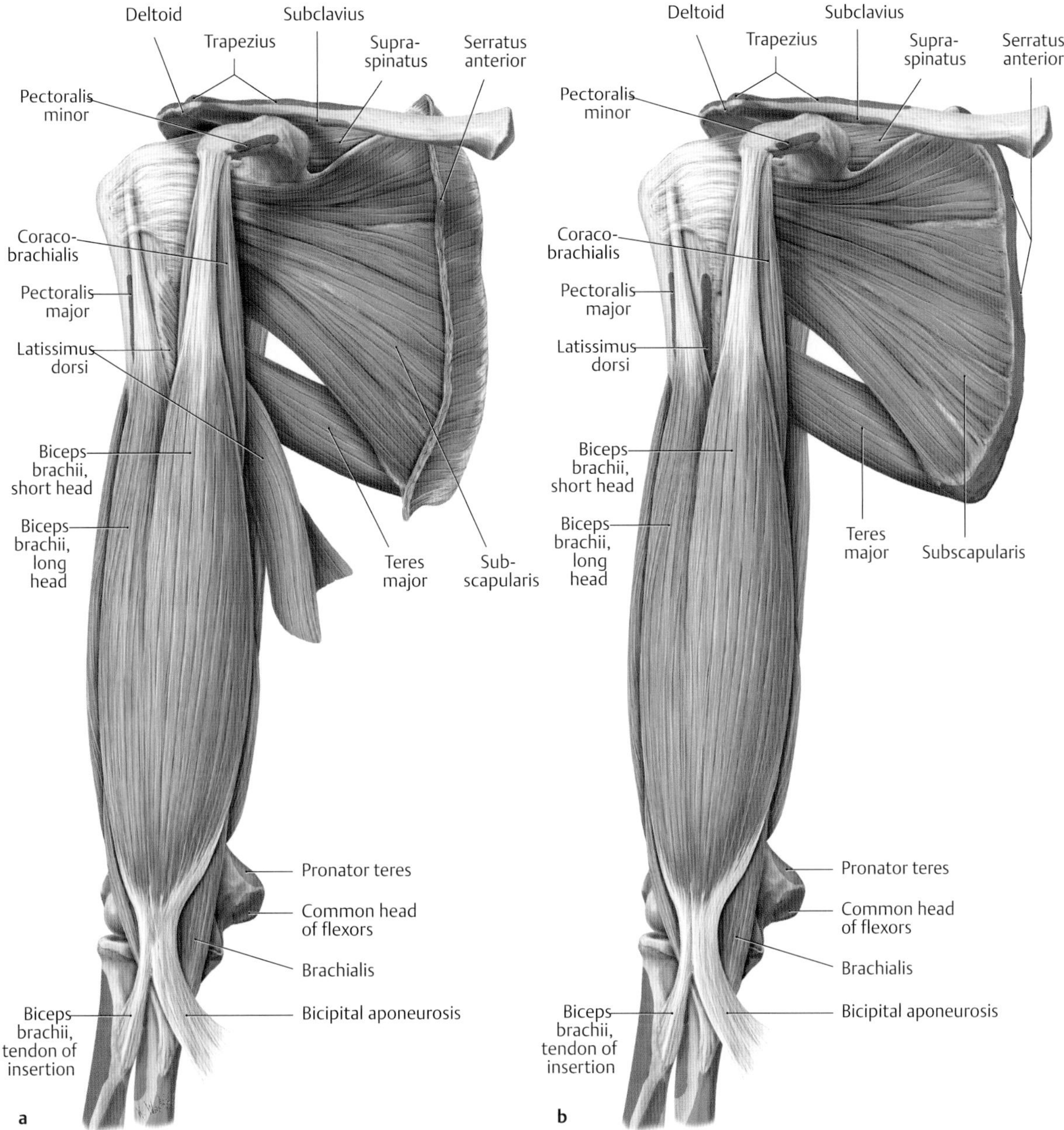

Fig. 7.19 Muscles of the right shoulder and right arm from the anterior view. The origins and insertions of the muscles are indicated by color shading: origin *(red)*; insertion *(blue)*. **(a)** After removal of the thoracic skeleton. Latissimus dorsi and serratus anterior have been removed to their insertions. **(b)** Latissimus dorsi and serratus anterior have been completely removed. (From Schuenke M, Schulte E. General Anatomy and the Musculoskeletal System: Thieme Atlas of Anatomy. New York: Thieme; 2005. Illustration by Karl Wesker.)

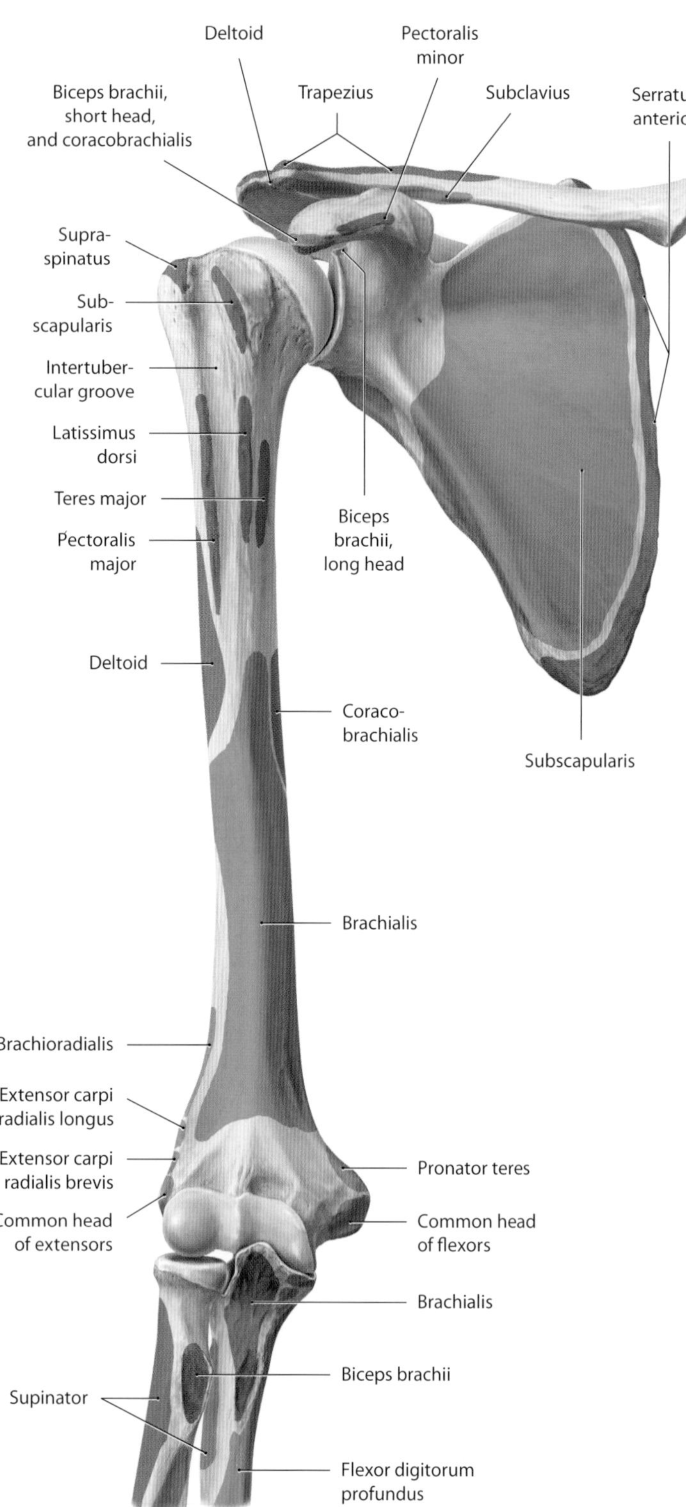

Fig. 7.20 Muscles of the right shoulder and right arm from the anterior view. All the muscles have been removed. (From Schuenke M, Schulte E. General Anatomy and the Musculoskeletal System: Thieme Atlas of Anatomy. New York: Thieme; 2005. Illustration by Karl Wesker.)

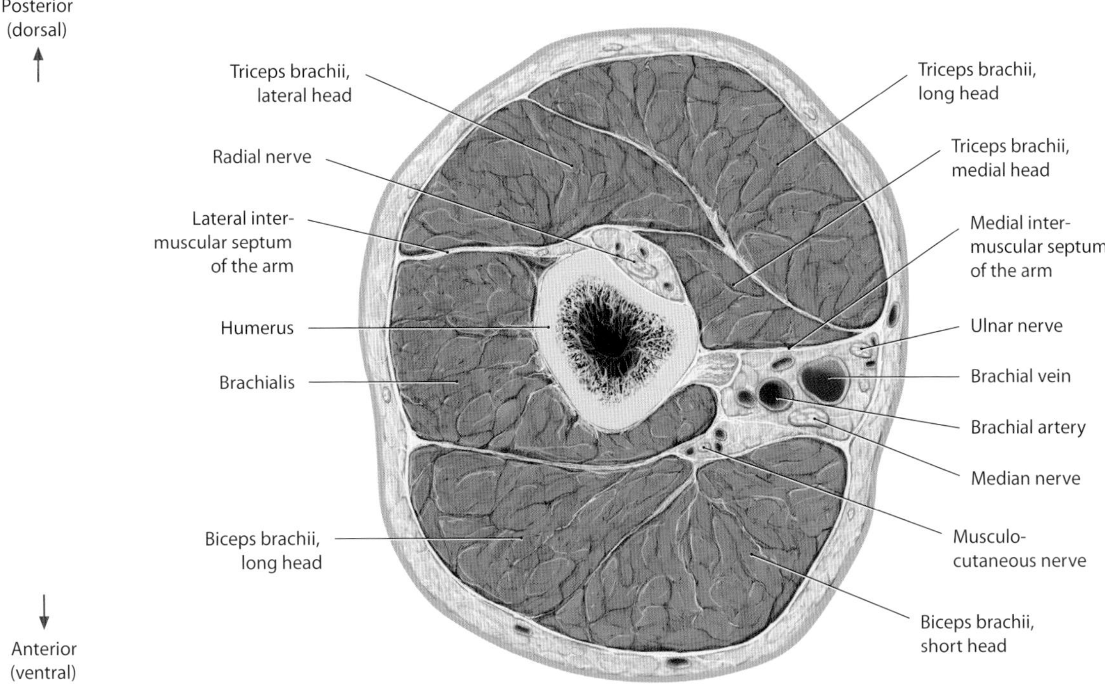

Fig. 7.21 Surgical approaches to humerus. (From Schuenke M, Schulte E. General Anatomy and the Musculoskeletal System: Thieme Atlas of Anatomy. New York: Thieme; 2005. Illustration by Karl Wesker.)

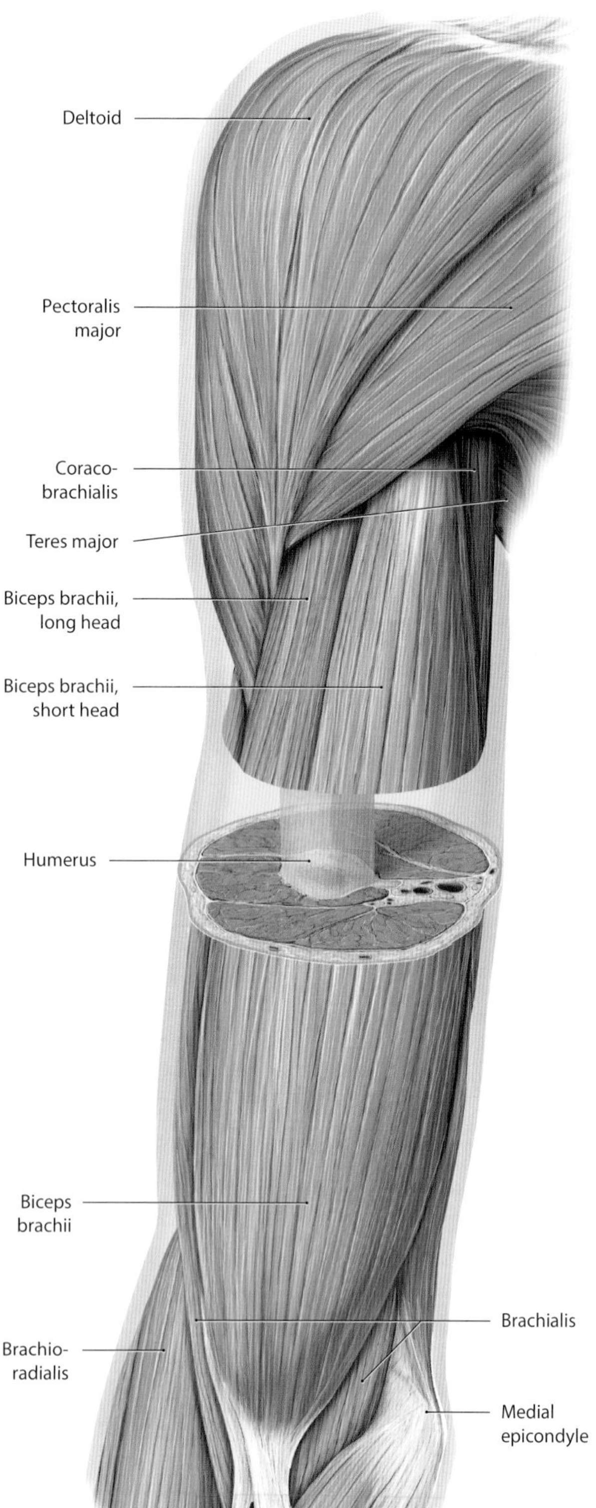

Fig. 7.22 "Windowed" dissection of the right arm. Anterior (ventral) view. (From Schuenke M, Schulte E. General Anatomy and the Musculoskeletal System: Thieme Atlas of Anatomy. New York: Thieme; 2005. Illustration by Karl Wesker.)

Table 7.2 Muscles of the Shoulder/Arm

Muscle	Origin	Insertion	Action	Innervation
Trapezius	Spinous process C7–T12	Clavicle, scapula	Scapular rotation	Cranial nerve XI
Latissimus dorsi	Spinous process T6–S5, ilium	Humerus	Extend, adduct, internal rotation of humerus	Thoracodorsal
Rhomboid major	Spinous process T2–T5	Medial border scapula	Adduct scapula	Dorsal scapular
Rhomboid minor	Spinous process C7–T1	Medial scapular spine	Adduct scapula	Dorsal scapular
Levator scapulae	Transverse process C1–C4	Superior medial scapula	Elevate and rotate scapula	C3, C4
Pectoralis major	Sternum, ribs, clavicle	Humerus	Adduct, internal rotation arm	Medial and lateral pectoral nerves
Pectoralis minor	Ribs 3–5	Coracoid	Protract scapula	Medial pectoral nerve
Subclavius	First rib	Inferior clavicle	Depresses clavicle	Subclavius
Serratus anterior	Ribs 1–9	Ventral medial scapula	Prevents scapular winging	Long thoracic
Deltoid	Lateral clavicle, scapula	Humerus	Abducts arm	Axillary
Teres major	Inferior scapula	Humerus	Adduct, internally rotate, extend arm	Lower subscapular
Teres minor	Dorsolateral scapula	Greater tuberosity	External rotation	Axillary
Subscapularis	Ventral scapula	Lesser tuberosity	Internal rotation	Upper and lower subscapular
Supraspinatus	Supraspinatus fossa of scapula	Greater tuberosity	Abduction, external rotation	Suprascapular
Infraspinatus	Infraspinatus fossa of scapula	Greater tuberosity	External rotation	Suprascapular
Coracobrachialis	Coracoid	Humerus	Flexion, adduction	Musculocutaneous
Biceps brachii	Coracoid (short head), supraglenoid tubercle (long head)	Radial tuberosity	Forearm supination, elbow flexion	Musculocutaneous
Brachialis	Humerus	Proximal ulna	Flex elbow	Musculocutaneous and radial
Triceps brachii	Infraglenoid tubercle (long head), posterior humerus (lateral and medial heads)	Olecranon	Extend elbow	Radial

3. Spaces/intervals **(Fig. 7.23)**
   - **Quadrangular space: teres minor (superior), teres major (inferior), long head of triceps (medial), humerus (lateral); contains axillary nerve and posterior circumflex humeral vessels**
   - **Triangular space: teres minor (superior), teres major (inferior), long head of triceps (lateral); contains circumflex scapular vessels**
   - **Posterior approach to the scapula is through the interval between infraspinatus and teres minor to avoid the triangular space**
   - Triangular interval: teres major (superior), long head of triceps (medial), lateral head of triceps/humerus (lateral); contains radial nerve and profunda brachii artery
   - Rotator interval: coracoid base (medial), supraspinatus (superior), subscapularis (inferior); contains coracohumeral ligament, superior glenohumeral ligament, biceps tendon, glenohumeral capsule

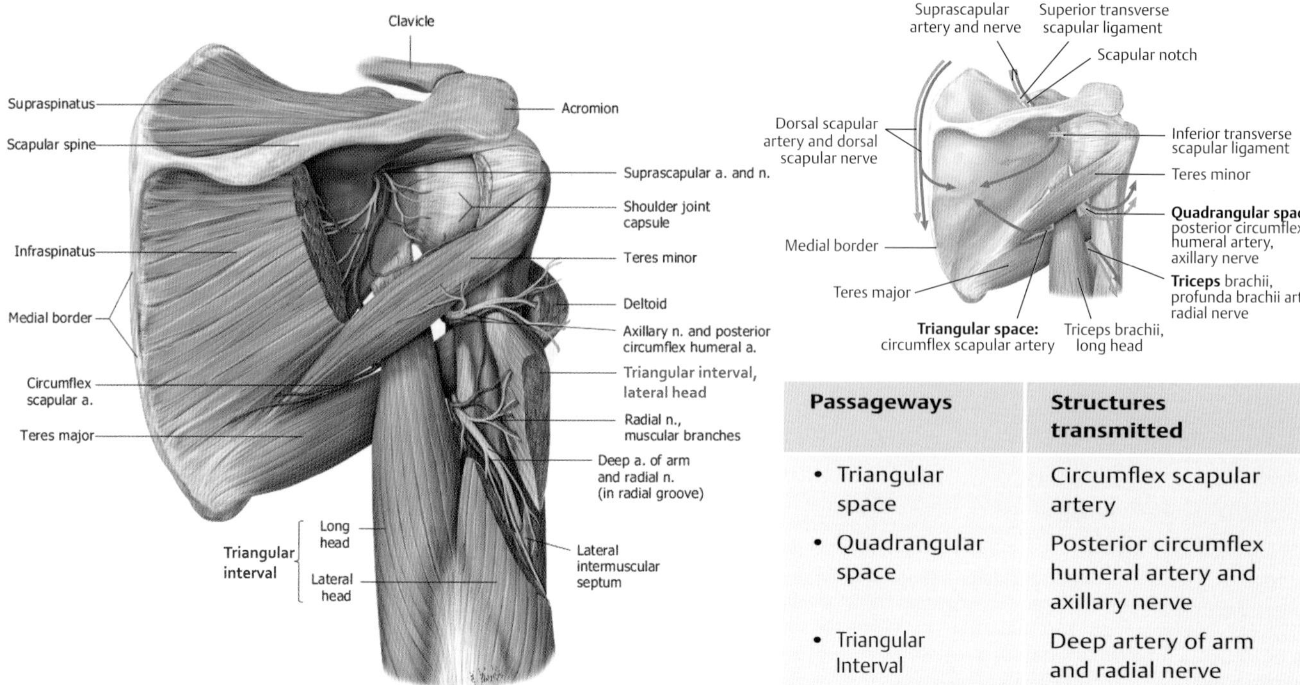

Passageways	Structures transmitted
• Triangular space	Circumflex scapular artery
• Quadrangular space	Posterior circumflex humeral artery and axillary nerve
• Triangular Interval	Deep artery of arm and radial nerve

Fig. 7.23 Posterior shoulder spaces and intervals. (Modified from Schuenke M, Schulte E. General Anatomy and the Musculoskeletal System: Thieme Atlas of Anatomy. New York: Thieme; 2005. Illustration by Karl Wesker.)

4. Nerves (also see Chapter 9) **(Figs. 7.24, 7.25, 7.26, 7.27, Table 7.3)**
   - Understanding anatomic relationships helps determine level of injury to brachial plexus; exits neck with subclavian artery between anterior and middle scalene muscles (interscalene groove)
   - Organized into roots (C5-T1), trunks, divisions, cords, and nerves; upper two roots (C5–C6) join to form the upper trunk at Erb's point, located 2–3 cm above the clavicle, just behind posterior edge of the sternocleidomastoid; divisions split above the clavicle; cords are named according to their relationship to the axillary artery
   - Supraclavicular branches: dorsal scapular, long thoracic, suprascapular, nerve to subclavius
   - Specific anatomic consideration **(Fig. 7.28)**
     a. Musculocutaneous: pierces coracobrachialis 2–8 cm (mean 5 cm) distal to coracoid
     b. Axillary: travels underneath deltoid 5 cm inferior to lateral edge of acromion
     c. Suprascapular nerve (passes through suprascapular notch): motor branches to supraspinatus located 3 cm from origin of long head of biceps, and motor branches to infraspinatus located 2 cm from superior glenoid rim
        - Infraspinatus branch passes in spinoglenoid notch and can be compressed by spinoglenoid notch cyst from posterior superior labral tear.
        - **Compression at suprascapular notch will weaken supraspinatus and infraspinatus; compression at spinoglenoid notch will only weaken infraspinatus.**
     d. Radial: in spiral groove 13 cm proximal to trochlea, pierces lateral intermuscular septum 7–10 cm proximal to trochlea
     e. Ulnar: medial to brachial artery in the arm
     f. Median: crosses brachial artery lateral to medial

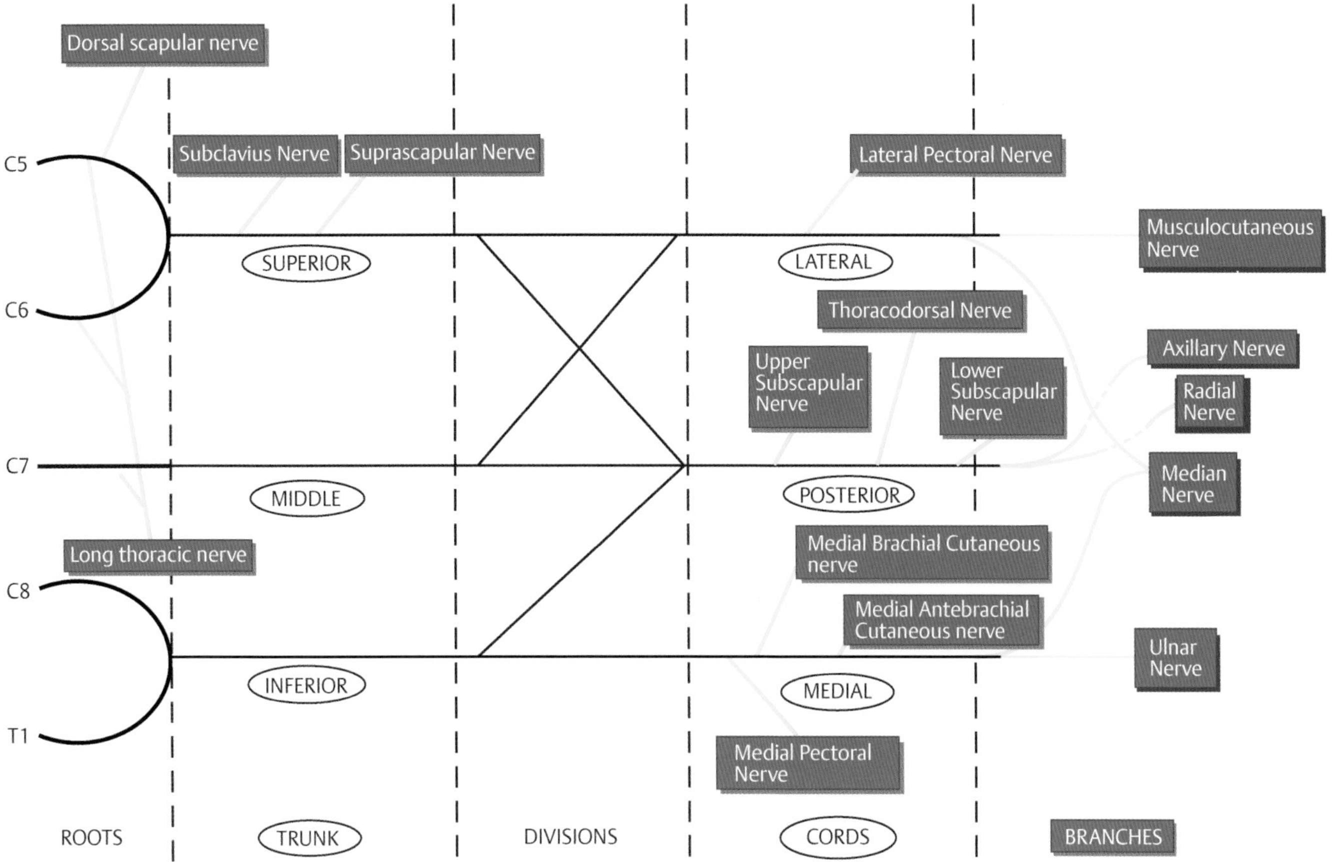

Fig. 7.24 Linear diagram of brachial plexus and branches.

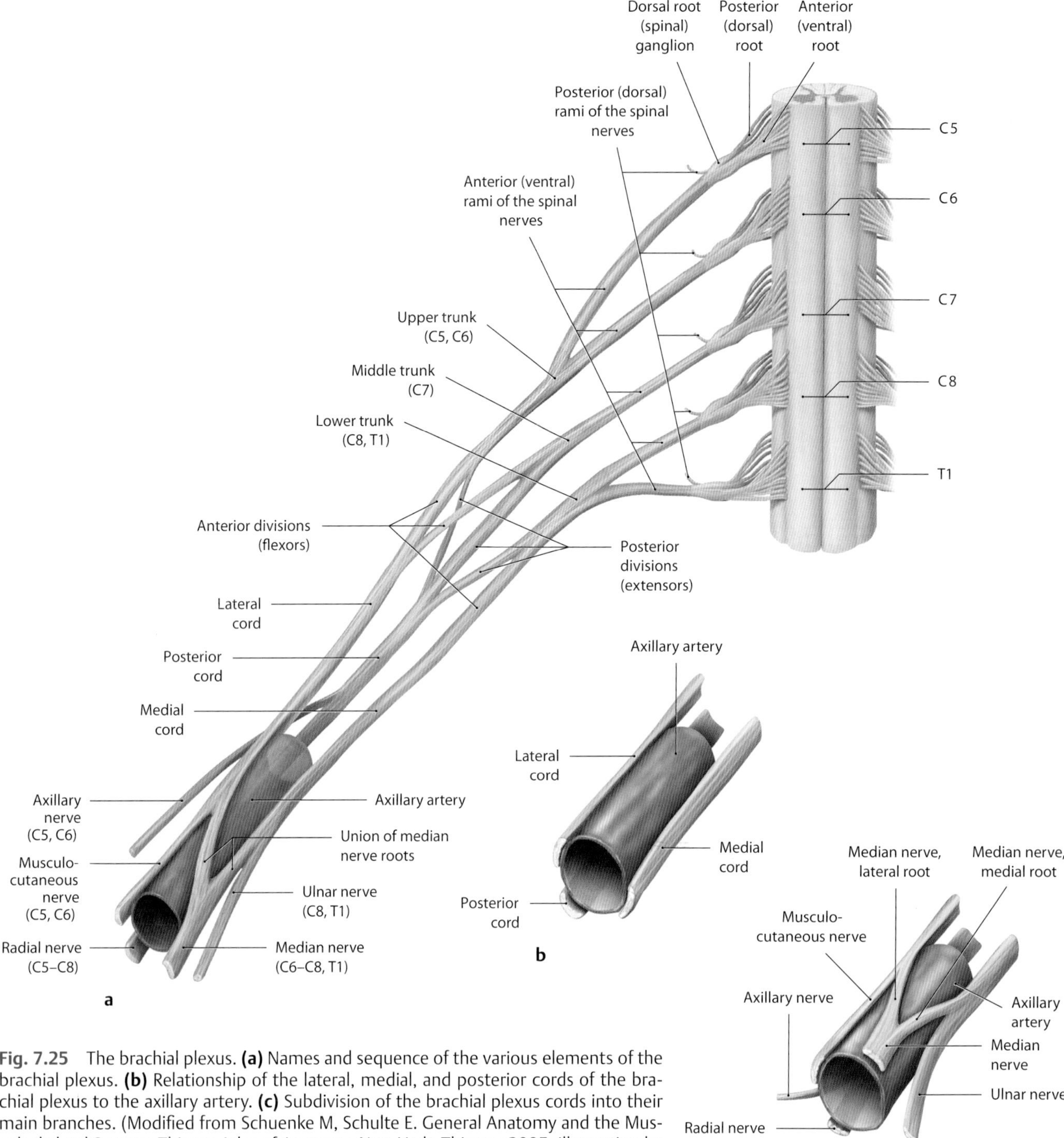

Fig. 7.25 The brachial plexus. **(a)** Names and sequence of the various elements of the brachial plexus. **(b)** Relationship of the lateral, medial, and posterior cords of the brachial plexus to the axillary artery. **(c)** Subdivision of the brachial plexus cords into their main branches. (Modified from Schuenke M, Schulte E. General Anatomy and the Musculoskeletal System: Thieme Atlas of Anatomy. New York: Thieme; 2005. Illustration by Karl Wesker.)

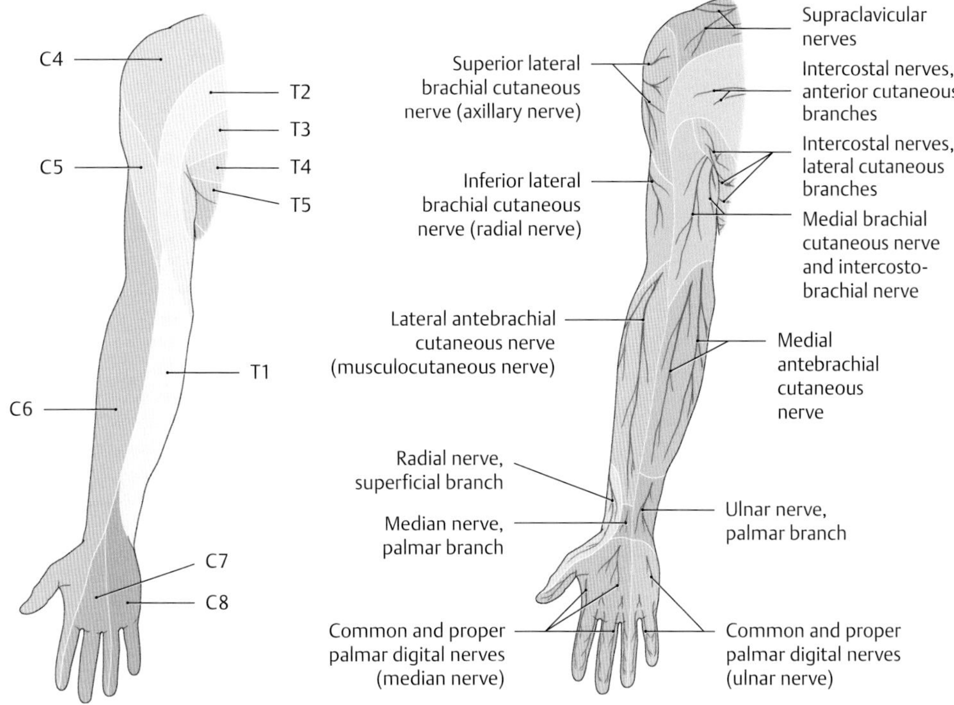

Fig. 7.26 Cutaneous innervation of the upper extremity. (From Schuenke M, Schulte E. General Anatomy and the Musculoskeletal System: Thieme Atlas of Anatomy. New York: Thieme; 2005. Illustration by Karl Wesker.)

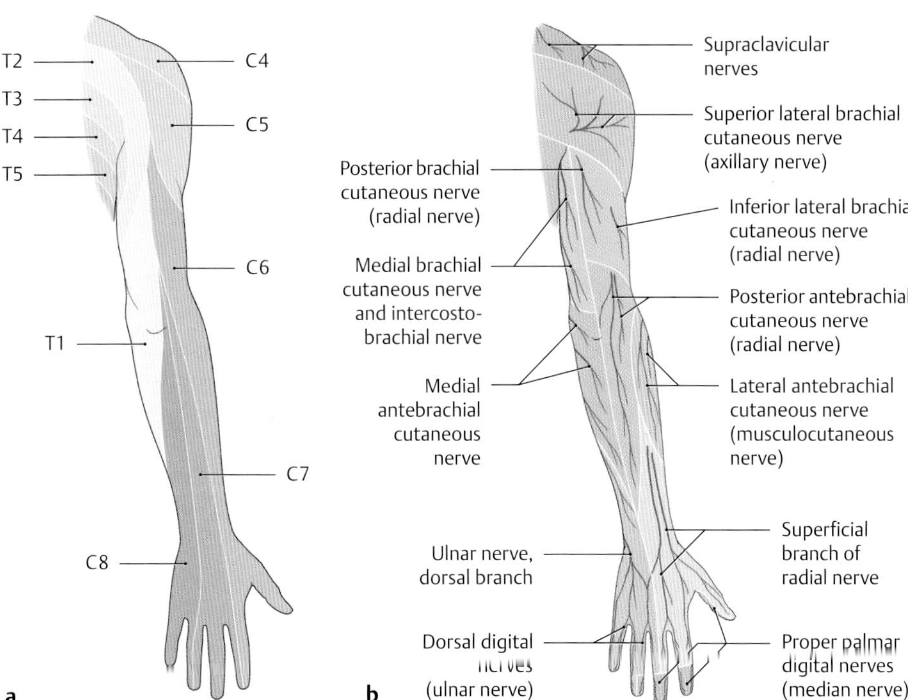

Fig. 7.27 **(a)** Segmental, radicular cutaneous innervation pattern (dermatomes) in the right upper limb. Posterior view. **(b)** Peripheral sensory cutaneous innervation pattern in the right upper limb. Posterior view. (From Schuenke M, Schulte E. General Anatomy and the Musculoskeletal System: Thieme Atlas of Anatomy. New York: Thieme; 2005. Illustration by Karl Wesker.)

Table 7.3 Number and Location of the Main Components of the Brachial Plexus

Components	Number	Location
1. Plexus roots (anterior rami of the spinal nerves from cord segments C5–T1)	5	Between scalenus anterior and scalenus medius (interscalene space)
2. The primary trunks: upper, middle, and lower	3	Lateral to the interscalene space and above the clavicle
3. The three anterior and three posterior divisions	6	Posterior to the clavicle
4. The lateral, medial, and posterior cords	3	In the axilla, posterior to pectoralis minor

Source: From Schuenke M, Schulte E. General Anatomy and the Musculoskeletal System: Thieme Atlas of Anatomy. New York: Thieme; 2005:314. Reprinted with permission.

5. Vessels **(Figs. 7.29** and **7.30)**
   - Subclavian artery: left subclavian arises from aorta, right from brachiocephalic trunk
   - Axillary artery: three parts based on relationship with pectoralis minor
     a. First part: medial to pectoralis minor; one branch (supreme thoracic)
     b. Second part: under pectoralis minor; two branches (thoracoacromial, lateral thoracic)
     c. Third part: lateral to pectoralis minor; three branches (subscapular, anterior humeral circumflex, posterior humeral circumflex)
        - Posterior humeral circumflex: dominant supply to humeral head ~ 60%), supplies posterior aspect of greater tuberosity, small area of posteroinferior humeral head
        - Anterior humeral circumflex artery supplies humeral head via anterolateral ascending branch
6. Surgical approaches to shoulder
   - Anterior deltopectoral (Henry approach) **(Fig. 7.31)**
     a. Interval: deltoid (axillary nerve) and pectoralis major (medial and lateral pectoral nerves)
        - Find cephalic vein and protect
     b. Structures at risk: axillary nerve (medial inferior to subscapularis muscle and lateral under deltoid, musculocutaneous nerve with dissection medial to or excessive medial retraction on coracobrachialis)
     c. Extensile approach: shoulder arthroplasty, anterior instability repair, open reduction and internal fixation (ORIF) proximal humerus
   - Lateral deltoid splitting
     a. Interval: deltoid splitting; between anterior and middle deltoid versus middle deltoid
     b. Structures at risk: axillary nerve (avoid deltoid split more than 5 cm inferior to lateral edge of acromion)
     c. Open rotator cuff repair; ORIF greater tuberosity; extended approach for ORIF proximal humerus
   - Posterior **(Fig. 7.32)**
     a. Interval: infraspinatus (suprascapular nerve) and teres minor (axillary nerve); also may split infraspinatus transversely rather than true internervous interval
     b. Structures at risk: quadrangular space structures (axillary nerve and posterior circumflex vessels) with dissection inferior to teres minor, suprascapular nerve with excess medial retraction
     c. Posterior instability repair, ORIF posterior glenoid/scapula

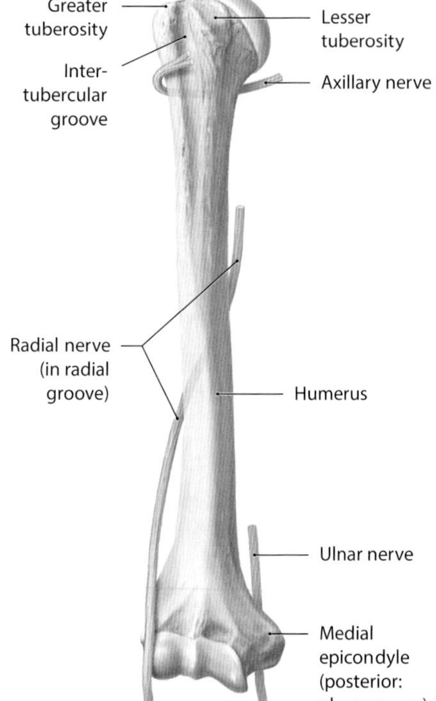

Fig. 7.28 Nerves that are closely related to the humerus. Right humerus, anterior view (From Schuenke M, Schulte E. General Anatomy and the Musculoskeletal System: Thieme Atlas of Anatomy. New York: Thieme; 2005. Illustration by Karl Wesker.)

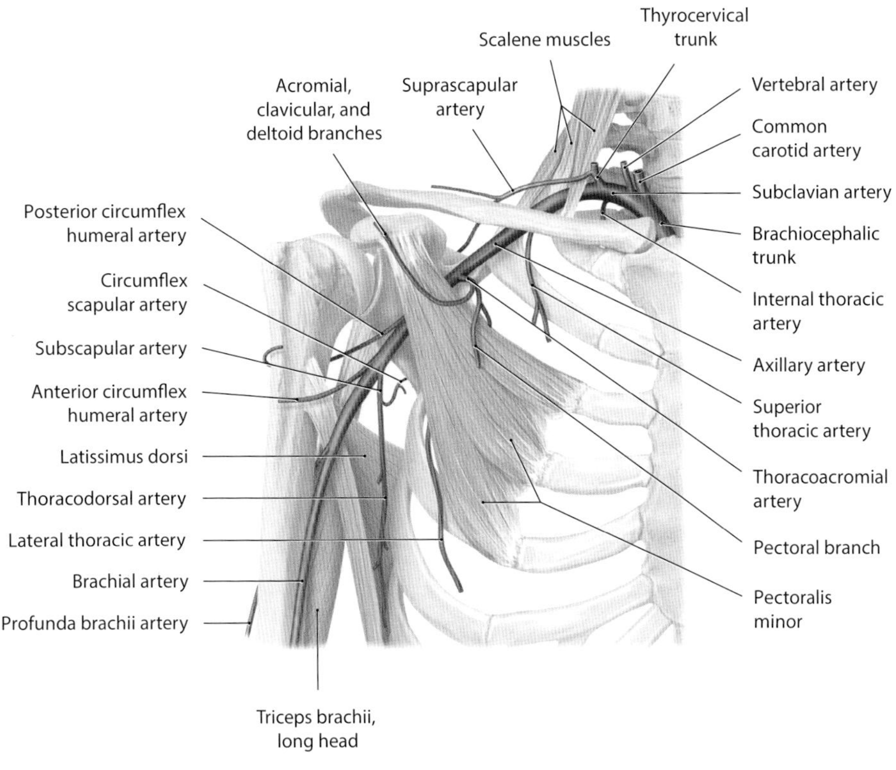

Fig. 7.29 Origin and branches of axillary artery. Right shoulder, anterior view. (From Schuenke M, Schulte E. General Anatomy and the Musculoskeletal System: Thieme Atlas of Anatomy. New York: Thieme; 2005. Illustration by Karl Wesker.)

- Arthroscopy **(Fig. 7.33)**
  a. Posterior portal: primary viewing portal into glenohumeral joint; 1 cm medial and 2 cm inferior to posterolateral border of acromion; axillary and suprascapular nerves potentially at risk
  b. Anterior superior portal: risks injury to musculocutaneous nerve
  c. Anterior inferior portal: do not go below subscapularis (risks axillary nerve and musculocutaneous nerve) or medial to conjoined tendon
  d. Lateral portal: 1–3 cm distal to lateral edge of acromion
  e. Inferior portals (anterior and posterior): risk injury to axillary nerve
  f. Supraspinatus (Neviaser portal): risks suprascapular nerve if portal placement is too medial

7. Surgical approaches to humerus
   - Proximal anterior/anterolateral

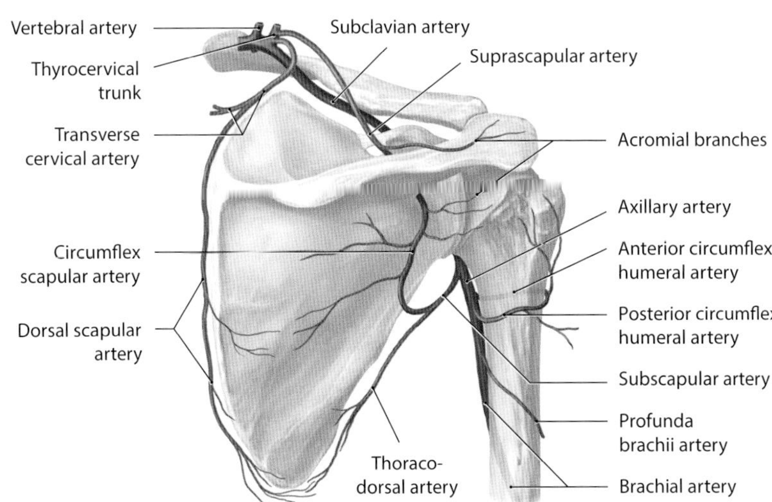

Fig. 7.30 Arterial supply to the scapular region. Right shoulder, posterior view. (From Schuenke M, Schulte E. General Anatomy and the Musculoskeletal System: Thieme Atlas of Anatomy. New York: Thieme; 2005. Illustration by Karl Wesker.)

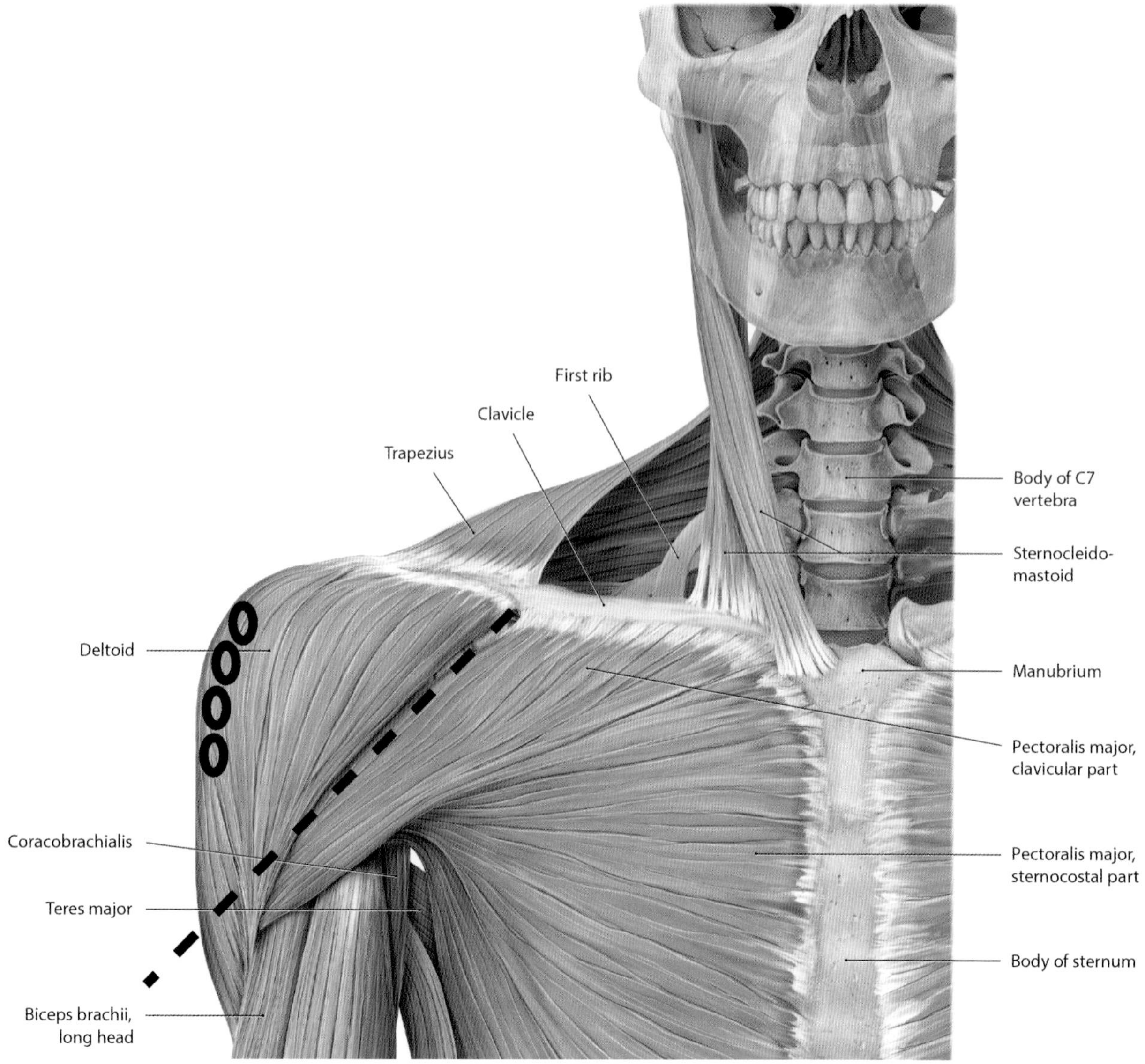

First rib
Clavicle
Trapezius
Body of C7 vertebra
Sternocleido-mastoid
Deltoid
Manubrium
Pectoralis major, clavicular part
Coracobrachialis
Pectoralis major, sternocostal part
Teres major
Body of sternum
Biceps brachii, long head

Fig. 7.31 Surgical approach to shoulder. *Dashed line*, deltopectoral; *line of circles*, deltoid split. (From Schuenke M, Schulte E. General Anatomy and the Musculoskeletal System: Thieme Atlas of Anatomy. New York: Thieme; 2005. Illustration by Karl Wesker.)

Rhomboid minor
Levator scapulae
Supra-spinatus
Trapezius
Deltoid, clavicular part
Deltoid, acromial part
Deltoid, spinal part
Teres minor
Infra-spinatus

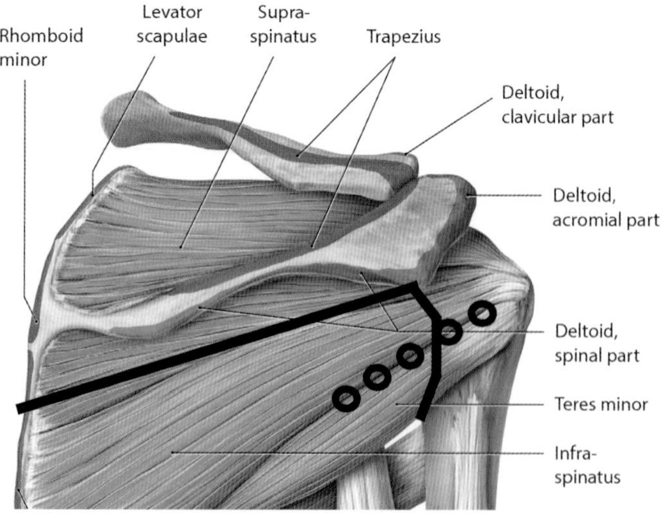

Fig. 7.32 Posterior approach to shoulder. *Solid line*, skin incision; *line of circles*, internervous plane. (From Schuenke M, Schulte E. General Anatomy and the Musculoskeletal System: Thieme Atlas of Anatomy. New York: Thieme; 2005. Illustration by Karl Wesker.)

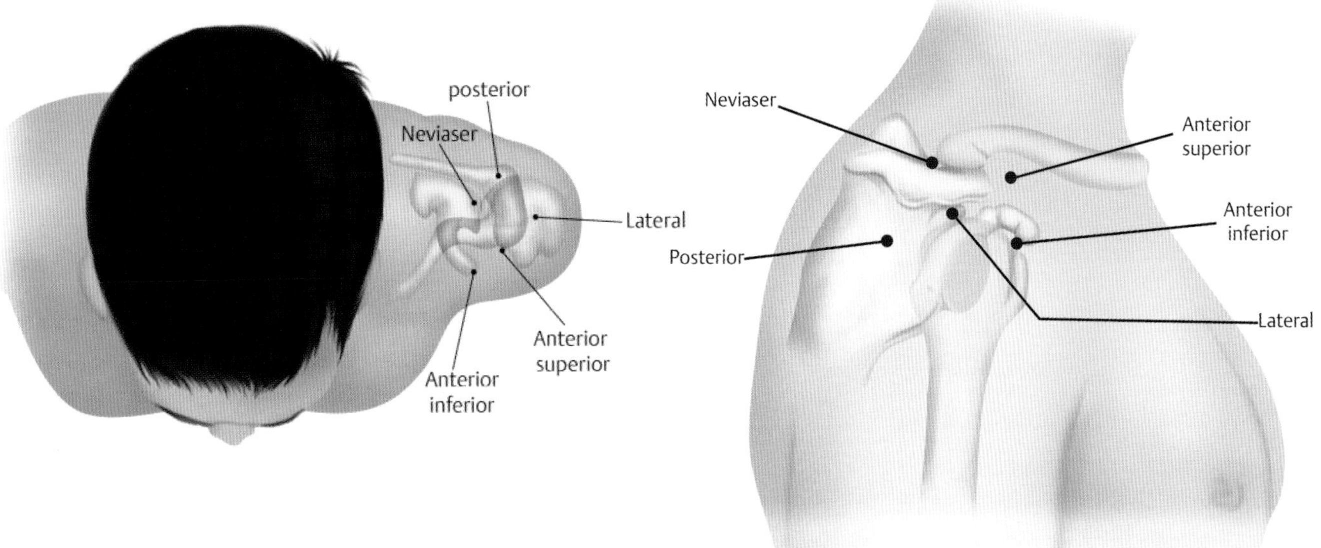

Fig. 7.33 Arthroscopic portals of the shoulder.

a. Interval: deltoid (axillary nerve) and pectoralis major (medial and lateral pectoral nerves) proximally
b. Structures at risk: axillary nerve, radial nerve, anterior circumflex humeral artery

- Distal anterolateral **(Fig. 7.34)**
  a. Interval: brachialis (radial and musculocutaneous nerves) and biceps (musculocutaneous nerve), or brachialis splitting (radial and musculocutaneous nerves); retract biceps medially
  b. Structure at risk: radial nerve
- Posterolateral
  a. Interval: triceps and brachioradialis (both radial nerve)
  b. Structure at risk: radial nerve at proximal extent
- Posterior
  a. Interval: lateral and long heads of triceps (radial nerve)
  b. Structures at risk: radial nerve and profunda brachii artery; can split triceps 15–16 cm proximal to lateral epicondyle (radial nerve crosses humerus at this point)

8. Surgical approaches to elbow
   - Posterior **(Fig. 7.35)**
     a. Approaches
        - Detach triceps: detach from olecranon with a thin wafer of bone
        - Olecranon osteotomy: apex-distal chevron osteotomy; reflect triceps tendon with osteotomized portion of olecranon
        - Triceps reflecting (Bryan-Morrey approach): triceps and anconeus elevated as one flap from medial to lateral
        - TRAP (triceps reflecting anconeus pedicle): extensile exposure that maintains triceps and anconeus continuity to protect neurovascular pedicle to anconeus; medial interval is along triceps proximally and between anconeus and flexor carpi ulnaris distally; lateral interval is between anconeus and extensor carpi ulnaris
        - Triceps on: attachment of triceps to proximal ulna is maintained
        - Triceps split: midline longitudinal incision through triceps fascia and tendon, split muscle and tendon longitudinally

     b. Structures at risk: ulnar nerve, radial nerve

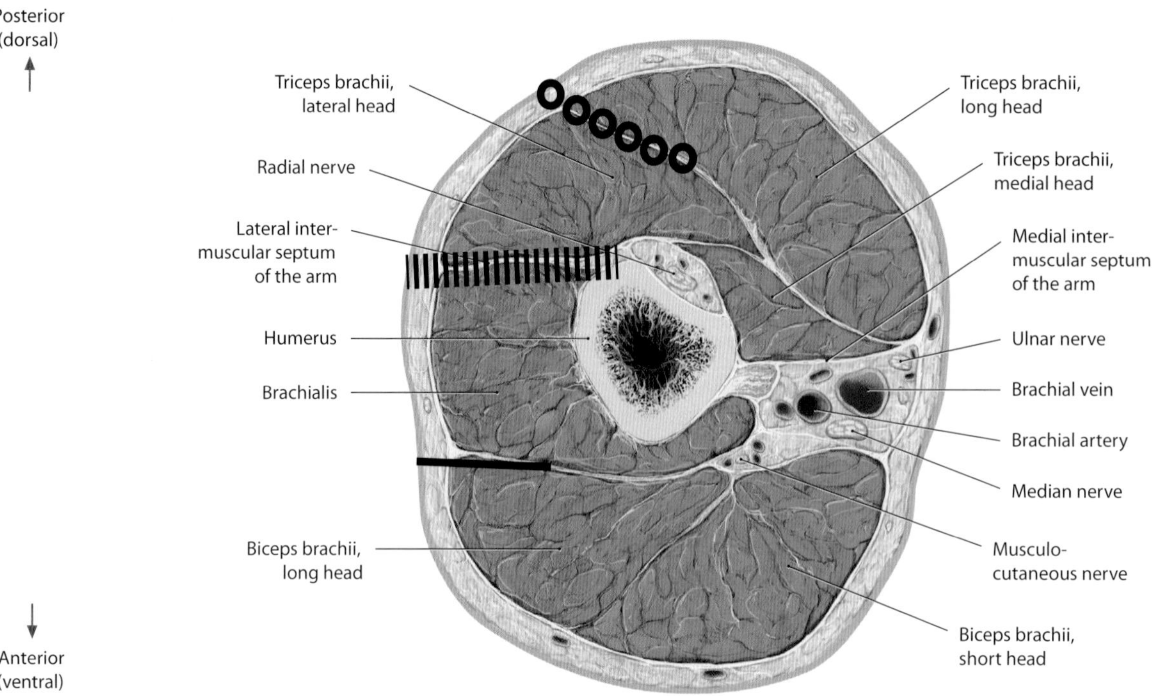

Fig. 7.34 Surgical approaches to humerus. *Solid line*, distal anterolateral; *hash line*, posterolateral; *line of circles*, posterior. (Modified from Schuenke M, Schulte E. General Anatomy and the Musculoskeletal System: Thieme Atlas of Anatomy. New York: Thieme; 2005. Illustration by Karl Wesker.)

- Medial **(Fig. 7.36)**
  a. Interval: brachialis (radial and musculocutaneous nerves) and triceps (radial nerve) proximally, brachialis and pronator teres (median nerve) distally
  b. Structures at risk: ulnar and medial antebrachial cutaneous nerves
- Medial splitting: split common flexor muscle bundle; used for ulnar collateral ligament reconstruction, coronoid fractures
- Lateral extensor splitting: between extensor digitorum communis and extensor carpi radialis brevis and longus superficially; deep dissection splits annular ligament anterior to lateral ulnar collateral ligament; approaches to capitellar, lateral condyle, and radial head fractures, as well as contracture releases
- Anterolateral (Henry approach)
  a. Interval: brachialis splitting proximally, pronator teres (median nerve) and brachioradialis (radial nerve) distally
  b. Structures at risk: lateral antebrachial cutaneous nerve, brachial artery, median nerve; may need to ligate radial recurrent artery
- Posterolateral (Kocher approach) **(Fig. 7.37)**
  a. Interval: anconeus (radial) and extensor carpi ulnaris [posterior interosseous nerve (PIN)]
  b. Structures at risk: PIN (pronate arm to move nerve anterior and radial to protect it)
- Arthroscopy
  a. Portals **(Fig. 7.38)**
    - Anterolateral: 1 cm distal and 1 cm anterior to lateral epicondyle; placed after joint distention; risks radial and lateral antebrachial cutaneous nerves
    - Proximal anteromedial: 2 cm distal and 2 cm anterior to epicondyle; risks medial antebrachial cutaneous and median nerves

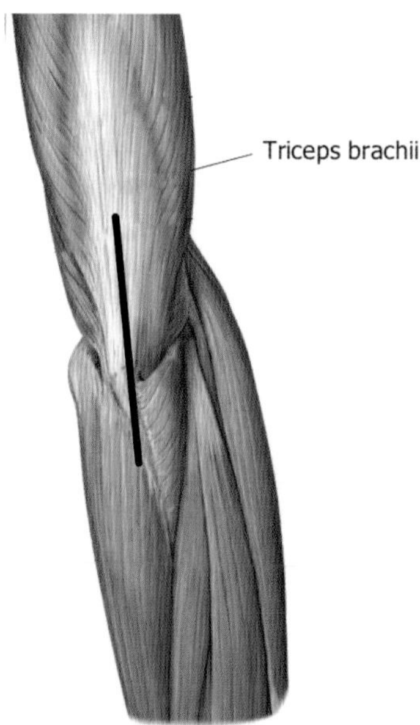

Fig. 7.35 Posterior approach to elbow. *Solid line*, skin incision. (Modified from Schuenke M, Schulte E. General Anatomy and the Musculoskeletal System: Thieme Atlas of Anatomy. New York: Thieme; 2005. Illustration by Karl Wesker.)

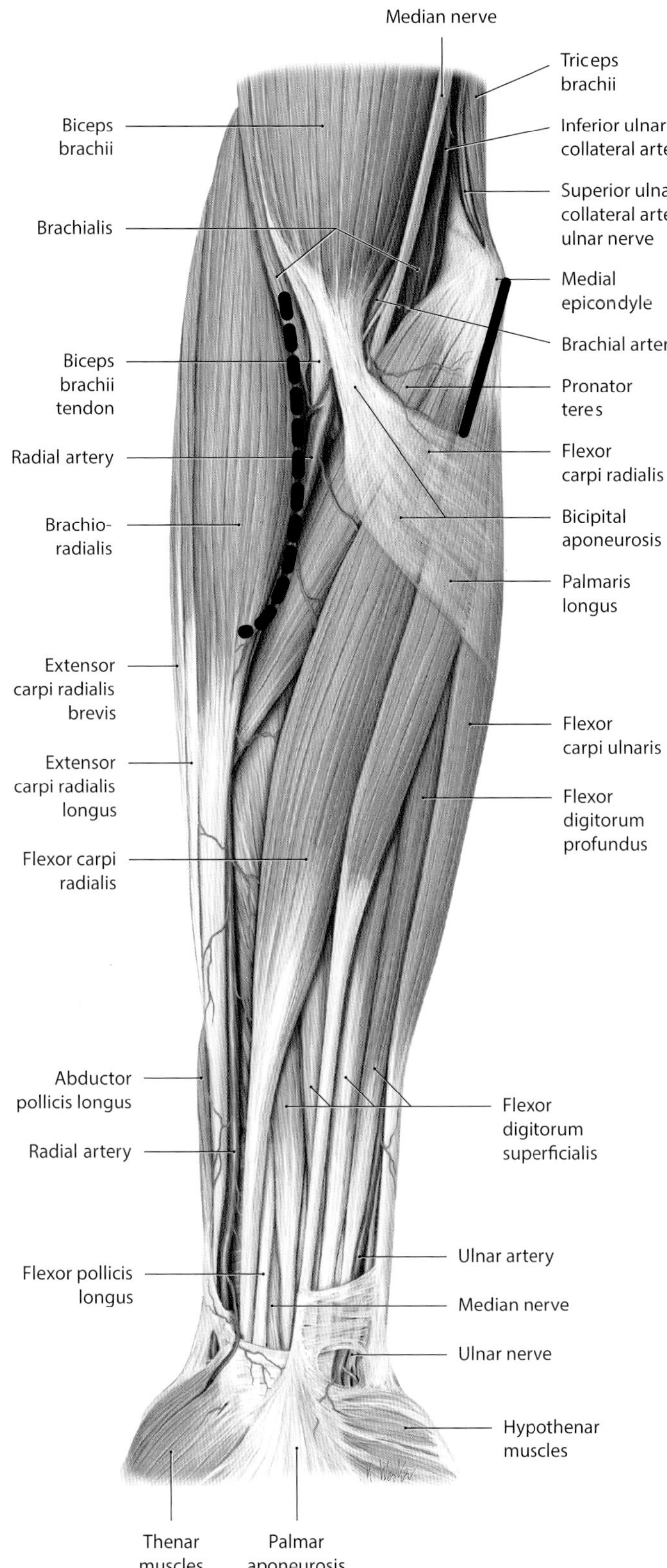

Fig. 7.36 Surgical approach to elbow. *Solid line*, medial; *dotted line*, anterolateral. (From Schuenke M, Schulte E. General Anatomy and the Musculoskeletal System: Thieme Atlas of Anatomy. New York: Thieme; 2005. Illustration by Karl Wesker.)

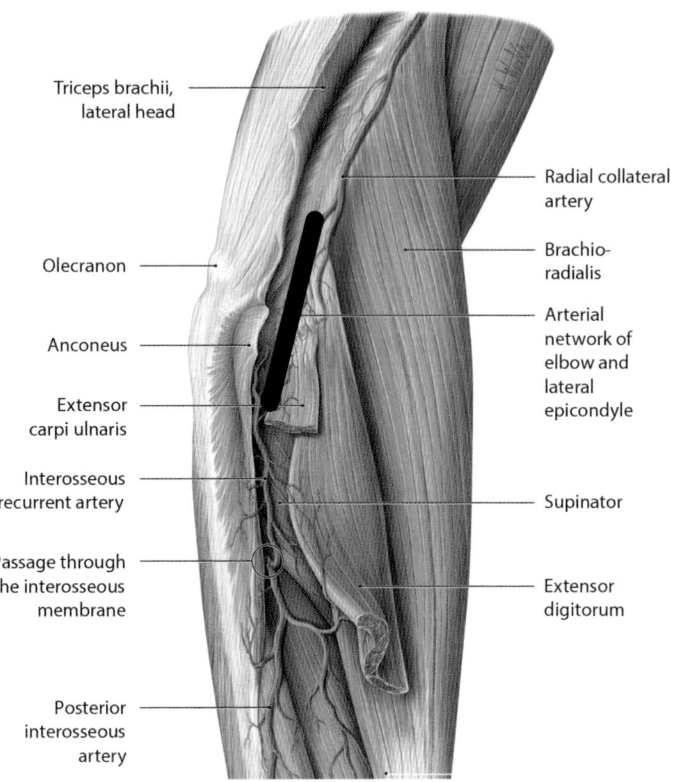

Fig. 7.37 Posterolateral approach to elbow. *Thick line*, interval. (From Schuenke M, Schulte E. General Anatomy and the Musculoskeletal System: Thieme Atlas of Anatomy. New York: Thieme; 2005. Illustration by Karl Wesker.)

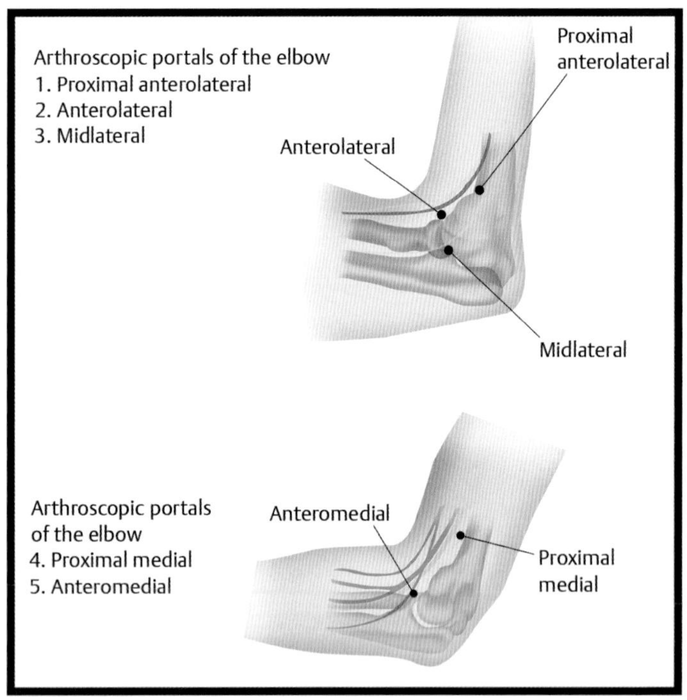

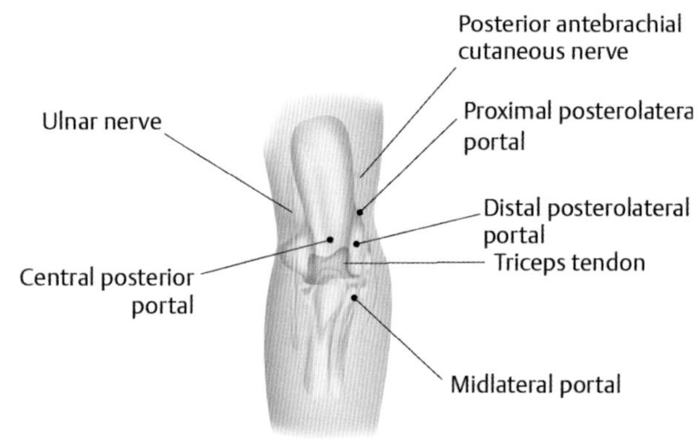

Fig. 7.38 Arthroscopic portals of the elbow.

- Lateral: through anconeus
- Posterior: 2–3 cm proximal to olecranon
- Posterolateral: 2–3 cm proximal to olecranon, lateral to triceps tendon
- Posteromedial: least safe; risks ulnar nerve; not recommended for use

b. Complications: most common nerve injury is transient ulnar nerve palsy

- Some consider ulnar neuropathy and a history of prior ulnar nerve transposition as contraindications to arthroscopy; alternatively, can find and protect nerve
- Posterior and posterolateral portals are safest for evaluation of posterior elbow

II. Shoulder Conditions

1. Physical examination **(Table 7.4)**
2. Radiographic views of shoulder
   - True AP (Grashey view): X-ray beam perpendicular to scapula; parallel to glenohumeral joint
   - 45-degree abduction true AP: glenohumeral joint space
   - Axillary lateral: arm abducted 70–90 degrees, beam directed at axilla; dislocation/subluxation, arthritis of glenohumeral joint
   - Outlet (y-view): patient stands with affected side rotated toward cassette; acromial morphology
   - Zanca: 10-degree cephalic tilt; acromioclavicular (AC) joint
   - Serendipity: 10-degree cephalic tilt; sternoclavicular (SC) joint
   - West Point: X-ray beam aimed 25 degrees medially from midline (toward axilla) and 25 degrees anterior of a prone patient; evaluate Bankart lesions
   - Stryker notch: X-ray beam 10 degrees cephalad of supine patient with shoulder forward elevated 120 degrees; evaluate Hill-Sachs defects
3. Shoulder instability: glenohumeral joint most commonly dislocated major joint in body
   - Traumatic glenohumeral dislocation

     a. Anterior

     - Mechanism: shoulder dislocation with arm abducted and externally rotated; direct blow to posterior shoulder
     - Clinical presentation: pain, limited internal rotation with anterior dislocation
     - Associated pathology
       - ♦ Bankart lesion: anterior labral tear; detachment of anteroinferior labrum and middle and inferior glenohumeral ligaments; most common finding during surgery for traumatic anterior shoulder dislocation in patients of ages < 40 years
         - Bony Bankart: anteroinferior glenoid rim fracture very common in younger patients
         - Labral injury variations
       - ♦ Perthes lesion: nondisplaced labral tear with intact medial scapular periosteum
       - ♦ ALPSA (anterior labroligamentous periosteal sleeve avulsion) lesion
       - ♦ Glenolabral articular disruption: labral tear extending into articular cartilage
       - ♦ Hill-Sachs defect: chondral impaction injury in posterosuperior humeral head, occurs with anterior dislocation

Table 7.4 Shoulder Exam Tests

Test Name	Technique	Associated Pathology
Neer impingement sign	Anterior superior shoulder pain with full passive forward elevation impingement	Impingement
Hawkins	Pain with passive forward flexion > 90 degrees in internal rotation	Impingement
Jobe	Pain with resisted elevation at 90 degrees with shoulder internally rotated and forearm pronated	Supraspinatus lesion
Drop-arm	Inability to maintain forward flexion in scapular plane	Large rotator cuff tear
Hornblower	Inability to actively externally rotate the arm in 90-degree abduction position	Massive posterior superior rotator cuff tear (supraspinatus, infraspinatus, possibly teres minor)
Liftoff	Inability to elevate hand off lower back or against resistance	Subscapularis injury
Belly press	Inability to keep hand on stomach against resistance	Subscapularis injury
Anterior apprehension	Pain/apprehension with abduction of 90 degrees and external rotation	Anterior instability
Relocation	Relief of pain/apprehension when applying posterior force during apprehension test	Anterior instability
Load and shift	Increased translation with anterior/posterior force on humeral head	Instability
Modified load and shift	Load and shift performed in supine position with elbow bent	Instability
Jerk	Clunk with posterior force on forward flexed/adducted arm and internally rotated (similar to Ortolani/Barlow),	Posterior glenohumeral instability
Sulcus	Increased acromiohumeral distance with inferior force on arm at side	Inferior laxity
Active compression (O'Brien)	Pain with resisted on arm in slight adduction/forward flexion 90 degrees/max pronation and relieved with supination/external rotation, pain located deep	SLAP lesion; AC pathology, rotator cuff pathology
Anterior slide	Pain with resistance with hand on hip	SLAP lesion
Crank	Pain with humeral loading and rotation in full abduction	SLAP lesion
Speed	Pain with resisted forward flexion in scapular plane	Biceps tendonitis
Yergason	Pain with resisted supination	Biceps tendinitis
Kim	Downward and posterior force on abducted shoulder while elevating shoulder	Posteroinferior labral lesion
Spurling	Pain/radicular symptoms with cervical spine lateral bending/extension/cervical loading	Cervical spine disease; use to differentiate shoulder pathology from cervical spine pathology
Wright	Loss of pulse/neurovascular symptoms with extension/abduction/external rotation of arm with neck rotated away	Thoracic outlet syndrome
Adson	Rotate head to ipsilateral side, extend neck, deep inspiration	Loss of radial pulse indicates thoracic outlet syndrome

Abbreviations: AC, acromioclavicular; SLAP, superior labral anteroposterior.

- ♦ Rotator cuff tear: more common in patients of ages > 40 years
  - ▪ Posterior superior: supraspinatus/infraspinatus
  - ▪ Anterior: subscapularis
- ♦ HAGL (humeral avulsion of inferior glenohumeral ligament) lesion: can contribute to recurrent instability; associated with subscapularis tears
- ♦ Axillary nerve injury: most common nerve injury with anterior glenohumeral dislocation

◦ Diagnostic evaluation

- ♦ Physical examination before and after closed reduction: assess rotator cuff strength; weakness suggests acute rotator cuff tear
- ♦ Neurovascular status
- ♦ Plain radiographs pre- and postreduction
- ♦ Rule out associated fractures of glenoid and proximal humerus.
- ♦ CT scan to evaluate bony pathology: glenoid fracture
- ♦ Magnetic resonance imaging (MRI) to evaluate for rotator cuff tear

◦ Treatment

- ♦ Closed reduction
  - ▪ Intra-articular local anesthetic, intravenous (IV) medications, conscious sedation
  - ▪ Gentle manipulative reductions
- ♦ Immobilization: simple sling versus 30-degree external rotation immobilizer; external rotation may reduce recurrence rate (controversial)
- ♦ Recurrence rate inversely correlates with age at initial dislocation/injury
- ♦ Primary repair: reduces recurrence rate in younger patients
  - ▪ Nonoperative treatment is first line for most patients
  - ▪ Acute glenoid fracture: arthroscopic or open repair

b. Posterior

◦ Mechanism of injury: posterior directed axial load; high-energy trauma, seizure, electric shock; seen in football linemen

◦ Clinical presentation: arm locked in internal rotation in posterior dislocation

◦ Associated pathology

- ♦ Posterior labral tear
  - ▪ Reverse Hill-Sachs defect: chondral impaction injury in anteromedial humeral head; occurs with posterior dislocation

◦ Diagnostic evaluation

- ♦ History of mechanism
- ♦ Physical examination: arm locked in internal rotation
- ♦ Imaging: posterior shoulder dislocations often missed
  - ▪ Humeral head overlaps glenoid rim on true AP X-ray axial imaging, plain radiographs or CT scan
  - ▪ Light bulb sign of humeral head seen with posterior dislocations; humerus internally rotated
  - ▪ Rule out associated proximal humerus fracture
  - ▪ CT to evaluate size of reverse Hill-Sachs lesion

◦ Treatment

- ♦ Closed reduction: internal rotation and traction to disengage humeral head from glenoid

    - ♦ < 20% head defect (reverse Hill-Sachs defect): reduce and treat conservatively; initial immobilization in external rotation
    - ♦ 20–40% head defect: McLaughlin procedure; lesser tuberosity transfer
    - ♦ > 40% head defect: humeral head allograft versus humeral head arthroplasty
      - ▪ Inferior: luxatio erecta: arm in full abduction with inferior dislocation

- Recurrent/chronic glenohumeral instability
  a. Pathogenesis
    - ∘ TUBS (traumatic unidirectional Bankart lesion): surgery often required
    - ∘ AMBRI (atraumatic multidirectional bilateral rehabilitation inferior) capsular shift

  b. Evaluation
    - ∘ History of mechanism of injury
      - ♦ Anterior: abduction external rotation
      - ♦ Traumatic (recurrent posterior subluxation in football linemen) versus atraumatic
      - ♦ Multidirectional: usually atraumatic; patients complain of pain more than instability
    - ∘ Physical examination
      - ♦ Provocative maneuvers
        - ▪ Anterior-load and shift, modified load and shift, anterior apprehension-relocation
        - ▪ Multidirectional sulcus sign
        - ▪ Posterior: jerk and Kim tests; load and shift
      - ♦ Grades of instability on physical exam
        - ▪ 0: normal, small amount of translation
        - ▪ 1: humeral head to glenoid rim
        - ▪ 2: humeral head over glenoid rim but spontaneously reduces
        - ▪ 3: humeral head over glenoid rim and locks
      - ♦ Sulcus sign: to test for multidirectional instability
        - ▪ Grading: acromiohumeral distance
          - 1: < 1 cm
          - 2: 1–2 cm
          - 3: > 2 cm

  c. Imaging
    - ∘ Plain X-ray: three views of shoulder (true AP, axillary lateral, scapular Y); West Point view for glenoid bone defects/bony Bankart, Stryker notch view for Hill-Sachs defect
    - ∘ MRI: MR arthrogram increases specificity of MRI in detecting labral pathology
    - ∘ CT scan/CT arthrogram: better to evaluate bony pathology
    - ∘ Glenoid bone deficit best evaluated on sagittal MRI or CT

  d. Pathological anatomy
    - ∘ Anterior
      - ♦ Anterior capsulolabral lesions
      - ♦ Glenoid rim fracture
      - ♦ Hill-Sachs
    - ∘ Multidirectional
      - ♦ Rarely labral tear; frequently hypoplastic labrum; increased capsular volume

- Generalized ligamentous laxity
- Posterior
  - Posterior labral tear in traumatic cases
  - Kim lesion: avulsion of posteroinferior labrum that is incomplete and concealed; associated with posterior and multidirectional instability

e. Nonoperative management
- Anterior: does not usually respond to rehab
- Multidirectional instability: rehab is first-line treatment; extended course, closed kinetic chain exercises
- Posterior: rehab more successful in atraumatic cases

f. Surgical management
- Anterior
  - Indications: recurrent instability (subluxation/dislocation), failure of conservative management
  - Bankart: repair of labrum, gold standard: open versus arthroscopic
  - Glenoid bone reconstruction/augmentation deficiency > 25%
    - Latarjet: transfer coracoid to anterior inferior glenoid, secured with screws, risks are nonunion, articular injury, migration, nerve injury
    - Glenoid bone graft
  - Historical procedures
    - Putti-Platt: subscapularis and anterior capsule overlapped to tighten; limits external rotation; late degenerative joint disease
    - Magnuson-Stack: transfer subscapularis lateral to the biceps groove; limits external rotation; late degenerative joint disease
    - Bristow: transfer tip of coracoid with attached tendons through subscapularis to anterior neck of scapula
  - Outcome: arthroscopic capsulolabral repair has equivalent outcomes to open Bankart repair
  - Complications
    - Open repair: overtightening; subscapularis rupture
    - Arthroscopic: overtightening; axillary nerve injury with inferior portal placement or inferior capsular suture
    - Anchor displacement
- Posterior
  - Indications: recurrent instability (subluxation/dislocation), failure of conservative management
  - Posterior Bankart: open or arthroscopic
    - Posterior labroplasty: Kim lesion after failed conservative treatment
    - Capsular shift if labrum intact of for associated multidirectional instability
    - Rotator cuff interval closure reduces posterior instability
  - Postoperative immobilization in gun-slinger position
  - Complications: axillary nerve injury with posteroinferior labral repair (nerve passes within 1 mm of inferior capsule)
- Multidirectional instability
  - Indications: persistent symptoms, failure of conservative management
  - Capsular shift: open versus arthroscopic; shift capsule superiorly; gold standard for multidirectional instability; risks overtightening
  - Closure of rotator interval
  - Thermal shrinkage no longer accepted treatment: associated with axillary nerve injury, chondrolysis, and capsular deficiency

4. Biceps tendon and superior labral anteroposterior (SLAP) pathology
   - Pathogenesis
     a. Classification of SLAP tears **(Fig. 7.39)**
        - Type I: biceps fraying, intact labral anchor
        - Type II: most common, detachment of biceps anchor
        - Type III: bucket-handle tear of superior labrum, biceps intact
        - Type IV: bucket-handle superior labral tear extends into biceps
        - Type V: anterior labral tear plus SLAP
        - Type VI: superior flap tear
        - Type VII: capsular injury plus SLAP

     b. Biceps tendinopathy: sometimes but not always associated with rotator cuff disease; can be isolated
     c. Biceps subluxation: associated with tears subscapularis tendon, coracohumeral and transverse humeral ligaments (hidden lesion)
   - Clinical Presentation
     a. SLAP: pain, biceps tenderness; positive O'Brien test and anterior slide, crank, and dynamic labral shear tests; cause of symptoms in younger patients, overhead athletes, axial load injuries
     b. Biceps tendinitis: pain, biceps tenderness, positive Speed and Yergason tests
     c. Biceps subluxation: palpable click with arm abduction/external rotation
   - Diagnostic workup
     a. MRI arthrogram: high sensitivity and specificity for labral pathology
   - Treatment: for symptomatic SLAP and/or biceps pathology
     a. SLAP
        - Patients of ages < 40: debridement for types I, III, VI; repair types II, V, VII; biceps tenodesis versus repair type IV
        - Patients of ages > 40: biceps tenodesis or tenotomy

     b. Biceps tendinitis/subluxation
        - Conservative: initial treatment; strengthening, corticosteroid injection
        - Surgical: refractory cases treated with tenotomy or tenodesis, with or without subscapularis repair in cases of subluxation
   - Rehabilitation
     a. SLAP repair: passive motion acutely postoperative to prevent stiffness, active motion in scapular plane at 4–8 weeks, strengthening last
   - Outcomes
     a. Biceps tenodesis with interference screw: strongest initial fixation, better prevents distal migration of tendon

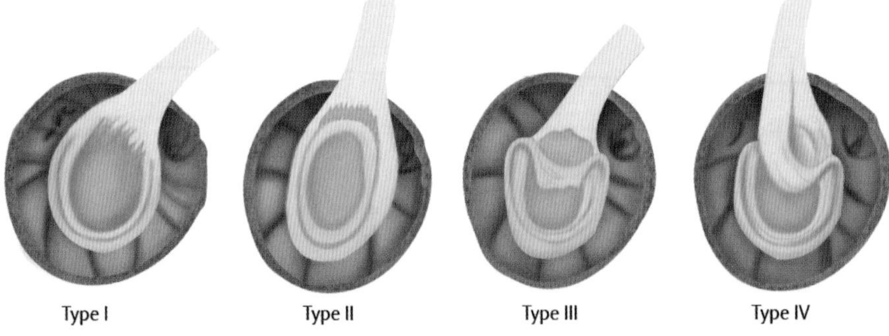

Fig. 7.39 Anterior and posterior lesion types I to IV.

b. Open versus arthroscopic tenodesis: theoretical advantage of being able to remove biceps tendon from groove (controversial as may not serve any benefit)

- Complications: tenotomy associated with "Popeye" deformity, subjective cramping, deformity after tenotomy is less than spontaneous rupture

5. Rotator cuff disease
   - Pathogenesis

a. Incidence increases with age: 30–60% of patients of ages > 70 years have full-thickness tear; of patients of ages > 60 years with rotator cuff tears, 50% have tears bilaterally, but the other side is asymptomatic 50% of the time.

b. Most tears result from degenerative processes.

c. External impingement syndrome (from acromion) contributes to bursal sided tears.

   - **External impingement of the rotator cuff causes bursal sided tears; internal impingement causes articular sided rotator cuff tears.**

d. Internal impingement syndrome (from posterosuperior rotator cuff between humerus and posterosuperior labrum) contributes to articular sided tears

e. Associated with shoulder dislocation in patients of ages > 40 years

f. Forced external rotation: traumatic subscapularis tear

g. Subcoracoid impingement: long or very lateral coracoid (less than 7 mm between coracoid and humerus is abnormal), posterior capsule tightness

- Clinical Presentation

a. Pain in the lateral shoulder; worse with overhead arm motions; night pain; weakness; difference between active and passive range of motion (rare); increased external rotation in extensive subscapularis tear

   - Elevated inflammatory markers and metalloproteinases in subacromial space may contribute to pain.

b. Positive provocative maneuvers for impingement: Neer impingement sign, Hawkins

c. Positive lag signs for cuff tear

d. Supra/infraspinatus: Jobe, drop-arm, Hornblower

e. Subscapularis: positive lift-off, modified lift-off, belly press, bear hug

- Diagnostic workup

a. X-ray: acromial spurring and ossification within coracoacromial ligament, degenerative and cystic changes in greater tuberosity, superior migration of humeral head with chronic large rotator cuff tear

b. Ultrasound

c. MRI: able to assess muscle quality atrophy and tendon retraction

   - **Subluxated biceps tendon with empty bicipital groove may be seen in the setting of a subscapularis tear.**

- Treatment

a. Conservative

   - Indications: initial treatment for most rotator cuff syndromes; impingement, chronic atraumatic tears, partial articular-sided tears
   - Modalities: physical therapy for stretching and rotator cuff strengthening and scapular stabilization, anti-inflammatories, subacromial corticosteroid injection, subcoracoid injection for subcoracoid impingement

b. Surgical

   - Subacromial decompression: failure of 4–6 months conservative treatment

- Massive irreparable tear: debridement, biceps tenotomy, greater tuberoplasty, preserve coracoacromial arch, latissimus dorsi transfer
- Rotator cuff repair: open, mini-open, arthroscopic
  - Techniques: single-row, double-row, suture bridge; double-row repair has higher ultimate tensile load than single row; combined double-row and suture bridge technique had lower re-tear rate compared with single and double row in some studies
  - Indications: chronic full-thickness rotator cuff tear, acute tears, partial-articular sided supraspinatus tendon avulsion (PASTA) tear with > 7 mm footprint bone exposed lateral to articular surface or > 50% tendon involvement; subscapularis repair with or without biceps tenodesis or tenotomy if subluxated
  - Partial rotator cuff repair can be performed for large tears, if possible.
- Latissimus dorsi transfer to greater tuberosity: indicated for irreparable supraspinatus and infraspinatus tears for active patients; subscapularis tear is a relative contraindication
- Pectoralis major transfer: chronic irreparable subscapularis tear
- Coracoid resection or arthroscopic coracoplasty: chronic subcoracoid impingement
- Arthroscopic debridement of partial articular-sided rotator cuff tear, labral repair: internal impingement

- Rehabilitation: early passive range of motion (controversial) transitioned to closed kinetic chain exercises (4–6 weeks) to stimulate safe co-contraction of scapular and rotator cuff muscles; delay strengthening to protect repair healing
- Outcomes
  a. Workers' compensation patients have worse outcomes after subacromial decompression and rotator cuff repair
  b. Subscapularis repair: better outcomes when biceps is tenodesed or tenotomized
  c. Latissimus dorsi transfer: better results if have good preoperative subscapularis and deltoid function and in men versus women; positive lift-off test most closely correlated with poor outcomes
- Complications
  a. Failure to heal: early failure due to tissue failure; increased age (> 65) is risk factor most often associated with failure to heal; larger tears, older age, increased severity of preoperative fatty degeneration of the rotator cuff muscles associated with higher re-tear rate
  b. Infection: *Propionibacterium acnes*
  c. Stiffness/loss of motion
  d. Suture anchor failure

6. Degenerative joint disease and arthroplasty
   - Pathogenesis: may be associated with shoulder instability (rare), rotator cuff disease, rheumatoid arthritis
     a. Primary osteoarthritis: etiology unknown, possible genetic factors
     b. Posttraumatic arthritis: nonunion, malunion, avascular necrosis, hardware complications
     c. Charcot arthropathy (rare): neuropathic such as result of syrinx
     d. Iatrogenic after capsule over-tightening, hardware
     e. Chondrolysis after thermal capsulorraphy or intra-articular local anesthetic pain pumps
     f. Osteonecrosis: steroids, sickle cell disease, trauma
     g. Inflammatory joint disease

- Clinical presentation: pain, decreased active and passive range of motion; painless loss of active motion in Charcot arthropathy; "pseudoparalysis" with loss of active elevation in advanced rotator cuff arthropathy
  a. Less than 10% of patients have concomitant rotator cuff tear in primary osteoarthritis.
- Diagnostic workup
- **Will see superior migration of humeral head in rotator cuff arthropathy, posterior wear and posterior humeral subluxation in osteoarthritis, and medialization with glenoid erosion in rheumatoid arthritis; can also see glenohumeral destruction in Charcot arthropathy from a syrinx**
  a. X-ray: posterior glenoid wear and increased glenoid retroversion in osteoarthritis, central glenoid wear and medialization of humeral head in rheumatoid arthritis, superior humeral head migration with rotator cuff arthropathy
  b. MRI: to evaluate rotator cuff preoperatively before total shoulder arthroplasty if there is concern about tear based on exam (5–10% incidence of full-thickness rotator cuff tear in patients undergoing total shoulder arthroplasty)
     - C-spine MRI if suspect Charcot arthropathy due to syrinx
  c. CT scan: to evaluate bony anatomy, glenoid bone loss and version, humeral malunion
- Treatment
  a. Conservative: physical therapy, nonsteroidal anti-inflammatory drugs (NSAIDs), intra-articular injections; initial treatment, especially in young laborers
  b. Surgical
     - Arthroscopy: debridement and capsular release; less severe cases, differentiate other etiologies of symptoms; temporizing measure
     - Arthroplasty indicated for progressive decreased range of motion and pain with inability to perform daily activities
     - Contraindications to arthroplasty: nonfunctioning deltoid and rotator cuff, active infection, Charcot arthropathy, intractable instability, poor compliance of patient; severe bone loss
     - Hemiarthroplasty indicated for early avascular necrosis of humerus with normal glenoid in younger patients
     - Humeral head replacement with glenoid reaming
     - Humeral head replacement with soft tissue glenoid resurfacing
     - Humeral head resurfacing: for end-stage rheumatoid arthritis and either cuff deficiency or glenoid bone stock deficiency. Alternative option for rotator cuff tear arthropathy in patients with preservation of active elevation to 90 degrees: preserve coracoacromial arch to prevent humeral head anterosuperior escape
     - Total shoulder arthroplasty: preferred procedure for primary glenohumeral osteoarthritis and inflammatory arthritis
       - Place humeral component in 20–30 degrees of retroversion
       - Evaluate preoperative CT for glenohumeral articulation and evaluate for posterior subluxation, glenoid bone stock (also see on axillary lateral)
       - Must have intact and functional rotator cuff
       - **Isolated supraspinatus tear without retraction not a contraindication and should be repaired at time of arthroplasty**
       - Options for glenoid deficiency: eccentric anterior glenoid reaming for mild posterior glenoid deficiency, posterior glenoid bone grafting if glenoid deficiency more severe, augmented glenoid component

- Reverse total shoulder arthroplasty
  - Indicated for rotator cuff tear arthropathy, low-demand patient, good glenoid bone stock, intact axillary nerve and deltoid
- Revision shoulder arthroplasty
  - Axillary nerve injury and deltoid dysfunction are contraindications.
  - **Must have active deltoid strength to have shoulder function after a reverse total shoulder arthroplasty**
  - Grammont-style humeral implant medializes center of rotation and increases humeral offset with distal positioning of the center of rotation, lengthens deltoid, increases deltoid moment arm, and improves deltoid power as shoulder elevator in absence of rotator cuff.
  - Lateral offset design positions center of rotation lateral to the glenoid.
- Arthrodesis: indicated with nonfunctioning rotator cuff and deltoid, failed total shoulder arthroplasty salvage
  - Best for younger laborers with intact hand and elbow function
  - Position of fusion: 20–30 degrees of abduction, 20–30 degrees of forward flexion, 20–30 degrees of internal rotation

- Outcomes
  a. Improved long-term pain relief, motion and function after arthroplasty for osteoarthritis or rheumatoid arthritis in most studies
  b. Hemiarthroplasty for osteoarthritis has inferior pain relief and higher early revision rate when compared with total shoulder arthroplasty.
  c. Preoperative rotator cuff integrity is most important factor affecting postoperative functional outcome of total shoulder arthroplasty.
  d. Rotator cuff tear is most common cause of poor outcomes late after total shoulder arthroplasty.
  e. Patients with sickle cell as cause of humeral head osteonecrosis have best outcomes for hemiarthroplasty.
- Rehabilitation
  a. Total shoulder arthroplasty: variable protocols transitioning from passive to active range of motion
     - Some suggest immediate active assisted range of motion, avoid excess external rotation to protect subscapularis repair, active strengthening not until 6 weeks
     - Strength of subscapularis repair most important determinant of postoperative rehab protocol
     - Options for anterior exposure of glenohumeral joint include subscapularis tenotomy, subscapularis peel, lesser tuberosity osteotomy; lesser tuberosity osteotomy stronger and more secure than tendon-to-tendon or tendon-to-bone healing
- Complications
  a. Infection: *Propionibacterium* species colonize shoulder more often than hip and knee and are more common in men
     - **Cultures should be held for at least 14 days; cause of clinical implant failure**
     - Early: < 6 weeks; treat with irrigation, debridement, IV antibiotics, retention of implant
     - Late: often result of *P. acnes*; treat with prosthetic removal, antibiotics, staged reconstruction
  b. Hemiarthroplasty: late glenoid pain
  c. Anatomic total shoulder arthroplasty
     - Brachial plexopathy is the most common neurologic injury.
     - Musculocutaneous nerve injury from excessive medial retraction against conjoined tendon

- Anterior instability secondary to pull-off of subscapularis; when occurs early, treat with subscapularis repair
- Glenoid loosening: increased rate with irreparable rotator cuff tear (total shoulder contraindicated with irreparable rotator cuff repair): common cause of late total shoulder failure
- Rotator cuff injury: can occur with humeral head cut that is excessively retroverted or too low; late rotator cuff deficiency is a common cause of failure

d. Reverse total shoulder arthroplasty
- Dislocation usually anterior
- Scapular notching: position glenoid component low to overhang the inferior native scapula (most important); some suggest tilting the glenosphere inferiorly, whereas others suggest increasing lateral offset; low-angle humerus lateralizes humerus and reduces notching
- **Positioning the glenosphere too low can cause scapular notching and failure after reverse total shoulder arthroplasty.**
- Higher complication rate when performed for failed shoulder arthroplasty
- Nerve injury
- Base plate failure
- Acromial fracture

7. Muscle ruptures
- Pathogenesis
  a. Pectoralis major: men, weight lifters, during eccentric contraction, avulsion of tendon of sternal head from humerus
  b. Deltoid: usually partial tear or strain, associated with acromial erosion in presence of chronic massive rotator cuff tear; iatrogenic during open rotator cuff repair
  c. Latissimus dorsi: rare; eccentric overload during follow-through of throwing
- Clinical presentation
  a. Pectoralis major: swelling, ecchymosis, palpable defect, weakness in adduction/internal rotation
  b. Latissimus dorsi: tenderness, pain with adduction and internal rotation
- Diagnostic workup: MRI
- Treatment
  a. Pectoralis major: surgical repair to bone for acute tear of tendinous insertion, allograft reconstruction (semitendinosus) for chronic
  b. Deltoid: repair to bone for complete deltoidplasty; usually poor outcome
  c. Latissimus dorsi: surgical repair in high-demand athletes
- Outcomes: open repair of pectoralis major tendon to bone after rupture has best long-term results compared with nonoperative treatment.

8. Calcific tendinitis
- Pathogenesis: self-limiting calcification of rotator cuff tendon most commonly supraspinatus; more common in women
  a. Three stages: precalcific, calcific, postcalcific
- Clinical presentation: pain; limited abduction if involves supraspinatus
- Diagnostic workup
  a. X-ray: calcification in supraspinatus tendon most common
- Treatment
  a. Conservative: initial treatment: heat, physical therapy for stretching, needling
  b. Surgical: debridement with or without rotator cuff repair

9. Adhesive capsulitis
   - Pathogenesis
     a. Distinguish idiopathic from other etiology; idiopathic has unknown etiology: more common in females, nondominant shoulder
     b. Posttraumatic, prolonged immobilization, postoperative, complex regional pain syndrome (CRPS), cervical spine disorder, cardiopulmonary
     c. Associated conditions: diabetes, thyroid disease,
     d. Myofibroplastic proliferation within glenohumeral joint capsule
     e. Clinical stages
        - Painful: diffuse pain; pain with reaching
        - Stiff: pain and decreased range of motion
        - Thawing: pain resolves, motion gradually improves
     f. Arthroscopic changes
        - Fibrous synovitis
        - Capsular contraction, adhesions, synovitis
        - Resolving synovitis, worse contraction
        - Severe contracture
   - Clinical presentation: loss of range of motion; pain felt at end range of motion
   - **Equivalent passive and active range of motion with pain at extremes of motion is commonly seen in adhesive capsulitis.**
   - Diagnostic workup
     a. Physical examination: equivalently decreased active and passive range of motion; pain at extreme of all motion; limited glenohumeral translation
     b. X-ray: usually normal except for variable osteopenia
     c. MRI thickening of inferior capsule and coracohumeral ligament: enhanced with IV gadolinium, decreased capsular volume (no pouch inferior with dye); not necessary done for initial evaluation and management
   - Treatment
     a. Conservative: physical therapy for stretching (avoid strengthening), anti-inflammatories, glenohumeral corticosteroid injection; conservative less effective in posttraumatic stiffness
     b. Arthrographic dilatation/distention
     c. Surgical: after failure to respond to at least 12–16 weeks of conservative therapy; lysis of adhesions with manipulation; arthroscopic capsular release, manipulation under anesthesia
   - Complications: fracture/dislocation after manipulation, rotator cuff tear
   - **Most common outcome after conservative treatment is decreased motion compared with nonaffected shoulder.**

10. Nerve disorders
    - Brachial plexus injuries/"burners"
      a. Pathogenesis: football players, compression of plexus between shoulder pad and superior-medial scapula
      b. Clinical presentation: unilateral upper extremity neurologic symptoms that are temporary and resolve completely
      c. Treatment: complete resolution of symptoms before returning to play; removal from play and cervical spine radiographs if occurs repeatedly
    - Brachial plexus neuritis (Parsonage-Turner syndrome)
      a. Pathogenesis: unknown etiology; possibly postviral syndrome similar to Bell's palsy
      b. Clinical presentation: initial onset of pain with subsequent weakness; burning shoulder pain, loss of active motion, full passive motion; motor deficit only; most commonly upper trunk, C5–6

c. Diagnostic workup: X-rays and MRI are normal
d. Treatment: observation, range of motion exercises
e. Outcome: most resolve with observation

- Thoracic outlet syndrome (see Chapter 9)
  a. Pathogenesis: compression of neurovascular structures; can be secondary to cervical rib, scapular ptosis, or scalene muscle abnormalities
  b. Clinical presentation: pain, ulnar paresthesias, positive Wright test
  c. Rule out compressive lesion, subclavian thrombosis, cervical rib
  d. Treatment
    - Conservative: scapular muscle strengthening and postural exercises
    - First rib resection occasionally needed; scalene muscle resection
- Serratus palsy (medial scapular winging)
- **The direction the scapula displaces in serratus palsy and spinal accessory palsy is based on the dysfunction of their innervated muscles and the loss of their normal pull on the scapula.**
  a. Pathogenesis
    - Long-thoracic nerve palsy (C5, C6, C7): serratus anterior palsy; seen in backpackers, weight lifters, trauma
  b. Clinical Presentation
    - Shoulder and scapular pain, weakness with overhead activities and forward flexion
    - Medial rotation of inferior scapular pole and elevation of scapula **(Fig. 7.40)**
  c. Treatment
    - Observation; most resolve in 18 months
    - Pectoralis major transfer in refractory cases to inferior border of scapula
- Trapezius palsy
  a. Pathogenesis
    - Spinal accessory nerve palsy: trapezius palsy; iatrogenic injury during surgery (most commonly dissection in posterior triangle of neck for lymph node biopsy)
  b. Clinical presentation
    - Shoulder and scapular pain, weakness with overhead activities and forward flexion
    - Shoulder drooping
    - Lateral rotation of inferior scapular pole and depression of scapula
  c. Treatment
    - Conservative: observation
    - Surgical repair of nerve: performed up to 1 year
    - Transfer of levator scapulae and rhomboids (Eden-Lange) for refractory cases or scapulothoracic fusion
- Suprascapular nerve compression
  a. Pathogenesis: compression by ganglion or fascial band in suprascapular notch (supraspinatus and infraspinatus branches) or spinoglenoid notch (infraspinatus branch only), SLAP tear in association with spinoglenoid notch cyst; repetitive overhead-motion athletes (baseball, volleyball)

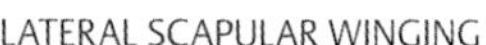

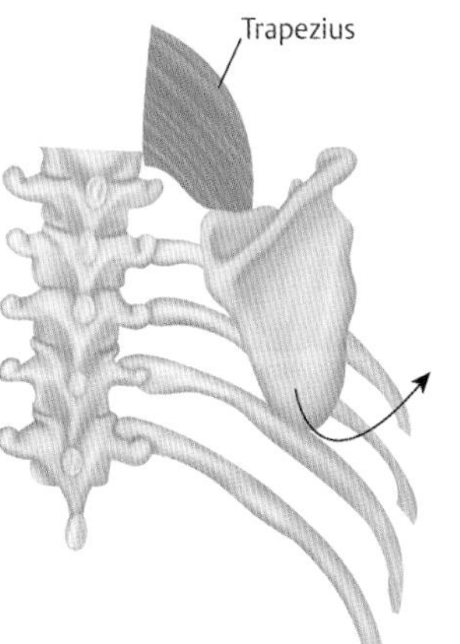

MEDIAL SCAPULAR WINGING

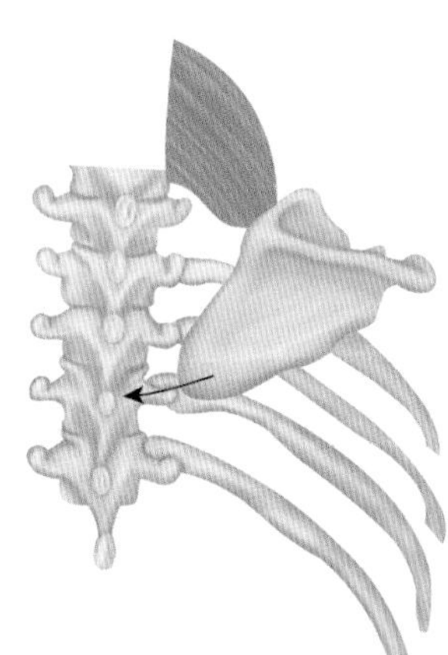

Fig. 7.40 Medial rotation of inferior scapular pole and elevation of scapula.

b. Clinical presentation: pain over dorsal aspect of shoulder, positive O'Brien test (when associated with SLAP tear), atrophy of posterior shoulder in infraspinatus fossa, weakness in external rotation (infraspinatus)
   - Suprascapular notch compression: weakness and atrophy of supraspinatus and infraspinatus
   - Spinoglenoid notch compression: weakness and atrophy of infraspinatus only

c. Diagnostic workup: MRI to localize mass effect; electromyogram (EMG)/nerve conduction velocity (NCV) test to evaluate neuropathy and affected musculature

d. Treatment
   - Ganglion cyst aspiration: high recurrence rate
   - Arthroscopic cyst decompression and labral repair: indicated for symptomatic nerve compression from ganglion cyst in association with labral tear
   - **Cyst typically seen from a tear in the labrum; treat the labral tear to address the etiology.**
   - Release of transverse scapular ligament: indicated for symptomatic nerve compression, performed when no structural lesion identified

- Quadrilateral space syndrome

a. Pathogenesis: seen in overhead-motion athletes during late cocking and acceleration phases; fibrous band between teres major and long head of triceps, compression of axillary nerve or posterior humeral circumflex artery

b. Clinical presentation: pain and paresthesias with overhead activities; weakness or atrophy of deltoid and teres minor

c. Diagnostic workup: arteriogram shows compression of posterior humeral circumflex artery

d. Treatment
   - Conservative: initial treatment; physical therapy
   - Surgical decompression and release of fibrous bands

- Fascioscapulohumeral muscular dystrophy

a. Pathogenesis: autosomal dominant disorder; onset between ages 6 and 20 years

b. Clinical presentation: facial muscle abnormalities, scapular winging
   - **They can't whistle.**

c. Treatment
   - Conservative: initial treatment; physical therapy
   - Scapulothoracic fusion

11. Other shoulder disorders

- Sternoclavicular joint infection

a. Pathogenesis: increased risk in IV drug abuse
   - **Can see pseudomonas in IV drug abuser**

b. Clinical presentation: pain, swelling, tenderness

c. Diagnostic workup
   - X-ray
   - CT of chest: rule out extension to chest and pericardial area prior to surgical intervention
   - MRI

d. Treatment: antibiotics first line; if fail, surgical debridement

- Osteitis condensans

a. Pathogenesis: bony sclerosis of medial end of clavicle, possibly traumatic etiology; occurs in middle-aged women
b. Clinical presentation: pain, swelling, tenderness; pain worse with forward elevation and abduction of shoulder
c. Diagnostic workup
  - X-ray: sclerotic patch at medial end of clavicle
d. Treatment
  - Conservative: initial treatment; NSAIDs
  - Surgical: if remains symptomatic despite nonoperative treatment; excision of medial clavicle

- Glenoid hypoplasia

a. Pathogenesis: bilateral, not associated with other syndromes
b. Clinical presentation: varied clinical findings including painless clicking, instability, or pain
c. Predisposed to develop glenohumeral osteoarthritis
d. Diagnostic workup
    - ♦ X-ray: inferior and posterior glenoid deficiency, enlarged distal clavicle
e. Treatment: physical therapy is initial management; surgical treatment to address symptoms refractory to therapy

- Os acromiale **(Fig. 7.41)**

a. Pathogenesis: unfused secondary ossification center; 3% incidence; most commonly at junction of meso and meta acromion; associated with rotator cuff pathology
b. Clinical presentation: pain, tenderness over acromion; most are identified incidentally
c. Treatment
  - Conservative: observation if asymptomatic
  - Surgical: for persistent symptoms; acromioplasty, ORIF versus excision (pre- and meso-acromion types)

- Glenohumeral internal rotation deficiency (GIRD)

a. Pathogenesis: multiple causes of lack of internal rotation
    - ♦ Internal impingement: often occurs in GIRD in young overhead-motion athletes; in late cocking phase have impingement of posterosuperior rotator cuff between humerus and posterosuperior labrum, causes articular-sided tears in some cases; associated with SLAP tears
f. Clinical presentation
  - Decreased internal rotation, increased external rotation, posterior capsular contracture
  - Internal impingement: pain in posterior shoulder and decreased throwing velocity; pain worse in 90 degrees of abduction and maximal external rotation
    - ♦ Decreased internal rotation, increased external rotation, posterior capsular contracture
b. Diagnostic imaging: Bennett lesion: mineralization of posterior inferior glenoid in internal impingement/overhead athletes
c. Treatment: posterior and posteroinferior capsular stretching; activity modification with cessation of throwing in athletes with partial articular-sided tears

- Distal clavicle osteolysis

a. Pathogenesis: weight lifters, traumatic injury
b. Diagnosis
  - X-ray: osteopenia, osteolysis of distal clavicle
  - MRI: increased signal distal clavicle

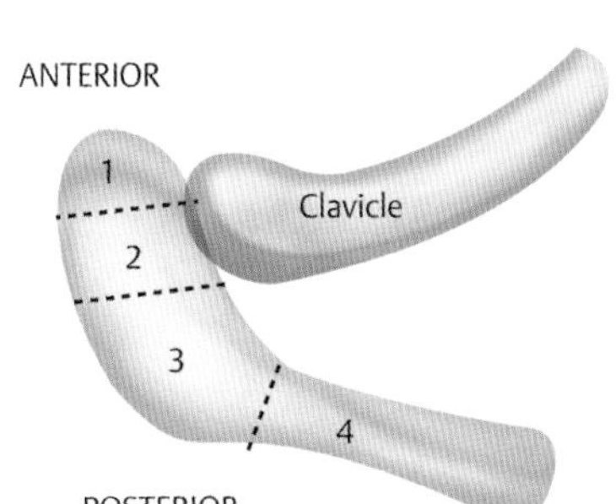

Fig. 7.41 Os acromiale.

7 Shoulder, Elbow, and Upper Extremity Sports

c. Treatment
  - Conservative: initial treatment: NSAIDS, activity modification, corticosteroid injections
  - Surgical: indicated for failure of conservative treatment; distal clavicle excision

- Little Leaguer's shoulder
  a. Pathogenesis: young overhead-motion athletes, overuse syndrome
  b. Diagnosis
    - Xray: Salter Harris I fracture, widen surgical neck of proximal humeral physis
    - MRI: if diagnosis unclear
  c. Treatment: nonoperative with rest, activity modification, return to play once asymptomatic
- Acromioclavicular degenerative joint disease
  a. Pathogenesis: typically idiopathic; repetitive overhead heavy work, rarely from chronic grade 1 or 2 AC joint separation
  b. Clinical presentation: activity-related pain, pain with overhead-motion and adduction activities, internal rotation and reaching behind back, and sleeping on affected side; tenderness over joint, positive cross-body adduction test, pain with O'Brien internal rotation at AC joint relieved by external rotation/supination
  c. Diagnosis
    - X-ray: AP of AC joint, Zanca view
    - MRI: AC joint edema
  d. Treatment
    - Conservative: initial treatment: NSAIDs, activity modification, corticosteroid injection
    - Surgical: indicated after failed course of conservative
      - ♦ Arthroscopic distal clavicle resection
      - ♦ Open distal clavicle resection (Mumford): resect less than 1 cm to prevent injury to coracoclavicular ligaments
  e. Complications
    - Superior-inferior AC instability: from excessive distal clavicle resection of > 1 cm, disrupts coracoclavicular ligaments
    - Anterior-posterior instability: from resection of posterior and superior acromioclavicular ligaments
    - Other: heterotopic ossification
- Sternoclavicular degenerative joint disease
  a. Clinical presentation: pain, localized tenderness, prominence and swelling
  b. Diagnosis: X-ray (serendipity view)
    - CT scan: clarify bony anatomy and pathology, evaluate for subluxation/dislocation
    - MRI: help evaluate for infectious etiology
  c. Treatment
    - Conservative: initial treatment; NSAIDs, activity modification, corticosteroid injection (consider ultrasound guidance)
    - Surgical: medial clavicle resection; preserve sternoclavicular and costoclavicular ligaments
  d. Complications
    - Excessive medial clavicle resection compromises costoclavicular ligaments, leading to clavicular instability; repair with graft reconstruction of SC joint
    - Injury to retrosternal structures, subclavian vessels

- Scapular disorders
  a. Scapular dyskinesis
    - Pathogenesis: abnormal scapular motion secondary to another primary shoulder pathology; also secondary to neurologic injury, thoracic kyphosis, poor throwing mechanics
    - Clinical presentation: shoulder pain and dysfunction, worse with overhead-motion activities; scapulothoracic crepitus, scapula protracted and more inferior; symptoms improve with scapular stabilization exercises; medial scapular winging
    - Treatment: conservative: physical therapy for scapular stabilization, NSAIDs
  b. Scapulothoracic crepitus
    - Clinical presentation: painful crepitus with arm elevation, scapular dyskinesia, pain relieved when scapula stabilized
    - Diagnosis: X-rays and CT to evaluate for skeletal anomaly such as scapular exostosis
    - Treatment
      - ♦ Conservative: initial treatment; physical therapy, NSAIDs, corticosteroid injection
      - ♦ Surgical: for failure to respond to conservative; bursectomy; resection of superomedial scapula

12. Other considerations
  - Respiratory insufficiency is relative contraindication for interscalene block for shoulder surgery
  - Most common complication after interscalene block is paresthesias for up to 6 months

III. Disorders of the Elbow

1. Elbow physical exam tests (**Table 7.5**)
2. Tendon disorders
  - Lateral epicondylitis (tennis elbow)
    a. Pathogenesis: overuse of extensor muscles; microtear of tendinous origin with angiofibroblastic hyperplasia at origin of extensor carpi radialis brevis (ECRB) tendon

Table 7.5 Elbow Physical Exam Tests

Test Name	Technique	Associated Pathology
Hook test	Patient actively supinates forearm, examiner attempts to hook finger under biceps tendon	Absence of cord-like structure to hook finger on indicative of distal biceps tendon rupture
Moving valgus stress test	Apply constant valgus stress to elbow while moving from flexion to extension	Medial elbow pain occurring maximally between 120 and 70 degrees indicative of medial collateral ligament injury
Milking test	Downward and valgus stress to supinated forearm with elbow flexed > 90 degrees	Medial collateral ligament injury
Lateral pivot shift test	Supinate forearm, valgus stress, and axial compression while flexing a fully extended elbow; radiocapitellar joint will reduce past 40 degrees of flexion	Lateral collateral ligament injury

- **Angiofibriblastic hyperplasia seen in the ECRB tendon in tennis elbow**

b. Clinical presentation: tenderness at lateral epicondyle/extensor origin; pain with resisted wrist extension; pain with middle finger extension

c. Diagnostic workup: diagnosis is clinical; plain radiographs to demonstrate calcification or spurring

d. Treatment
   - Conservative: mainstay of treatment; activity modification, physical therapy for eccentric strengthening and passive stretching, NSAIDs, cock-up splint, counterforce bracing, corticosteroid injection, platelet-rich plasma (PRP) injection (controversial)
   - **Conservative management is the gold standard for tennis elbow; in refractory cases, surgery is indicated. Corticosteroid injections may change the natural history of tennis elbow, which takes longer to resolve.**
   - Surgical: open or arthroscopic debridement/release of ECRB origin; indicated for refractory cases

e. Complications: excessive resection can disrupt LUCL, causing posterolateral rotatory instability.
   - **Beware of posterolateral rotatory instability after elbow dislocation or overaggressive tennis elbow debridement.**

- Medial epicondylitis (golfer's elbow)
  a. Pathogenesis: overuse of flexor/pronator muscles
  b. Clinical presentation: tenderness over medial epicondyle/flexor pronator origin, pain with resisted wrist flexion and forearm pronation
  c. Diagnostic workup: diagnosis is clinical; plain radiographs to evaluate for calcification or spurring
  d. Treatment
     - Conservative: mainstay of treatment; activity modification, NSAIDs, corticosteroid injection, passive stretching, splinting
     - Surgical: open or arthroscopic debridement; indicated for refractory cases
  e. Complication: ulnar nerve injury
- Distal biceps tendon rupture/tear
  a. Pathogenesis: more common in men; forced eccentric load on partially flexed elbow; partial tear is rare and usually occurs at radial border of insertion
  b. Clinical presentation: biceps muscle deformity, pain in antecubital fossa, ecchymosis anterior forearm, tenderness at biceps insertion; Hook test
  c. Diagnostic workup
     - X-ray: usually normal
     - MRI: to diagnose suspected partial tear, determine location of tear and degree of retraction; not necessary to make diagnosis in acute complete tear
  d. Treatment
     - Nonoperative: partial tear
     - Surgical: indicated to restore supination strength; two-incision (Boyd-Anderson) or one-incision technique
       - ♦ Detachment and repair of partial tear that fails conservative treatment
  e. Complications
     - Conservative treatment: up to 50% weakness of supination, up to 50% elbow flexion weakness
     - Nerve injury: neurapraxia of lateral antebrachial cutaneous (LABC) nerve is most common nerve injury and most common complication

of anterior single-incision approach; PIN injury more often with two-incision technique

- **An LABC injury can occur with one incision, and a PIN injury with two incisions**
- Heterotopic ossification: radioulnar synostosis with two-incision technique; anterior with single incision
- Synostosis: increased rate in two-incision technique
- Loss of terminal extension; loss of pronation

• Distal triceps tendon rupture/tear

a. Pathogenesis: deceleration of extended elbow, chronic olecranon bursitis, multiple corticosteroid injections, anabolic steroids, renal osteodystrophy, fluoroquinolone

b. Clinical presentation: pain, inability to actively extend elbow

c. Diagnostic workup

d. Physical examination: palpable defect, weak elbow extension
- X-ray: "flake sign" showing avulsion fracture, pathognomonic; fractured olecranon spur
- MRI: confirms injury, determines severity

e. Treatment
- Surgical: repair with transosseous sutures versus suture anchor

3. Ligament injuries **(Figs. 7.13b,c** and **7.42)**

• Medial collateral ligament (MCL); ulnar collateral ligament (UCL)

a. Pathogenesis: repetitive valgus stress, late cocking and acceleration phases of pitching; increased internal rotation torque during pitching increases elbow valgus load
- Anterior band of UCL is most important medial stabilizer of flexed elbow

b. Clinical presentation: medial elbow pain and tenderness from medial epicondyle to sublime tubercle; valgus instability in 25–50%
- Dynamic valgus instability: detected by moving valgus stress test, milking test

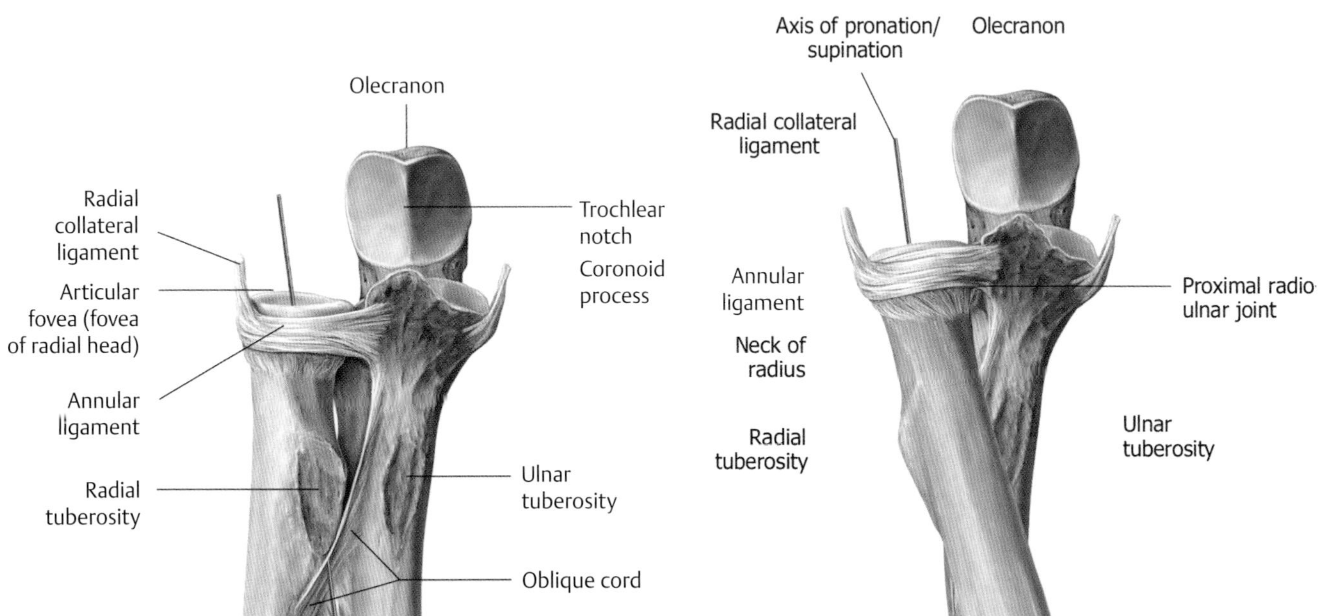

Fig. 7.42 Proximal radioulnar joint. (From Schuenke M, Schulte E. General Anatomy and the Musculoskeletal System: Thieme Atlas of Anatomy. New York: Thieme; 2005. Illustration by Karl Wesker.)

c. Diagnostic workup
   - X-ray: posteromedial olecranon fossa osteophytes
   - MR arthrogram: confirms diagnosis; imaging modality of choice

d. Treatment
   - Conservative: initial treatment; rest, physical therapy for flexor/pronator strengthening; specifically of flexor carpi ulnaris (FCU) as is important dynamic medial elbow stabilizer
   - Surgical: indicated in high-level athletes desiring return to play, failure of conservative treatment
     - ♦ Ligament reconstruction: palmaris longus, hamstring autograft, or allograft in figure of eight configuration (Tommy John surgery) or by docking technique; ulnar nerve transposition if ulnar nerve symptoms present preoperatively

e. Outcomes: 75% return to same or better level of activity at 1 year; reconstruction favored over direct repair; better results for treatment of chronic rather than acute injuries

f. Complications: loss of motion, graft harvest site morbidity

- Lateral collateral ligament **(Fig. 7.13a)**
  a. Pathogenesis
     - Acute injury: first ligament injured in elbow dislocation (see Chapter 3)
     - Chronic incompetence: ulnar portion (LUCL) results in posterolateral rotatory instability
  b. Clinical presentation (posterolateral rotatory instability): pain, clicking or locking during elbow extension, i.e., when pushing off from chair
     - **Patient will be unable to push up out of a chair with this arm due to instability.**
     - Lateral pivot shift test
  c. Diagnostic workup
     - MRI: insufficiency in chronic injuries
  d. Treatment: chronic incompetence
     - Conservative: activity modification in older/infirm patient
     - Surgical: ligament reconstruction and capsule plication

4. Osteochondritis dissecans (OCD) and Panner's disease
   - Pathogenesis
     a. OCD: involves capitellum; occurs in adolescents and athletes involved in weight bearing of upper extremities or overhead-motion sports (gymnasts and throwers) causing repetitive microtrauma and vascular insufficiency
     b. Panner's disease: osteochondrosis of capitellum, in ages <1 2 years; more benign and self-limiting
   - Clinical presentation: pain in lateral elbow, catching, locking, loss of elbow extension early
   - Diagnostic workup
     a. X-ray: irregularity and fragmentation of capitellum
     b. MRI
        - OCD: separation of cartilage from capitellum, chondral fissures
        - Panner's: chondral injury with involvement of entire ossific nucleus of capitellum
   - Treatment
     a. Conservative
        - Panner's disease: observation; will resolve without residual sequelae; rest for 3–6 weeks with gradual return to activities; initial management for stable OCD lesions

- OCD: observation initially with rest for 3–6 weeks with gradual return to activities

b. Surgical: failed conservative management with continued symptoms
   - Symptomatic lesion with intact articular surface: arthroscopic in-situ drilling
   - Large fragment partially displaced: reduction and stabilization
   - Unstable or loose fragment: excision and drilling of defect
   - Large defect not amenable to fixing: osteochondral graft [osteochondral autograft transplantation surgery (OATS)]

- Outcomes: 90% good results with conservative treatment for stable OCD lesions

5. Little Leaguer's elbow
   - Pathogenesis: stress fracture of medial epicondyle; throwing athletes, repetitive valgus stress
   - Clinical presentation: elbow pain with decreased pitching performance; pain medially and with valgus stress
   - Diagnostic workup
     a. X-ray: widened physis of medial epicondyle; enlarged and fragmented medial epicondyle
   - Treatment
     a. Conservative: mainstay of treatment; rest, activity modification, limit number of pitches
     b. Operative: in-situ fixation of medial epicondyle for refractory cases
6. Valgus extension overload (pitcher's elbow)
   - Pathogenesis: combination of medial tension, lateral compression, posterior extension overload
   - Clinical presentation: pain in the posteromedial elbow during deceleration phase, pain with forced elbow extension, increased valgus, hypertrophy of pronator mass, lack of elbow extension
   - Diagnostic workup
     a. X-ray: posteromedial olecranon osteophytes, chondromalacia in medial wall of olecranon fossa
   - Treatment
     a. Conservative: first-line treatment; NSAIDs, pitching instruction to improve mechanics, activity modification
     b. Surgical: persistent symptoms despite conservative treatment; intra-articular debridement, resection of posteromedial osteophytes and loose body removal; contraindicated in elbows with MCL insufficiency
   - Complications: valgus instability with excessive olecranon resection (creating MCL insufficiency)
   - **Beware of creating valgus instability from overzealous medial debridement.**
7. Olecranon stress fracture
   - Pathogenesis: overhead-motion athletes, traction from triceps contraction during deceleration phase of throwing
   - Clinical presentation: posterior elbow pain
   - Diagnostic workup
     a. X-ray: may see oblique or transverse fracture line
   - Treatment
     a. Conservative: initial treatment; rest, temporary splinting
     b. Surgical: indicated when nonoperative treatment fails; ORIF with compression screw

8. Congenital radial head dislocation
    - Pathogenesis: dislocation of radial head from birth, leading to dome-shaped radial head with hypoplastic capitellum
    - Clinical presentation: limitation of elbow flexion and supination; pain not necessarily present
    - Diagnostic workup: elbow X-rays: abnormally shaped radial head (bullet or dome-shaped) and abnormally shaped capitellum; posterior subluxated radial head
    - Treatment
        a. Conservative: for asymptomatic patients with adequate range of motion
        b. Surgical: radial head resection for pain control; may not affect elbow range of motion
9. Osteoarthritis: primary degenerative arthritis
    - Pathogenesis: laborers, predominantly males
    - Clinical presentation: limited motion, pain at extremes of motion
    - Diagnostic workup
        a. X-ray: osteophytes especially on tip of coronoid and olecranon as well as the coronoid and olecranon fossae; narrowed joint space; radial neck spurring; ulnohumeral joint space/articular surface usually spared
    - Treatment
        a. Conservative: activity modification, NSAIDs, injections
        b. Surgical management
            - Arthroscopic debridement, removal of loose bodies, release of soft tissues to increase range of motion; early arthritis; younger age, heavy laborer
            - Distraction/interposition arthroplasty in those where total elbow arthroplasty is contraindicated; young active patients with severe pain and end-stage arthritis with normal joint architecture intact
            - Ulnohumeral arthroplasty (open/Outerbridge-Kashiwagi, or arthroscopic osteocapsular osteoplasty); young active patients
            - Total elbow arthroplasty (TEA): rarely required; low-demand elderly patients
        c. Rehabilitation: physical therapy to maintain range of motion (see Rehabilitation in the next subsection)
10. Rheumatoid arthritis (RA)
    - Pathogenesis: unclear cause; cell-mediated immune response thought to be involved
    - Clinical presentation: pain throughout arc of motion, loss of motion, instability depending on severity of disease
    - Diagnostic workup
        a. X-ray
            - Rheumatoid: Larsen grading system **(Fig. 7.43)**
                - ♦ Larsen 1: near-normal radiographs
                - ♦ Larsen 2: periarticular erosion and mild cartilage loss, soft tissue swelling, osteopenia
                - ♦ Larsen 3: marked joint space narrowing
                - ♦ Larsen 4: advance erosions that penetrate subchondral bone
                - ♦ Larsen 5: advanced joint damage, loss of articular contour
    - Treatment
        a. Nonoperative: medical management, splinting, injections
        b. Surgical
            - Larsen 1, 2: arthroscopic synovectomy, open synovectomy with radial head excision

- Larsen 3–5: total elbow arthroplasty
    - ♦ Indications: persistent symptoms despite conservative treatment or limited surgical intervention
    - ♦ Contraindications: Charcot arthropathy, active infection

- Rehabilitation: total elbow arthroplasty with triceps-reflecting Bryan-Morrey approach; limit weight bearing to 5 pounds or less; splint for 5–10 days to allow soft tissue healing; start active flexion and passive extension; no strengthening for 6–8 weeks
- Outcomes: best survivorship for total elbow when performed for rheumatoid arthritis

- **Outcomes from TEA best in RA; likely from low demand, infirm lifestyle**

- Complications
  a. Failure of extensor mechanism after Bryan-Morrey approach
    - Loosening: linked total elbow arthroplasty implants
    - Instability: unlinked total elbow arthroplasty implants
    - Infection: treat chronic infection with staged revision if adequate bone stock remains

11. Elbow contracture
- Pathogenesis: trauma, degenerative joint disease; differentiate intra-articular, extra-articular, and combined
- Clinical presentation: decreased motion
- Diagnostic workup
  a. X-ray: fossa overgrowth (radial, olecranon, coronoid), heterotopic ossification
- Treatment
  a. Conservative
    - Observation: indicated for loss of terminal extension after dislocation; physical therapy; static progressive splinting
    - Goal of motion from 30–130 degrees (100-degree arc of motion for functional activities)

  b. Surgical
    - Ligament sparing open surgical capsular release and capsular excision; lateral or medial column approaches
    - Release of posterior oblique band of MCL to restore flexion
    - **Release/excise anterior capsule to gain extension**
    - Ulnar nerve release or transposition if severe loss of flexion to avoid postoperative ulnar neuropathy
- Outcomes: success dependent on etiology and patient compliance in therapy

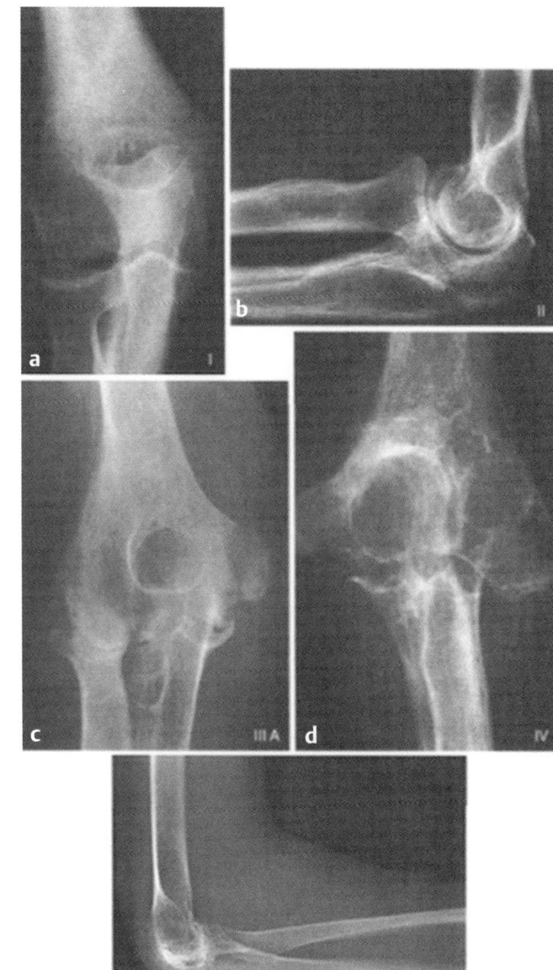

Fig. 7.43 Rheumatoid: Larsen grading system. (From Morrey BF. Linked total elbow arthroplasty in patients with rheumatoid arthritis. In: Morrey's The Elbow and Its Disorders, 4th ed. New York: Elsevier; 2009. Reprinted with permission.)

8

Sports Medicine and Lower Extremity Sports

Stephen Klinge, Gregory A. Sawyer, and Paul Fadale

I. Hip

A. Anatomy

1. Acetabulum is 15–20 degrees anteverted (flexed) and 45 degrees abducted
2. Femoral neck is anteverted 15 degrees relative to femoral condyle with average neck shaft angle of 126 degrees
3. Hip is a ball-and-socket joint and innately stable secondary to bony architecture; however, secondary stabilization is provided by fibrocartilaginous labrum and capsule; capsule composed of iliofemoral (ligament of Bigelow), ischiofemoral, and pubofemoral ligaments **(Fig. 8.1)**
4. Normal hip range of motion (ROM) **(Fig. 8.2)**
   - 140 degrees' flexion
   - 20 degrees' extension
   - 80 degrees' abduction
   - 20 degrees' adduction
   - 40 degrees' internal rotation
   - 50 degrees' external rotation
5. Hip musculature and innervation **(Table 8.1)**
6. Greater trochanter is insertion site of hip's short external rotators and abductors, and is a lateral structure; lesser trochanter is insertion site of iliopsoas and is a posterior-medial structure
7. Femoral head receives blood supply contributions from the medial femoral circumflex (branch of profunda femoris), lateral femoral circumflex (branch of

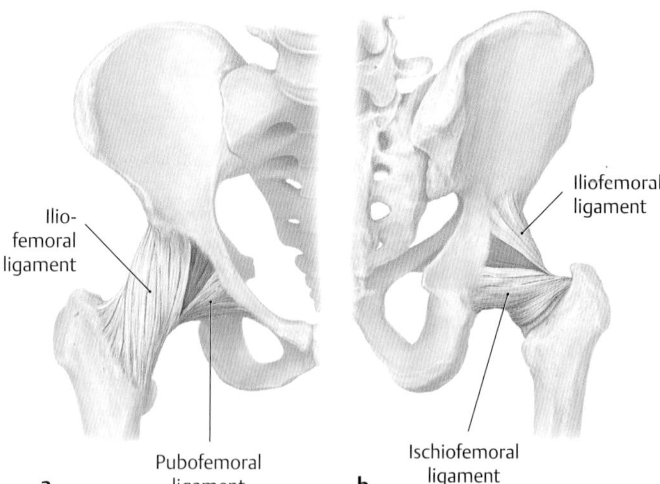

Fig. 8.1 Hip capsule consisting of **(a)** iliofemoral, pubofemoral, and **(b)** ischiofemoral ligaments. (From Schuenke M, Schulte E. General Anatomy and the Musculoskeletal System: Thieme Atlas of Anatomy. New York: Thieme; 2005. Illustration by Karl Wesker.)

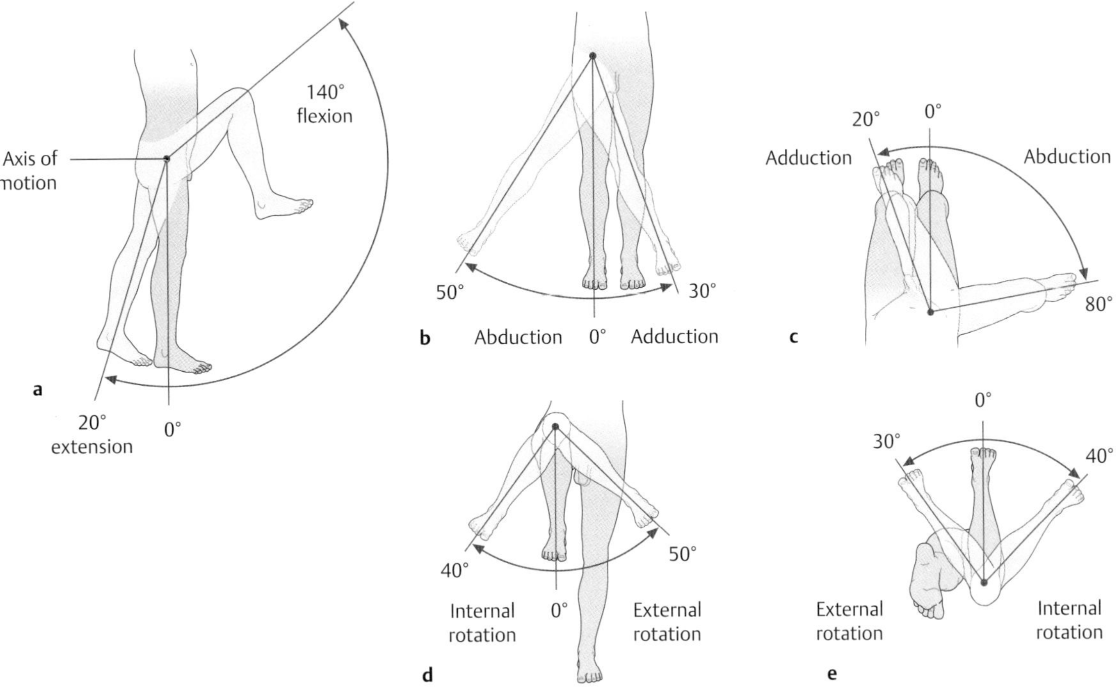

Fig. 8.2 (a–e) Hip ranges of motion, using the neutral-zero method. (From Schuenke M, Schulte E. General Anatomy and the Musculoskeletal System: Thieme Atlas of Anatomy. New York: Thieme; 2005. Illustration by Karl Wesker.)

profunda femoris), and artery of the ligamentum teres (branch of obturator artery)

8. Primary blood supply in adulthood is from medial femoral circumflex, which provides retrograde flow to head from posterior
   - **Protect medial femoral circumflex artery with medial and posterior hip approaches**
9. In adulthood, contributions from lateral femoral circumflex and ligamentum teres are negligible

B. Physical Examination (Table 8.2)

1. Ischial tuberosity is a posterior structure, and tenderness to palpation can indicate a hamstring origin injury.
2. Adductor longus is a palpable groin structure and tenderness is consistent with a strain ("groin pull").
3. Positive Trendelenburg sign indicates hip abductor weakness; when the patient is standing on the affected limb, the contralateral pelvis will drop below the horizontal **(Fig. 8.3)**.

C. Hip Arthroscopy

1. Indications: labral tears, intra-articular loose bodies, femoroacetabular impingement (FAI), septic arthritis, chondral injuries, synovial disorders
2. Common portals: anterior, anterolateral, and posterolateral
   - Anterior portal at junction of vertical line drawn from anterior superior iliac spine (ASIS) and horizontal line from tip of greater trochanter; lateral femoral cutaneous nerve and femoral vessels at risk
   - Anterolateral portal on anterior surface of greater trochanter; superior gluteal nerve at risk

Table 8.1 Hip Musculature and Innervation

	Origin	Insertion	Innervation	Action at Hip[1]
Anterior				
Iliopsoas	Verterbal bodies T12–L5/ iliac fossa	Lesser trochanter	Femoral	Flexion
Rectus femoris	Anterior-inferior iliac spine/ anterior hip capsule	Patella	Femoral	Flexion
Sartorius	Anterior superior iliac spine	Pes anserinus superficial	Femoral	Flexion, abduction, external rotation
Posterior				
Piriformis	Anterior sacral spine	Greater trochanter	Branches sacral plexus L5–S2	External rotation
Superior/inferior gemelli	Ischial spine/tuberosity	Greater trochanter	Branches sacral plexus L4–S3	External rotation
Obturator internus	Inferior pubic ramus/ obturator membrane	Greater trochanter	Branches sacral plexus L5–S2	External rotation, abduction
Obturator externus	Obturator foreman/ membrane	Trochanteric fossa	Obturator	External rotation, adduction
Quadratus femoris	Ischial tuberosity	Intertrochanteric crest	Branches sacral plexus L4–S1	External rotation, adduction
Gluteus maximus	Ilium/lumbar fascia/sacrum	Gluteal tuberosity/iliotibial tract	Inferior gluteal	Extension, external rotation ER
Biceps long head	Medial ischial tuberosity	Proximal fibula	Tibial	Extension
Semimembranosus	Proximal/lateral ischial tuberosity	Multiple insertions[2]	Tibial	Extension
Semitendinosus	Distal/medial ischial tuberosity	Pes anserinus deep/distal	Tibial	Extension
Lateral				
Gluteus medius	Ilium, below gluteus maximus	Greater trochanter	Superior gluteal	Abduction, internal rotation
Gluteus minimus	Ilium, below gluteus medius	Greater trochanter	Superior gluteal	Abduction, internal rotation
Iliotibial tract	Anterior iliac crest	Gerdy's tubercle	Superior gluteal	Flex, abduction, internal rotation
Medial				
Adductor longus	Pubic body/below crest	Linea aspera/middle third	Obturator	Adduction, flexion
Adductor brevis	Inferior pubic ramus/body	Linea aspera/lesser trochanter	Obturator	Adduction
Adductor magnus	Pubis/ischial tuberosity	Linea aspera/adductor tubercle	Obturator	Adduction, flexion/ extension[3]
Gracilis	Inferior public arch	Pes anserinus (deep/proximal)	Obturator	Adduction, flexion, internal rotation

[1]Several muscles about the hip have multiple actions, depending on their relation to the hip axis of rotation.
[2]Insertions include posterior oblique ligament, posterior capsule, posterior-medial tibia, popliteus and medial meniscus.
[3]Adductor part of adductor magnus flexes hip, while hamstring part extends hip.

Table 8.2 Physical Examination of the Hip

Test Name	Technique	Importance
Anterior impingement	Passive hip flexion/adduction/internal rotation reproduces symptoms	Indicative of femoroacetabular impingement
External snapping	Hip flexion (in adducted position)	Iliotibial tract catching/irritation over the greater trochanter
Internal snapping	Passive movement from external rotation/flexion to extension/internal rotation	Iliopsoas tendon catching/irritation over lesser trochanter[1]
Ober	Inability to adduct past midline with hip extended/abducted in lateral position	Tightness of iliotibial tract
FAIR	Hip FAIR	Stretch of piriformis may exacerbate symptoms of piriformis syndrome

Abbreviation: FAIR, flexion/adduction/internal rotation.
[1]Iliopsoas tendon can also catch on the anterior inferior iliac spine or the iliopectineal ridge

- Posterolateral portal on posterior surface of greater trochanter; sciatic nerve at risk; internally rotate leg to avoid neurologic injury

3. Complications: most common are pudendal nerve palsy from perineal post and neurovascular injury from portals

D. Hip Pathology

1. Bursitis
   - Greater trochanteric bursitis
     a. Demographic: middle-aged females or female runners training on banked surfaces
     b. Presentation: lateral hip pain with tenderness, normal passive ROM, pain with resisted abduction and internal rotation
        - Associated with tightness of iliotibial (IT) band and positive Ober test. The Ober test is performed with the patient in the lateral position, with the affected hip abducted and extended, with knee extension (or flexion).

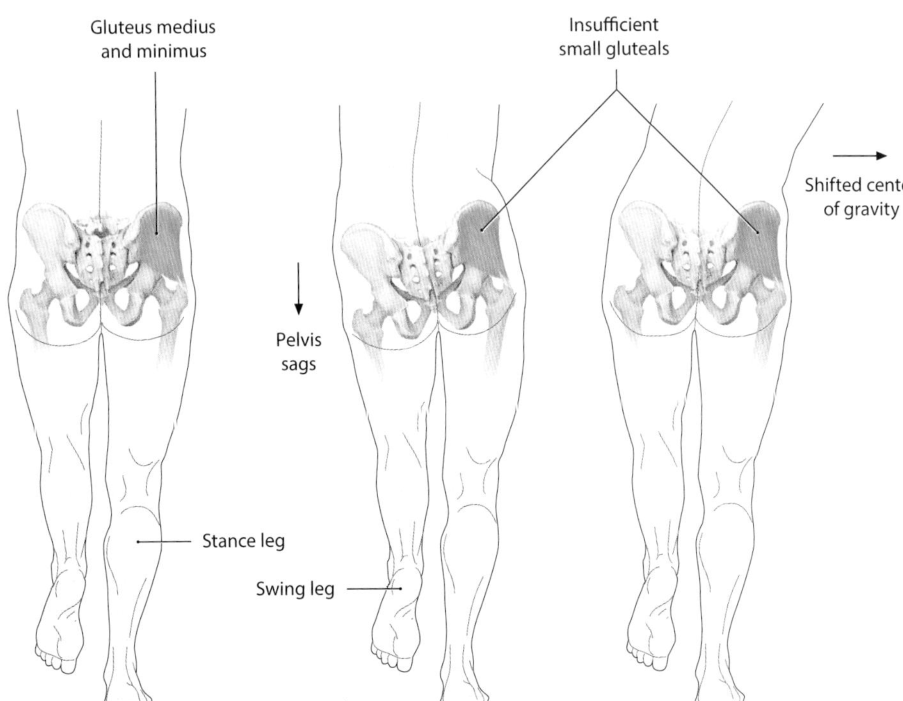

Fig. 8.3 **(a)** Normal gait. **(b)** Contralateral hip drop observed with Trendelenburg gait pattern. **(c)** Compensatory ipsilateral trunk shift observed with Trendelenburg gait. (From Schuenke M, Schulte E. General Anatomy and the Musculoskeletal System: Thieme Atlas of Anatomy. New York: Thieme; 2005. Illustration by Karl Wesker.)

The test is positive when the patient cannot adduct the hip past the midline from this position.

- Tightness of IT band can result in "external" snapping hip
- **External snapping hip can be palpated over trochanter as IT band slides over it; internal snapping hip produced by passively moving hip from flexed/externally rotated to extended/internally rotated**
- Coxa saltans

c. Pathology: tendinosis of gluteus medius or minimus tendon

d. Imaging: none, clinical diagnosis

e. Treatment: conservative with nonsteroidal anti-inflammatory drugs (NSAIDs), stretching, rest, corticosteroid injection

- Surgical management with debridement of tendon and reattachment ("hip rotator cuff repair")
- In coxa saltans, treat with a Z-plasty of the IT band.

• Iliopsoas bursitis

a. Demographic: young athletes (gymnasts, track athletes) and ballet dancers

b. Presentation: anterior hip pain after repetitive hip flexion/extension

- Can result in "internal" snapping (audible snap is heard) and pain when moving hip from flexed/externally rotated to extended/internally rotated

c. Pathology: bursitis between hip capsule and iliopsoas tendon; snapping caused by tendon gliding over iliopectineal line or femoral head

d. Imaging: conventional and dynamic ultrasonography to identify the snapping iliopsoas tendon

e. Treatment: conservative with rest, NSAIDs, hip flexor stretching/strengthening, corticosteroid injection

- Surgery rarely indicated; arthroscopic release of iliopsoas tendon
- Zona orbicularis is a ring of capsular tissue that provides an arthroscopic landmark for identification of the iliopsoas

2. Musculotendinous injuries (strains/tears)

• Hamstring

a. Consist of semimembranosus, semitendinosus, biceps femoris (long head and short head)

b. Demographic: common injury in all ages; frequent during sprinting

c. Presentation: pain with hip flexion and knee extension, ecchymosis in posterior thigh

d. Pathology: strain or tear, frequently at myotendinous junction

3. Imaging: X-ray—ischial tuberosity avulsion seen in pediatric population; MRI for diagnosis and grading of injury

f. Treatment

- Conservative management is the gold standard; protected weight bearing with crutches; stretching and strengthening
- Surgical repair considered for high-level athletes with proximal tendon ruptures

• Rectus Femoris

a. Consists of direct and indirect heads; direct (straight) head originates from anterior inferior iliac spine (AIIS), whereas indirect (reflected) head originates from superior acetabular ridge and hip capsule

b. Demographic: young athletes, particularly soccer and football players

c. Presentation: anterior thigh pain (proximal or distal) reproduced with resisted hip flexion

d. Pathology: strains/tears at proximal origin, midsubstance, or at distal insertion

e. Imaging: X-ray useful for identification of bony avulsion at AIIS, common in adolescents

f. Treatment: conservative with rest, NSAIDs, stretching for 4–6 weeks

- Adductor

a. Consists of adductor longus, adductor brevis, adductor magnus

b. Demographic: any athlete

c. Presentation: injury occurs with forced external rotation of an abducted leg; presents with significant groin pain and tenderness to palpation along pubic ramus

d. Pathology: strain of the musculotendinous junction or tear of the origin

e. Imaging: magnetic resonance imaging (MRI): signal at pubis signifying tendinous avulsion

f. Treatment: conservative with rest, ice, NSAIDs, and protected weight bearing; rehabilitation follows with stretching and strengthening

3. Sports Hernia/Athletic Pubalgia

- Demographic: athletes of any age, especially soccer and hockey players, males > females
- Presentation: anterior pelvic or groin pain, without physical exam evidence of inguinal hernia; exacerbated with activities that increase intra-abdominal pressure (Valsalva maneuver, sit-ups, etc.); tenderness over adductor longus origin

a. Secondary to sports with frequent abdominal hyperextension and hip abduction

b. Can be confused with osteitis pubis, where patients have focal tenderness over pubic symphysis and pain with resisted rectus abdominis testing

- Pathology: poorly understood and controversial; due to chronic overuse with microtearing of the anterior abdominal wall (rectus abdominis, obliques, or transversalis fascia) and adductor involvement with associated pubis changes
- Imaging: diagnosis of exclusion; X-ray and MRI are useful to rule out other etiologies, such as osteitis pubis.
- Treatment: conservative with 6–8 weeks of rest and rehabilitation

a. Surgery focused on the site of complaint can be indicated, with pelvic floor reconstruction, adductor release, or rectus reattachment.

b. In patients with chronic adductor pain and normal MRI scans, a single corticosteroid shot has been shown to provide relief.

4. Femoral neck stress fractures

- Demographic: young female athletes, particularly runners
- Presentation: groin pain with weight bearing in athletes who have a history of overuse or recent increase in training; physical exam usually benign
- Pathology: chronic, repetitive loading results in microfractures in femoral neck; seen on tension side (superior-lateral) or compression side (inferior-medial)
- Imaging: X-ray can identify fracture line late in process; MRI is study of choice for identification in patients with normal X-rays
- Treatment

a. Compression-side stress fracture: in compliant patients can be managed conservatively with weight bearing with crutches until pain free and cessation of running for 8–12 weeks.

b. Compression side: conservative management; tension side: surgery

c. Tension-side fracture and injuries spanning > 50% of neck: have a higher propagation rate and surgically treated with percutaneous screw fixation

5. Femoroacetabular impingement (FAI)

- Hip impingement syndrome secondary to abnormal contact between femur and acetabulum
- Demographic: young and middle-aged adults, leading to early-onset hip dysfunction, labral pathology, and secondary arthritis
- Three types of FAI: cam, pincer, and combined
  a. Cam: abnormality of the proximal femur including asymmetric femoral head, decreased femoral offset, abnormal head/neck ratio, and retroversion of femoral neck [secondary to old fracture or slipped capital femoral epiphysis (SCFE)]; seen in young athletes
  b. Pistol grip deformity is an irregularity of the contour of the superolateral femoral head/neck junction, indicating cam impingement
  c. Pincer: abnormality of the acetabulum from acetabular retroversion, acetabular protrusion ("protrusio acetabuli"), coxa profunda (deep acetabulum), and excess anterior-superior acetabular rim; seen in active middle-aged patients
  d. The crossover sign on X-ray indicates acetabular retroversion, seen in pincer impingement
  e. Combined: involvement of both the femur and acetabulum
- Presentation: activity-related groin pain, particular with deep hip flexion; can report mechanical symptoms; exam reveals limited hip flexion and internal rotation
  a. Positive anterior impingement test: reproduction of symptoms with flexion, adduction, and internal rotation
  b. Pathology: cam, pincer, or combined mechanisms resulting in labral pathology or chondral degeneration
     - Labral tears observed within the anterosuperior quadrant of the acetabulum
  c. Imaging: X-rays useful in assessment of proximal femur and acetabular anatomy
     - On anteroposterior (AP) views of the pelvis, evaluate for crossover sign, indicating acetabular retroversion and pincer impingement; assess for pistol-grip deformity of femoral neck/head, indicating cam impingement
     - False-profile view: important and frequently tested **(Fig. 8.4)**
       - ♦ Assesses the anterior acetabulum coverage for pincer impingement; performed with 65-degree angle between pelvis and X-ray cassette
     - Computed tomography (CT): to evaluate bony anatomy
     - MR arthrogram: to assess labrum
     - MRI: test of choice to evaluate tear location and pattern; use caution, as false-positive results are common
  d. Treatment
     - Conservative management: most successful for patients with minimal symptoms and no mechanical complaints
     - Surgical management: open or arthroscopic; open is considered gold standard; however, recent literature indicates similar results with arthroscopic procedures; surgery directed at correcting pathology
     - Cam: osteochondroplasty of femoral head/neck, possible femoral osteotomy
     - Pincer: osteochondroplasty of acetabular rim, labral debridement/repair

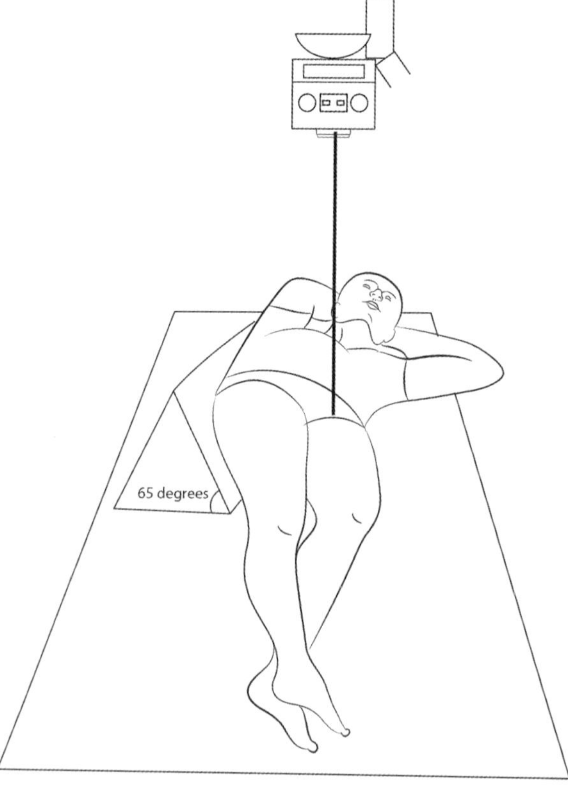

Fig. 8.4 Depiction of patient position and X-ray beam angle for obtaining false-profile radiographic view.

- For patients with significant arthritic changes, hip arthroplasty is indicated.

6. Hip nerve entrapment syndromes
   - Ilioinguinal nerve entrapment
     a. Pathology: hypertrophied abdominal muscles that results in hyperesthesia and pain
     b. Presentation: dysesthesia in groin; numbness exacerbated with hip hyperextension
     c. Treatment: conservative, stretching/activity modification; surgical release indicated if symptoms persist
   - Obturator nerve entrapment
     a. Pathology: adductor muscle hypertrophy, resulting in chronic medial thigh pain
     b. Nerve conduction studies can aid in diagnosis
     c. Treatment: conservative, stretching
   - Lateral femoral cutaneous nerve entrapment ("meralgia paresthetica")
     a. Presentation: pain and dysesthesia in the proximal lateral thigh; symptoms exacerbated with prolonged hip flexion and tight lap belts
     b. Treatment: conservative, stretching
   - Sciatic nerve entrapment
     a. Pathology: occurs at the level of the ischial tuberosity or the piriformis ("piriformis syndrome"), causing pain in the buttocks and posterior thigh
     b. Treatment: conservative, stretching; surgical release is rarely needed

E. Miscellaneous

1. Anterior superior iliac spine avulsion fractures
   - Demographic: adolescent athletes secondary to sudden contractions of sartorius or tensor fascia lata
   - Treatment: conservative, protected weight bearing
     a. Surgery considered in painful nonunions and displacement > 3 cm
2. Quadriceps contusion
   - Can result in intramuscular hemorrhage and carries a low risk of compartment syndrome
   - **Acute management requires icing and immobilization in flexion (120 degrees)**

II. Knee

A. Anatomy (Fig. 8.5)

1. Femoral condyles, both convex **(Fig. 8.6)**
   - Lateral: wider medial-lateral, projects more anteriorly
   - Medial: larger/more curved, projects more distally/posteriorly
2. Tibia plateau, 7- to 10-degree posterior slope
   - Medial: oval, larger, biconcave **(Fig. 8.7)**
   - Lateral: circular, smaller, convex (sagittal)/concave (coronal)
3. Proximal tibia
   - Tibial tubercle anterior, patellar tendon attachment
   - Gerdy's tubercle 2–3 cm lateral, insertion IT band
   - Joint capsule 1.5 cm below joint line at posterior recesses
   - **Fixator pins should not be within 15 mm of the joint due to the risk of being intracapsular.**

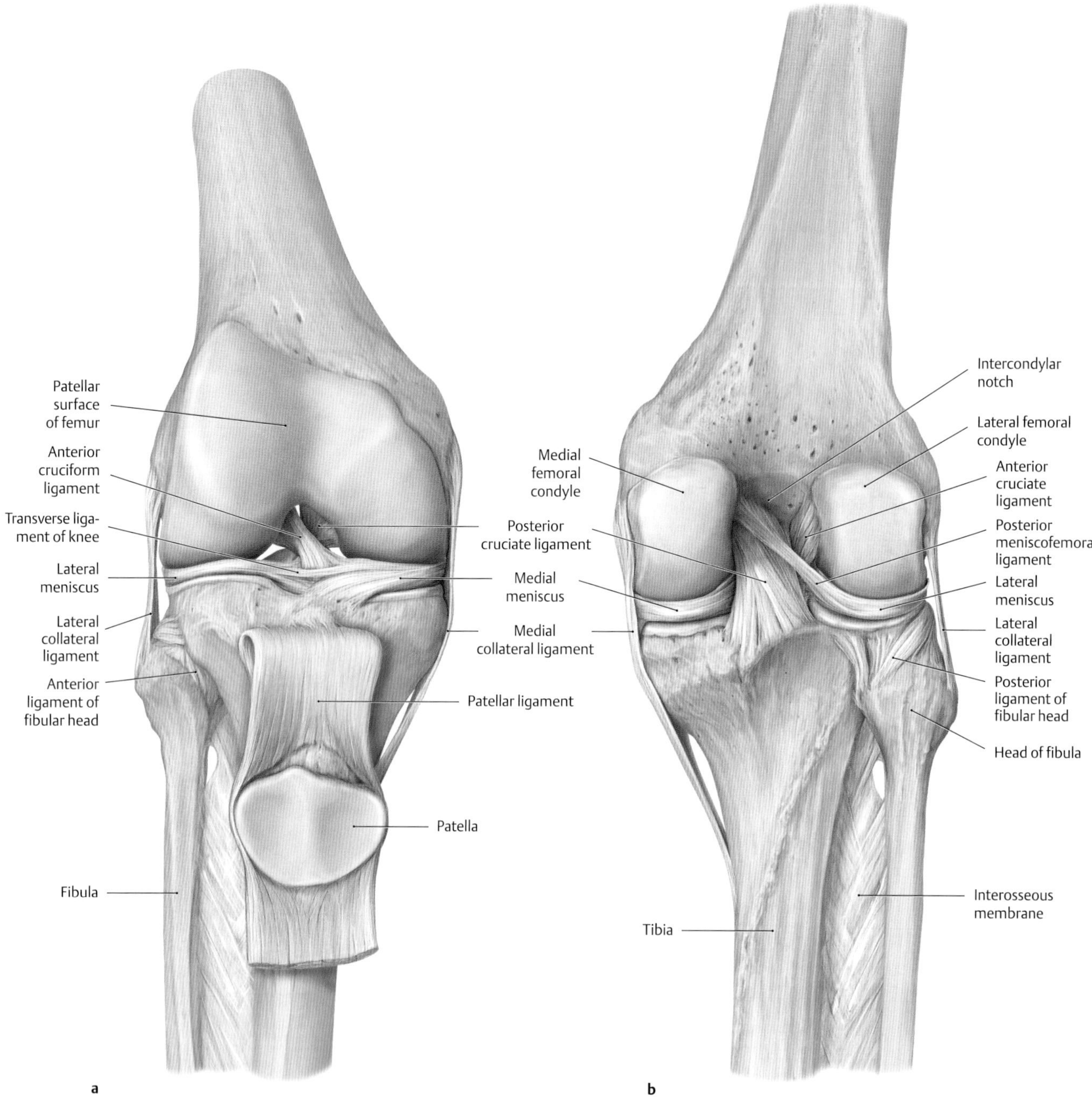

Fig. 8.5 Knee anatomy. **(a)** Anterior. **(b)** Posterior. (From Schuenke M, Schulte E. General Anatomy and the Musculoskeletal System: Thieme Atlas of Anatomy. New York: Thieme; 2005. Illustration by Karl Wesker.)

4. Proximal fibula
   - Proximal tibiofibular articulation distal to knee joint
   - Styloid process, attachment lateral knee stabilizers **(Fig. 8.8)**
     a. Insertions from anterior to posterior: lateral collateral ligament (LCL), popliteofibular ligament, biceps tendon
5. Patella, largest sesamoid, thickest cartilage (5 mm midportion)
   - Fulcrum to increase quadriceps strength, protective
   - Bipartite patella (superolateral), differentiate from fracture
6. Patellofemoral stabilizers
   - Conforming bony/cartilaginous anatomy **(Fig. 8.9)**

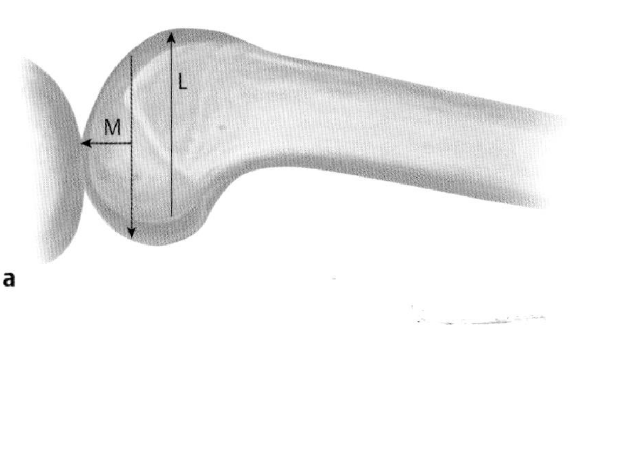

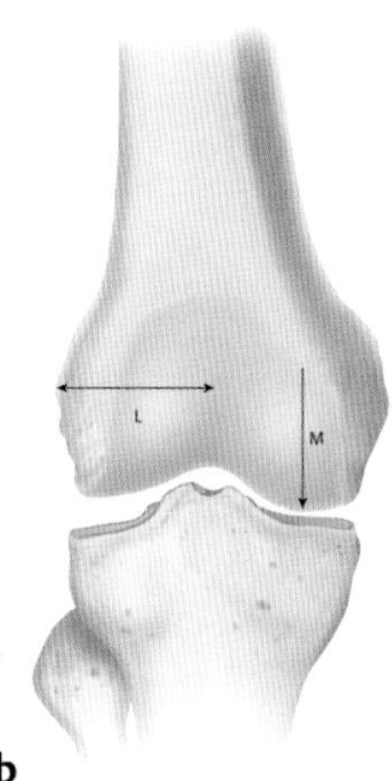

Fig. 8.6 Femoral condyle anatomy. **(a)** lateral view and **(b)** anteroposterior view. M refers to the dimensions of the medial condyle and L refers to the dimensions of lateral condyle.

Fig. 8.7 Differences in medial/lateral tibial plateau anatomy as demonstrated in axial view. **(a)** The medial plateau is larger, oval-shaped and biconcave. **(b)** The lateral plateau is smaller, circular and convex (sagittal)/concave (coronal).

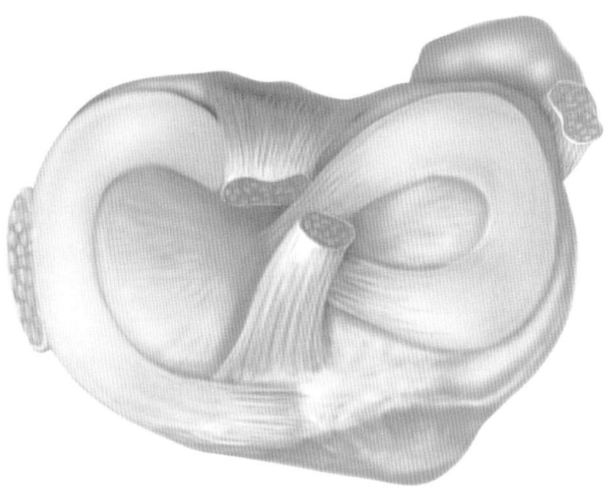

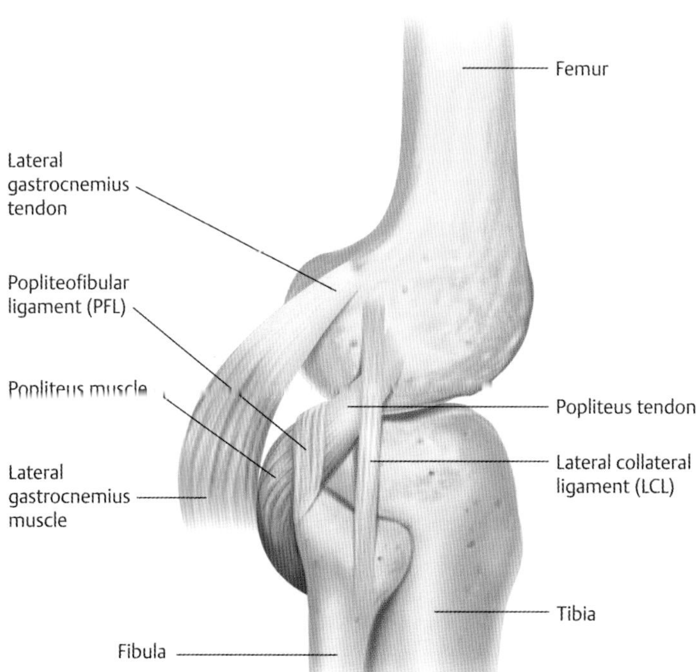

Fig. 8.8 Origin/insertions of the lateral knee stabilizers. (Modified from Schuenke M, Schulte E. General Anatomy and the Musculoskeletal System: Thieme Atlas of Anatomy. New York: Thieme; 2005. Illustration by Karl Wesker.)

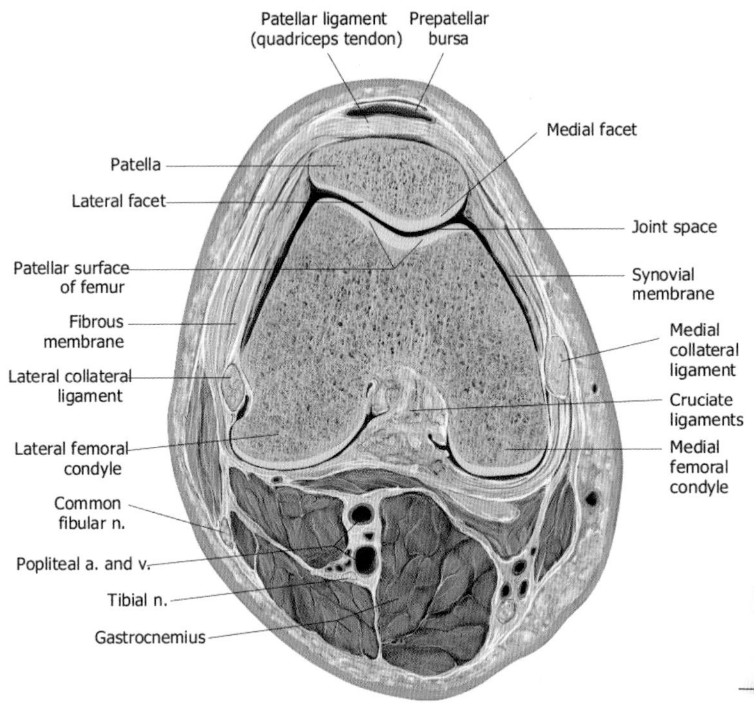

Fig. 8.9 Transverse section at the level of the patellofemoral joint. (From Schuenke M, Schulte E. General Anatomy and the Musculoskeletal System: Thieme Atlas of Anatomy. New York: Thieme; 2005. Illustration by Karl Wesker. Drawn from a specimen in the Anatomical Collection of Kiel University.)

- Retinaculum and extensor mechanism musculature
- Patellofemoral ligaments: medial patellofemoral ligament (MPFL) most important
- **Medial patellofemoral ligament provides > 50% of total medial restraint to lateral patellar instability.**
  a. Origin: intersection of point just anterior to posterior femoral shaft and proximal to Blumensaat's line **(Fig. 8.10)**, just anterior and distal to adductor magnus insertion, between medial epicondyle and adductor tubercle
  b. Inserts onto junction of upper and middle aspect of medial patella

7. Anterior cruciate ligament (ACL)
   - Attachment/insertion, dimensions **(Fig. 8.11)**
   - Bundles: anteromedial and posterolateral
   - **Anteromedial bundle tight in flexion; posterolateral bundle tight in extension**
     a. Anteromedial (AM): stronger, anterior tibial stability, tight in flexion
     b. Posterolateral (PL): rotatory stability, tight in extension
        - Isolated AM tear: increased anterior translation at 90 degrees' flexion
        - Isolated PL tear: increased anterior tibial translation and rotatory instability at 30 degrees' knee flexion
   - Native strength: 2,200 N (maximum tension in full knee extension)
8. Posterior cruciate ligament (PCL)
   - Attachment/insertion, dimensions **(Fig. 8.12)**
   - Bundles: anterolateral and posteromedial
   - **Bundles are opposite those of the ACL.**

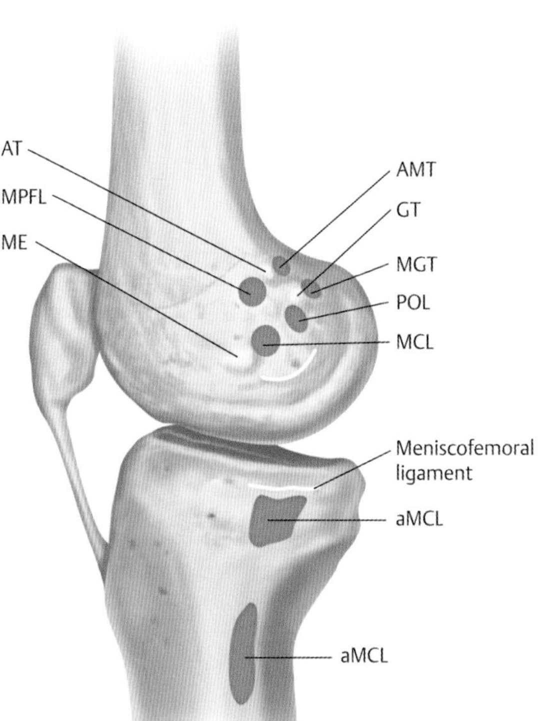

Fig. 8.10 **(a)** Depiction of medial patellofemoral ligament (MPFL) insertion at the intersection of a point just anterior to the posterior femoral shaft and proximal to Blumensaat's line. **(b)** Other relevant anatomy of the medial knee. aMCL, anterior medial collateral ligament. AMT, adductor magnus tendon; AT, adductor tubercle; GT, gastrocnemius tubercle; MCL, medial collateral ligament; ME. medial epicondyle; MGT, medial gastrocnemius tendon; POL, posterior oblique ligament.

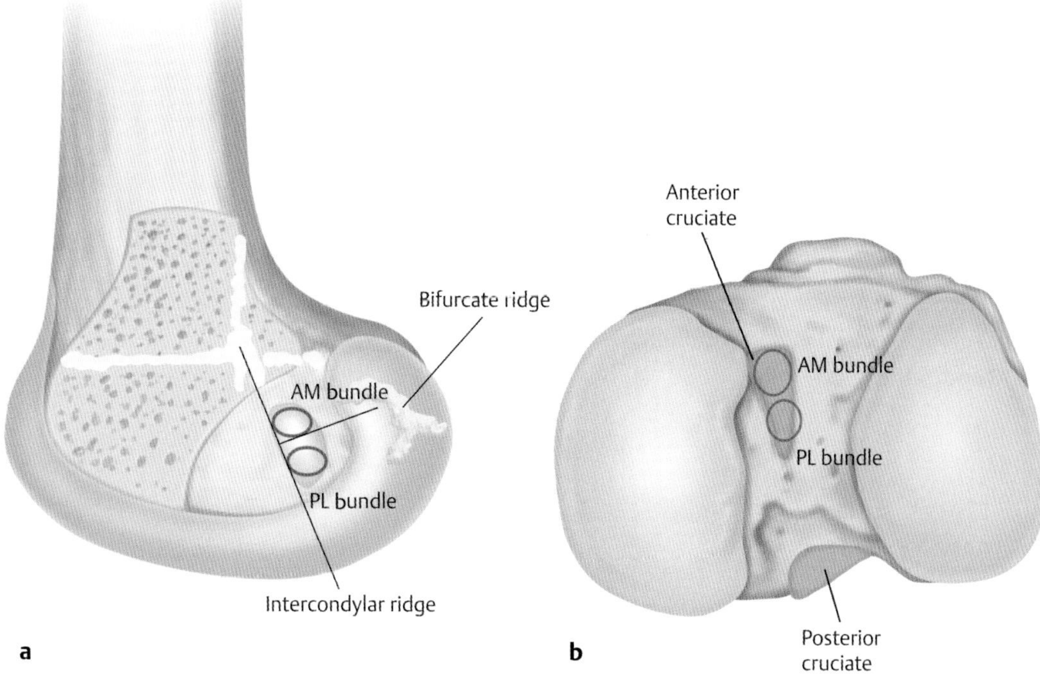

Fig. 8.11 (a,b) Anterior cruciate ligament anatomy: footprint dimensions and bundle origins/insertions. AM, anteromedial; PL, posterolateral.

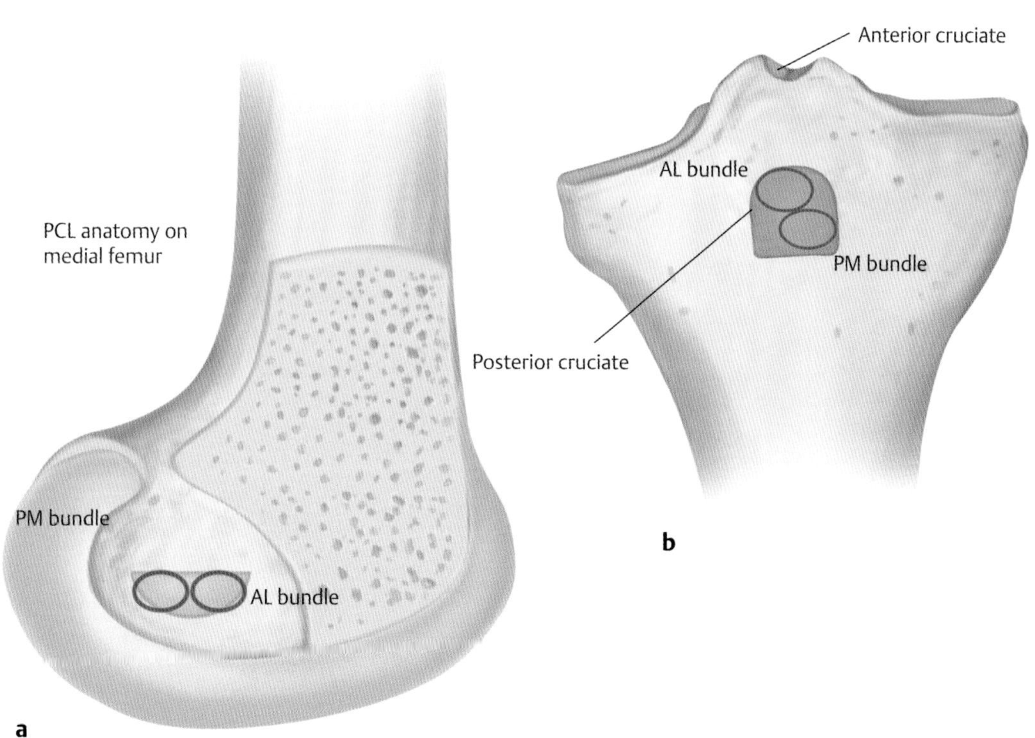

Fig. 8.12 (a,b) Posterior cruciate ligament (PCL) anatomy: footprint dimensions and bundle origins/insertions. AL, anterolateral; PM, posteromedial.

a. Anterolateral (AL): posterior tibial stability, tight in flexion (reconstruct this in single bundle reconstruction)

b. Posteromedial (PM): rotatory stability

- Strength: 2,500–3,000 N

9. Common ACL/PCL characteristics
   - **Anterior bundles: tight in flexion; posterior bundles: tight in extension**
   - Both secondary stabilizers to knee varus/valgus stress
   - Composition: 90% type I, 10% type III collagen
   - Vascular supply: primarily middle genicular artery
   - Innervation: tibial (sciatic) nerve (posterior articular branch)
10. Medial stabilizers **(Fig. 8.13** and **Table 8.3)**

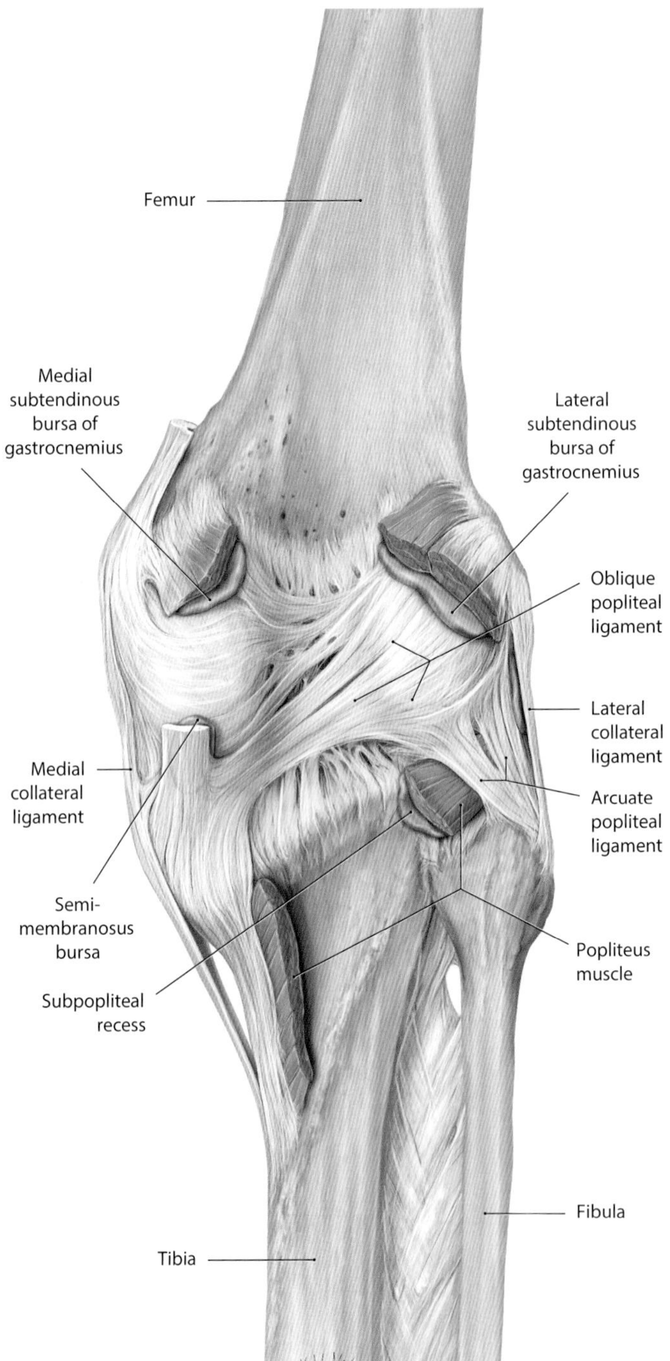

Fig. 8.13 Medial and lateral posterior knee stabilizers. (From Schuenke M, Schulte E. General Anatomy and the Musculoskeletal System: Thieme Atlas of Anatomy. New York: Thieme; 2005. Illustration by Karl Wesker.)

Table 8.3 Medial Knee Layers/Dynamic Stabilizers

Medial layer	
I	Sartorial/vastus medialis fascia
II	Superficial MCL, posterior oblique ligament, semimembranosus, MPFL
III	Deep MCL and capsule
Dynamic stabilizers	Semimembranosus, gracilis, semitendinosus, sartorius, vastus medialis
PMC	Posterior oblique ligament (originates from adductor tubercle), oblique popliteal ligament (posterior capsular thickening, continuous with deep MCL), semimembranosus (multiple tendinous insertions)

Abbreviations: MCL, medial collateral ligament; MPFL: medial patellofemoral ligament; PMC, posteromedial corner.

- Three anatomic layers of medial knee; static and dynamic stabilizer of medial collateral ligament (MCL)
  a. Superficial MCL**:** vertical sheet, deep to pes anserinus that originates 3 mm proximal and 5 mm posterior to medial femoral epicondyle; inserts distal to joint line (4–6 cm)
    - Primary function valgus stability; anterior portion tight in flexion, posterior tight in extension
  b. Deep MCL: capsular thickening with meniscofemoral and meniscotibial components
- Posteromedial corner (PMC) components **(Table 8.3)**
  a. Function: internal knee rotatory stability

11. Lateral stabilizers **(Fig. 8.13** and **Table 8.4)**
- Lateral (or fibular) collateral ligament (LCL)
  a. Cord like structure; 3–4 mm in diameter, 6 cm in length
  b. Varus knee stabilizer; isolate at 30 degrees' flexion; also secondary anterior-posterior stabilizer (along with MCL)
- Other lateral stabilizers **(Fig. 8.8)**
  a. Three anatomic layers of lateral knee; static and dynamic stabilizers
  b. Popliteus: internal rotator of tibia
    - Originates posterior tibia; inserts anterior, inferior, and deep to LCL origin
    - Intra-articular segment passes through popliteal hiatus (posterolateral aspect of lateral meniscus)
    - Popliteofibular ligament branches off popliteus

Table 8.4 Lateral Knee Layers/Dynamic Stabilizers

Lateral layer	
I	Iliotibial band, long head biceps femoris, fascia
II	Lateral patellar retinaculum/patellofemoral ligament
III	LCL, fabellofibular ligament, arcuate/coronary ligaments, popliteus tendon/popliteofibular ligament, capsule
Dynamic stabilizers	Long head biceps, popliteus, iliotibial band, lateral gastrocnemius
PLC components	Popliteus/popliteofibular ligament, long head biceps femoris, lateral capsule, iliotibial band, fabellofibular ligament, arcuate ligament

Abbreviations: LCL, medial collateral ligament; PLC, posterior lateral corner.

- Posterolateral corner (PLC) components **(Table 8.4)**
  a. Function: external knee rotatory stability

12. Menisci
  - Crescents, triangularly shaped in cross section
  - Connected anteriorly via intermeniscal ligament, peripherally by coronary ligaments
  - Variably present meniscofemoral ligaments (MFLs), 70%
    a. Ligament of Humphrey (anterior to PCL), ligament of Wrisberg (posterior to PCL), originate on posterior horn, insert into medial femoral condyle/PCL
  - Meniscal fiber types (circumferential, radial, and oblique)
    a. Circumferential most abundant, dissipates hoop stress
    b. Fibrocartilaginous material, primarily type I collagen
  - Vascular supply (genicular arteries)
    a. Peripheral third well-vascularized (red zone), middle third relatively avascular (red-white zone), inner third nonvascular (white zone; nourishment by diffusion) **(Fig. 8.14)**
      - Posterior horns fed by middle genicular artery
      - Posterolateral meniscus at the popliteal hiatus has minimal to no vascular supply

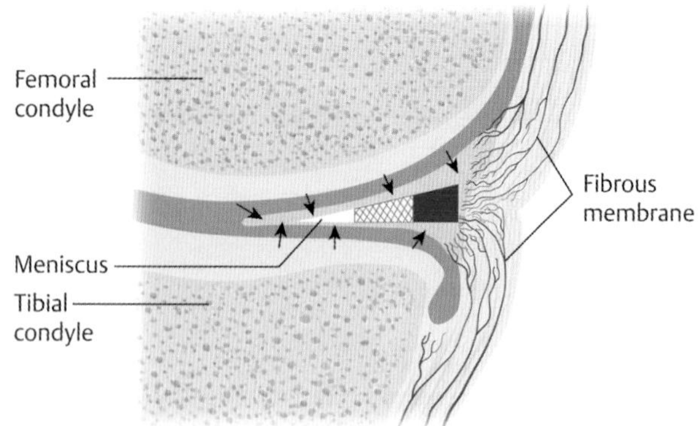

Fig. 8.14 Medial and lateral menisci dimensions. Blood supply to the menisci divided into the outermost/highly vascular **(a)** red–red, **(b)** red–white, and the innermost/avascular **(c)** white–white zones. Arrows indicate joint forces. (Modified from Schuenke M, Schulte E. General Anatomy and the Musculoskeletal System: Thieme Atlas of Anatomy. New York: Thieme; 2005. Illustration by Karl Wesker.)

  - Medial versus lateral meniscus **(Fig. 8.15)**
    a. Dimensions
      - Medial: C-shaped, less mobile (5 mm), more soft tissue attachments/joint conformity
      - Lateral: circular, broader, more mobile (11 mm), fewer soft tissue attachments
    b. Vascular supply
      - o Medial: peripheral 20–30%
      - o Lateral: peripheral 10–25%
  - Function/biomechanics
    a. Decrease knee joint contact pressure by increasing area; enhances knee stability and deepens joint concavity
    b. Resists tensile hoop stresses associated with weight bearing
  - **Medial meniscus becomes secondary restraint to anterior tibial translation in ACL-deficient knee**

B. Knee Musculature and Innervation (Table 8.5)

C. Physical Examination of the Knee (Table 8.6)

D. Knee Open Surgical Approaches

1. MPFL/medial ligament complex approach
   - Superficial interval: sartorius (femoral nerve) and medial patellar retinaculum
   - Deep: semimembranosus (sciatic nerve) and MCL
2. Hamstring graft harvest/open medial meniscal repair approach
   - Tendon orientation: gracilis/semitendinosus run obliquely across MCL deep to sartorial fascia (between medial layers I and II)
   - Saphenous neurovascular bundle at risk
     a. Sartorial branch anterior to semitendinosus during knee extension; infrapatellar branch continues to anteromedial knee

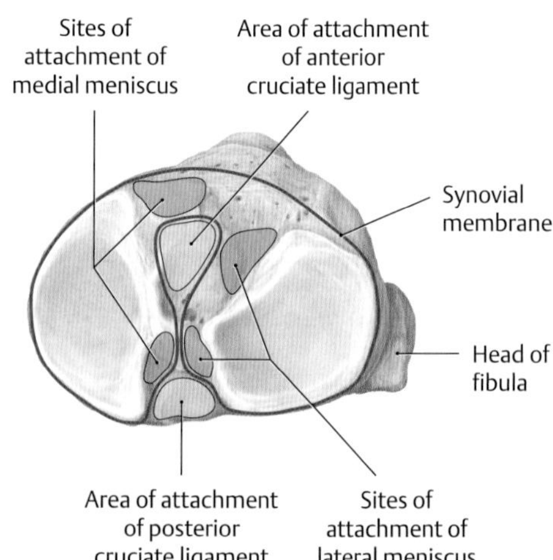

Fig. 8.15 The sites of attachment of the menisci and cruciate ligaments. (From Schuenke M, Schulte E. General Anatomy and the Musculoskeletal System: Thieme Atlas of Anatomy. New York: Thieme; 2005. Illustration by Karl Wesker.)

Table 8.5 Table Muscles about the Knee

	Origin	Insertion	Innervation	Action at Knee
Anterior thigh				
Vastus lateralis	Lateral linea aspera	Lateral patella	Femoral	Knee extension
Vastus medialis	Medial linea aspera	Medial patella	Femoral	Knee extension[2]
Vastus intermedius	Anterior/proximal femur	Patella	Femoral	Knee extension
Posterior thigh				
Biceps long head	Medial ischial tuberosity	Proximal fibula	Tibial	Knee flexion[1]
Biceps short head	Distal lateral linea aspera	Lateral tibial condyle	Peroneal	Knee flexion
Semimembranosus	Proximal/lateral ischial tuberosity	Multiple insertions[3]	Tibial	Knee flexion[2]
Semitendinosus	Distal/medial ischial tuberosity	Pes anserinus deep/distal	Tibial	Knee flexion[2]
Medial thigh				
Gracilis	Inferior public arch	Pes anserinus deep/proximal	Obturator	Medial stability
Sartorius	Anterior superior iliac spine	Pes anserinus superficial	Femoral	Medial stability
Anterior thigh				
Iliotibial band (tensor fascia lata)	Anterior iliac crest	Gerdy's tubercle	Superior gluteal	Knee flexion[1,4]
Posterior calf				
Lateral/medial Gastrocnemius	Posterior femoral condyles (medial/lateral)	Calcaneus	Tibial	Knee flexion[1,2]
Popliteus	Lateral femoral condyle[5]	Proximal/posterior tibia	Tibial	Internal rotation of tibia[1]

[1]Also contributes to dynamic lateral knee stability.
[2]Also contributes to medial knee stability.
[3]Insertions include posterior oblique ligament, posterior capsule, posterior-medial tibia, popliteus and medial meniscus.
[4]Iliotibial band also extends knee at < 20–30 degrees knee flexion.
[5]Popliteofibular ligament attaches popliteus to proximal fibula.

b. Horizontal incision, knee flexion/hip internal rotation decreases risk of nerve damage (relaxes structures)

3. LCL/popliteus/PLC complex/open lateral meniscal repair approach
   - Interval: IT band (superficial gluteal nerve) and long head of biceps femoris (sciatic), retract lateral gastrocnemius posteriorly
   - Common peroneal nerve at risk, runs along posterior border biceps between lateral layers I and II; inferolateral geniculate artery runs between lateral gastrocnemius and posterolateral knee capsule
4. Patellar tendon graft/tibial tubercle approach (midline anterior)
   - Structures at risk: terminal branches of infrapatellar branch saphenous nerve, results in anesthesia lateral to incision
5. Posterior knee/PCL
   - Small saphenous vein important landmark during incision
   - Remember to stay medial to avoid medial sural cutaneous nerve
   - Popliteal vessels/tibial nerve run between heads of gastrocnemius

E. Knee Arthroscopy

1. Gold standard for diagnosis of intra-articular knee pathology (versus open)
2. Small incisions, low morbidity, rapid recovery, better visualization
3. Portals **(Fig. 8.16)**
   - Inferomedial/inferolateral: standard working portals
     a. Just below and adjacent to patella; perform in flexion

Table 8.6 Physical Examination of the Knee

Test Name	Technique	Importance
Anterior cruciate ligament (ACL)		
Lachman	Anterior tibial translation 30 degrees of knee flexion	ACL tear (most sensitive)
Pivot shift	Valgus/internal rotation, extension to flexion	ACL tear (most specific)
Posterior cruciate ligament (PCL)		
Posterior drawer	Posterior tibial translation 90 degrees of knee flexion	PCL tear
Reverse pivot	Valgus/external rotation, flexion to extension	PCL tear
Tibial sag	Posterior translation 90 degrees of knee flexion	PCL tear
Quadriceps active	Sag improves with quadriceps fire	PCL tear
Meniscus		
Joint line palpation	Tenderness upon palpation of medial/lateral joint line	Meniscal injury
McMurray (medial)	Full knee flexion to extension while externally rotating leg (valgus knee force)	Medial meniscal injury (pain or click)
McMurray (lateral)	Full knee flexion to extension while internally rotating leg (varus knee force)	Lateral meniscal injury (pain or click)
Apley	McMurray technique, prone/90 degrees of knee flexion	Meniscal injury, or arthritis
Medial collateral ligament (MCL)/lateral collateral ligament (LCL)/posterolateral corner (PLC)		
Varus/valgus stress at 30 degrees	Medial/lateral joint opening at 30 degrees of knee flexion	MCL/LCL injury
Varus/valgus stress at 0 degrees	Medial/lateral joint opening in full extension	MCL/LCL, and ACL or PCL injury
Dial at 30 degrees	Prone, increased external rotation compared with uninjured side (> 10 degrees)	PLC injury
Dial at 90 degrees	Prone, increased external rotation compared with uninjured side (> 10 degrees)	PCL tear
Patellar		
Apprehension	Lateral push at 20–30 degrees of knee flexion	Discomfort, stability concerns
Crepitus	Palpating crepitus with passive range of motion	Patellofemoral pathology
Grind	Posterior force with active knee extension	Patellofemoral pathology
Glide	Passive push laterally at 20–30 degrees of knee flexion, normal translation of two quadrants	Lateral patellar instability (if translates three or more quadrants)

  b. Transverse portals decrease risk of infrapatellar saphenous nerve injury
- Superolateral/medial for accessory work, uncommonly inflow
  a. Perform in extension
  b. Other accessory portals
    - Accessory posteromedial: 1 cm behind MCL; saphenous nerve/vein at risk
    - Accessory posterolateral: between LCL and biceps (as above, lateral approach)
    - Transpatellar: 1 cm below inferior pole patella, central access
    - Low anteromedial medial (for ACL reconstruction) and far medial or lateral for loose body removal, etc.

4. Diagnostic technique: perform complete examination
   - Evaluate posteromedially through notch utilizing Gillquist maneuver, 70-degree scope can aid in visualization; interval between PCL and medial femoral condyle
   - Avoid iatrogenic cartilage damage (number one complication), infection, instrument breakage

- Popliteal artery lies anterior to vein, 9 mm from posterior tibial plateau in 90 degrees of knee flexion

F. Knee Pathology

1. ACL injury
   - Diagnosis of ACL tear may be subtle, and therefore a high index of suspicion must be maintained.
   - Mechanism: usually sports-related injury; noncontact, hyperextension, deceleration; often audible "pop"
     a. Direct blow less common
   - Demographics: female > male (2–10:1)
     a. Number one risk factor: altered neuromuscular control and landing biomechanics, especially greater dynamic valgus; but ACL injury has many proposed etiologies, such as higher quadriceps relative to hamstring activation
     b. Presentation: acute pain, swelling (> 70%) and "giving way"; acute effusion (hemarthrosis); both anterior and rotational laxity
        - Lachman test (most sensitive): anterior tibial translation with femur held fixed at 20–30 degrees of knee flexion
        - Pivot shift (most specific): internal rotation and valgus tibial stress from full knee extension to 30–40 degrees of flexion
          - ♦ Positive when anteriorly subluxed tibia reduces, most discernible under anesthesia
        - Perform dial test to rule out posterolateral corner injuries
   - Imaging/supplementary tests
     a. X-ray: Segond fracture-lateral tibial capsular avulsion (meniscotibial ligament); pathognomonic for ACL tear
        - Tibial avulsion fracture rare, pediatric population
     b. MRI: not required but can confirm diagnosis, especially in subtle cases and assess concomitant pathology (see Associated injuries, below)
     c. KT-1000/2000 arthrometers: anterior force (30 lb) in 20–30 degrees of knee flexion
        - > 3 mm difference significant (versus normal side)
   - Associated injuries
     a. Trabecular microfractures ("bone bruise") in > 50%
        - Located at posterolateral tibial plateau and mid-aspect lateral femoral condyle (sulcus terminalis)
        - **Trabecular bone bruising pattern corresponds to initial "pivot shift" during injury**
     b. Meniscal tear (in up to 70%)
        - Lateral tears most common for acute ACL tears, often repairable
        - Medial tears (degenerative posterior horn, usually unrepairable) typical from chronic ACL injury, as meniscus recruited for translational restraint
     c. Differentiate from osteochondral fracture or patella fracture/dislocation, quadriceps/patellar ruptures
        - Some similar signs/symptoms
   - Treatment
     a. Initial management: physical therapy (PT)/mobilization to achieve full ROM, effusion resolution, normal gait
     b. Individualized based on age, activity level, instability, associated injuries/comorbidities

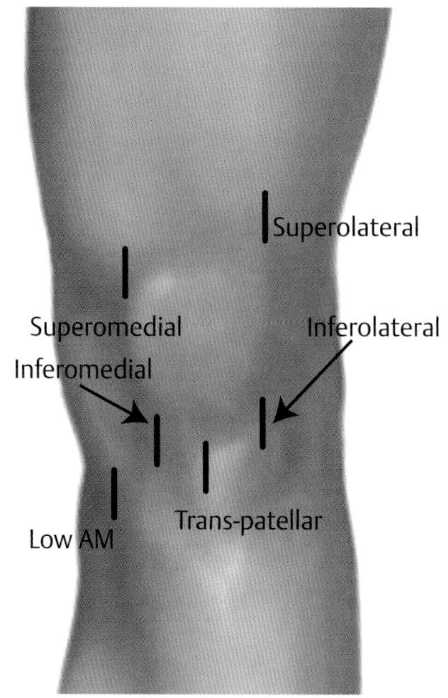

Fig. 8.16 Knee arthroscopy portal locations. AM, anteromedial.

c. Conservative management
   - Indications: isolated ACL injury, relatively asymptomatic, sedentary or low activity level
   - Rehabilitation: similar to operative (below), emphasize hamstring strengthening, proprioceptive training, bracing controversial

d. Surgical management:
   - Indications: symptomatic instability, particularly competitive/recreational athletes to improve function and avoid secondary injury
   - Contraindications: quadriceps dysfunction, medically unstable, significant osteoarthritis
   - Surgical technique: ligament reconstruction with anatomic single-bundle (currently most commonly performed)
     - Separate low anteromedial portal for femoral tunnel drilling
     - Horizontal graft placement (2 or 10 o'clock position) in center of anatomic footprint
     - Versus transtibial drilling, tendency for vertical graft placement (12 o'clock position)
     - Tension all strands equally at 30 degrees' flexion
     - Double-bundle (less commonly performed)
       - Separate AM/PL bundles/tunnels
       - Improved biomechanical testing results, but currently not significantly improved clinical outcomes from anatomic single bundle

e. Graft selection—autograft
   - Bone–patellar tendon–bone (BTB) autgraft
     - Choice for young contact/pivoting athlete
     - Strong; 10-mm BTB 2,900 N (versus 2,200 N native ACL)
     - Quickest return to athletics, bone-to-bone healing
     - Higher incidence anterior knee pain (especially kneeling)/loss terminal extension (versus hamstring)
     - Rare risk patella fracture/tendon rupture and infrapatellar contraction syndrome (global stiffness)
   - Quadrupled hamstring autograft (looped gracilis and semitendinosus)
     - Greatest maximal strength (up to 4,000 N) versus native ACL, 10-mm BTB or 10-mm quadriceps graft
     - **Quadrupled hamstring autograft has greatest maximal strength, though clinically equivalent outcomes.**
     - Semitendinosus stronger than gracilis
     - Bone in-growth into tendon limiting factor
     - Increased failures versus BTB in young athletes
   - Overall similar clinical success with various autografts
   - Allografts
     - Good outcomes in older/revision patients
     - Increased failure rate shown in young, active patients
     - Infection/immune risk
       - HIV risk is 1:1.6 million (not eliminated with standard 3 Mrad dose, and higher dose compromises strength)
       - *Clostridium difficile* reported within past 20 years; hepatitis B, tuberculosis, HIV all reported more than 20 years ago
       - Routine preimplantation culturing not useful
       - Antigenicity highest for bone plug grafts

f. Rehabilitation
  - Early physical therapy:
    - 0–90 degrees in 2 weeks, minimize immobilization; aspirate persistent postoperative hemarthrosis, no open-chain exercises
  - Graduated strengthening/endurance (2 weeks to 3 months)
    - Early co-contraction/closed chain (fixed distal extremity) exercises; compressive/predictable forces; protect healing graft
      - Lowest strain during isometric hamstring contractions at 60 degrees of knee flexion
    - Open-chain exercises introduced at 6 weeks (avoid any earlier), high shear forces with terminal knee movements 0- to 60-degree
    - Running and sports-specific after 3–4 months
      - Include eccentric strengthening/functional exercises
    - Return to sports at 6–12 months
      - Requires strength return ≥ 80% versus normal side
    - Postoperative bracing controversial (benefits skiers)

- Outcomes
  a. Clinical outcomes generally excellent
    - 75–97% < 3 mm on KT-1000 (versus normal side), two thirds of patients return to preinjury levels, half return competitively
    - **Elimination of pivot shift postoperatively correlates with positive outcomes.**
- Complications
  a. Graft failure (2–5%): over two thirds due to aberrant tunnel/hardware placement **(Fig. 8.17a)**
    - Number one error: anterior femoral tunnel placement; limited flexion, graft stretch (need clear visualization of posterior notch)
    - Vertical or nonanatomic graft placement on the femur
    - Tibial tunnel: too anterior leads to notch impingement; too posterior leads to PCL impingement
      - Failure to place tibial tunnel posterior to Blumensaat's line, causes extension impingement
    - Femoral tunnel: too anterior is tight in flexion, loose in extension; too posterior is tight in extension
    - Overly divergent interference screws > 15–30 degrees associated with poor fixation
  b. Instability or stiffness
    - Vertical graft limits rotational stability, especially with cutting movements (pivot shift positive postoperatively) **(Fig. 8.17b)**
    - Cyclops lesion: anterior scarring limits extension
    - ACL (ganglion) cyst rare cause of pain/loss motion; MRI for diagnosis; may require debridement
    - Arthrofibrosis: early, aggressive rehabilitation key
  c. Deep infection: < 1%; aspirate if any suspicion
  d. Bone–tendon–bone harvest from patella can lead to fracture 8–12 weeks postoperative
  e. Hamstring harvest can damage saphenous nerve (anterior to gracilis, between gracilis and sartorius)
- Pediatric ACL injury considerations
  a. Increased incidence due to sports participation and awareness
  b. Skeletal maturity influences treatment (techniques controversial)

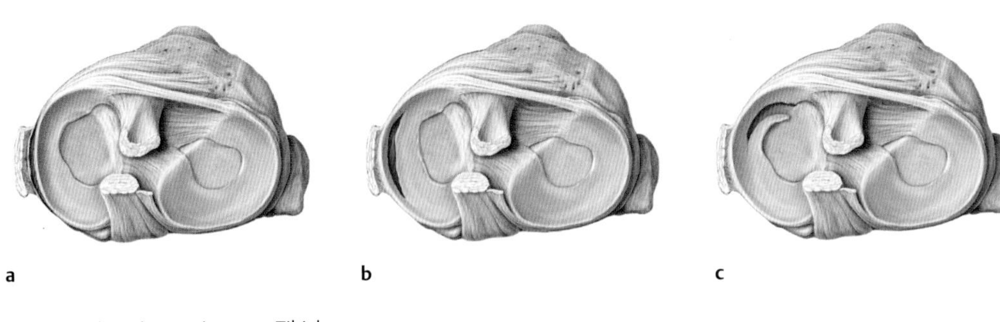

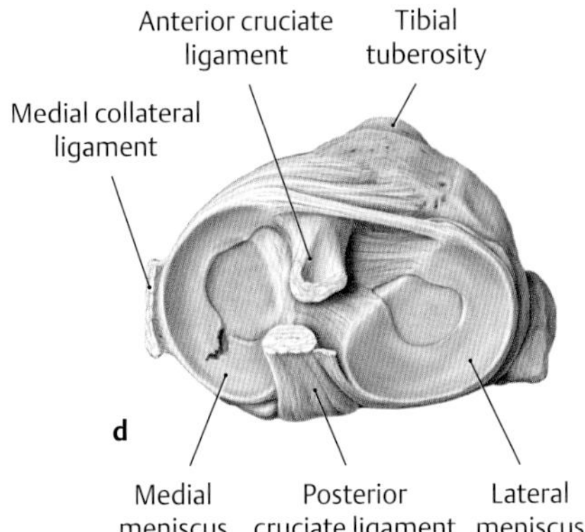

Fig. 8.17 Different patterns of meniscal tears. Right tibial plateau, proximal view. **(a)** Peripheral tear. **(b)** Bucket-handle tear. **(c)** Longitudinal or flap tear of the anterior horn. **(d)** Radial tear of the posterior horn.

c. Tanner stages I and II: physical sparing techniques recommended

d. Tanner stages III and IV: various transphyseal techniques with excellent results, no significant growth disturbances

- Prevention
  a. Neuromuscular control/proprioceptive regimens may be effective (especially for female athletes); minimum 6 weeks plyometrics/knee flexor exercises
  b. No proven scientific protocols available to reduce reinjury risk

2. PCL injury
- Mechanism: anterior force on hyperflexed (dashboard) or extended knee; fall onto flexed knee with plantar-flexed foot
- Presentation: pain, swelling, less often instability (versus ACL)
  a. Posterior drawer test (most accurate): posterior tibial translation at 90 degrees of knee flexion; increased external rotation at 90 degrees (dial test)
- Imaging: X-ray/CT scan may reveal posterior tibial avulsion fracture
  a. Chronic PCL deficiency is associated with medial compartment/patellofemoral arthritis
  b. MRI: confirmatory, and assesses concomitant pathology
- Classification: based on degree of posterior subluxation of tibia on femur (normal: 1 cm at medial tibial plateau) at 90 degrees
  a. Grade I: isolated PCL, tibia remains anterior (to the femoral condyle)
  b. Grade II: isolated PCL, tibia in line with femur
  c. Grade III: often multiligamentous injury, tibia posterior to femur
- Treatment
  a. Initial: PT/mobilization to achieve full range of motion, effusion resolution, normal gait (similar to ACL)
  b. Conservative management: indicted for most isolated grade I–II tears
  c. Surgical management: for persistent instability, grade III or combined injuries

- Transtibial reconstruction technique: 180-degree "killer turn," possible graft attenuation/damage
- Tibial inlay: risks injury to popliteal vessels and tibial nerve, but avoids "killer turn"
- Single bundle construct reconstructs AL bundle, and should be tensioned at 90 degrees (double bundle tension AM bundle at 30 degrees of flexion)
- Achilles allograft typically used

d. Rehabilitation: immediate active extension 0 to 90 degrees (quadriceps protective); no active knee flexion until graft healed

- **Quadriceps strengthening is the number one factor in protecting the graft.**

- Outcomes: often greater residual postoperative laxity (versus ACL); address concomitant ligament injuries

3. Meniscal injury

- Most common knee injury requiring surgery
- Pathology: acute traumatic tears in young; degenerative tears in older individuals

a. Medial > lateral (3:1): lateral associated with horizontal cleavage tear and cysts (middle third) and discoid meniscus

b. Lateral more common with acute ACL tears

c. Posterior horn medial more common in chronic ACL-deficient knee

- Presentation: subacute swelling, pain/locking with flexion (posterior horn tear) or extension (anterior horn); effusion; positive joint line tenderness

d. Positive McMurray: palpable pop or pain over joint line while flexing/extending and rotating the tibia on the femur, along with a varus or valgus stress, pinching the meniscus in the affected compartment)

- Imaging: X-rays negative
- MRI is utilized to confirm physical exam
- **"Double PCL sign": bucket-handle tear medial meniscus**
- T2 MRI images may reveal parameniscal cyst (synovial fluid collection adjacent to meniscus) or Baker's cyst (fluid collection between semimembranosus and medial gastrocnemius muscles)

- Classification **(Fig. 8.17b)**
- Treatment

a. Conservative management: PT, strengthening for asymptomatic tears, especially degenerative tears

b. Surgical management: bucket-handle tears/locked knee, mechanical symptoms (catching/locking), failure of conservative management, cruciate injury

- Partial meniscectomy for tears that cannot be repaired
  - Goal: minimal resection, stable contour
  - Symptomatic Baker's cysts resolve after meniscectomy
- Meniscal repair for peripheral/longitudinal tears in red zone (peripheral), and for younger patients
  - Concomitant ACL tear and synovial rasping; trephination augments healing
  - Large acute peripheral bucket-handle tears often repairable

- **Gold standard is the inside-out vertical mattress, but the all-inside method is increasingly popular.**

- Superior outcomes when done in conjunction with ACL reconstruction

- Allograft transplantation
  a. Option for younger patients requiring total to near-total meniscectomy
  b. Utilize bone plugs, typically fresh frozen
    - **Meniscus graft size must match native meniscus within 5–10%. This is the number one factor relating to success.**
    - Requires intact ACL/PCL, normal axial alignment to preserve graft
    - Contraindications: advanced (grade III–IV) osteoarthritis or inflammatory arthritis
- Outcomes: increased osteoarthritis observed with tear with or without meniscectomy; increased contact pressure proportional to amount excised
- Discoid (lateral) meniscus
  a. Presentation: may be asymptomatic or cause pain or mechanical symptoms
  b. Imaging
    - X-ray: widened lateral joint space, lateral femoral condyle squaring, lateral plateau cupping
    - MRI: three or more contiguous 5-mm sagittal slices with meniscus still in continuity; "bow-tie" sign
  c. Treatment: observe if asymptomatic; arthroscopic meniscectomy
    - Saucerization or repair if symptomatic (and peripheral)
  d. Complications
    - Meniscal repair: medial approach can injure saphenous nerve (stay anterior to sartorius); lateral approach can injure peroneal nerve, popliteal artery (stay anterior to biceps)

4. MCL injury
- Mechanism: sudden valgus stress; injured most often on femoral side
  a. Most commonly injured knee ligament
- Presentation: pain or instability with valgus stress at 30 degrees
  a. Valgus instability at full extension indicates posteromedial capsular and cruciate injury (isolate collateral by flexing to 30 degrees)
  b. Effusion large for grade II injuries but may be minimal for grade III due to fluid extravasation through capsular tear
    - A distinction between medial meniscal pathology and MCL injury is that there is often no effusion with MCL injury but considerable extra-articular swelling.
  c. Imaging
    - X-rays: medial joint space widening; "Pellegrini-Stieda" lesion is sign of chronic tear, with calcification at femoral origin; stress views can differentiate physeal injury
    - MRI: location/extent injury, concomitant pathology
- Classification **(Table 8.7)**
- Treatment
  a. Conservative management
    - Grade I/II or III injuries that are stable in extension, with no associated cruciate injury
    - Progressive ROM in hinged knee brace; quadriceps and straight leg raise exercises
    - Better healing with proximal/midsubstance tears
      - ♦ Use caution and monitor closely as proximal medial collateral ligament injuries can frequently result in stiffness.
    - Prophylactic bracing effective in preventing MCL injuries (e.g., football offensive linemen)
  b. Surgical management

Table 8.7 Collateral Ligament Injury Classification

Medial Collateral Ligament (MCL)/Lateral Collateral Ligament (LCL) Injury Grade[1]	Findings
I (mild)	1–5 mm
II (moderate)	6–10 mm
III (severe)[2]	> 10 mm

[1]Laxity versus normal side.
[2]Gross laxity with lack of end point.

- Rare; indicated for persistently unstable grade III MCL tears or if valgus laxity in full extension also present (concomitant cruciate or capsular injury with posteromedial instability)
- Ligament can become entrapped in joint or have tissue interposed ("Stener lesion"), requiring repair
- Acute avulsions can be reattached with suture anchors versus direct repair of midsubstance tears, may require posterior oblique ligament (POL) advancement
- Chronic injuries or injuries that cannot be repaired are reconstructed with autograft (e.g., semitendinosus).

5. LCL injury
   - Mechanism: sudden varus stress; isolated injury rare
   - Presentation: pain or instability with varus stress at 30 degrees (isolates LCL)
     a. Varus instability at full extension indicates concomitant cruciate or posterolateral capsular injury
   - Imaging
     a. X-rays: lateral joint space widening
     b. MRI: to assess injury pattern
   - Classification **(Table 8.7)**
   - Treatment
     a. Conservative management: isolated partial injuries; PT
     b. Surgical management: complete ruptures and combined injuries; acute repair or chronic reconstruction
6. Posterolateral corner (PLC) injury
   - Mechanism: knee hyperextension, varus angulation, and external rotation
     a. Typically athletic injuries or vehicle accidents
     b. Usually part of multiligamentous injury, often PCL
   - Presentation: pain and instability; dial test positive when side-to-side difference > 10 degrees of external rotation (while lying prone) compared with uninjured side
     a. Positive at 90 degrees indicates PCL injury
     b. Positive at 30 degrees indicates isolated PLC injury
     c. Positive at both 90 and 30 degrees indicates injury to both PCL/PLC
     d. Nearly 30% have peroneal nerve injuries
     e. Chronically, may see varus or hyperextension thrust during gait
   - Imaging
     a. X-ray: long-leg films to measure mechanical axis
     b. MRI: signal at PLC, assess injury
   - Treatment
     a. Conservative management: low-grade injuries with stable knee: PT
     b. Surgical management: acute repair early, direct suturing midsubstance tear versus anchor fixation of avulsions
     c. Must address any malalignment (varus) with concomitant procedure
     d. Reconstruct concomitant cruciate injuries
     e. Chronic tears with instability: anatomic reconstruction of LCL and popliteus/popliteofibular ligament
        - **Correcting varus malalignment prevents failure of PLC reconstructions.**
7. Multiligamentous knee injury
   - Mechanism: high-energy trauma, or lower energy in obese patient
   - **Have high suspicion for knee dislocation if three or more ligaments are injured**

- Presentation: pain; high risk of associated neurovascular injury
- Classification (**Table 8.8**)
- Imaging
  a. X-rays: diagnose and confirm relocation
  b. MRI: assess all associated ligamentous and soft tissue injuries
- Treatment
  a. Early closed reduction and monitoring of vascular status, 48–72 hours recommended
  b. Conservative management: elderly, low-demand, medically ill
  c. Surgical management: open injury, vascular injury, compartment syndrome
     - Delayed ligamentous reconstruction after PT
     - Fix associated fractures first, early motion key to decrease high rate of associated arthrofibrosis

8. Extensor mechanism tendinitis
   - Pathology: tendon degeneration or "tendinosis"; "jumper's knee"
     a. Mechanism: repetitive, forceful eccentric loading
     b. Demographic: patella affected in younger individuals; quadriceps affected in middle-aged to older individuals
     c. Presentation: patellar pole tenderness/swelling
        - Quadriceps/hamstring inflexibility associated with higher rates of chronic patellar tendonitis
     d. Imaging: MRI: tendon thickening
     e. Treatment
        - Conservative management: activity modification, physical therapy, off-loading straps, eccentric exercises (most important)
        - Surgical management: rare; midline debridement of degenerative tendon
     f. Complication: avoid corticosteroid injections, risk rupture
9. Extensor mechanism apophysitis
   - Pathology: pediatric overuse/traction injury
     a. Osgood-Schlatter (tibial tubercle), Sinding-Larson-Johansson disease (inferior patellar pole)
   - Treatment: conservative; symptomatic, rare ossicle excision if fails conservative
10. Extensor mechanism tendon rupture (**Fig. 8.18**)
    - Mechanism: eccentric loading on planted, partially flexed knee
    - Presentation: pain, palpable defect, loss of extension or lag
      a. Quadriceps (age > 40 years) versus patella (age < 40 years)
      b. Risks: obesity, diabetes, other systemic disease, anabolic steroids, local corticosteroids, prior BTB harvest
    - Imaging
      a. X-rays: patella alta (patellar rupture) versus patella baja (quadriceps rupture) (**Fig. 8.19**)
      b. MRI: partial versus complete tear, underlying tendinosis
    - Treatment
      a. Conservative management: immobilization/PT for partial tear, intact extension
      b. Surgical management: complete tear; perform early; suture fixation with locked sutures through patellar drill holes
    - Rehabilitation (goal to protect repair)

Table 8.8 Knee Dislocation (KD) Classification

Injury Grade[1]	Injury Pattern
I[2]	ACL or PCL (one intact) ± MCL or LCL
II	ACL and PCL (both cruciates torn)
III	ACL and PCL and MCL or LCL
IV	ACL and PCL and MCL and LCL
V	Fracture/dislocation (periarticular)

Abbreviations: ACL, anterior cruciate ligament; PCL, posterior cruciate ligament; MCL, medial collateral ligament; LCL, lateral collateral ligament.
[1]Classifed by direction of tibial displacement.
[2]Rare.

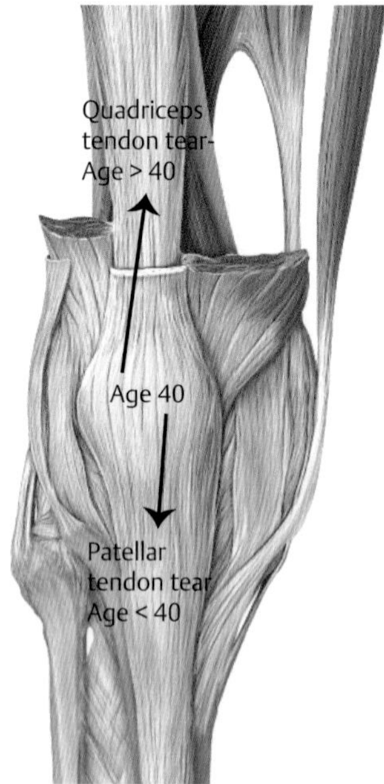

Fig. 8.18 Typical age range of quadriceps versus patella tendon ruptures.

a. Immobilization, progressive ROM/strengthening
b. Initial non–weight bearing, active knee flexion (heel slides)
c. Passive extension, no active extension for 4–6 weeks

11. Lateral patellar instability (subluxation/dislocation)
   - Demographics: age teens to 20s, more likely female if recurrent, equal gender likelihood if first episode
   - Risk factors/pathology
     a. High Q-angle, (normal female average, 17 degrees), genu valgum, patella alta, trochlea dysplasia (shallow), ligamentous laxity
     b. Lateral patellar tilt, femoral anteversion, tibial torsion, "miserable malalignment"
     c. Abnormal tibial tubercle offset from trochlear groove (> 15 mm)
     d. Previous instability episode (highest risk recurrence)
   - Mechanism: typically noncontact pivot; external rotation leg/foot
   - Presentation: swelling (acute), medial pain, "giving out"; patellar "apprehension," excessive lateral patellar displacement; no effusion if chronic or congenital
   - Imaging
     a. X-rays: rarely reveal avulsion or impaction fracture
     b. MRI: bone bruising versus osteochondral injury to medial patellar facet, and anterior aspect lateral condyle
     c. Delineation of MPFL injury (in order of frequency):
        - Pattern femoral-sided soft tissue avulsion (most common)
        - Midsubstance or patellar-sided soft tissue injury
        - Medial bony avulsions (least common)
   - Treatment
     a. Conservative management: extensive limb, core and vasti strengthening
     b. Surgical management: controversial; currently MPFL reconstruction gaining popularity
        - Arthroscopy for removal of bony fragments
        - Tibial tubercle distal realignment for excessive patella alta; tubercle medial realignment for excessive patella lateralization (> 15 mm offset)
        - Anteromedial realignment contraindicated if significant medial patellar facet arthritis
        - o Surgery most likely beneficial for instability over pain

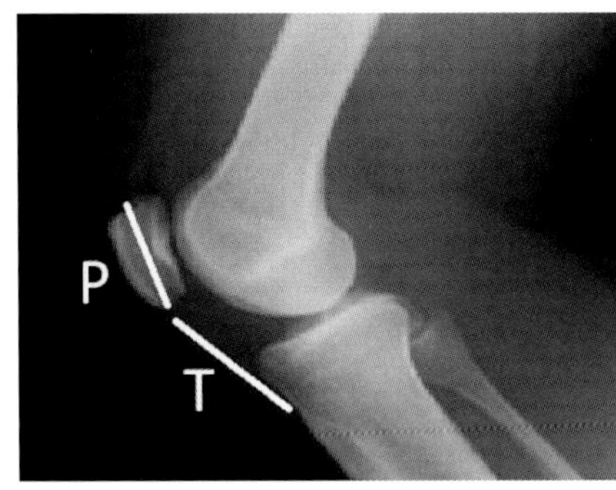

Fig. 8.19 Insall-Salvati ratio: alta (T/P ≥ 1.2, patellar rupture) versus baja (T/P ≤ 0.8, quadriceps rupture). P, patella; T, tendon.

12. Lateral patellar facet compression syndrome
   - Pathology: tight lateral patellar retinaculum or medial laxity
   - Presentation: lateral tenderness, but normal patellar mobility
   - Imaging: X-ray: sunrise view shows elevated lateral patellar tilt, which normally is 5 degrees or less (**Fig. 8.20**)
   - Treatment
     a. Conservative management: initially with PT, focus on medial strengthening, vastus medialis obliquus
     b. Surgical management: if refractory, and lateral patellar tilt is present (with lack of lateral opening), either open or arthroscopic lateral release

13. Patellofemoral degenerative disease (term "chondromalacia patellae" no longer used)

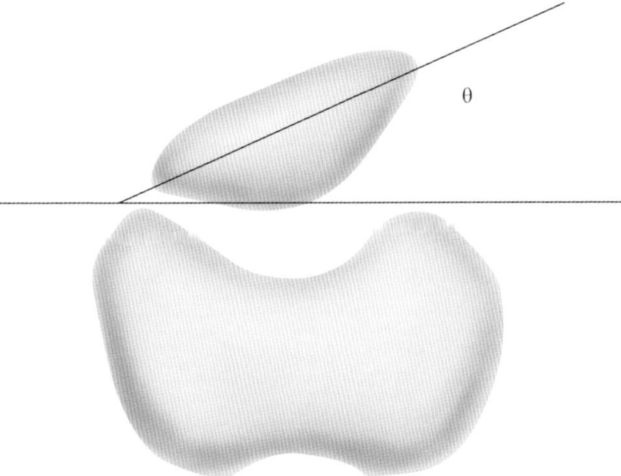

Fig. 8.20 Lateral patellar tilt. Normal lateral patellar tilts 5 degrees or less. **(Left)**, lateral; **(right)**, medial. Θ, tilt angle.

- Presentation: anterior knee pain, worse with sitting/stair-climbing where knee gets stiff/stuck in flexion ("theater sign")
- Imaging
  a. X-rays: joint space narrowing seen in severe disease
  b. MRI: more sensitive for patellar chondral injury
- Treatment
  a. Conservative management: PT for isometrics and closed chain exercises; strengthen but limit further wear
  b. Surgical management: if refractory, arthroscopy/debridement, realignment, patella-femoral arthroplasty, patellectomy (salvage)
  c. Outcomes: inconsistent results for cartilage restorative procedures

14. Other pathologies around knee
- Pre-patellar bursitis: common with prolonged kneeling
  a. Treatment: protective pads, aspiration (rule out infection)
- Pes anserine bursitis: inflammation over sartorius fascia and underlying gracilis/semitendinosus tendons
  a. Treatment: therapy, anti-inflammatory meds, injections
  b. IT band friction syndrome
     - Common irritation over lateral femoral condyle (runners)
     - Treatment: cross-training/stretching, rare partial excision
  c. Anterior fat pad syndrome (Hoffa disease)
     - "Pinching" pain/fibrosis anterior-inferior knee
     - Related to trauma-related change of fat pad
     - Conservative treatment, injection; surgical excision if refractory
  d. Gastrocnemius injury ("tennis leg")
     - Acute midcalf pain swelling; musculotendinous tear of medial head of the gastrocnemius
     - Treatment: conservative; many patients need immobilization initially for pain control
     - Less common is plantaris rupture

15. Osteochondritis dissecans (OCD)
- Pathology: etiology unknown, vascular/traumatic injury; separation of articular cartilage from underlying subchondral bone
- Demographics: juvenile form entails open physis; adult form entails closed physis
- **Juvenile OCD cases tend to resolve.**
- Presentation: pain (not always localizable); may have effusion and/or crepitus
- Imaging
  a. X-rays: subchondral lucency, classically located posterolateral aspect medial femoral condyle (minority 15–20% on lateral condyle); seen best on weight-bearing 30-degree posteroanterior (PA) view (tunnel view)
  b. MRI: best delineates lesion; fluid surrounding entire lesion is a poor prognostic indicator
- Treatment
  a. Conservative management: protected weight bearing for young patients, typically successful when physes open
  b. Surgical management: for mechanical symptoms, displaced fragment, failed conservative
  c. Retrograde drilling if stable articular surface
  d. Excision/debridement: damaged cartilage with < 3 mm subchondral bone

e. Outcomes: vast majority of juvenile OCD lesions resolve with nonsurgical management (50% chance of spontaneous resolution in adolescents, rare in adults)

16. Osteochondral injury/defect
    - Mechanism: acute trauma with shearing/rotational forces
    - Presentation: pain (not always localizable); may have effusion and/or crepitus
    - Treatment
      a. Conservative management: for non–weight-bearing lesions
      b. Surgical management: indicated for weight-bearing symptomatic lesions
        - In-situ drilling: for stable/intact lesions
        - Low-profile screw fixation: for unstable/displaced but intact lesions (≥ 3 mm subchondral bone)
        - Excision/debridement: damaged cartilage with < 3 mm subchondral bone
        - Cartilage restoration: options for full-thickness loss (requires debridement to stable base)
          - Small to medium-sized (< 2 cm^2)
            - Microfracture: drilling into subchondral bone; fibrocartilaginous repair tissue (type I collagen); up to 80% early clinical success
            - Autograft osteochondral plugs/mosaicplasty: for cartilage and bone loss; limited by donor site size/morbidity
          - Large (> 2 cm^2)
            - Autologous chondrocyte implantation (ACI): method of culturing explanted native cartilage that produces hyaline-like cartilage (type II collagen); intact bone required; limited by cost and requirement of multiple procedures
            - Osteochondral allografts: for larger defects with bone loss; limited by risk of infection and graft incorporation
        - Other considerations: these cartilage restoration procedures are evolving treatment options and long-term; sustained success replacing native type II cartilage remains elusive

17. Synovial pathologies
    - Plicae: embryologically derived folds; considered normal anatomy; rarely symptomatic clinically
    - Synovial chondromatosis: proliferative cartilage metaplasia, multiple loose bodies (see Chapter 2)
      a. Treatment: debride/excise if symptomatic

G. Sports-Related Leg Pathology

1. Chronic exertional compartment syndrome
    - Pathology: typical for athletes with muscular leg; usually anterior compartment
    - Presentation: similar to acute compartment syndrome, but nonacute, gradual onset, subsides with rest
    - Diagnosis: compartment pressure testing after exercise, positive result if
      a. > 15 mm Hg at rest
      b. > 20 mm Hg at 5 minutes postexercise
      c. > 30 mm Hg at 1 minute postexercise
    - Treatment: compartment fasciotomies if refractory to activity modification
    - Differential diagnosis
      a. Popliteal artery entrapment: pedal pulses reduced by ankle plantar/dorsiflexion; treat with medial gastrocnemius release

b. Superficial peroneal nerve entrapment: painful passive ankle plantar flexion/inversion; treat with fascial release ± neurolysis
c. Saphenous nerve entrapment: anterior-medial knee pain

2. Tibial stress fracture
   - Pathology: due to repetitive microtrauma; common in running athletes, especially in females and after altered or increased training
   - Presentation: slow onset of activity-related anterior leg pain, with focal tenderness
   - Imaging
     a. X-ray: may be unrevealing
        - **Persistent lucent line indicates impending tibial stress fracture.**

     b. Bone scan: highly sensitive for lesion
     c. MRI: modality of choice (increased signal on T1 and T2); reveals edema and fracture
   - Treatment: protected weight bearing initially; cross-training if symptom-free; intramedullary fixation for persistent anterior midshaft lucent line
   - Other considerations
     a. Stress injury has bony point tenderness and a focal area of uptake on bone scan versus more diffuse distal third shin tenderness and diffuse bone scan uptake with tibial periostitis or "shin splints"
     b. Anterior tibial diaphysis: high-risk area for delayed or nonunion due to tremendous tensile stress, more proximal posteromedial stress injuries lower risk

3. Achilles injury
   - Pathology: degeneration secondary to avascular region of tendon
   - **Injury is related to tenuous blood supply (watershed area) at ~ 4 cm from calcaneal Achilles insertion.**
   - Injury types
     a. Tendinitis versus tendinosis: painful overuse injury versus degeneration
        - Treatment: eccentric strengthening, may need debridement/repair
     b. Partial tear treatment: eccentric strengthening, debridement/repair as needed
     c. Complete tear
        - Presentation: acute distal calf pain; abnormal Thompson test (normally observe plantar-flexion with calf compression)
        - Treatment: compared to nonoperative management surgical repair is associated with decreased rerupture rates and earlier mobility/stronger plantar-flexion but also more frequent complications (wound/skin healing issues and infection)
     d. American Academy of Orthopaedic Surgeons (AAOS) Clinical Practice Guideline: Strong evidence: use of protective device that allows for mobilization within 2–4 weeks postoperatively. Moderate evidence: operative treatment should be approached cautiously in patients with diabetes mellitus (DM), neuropathy, immunocompromised, age > 65 years, smoker, sedentary, body mass index (BMI) > 30, peripheral vascular disease; < 2 weeks protected weight bearing postoperatively

H. Other Aspects of Sports Medicine

1. Concussion
   - Pathology: represents a spectrum of diffuse brain/axonal injury
   - Presentation: confusion, headache, irritability, concentration problems or frank loss of consciousness

- Diagnosis:
  a. CT: recommended for prolonged loss of consciousness (> 5 minute)
  b. Neuropsychological testing (baseline and postinjury): measures that assess cognition (e.g., attention, orientation, and memory):
     - Standardized Assessment of Concussion (SAC)
     - Immediate Post-concussion Assessment and Cognitive Testing (ImPACT) battery, computer-based
  c. Current evaluation techniques inadequate for accurate grading of concussion
- Classification **(Table 8.9)**
- Return to play
  a. Physician must keep athlete's best interests in mind
     - Requirements: patient needs to be completely symptom-free with progressive activities, return to baseline on neuropsychological testing
  b. Return same day: not recommended
     - Particularly if amnesia, symptoms > 15 minutes, history of prior concussion, or return of symptoms with exertion
     - Some advocate return if above negative and patient returns to baseline on testing
  c. Return at 7–30 days: after first concussion, mild-moderate grade
  d. Return at 30 days: after first concussion, severe grade
  e. Return next season: repeat concussion, any grade
  f. Treatment and return-to-play recommendations constantly evolving as epidemiological data are reviewed
- Other considerations
  a. **Head protection recommended; lowers head injury rates significantly, especially in equestrian and contact sports**
  b. Severe diffuse axonal injury: loss consciousness > 6 hours, lifetime cessation of sport recommended
  c. "Second-impact" syndrome: rare; associated with second hit after recent concussion; brain herniation and autoregulatory dysfunction possible; high mortality (50%) and careful adherence to return guidelines key

2. On-field spine injury management
- Initial treatment: careful management for all suspected spine injuries
  a. Leave shoulder pads/helmet in place
  b. Stabilize head–cervical spine, log-roll onto backboard
  c. Remove facemask only if cardiopulmonary resuscitation needed
- Burner/stinger (brachial plexus traction injury/neurapraxia)
  a. Mechanism: ipsilateral shoulder depression and opposite shoulder lateral bend, versus direct blow
  b. Presentation: transient (most < 1 minute, not > 15 minute), unilateral, upper extremity, nondermatomal burning pain (± weakness); no neck pain
  c. Treatment: conservative/supportive
  d. Return to play: once symptom-free, normal function and strength; after three episodes or the season, requires a workup prior to return to play
  e. Atypical symptoms: axial neck pain, persistent or bilateral symptoms
     - Workup with radiographs, electromyogram (EMG), or MRI (for bilateral; also to rule out disk herniation)
  f. Recurrence: threefold risk recurrence after first stinger
- Transient quadriplegia
  a. Mechanism: axial neck loading while hyperflexed/extended

Table 8.9 Concussion Classification of the American Academy of Neurological Surgeons

Grade	Findings
I	No LOC, amnesia absent or < 30 minutes
II	LOC < 5 minutes, amnesia 30 minutes to 24 hours
III	LOC ≥ 5 minutes or amnesia > 24 hours

Abbreviation: LOC, loss of consciousness.

b. Presentation: similar to burner but bilateral symptoms, or complete paralysis

c. Imaging: X-ray and MRI to rule out associated injury/conditions

d. Treatment: spine immobilization, log rolling, backboard (cannot return to play until workup is negative)

e. Contraindications to sports return
   - Congenital cervical fusion or stenosis (canal < 13 mm, "relative stenosis," versus < 10 mm, "absolute stenosis")
   - Prolonged symptoms
   - Contraindications to return remain controversial

3. Medical management issues

- Cardiac abnormalities

  a. Pathology: hypertrophic cardiomyopathy (HCM) number one cause of sudden cardiac death in young athlete

  b. Preparticipation history/physical exam
     - Most cost-effective screening tool
     - Ask about chest pain, dizziness, syncope, or dyspnea
     - Ask if any family history of sudden death at young age
     - Murmur: diastolic or increased intensity with Valsalva; think HCM

  c. Formal cardiac evaluation (if prescreen positive)
     - Electrocardiogram; echocardiogram most sensitive
     - **HCM is an absolute contraindication to vigorous activity/sports.**

- Commotio cordis (sports-related cardiac contusion)

  a. Mechanism: due to blunt trauma in ball sports; poor prognosis

  b. Treatment: cardiopulmonary resuscitation, emergent cardioversion

- Splenic injury/splenomegaly

  a. Most commonly injured solid organ, blunt trauma

  b. Splenomegaly in mononucleosis
     - Treatment: return 4 weeks after infectious mononucleosis
     - Teammates should avoid sharing drinking dispensers, etc.

- "Female athlete triad" **(Fig. 8.21)**

  a. Pathology: amenorrhea, stress fractures, and eating disorders

  b. Secondary amenorrhea (> 6 months) common (50% elite runners)
     - Usually due to insufficient caloric intake (number 1 cause), or overtraining
     - If > 1 year, significantly increased risk of stress fracture

  c. Treatment: Workup of all three components, clinical counseling required (menstrual history, dietary issues)

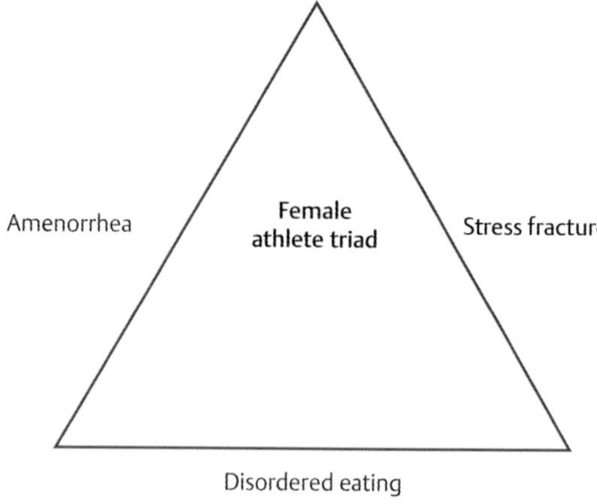

Fig. 8.21 Female athlete triad.

9

Hand and Microvasculature

Eric Cohen, Byung J. Lee, and Arnold-Peter Weiss

I. Anatomy

1. Bony and articular anatomy
   - Forearm
     a. Osteology **(Figs. 9.1** and **9.2)**
        - Radius and ulna
        - Radial head is intra-articular at the elbow
        - Anterolateral portion of radial head has less subchondral bone, making it more susceptible to fracture
        - Radial tuberosity is site of biceps tendon insertion, and it points ulnarly in supination
        - Radial bow allows rotation around the ulna; restoration of radial bow and length is critical when fixing the radius
        - Radius and ulna stabilized by the proximal and distal radioulnar joints and the interosseus membrane

     b. Interosseus membrane: transfers compressive load from wrist to elbow
        - Composed of interosseus ligament proper, proximal interosseus bands, and accessory bands
        - Lister's tubercle on dorsal surface of distal radius; extensor pollicis longus (EPL) travels around Lister's tubercle to attach to distal phalanx of thumb
        - **Just ulnar to Lister's is the third dorsal compartment/EPL tendon. This is also the landmark used to create the 3/4 portal for wrist arthroscopy.**

     c. Range of motion (ROM): supinate 80–90 degrees, pronate 75–90 degrees
        - **About 10–15 degrees of rotation occurs at the wrist.**

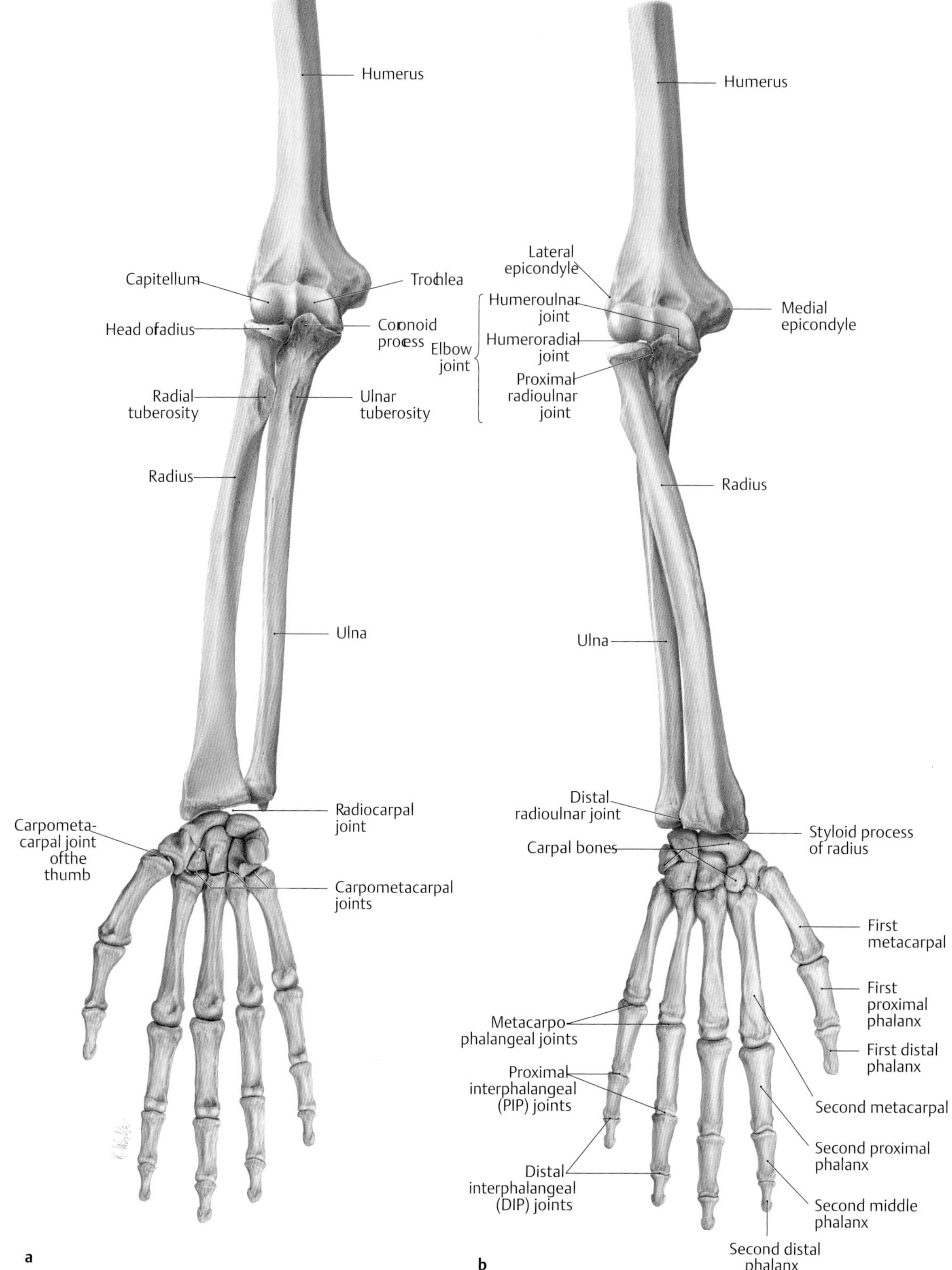

Fig. 9.1 The radius and ulna of the right arm in **(a)** supination and **(b)** pronation. (From Schuenke M, Schulte E. General Anatomy and the Musculoskeletal System: Thieme Atlas of Anatomy. New York: Thieme; 2005. Illustration by Karl Wesker.)

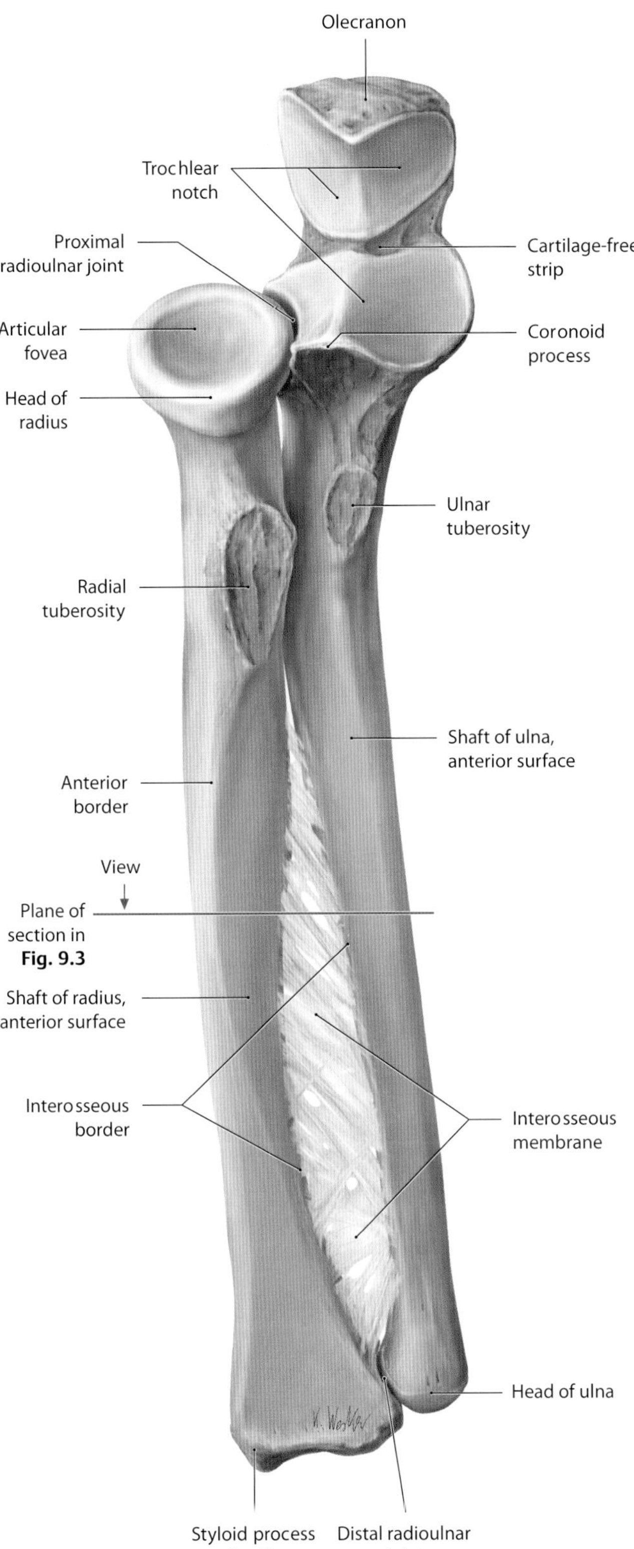

Fig. 9.2 The radius and ulna of the right forearm. Anterosuperior view. The proximal and distal radioulnar joints are functionally interlinked by the interosseous membrane between the radius and ulna. (From Schuenke M, Schulte E. General Anatomy and the Musculoskeletal System: Thieme Atlas of Anatomy. New York: Thieme; 2005. Illustration by Karl Wesker.)

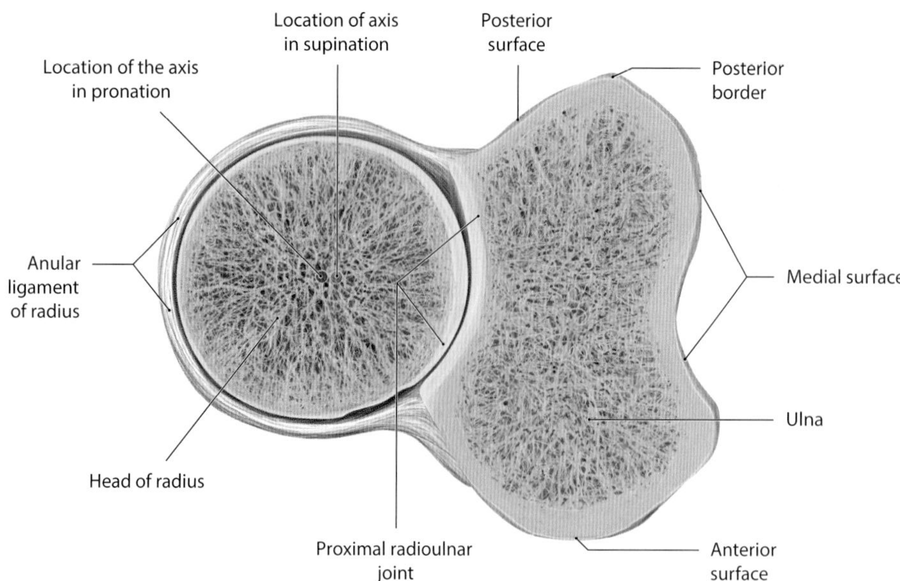

Fig. 9.3 Cross section through the right proximal radioulnar joint in pronation. Owing to the slightly oval shape of the radial head, the pronation/supination axis that runs through the radial head moves ~ 2 mm radially during pronation. This ensures that when the hand is pronated, there will be sufficient space for the radial tuberosity. (From Schuenke M, Schulte E. General Anatomy and the Musculoskeletal System: Thieme Atlas of Anatomy. New York: Thieme; 2005. Illustration by Karl Wesker.)

- Distal Radioulnar Joint (**Figs. 9.3, 9.4, 9.5**)
- **Distal radioulnar articulation is most stable in supination.**
- The ulnar sigmoid notch on the distal radius is a groove for the ulnar head and the site of the distal radioulnar joint.
    a. Distal radius has two facets separated by an anterior/posterior ridge: scaphoid and lunate.

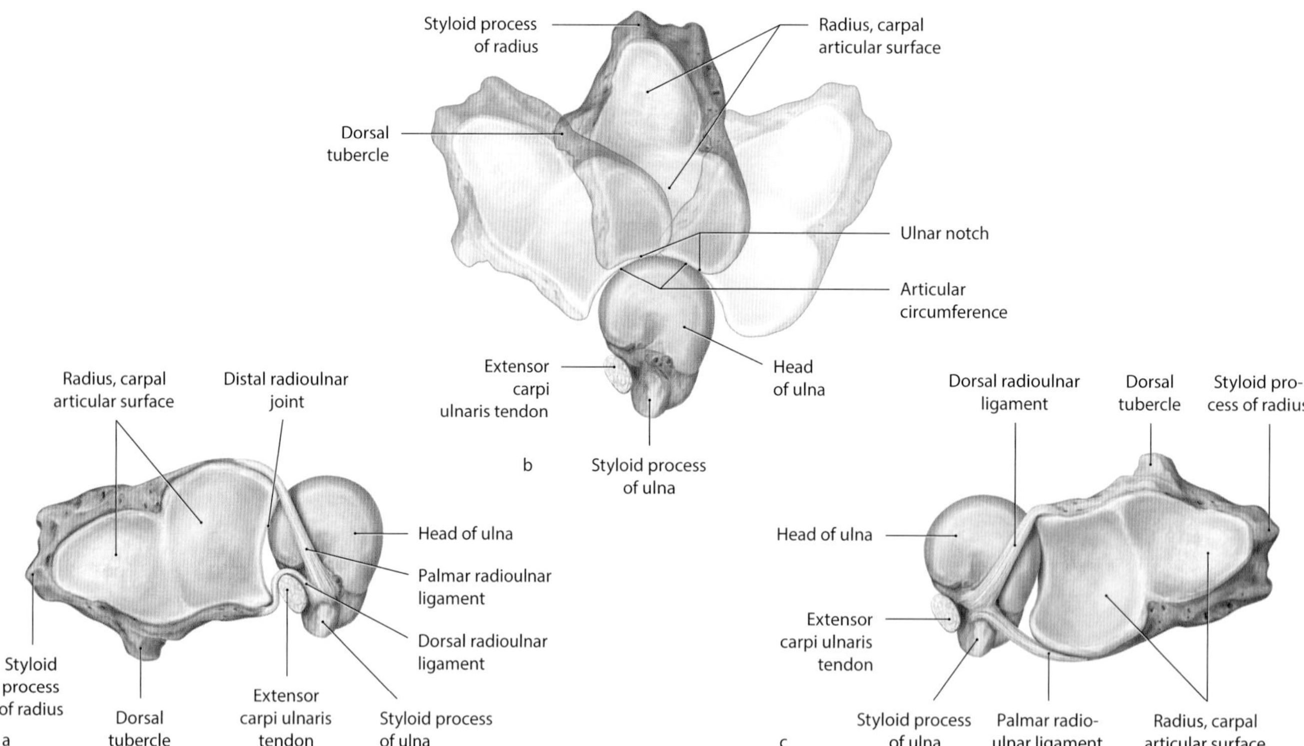

Fig. 9.4 Rotation of the radius and ulna during **(a)** supination, **(b)** semipronation, and **(c)** pronation. The dorsal and palmar radioulnar ligaments are part of the "ulnocarpal complex," which serves to stabilize the distal radioulnar joint. The mode of contact between the two distal articular segments varies with the position of the radius and ulna. (From Schuenke M, Schulte E. General Anatomy and the Musculoskeletal System: Thieme Atlas of Anatomy. New York: Thieme; 2005. Illustration by Karl Wesker.)

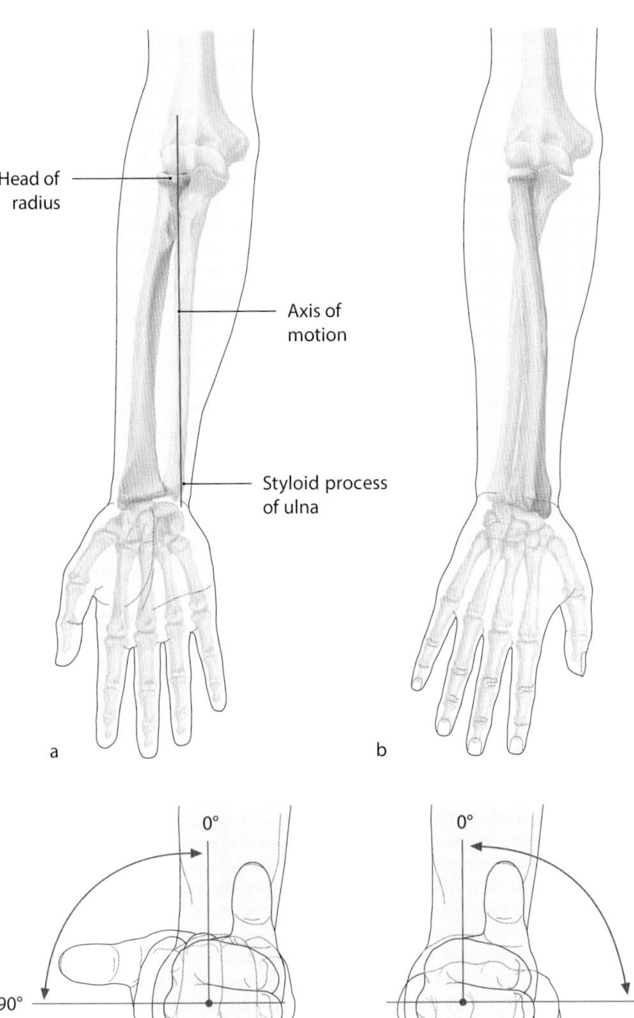

Fig. 9.5 Range and axis of pronation/supination of the right hand. The neutral (0-degree) position of the hand and forearm is called semipronation. The axis of pronation/supination extends through the head of the radius and the styloid process of ulna. **(a)** Supination. **(b)** Pronation. **(c)** Supination of the hand with the elbow flexed. **(d)** Pronation of the hand with the elbow flexed. (From Schuenke M, Schulte E. General Anatomy and the Musculoskeletal System: Thieme Atlas of Anatomy. New York: Thieme; 2005. Illustration by Karl Wesker.)

b. At the base of the ulnar styloid is the fovea, the insertion of the deep fibers of the radioulnar ligaments, which make up part of the triangular fibrocartilage complex (TFCC).

c. Only 10 to 15 degrees of pronation and supination from wrist

- Carpus
  a. Radiocarpal joint **(Figs. 9.6, 9.7, 9.8)**
    - Composed of distal radius, and scaphoid, lunate, and triquetrum
    - Composed of volar and dorsal radiocarpal ligaments and radial and ulnar collateral ligaments
    - **Volar radiocarpal ligaments are strongest supporting ligaments**
    - Range of motion **(Fig. 9.9)**
      - ♦ Extend ROM 75 degrees, flexion 80 degrees
      - ♦ Radial deviation 15–25 degrees, ulnar 30–45 degrees

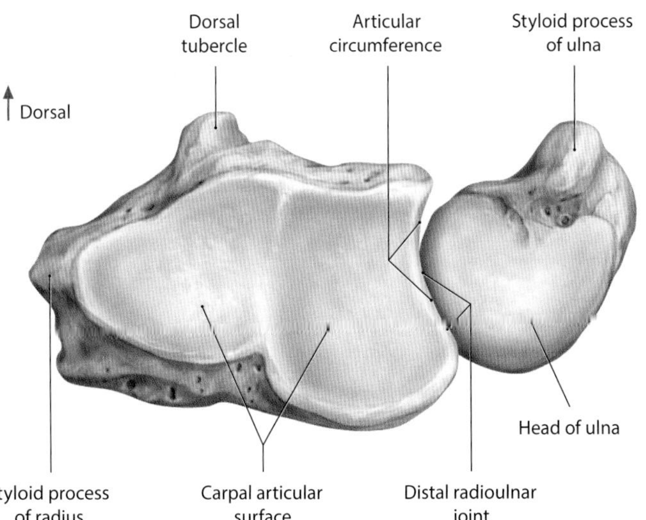

Fig. 9.6 The distal articular surfaces of the radius and ulnar of right forearm. (From Schuenke M, Schulte E. General Anatomy and the Musculoskeletal System: Thieme Atlas of Anatomy. New York: Thieme; 2005. Illustration by Karl Wesker.)

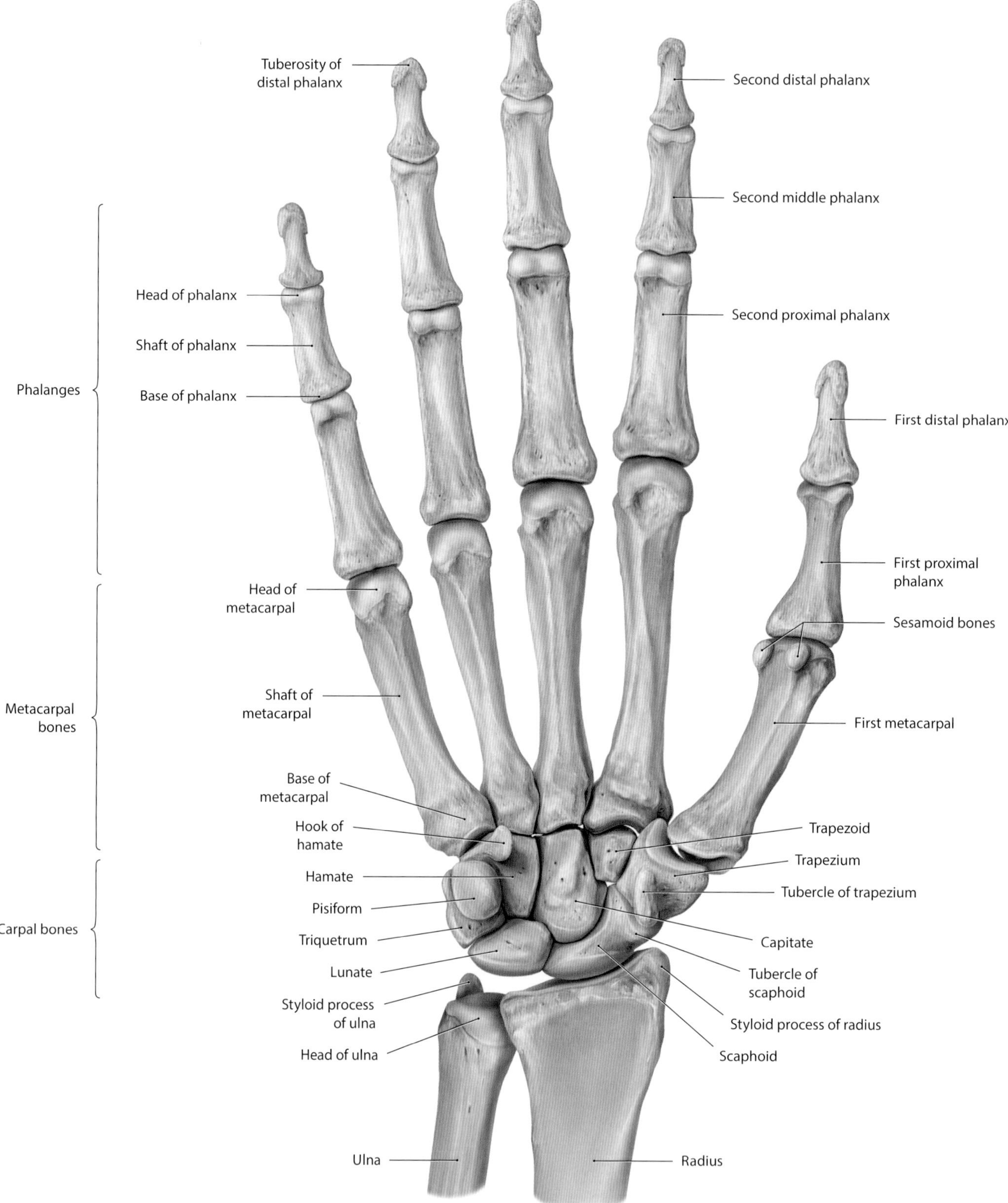

Fig. 9.7 The bones of the right hand. Palmar view. (From Schuenke M, Schulte E. General Anatomy and the Musculoskeletal System: Thieme Atlas of Anatomy. New York: Thieme; 2005. Illustration by Karl Wesker.)

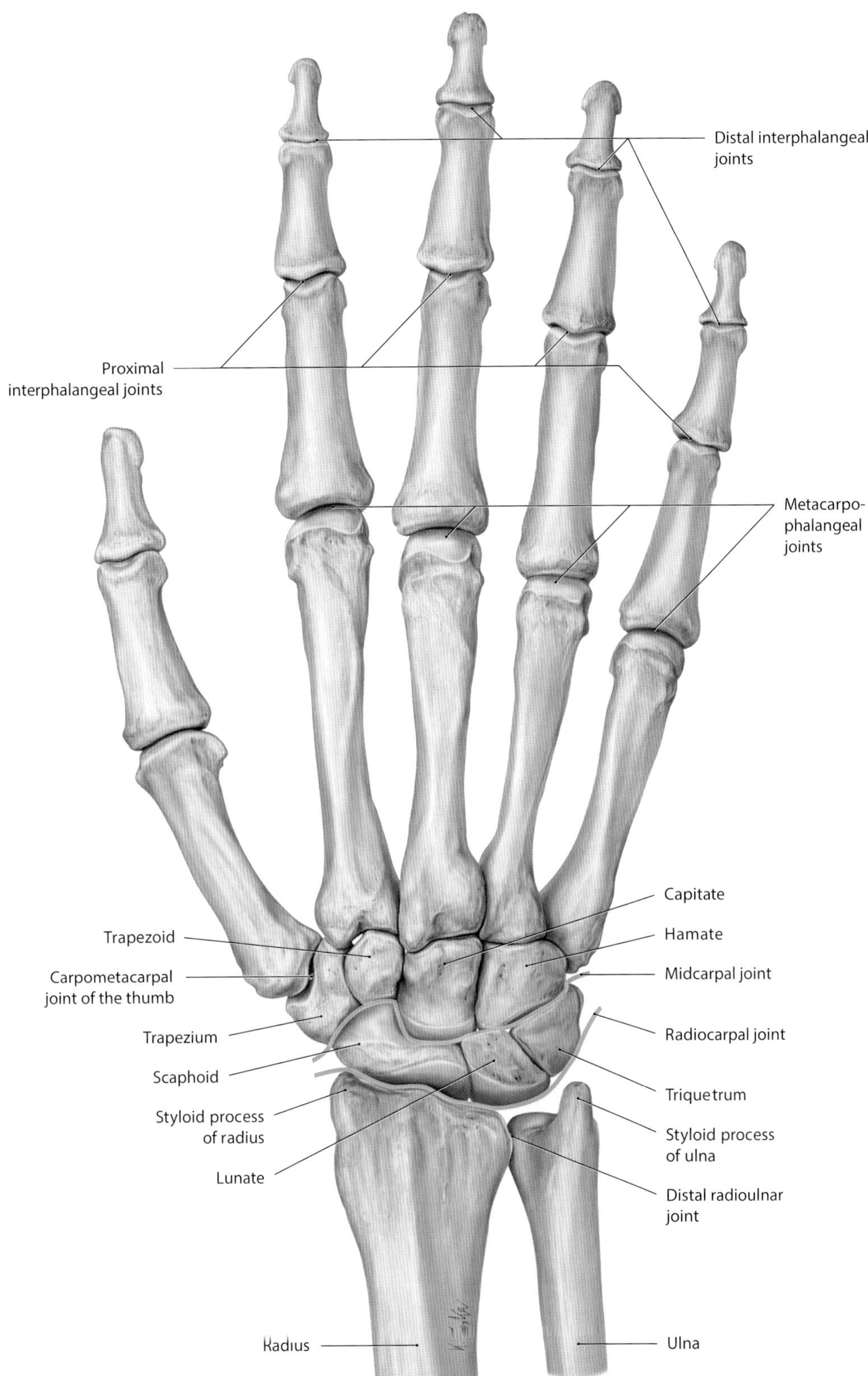

Fig. 9.8 The bones of the right hand. Dorsal view. The radiocarpal and mid carpaljoints are indicated by *green* and *blue lines* respectively. (From Schuenke M, Schulte E. General Anatomy and the Musculoskeletal System: Thieme Atlas of Anatomy. New York: Thieme; 2005. Illustration by Karl Wesker.)

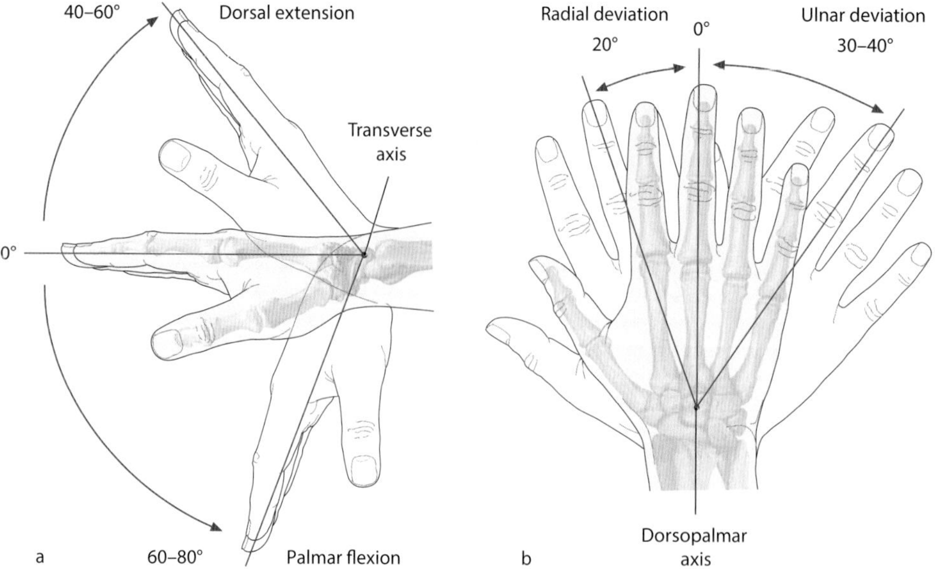

Fig. 9.9 Movement of the radiocarpal and midcarpal joints. Starting from the neutral (0-degree) position: **(a)** palmar flexion and dorsal extension are performed about the transverse axis, while **(b)** radial and ulnar deviation occur about a dorsopalmar axis. The transverse axis runs through the lunate for the radiocarpal joint and through the capitate for the midcarpal joint. The dorsopalmar axis runs through the capitates bone. Thus, although palmar flexion and dorsal extension can occur in both the radiocarpal and midcarpal joints, radial and ulnar deviation occurs in the radiocarpal joint. (From Schuenke M, Schulte E. General Anatomy and the Musculoskeletal System: Thieme Atlas of Anatomy. New York: Thieme; 2005. Illustration by Karl Wesker.)

b. Proximal row: scaphoid, lunate, triquetrum (sesamoid, pisiform)
   - The proximal row has no muscular or tendinous attachments. It is an intercalary segment.
   - **Scaphoid primary blood supply is from the radial artery at the dorsal ridge just distal to waist; proximal pole perfused in retrograde fashion**

- Transverse carpal ligament attaches to the volar tubercle
  a. Distal row: trapezium, trapezoid, capitates, hamate
  b. Pisiform is a sesamoid bone within the flexor carpi ulnaris (FCU) tendon; also the origin for abductor digit quinti
  c. Significant carpal ligaments
     - Scapholunate ligament: strongest dorsally, and rupture leads to dorsal intercalated segment instability (DISI) deformity
     - Lunotriquetral ligament: strongest volarly and rupture leads to volar intercalated segment instability (VISI) deformity
  d. Carpal ossification **(Fig. 9.10)**
     - First to ossify is the capitate, at 1 year; last to ossify is the pisiform, by 12 years; ossification occurs in characteristic counterclockwise pattern
- Fingers
  a. Functional position of hand **(Fig. 9.11)**
  b. Thumb carpometacarpal (CMC) (trapeziometacarpal) joint
     - Saddle shaped, allowing a large degree of motion
     - Thumb CMC joint stabilized by capsule, dorsoradial ligament, ulnar collateral ligaments, posterior oblique and anterior oblique ligament

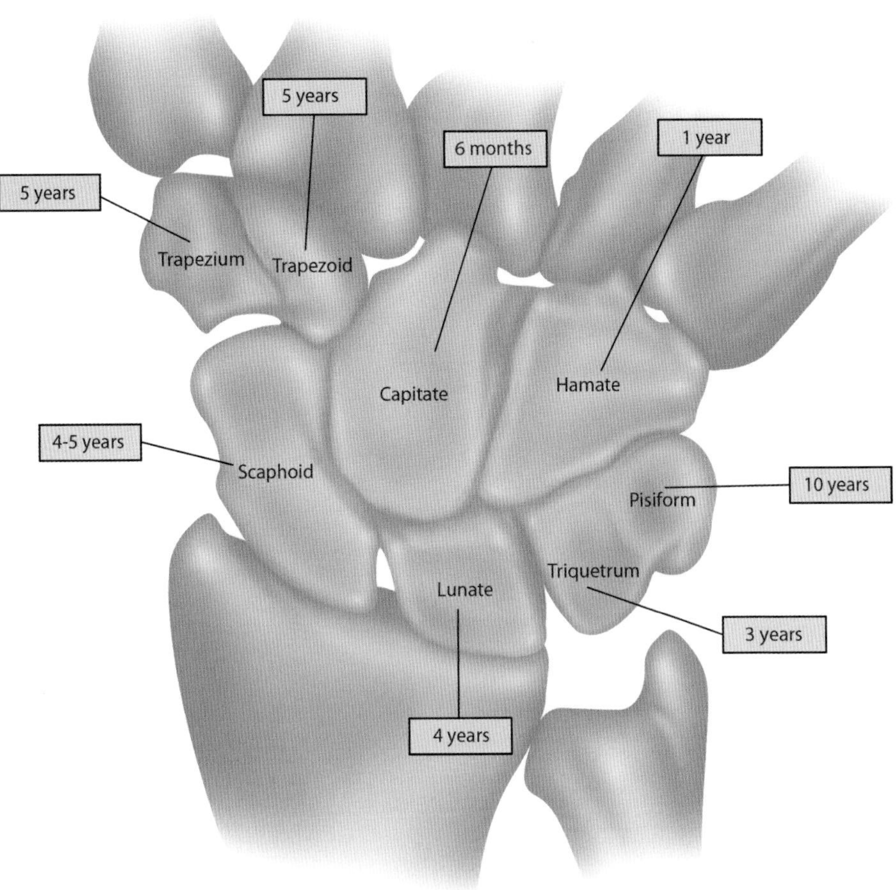

Fig. 9.10 Carpal ossification. Eight bones that ossify in characteristic counterclockwise order (when looking at volar aspect of right wrist) beginning with the hamate and ending with the pisiform.

- **Primary stabilizer is anterior oblique ligament (beak ligament)**

c. Finger CMC joint (**Figs. 9.12** and **9.13**)
- Gliding joint
- Stabilized by capsule, dorsal, and volar CMC and interosseous ligaments
- Dorsal CMC ligament strongest

d. Metacarpophalangeal (MCP) joint
- Ellipsoid, creating a cam effect on ROM
- Stabilized by volar plate, collateral and deep transverse metacarpal ligaments
- ROM: extend/flex 0–90 degrees, adduct/abduct 0–20 degrees (**Fig. 9.14**)

e. Interphalangeal (IP) joints
- Hinge joint, no cam effect on ROM
- Capsule and oblique collateral ligaments
- ROM:
  - Proximal interphalangeal (PIP): extend/flex 0–110 degrees
  - Distal interphalangeal (DIP): extend/flex 0–80 degrees

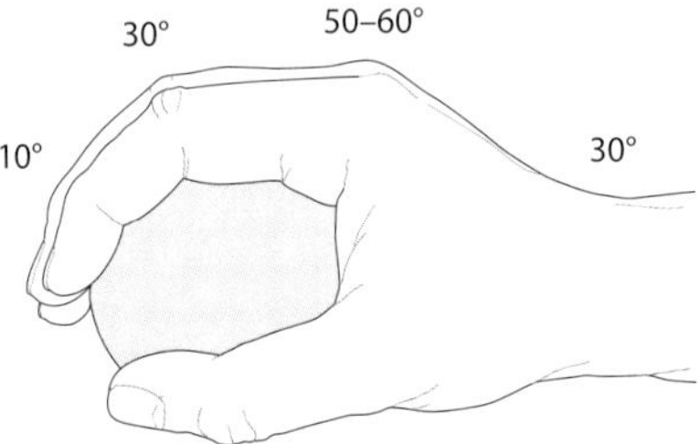

Fig. 9.11 Functional position of the hand. For postoperative immobilization of the hand, the desired position of the wrist and fingers should be considered when the cast, splint, or other device is applied. Otherwise the ligaments may shorten and the hand can no longer assume a resting position. (From Schuenke M, Schulte E. General Anatomy and the Musculoskeletal System: Thieme Atlas of Anatomy. New York: Thieme; 2005. Illustration by Karl Wesker.)

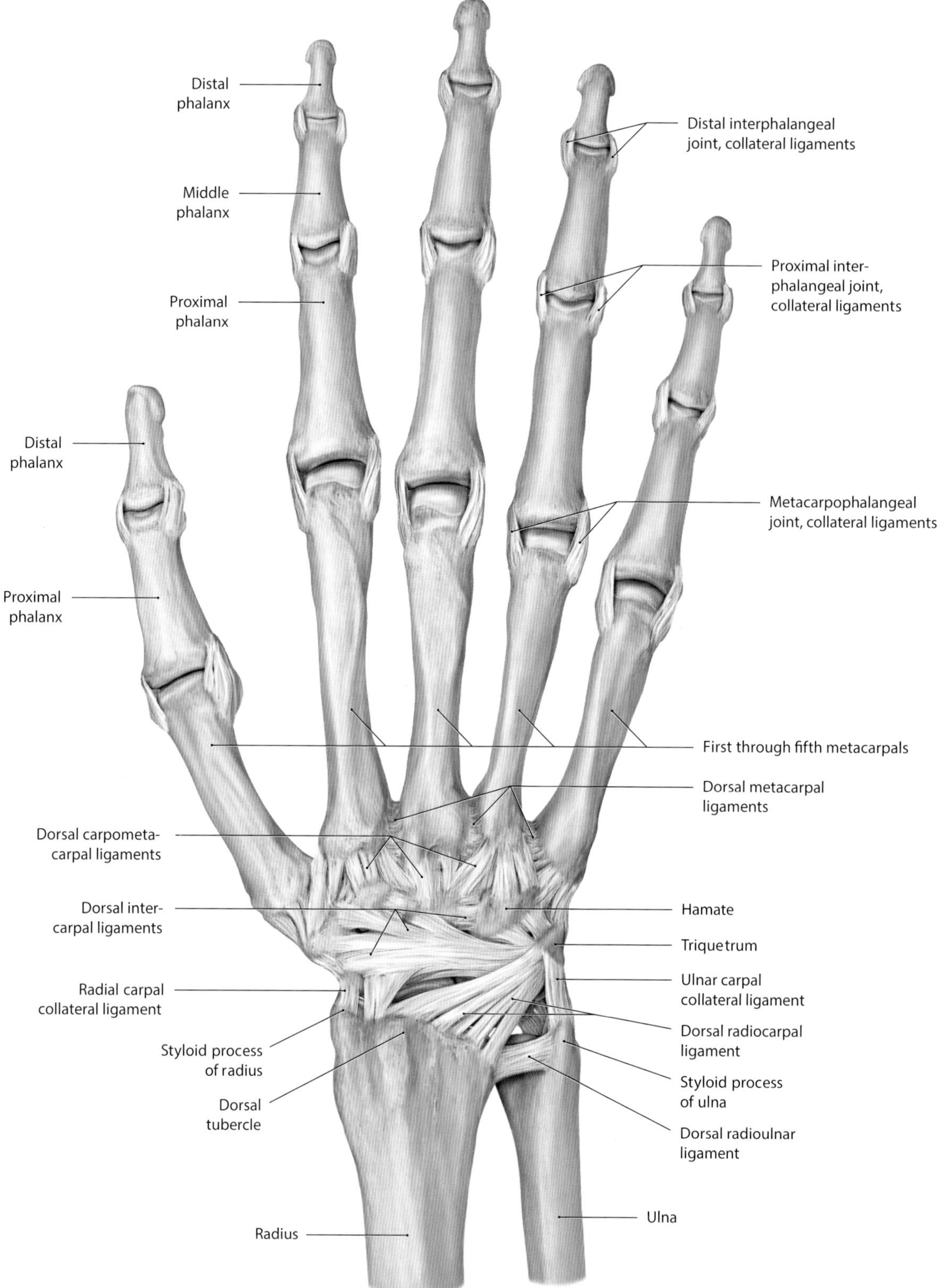

Fig. 9.12 The ligaments of the right hand. Posterior view. The various ligaments in the carpal region form a dense network that strengthens the joint capsule of the wrist. Four groups of ligaments can be distinguished based on their location and arrangement ((From Schuenke M, Schulte E. General Anatomy and the Musculoskeletal System: Thieme Atlas of Anatomy. New York: Thieme; 2005. Illustration by Karl Wesker.)

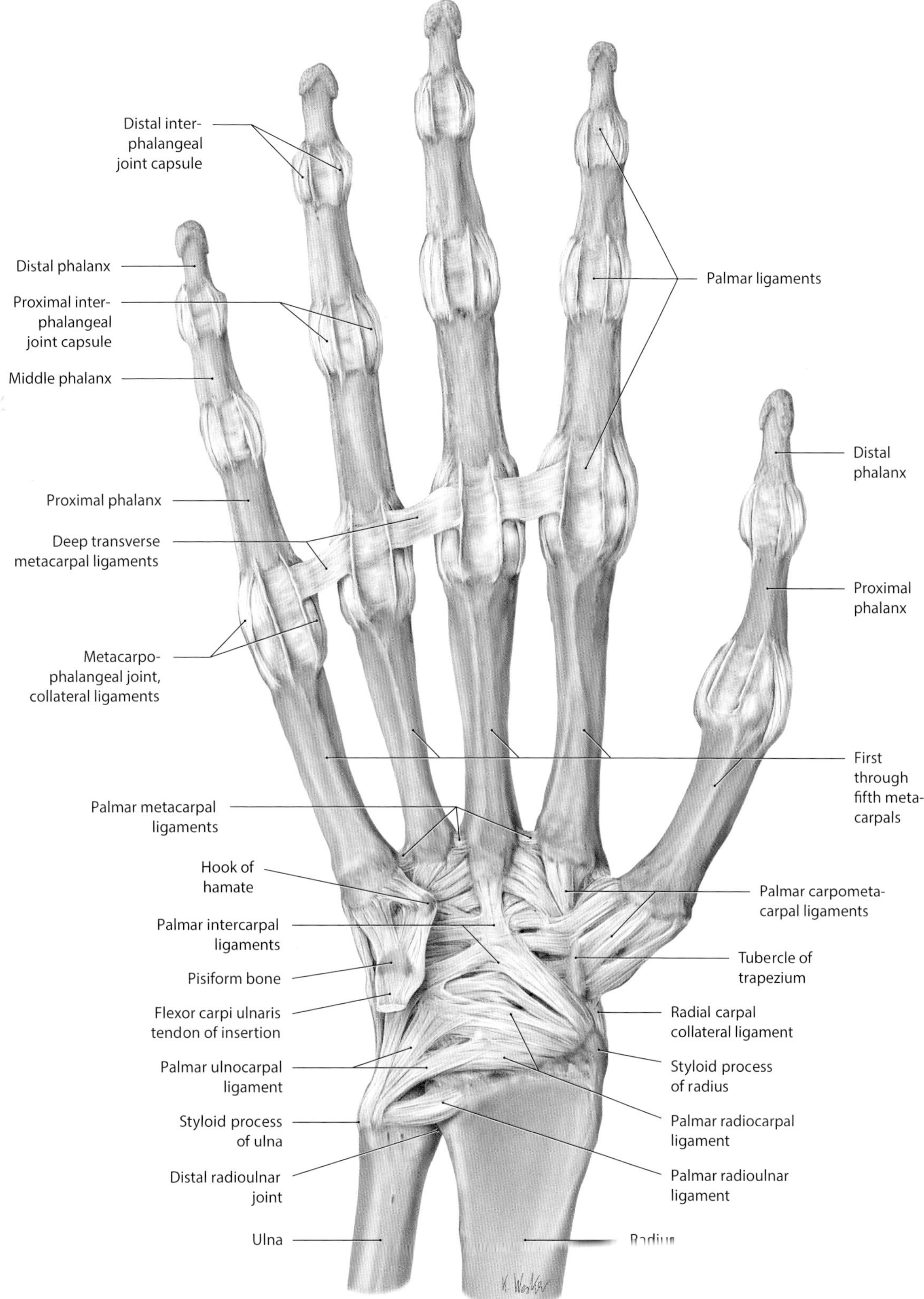

Fig. 9.13 The ligaments of the right hand. Anterior view. Among the ligaments that bind the carpal bones together (intercarpal ligaments),a distinction is made between internal ligamentsandsurfaceligaments. The internal ligaments interconnect the individual bones ata deeper level and include the interosseous intercarpal ligaments (notshown here). The surface ligaments consist of the dorsal (see A) andpalmar intercarpal ligaments. (From Schuenke M, Schulte E. General Anatomy and the Musculoskeletal System: Thieme Atlas of Anatomy. New York: Thieme; 2005. Illustration by Karl Wesker.)

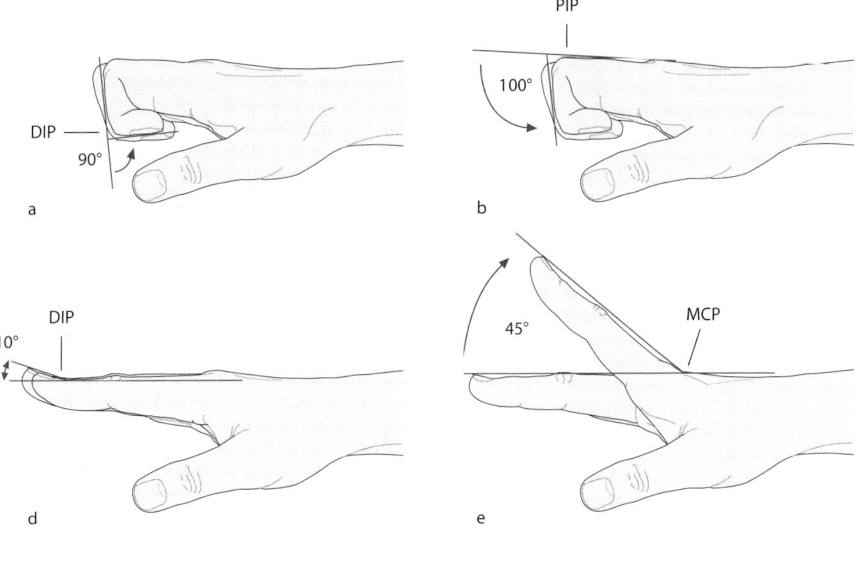

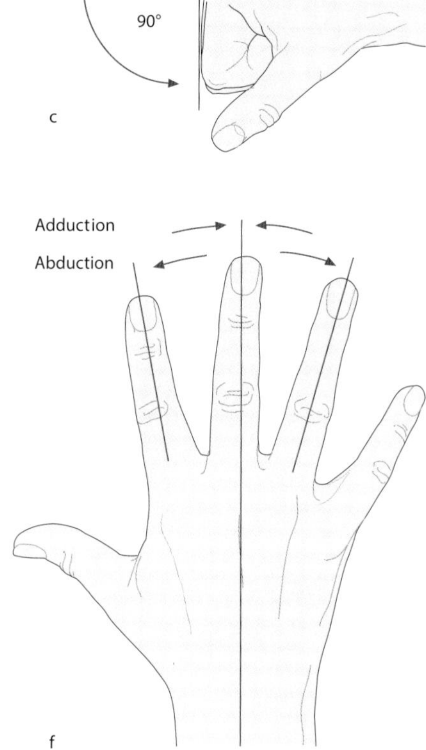

Fig. 9.14 Range of motion of the finger joints. **(a)** Flexion in the distal interphalangeal (DIP) joint. **(b)** Flexion in the proximal interphalangeal (PIP) joint. **(c)** Flexion in the metacarpophalangeal (MCP) joint. **(d)** Extension in the distal interphalangeal (DIP) joint. **(e)** Extension in the metacarpophalangeal (MCP) joint. **(f)** Abduction and adduction in the MCP joint. (From Schuenke M, Schulte E. General Anatomy and the Musculoskeletal System: Thieme Atlas of Anatomy. New York: Thieme; 2005. Illustration by Karl Wesker.)

2. Extensor compartments **(Figs. 9.15** and **9.16)** (six compartments)
   - **Be able to recognized which tendons are in which compartment on an axial magnetic resonance imaging (MRI)**
   - Covered by extensor retinaculum on dorsum of wrist
   - I: Abductor pollicis longus (APL), extensor pollicis brevis (EPB)
     a. De Quervain's tenosynovitis
     b. **APL has multiple tendon slips; need to evaluate whether EPB has a distinct separate tendon sheath that needs to be released during surgery.**
   - II: Extensor carpi radialis longus (ECRL) and brevis (ECRB)
     a. Intersection syndrome: at intersection of first and second compartment, often with palpable crepitus on wrist motion
   - III: Extensor pollicis longus (EPL)
     a. Rupture at Lister's tubercle after distal radius fracture
     b. **Treat with extensor indicis proprius (EIP) to EPL transfer.**
   - IV: Extensor digitorum communis, extensor indicis proprius (EIP)
     a. **EIP is last muscle to be reinnervated in radial nerve injuries**
     b. Posterior interosseous nerve (PIN) is located on the floor of the fourth compartment
   - V: Extensor digiti minimi
     a. **Vaughan-Jackson syndrome in rheumatoid arthritis, rupture of extensors in ulnar to radial direction; extensor digiti minimi (EDM) first to rupture**
   - VI: Extensor carpi ulnaris (ECU)
     a. Pathology: can have instability at ulnar styloid

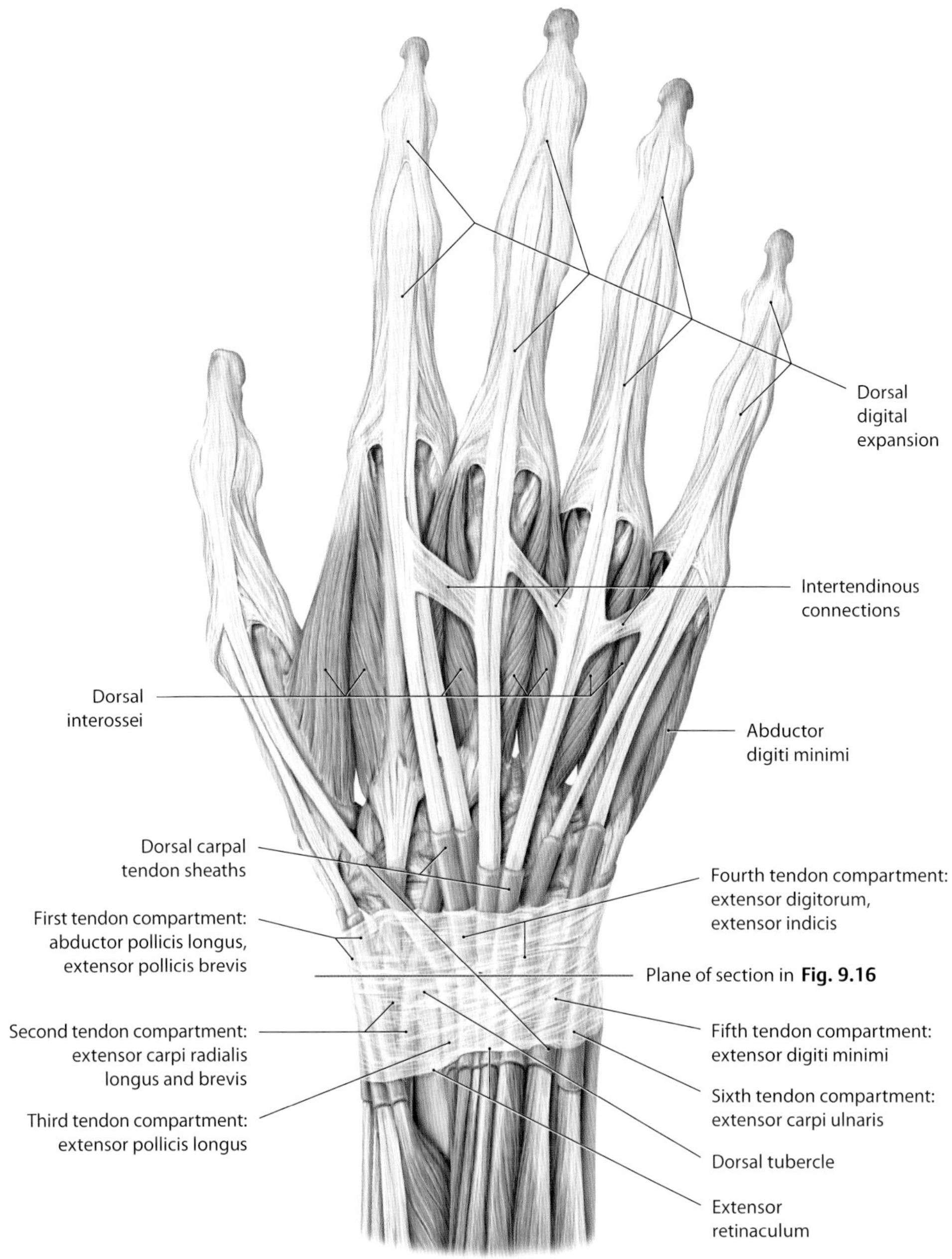

Dorsal digital expansion
Intertendinous connections
Dorsal interossei
Abductor digiti minimi
Dorsal carpal tendon sheaths
Fourth tendon compartment: extensor digitorum, extensor indicis
First tendon compartment: abductor pollicis longus, extensor pollicis brevis
Plane of section in **Fig. 9.16**
Second tendon compartment: extensor carpi radialis longus and brevis
Fifth tendon compartment: extensor digiti minimi
Sixth tendon compartment: extensor carpi ulnaris
Third tendon compartment: extensor pollicis longus
Dorsal tubercle
Extensor retinaculum

Fig. 9.15 Extensor compartments. Dorsal view. There are total of six compartments, numbered 1 to 6, from the radial to the ulnar side of the wrist. (From Schuenke M, Schulte E. General Anatomy and the Musculoskeletal System: Thieme Atlas of Anatomy. New York: Thieme; 2005. Illustration by Karl Wesker.)

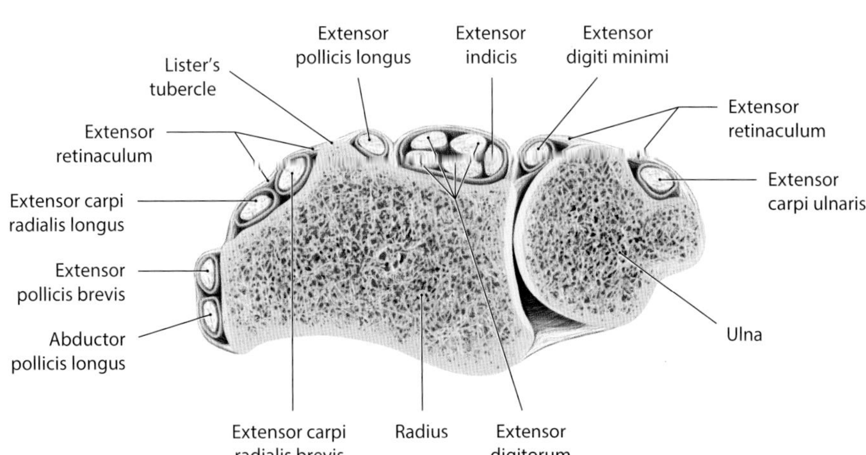

Fig. 9.16 Axial view of the distal radioulnar joint and extensor compartments of the wrist. There are six fibro-osseus tunnels created by the extensor retinaculum and intervening septa that divide the extensor tendons. Note Lister's tubercle redirects the extensor pollicis longus to the thumb. (Modified from Schuenke M, Schulte E. General Anatomy and the Musculoskeletal System: Thieme Atlas of Anatomy. New York: Thieme; 2005. Illustration by Karl Wesker.)

3. Tendons
   - Flexor tendons
     a. Flexor digitorum profundus (FDP): action is flexion at the DIP joint; FDP inserts on the distal phalanx
     b. Flexor digitorum superficialis (FDS): action is flexion at the PIP joint. Prior to FDS insertion to the middle phalanx it splits to form Camper's chiasm. The FDP travels through Camper's chiasm to insert on the distal phalanx.
     c. Flexor tendon zones **(Fig. 9.17)**
   - Flexor tendon sheaths
     a. Provide nourishment to tendons via vincula
     b. Provide protection to tendon
   - Pulleys
     a. Five annular pulleys (A1–A5) and three cruciate pulleys (C1–C3)
     b. A2, A4: arise from periosteum of P1 and P2, respectively; important to conserve to prevent bowstringing
     c. A1, A3, A5: arise from volar plate of MCP, PIP, and DIP joint, respectively
     d. A1 pulley involved in trigger digits
        - Tendon blood supply from two sources: direct vascular supply and diffusion through synovial sheath **(Fig. 9.18)**
        - **In zone II (see Fig. 9.17), tendon blood supply primarily through diffusion**

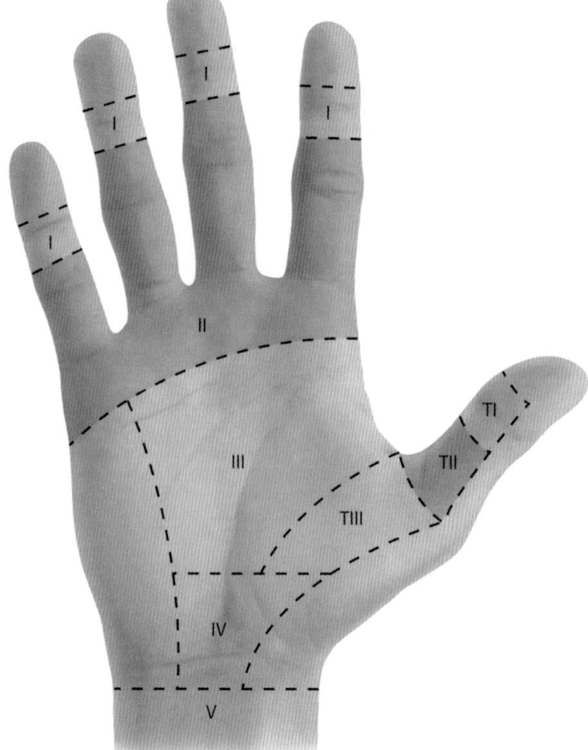

Fig. 9.17 Flexor tendon zones of the hand. Zones of the hand are used to help guide flexor tendon injury and repair. Zone I is distal to the flexor digitorum superficialis (FDS) insertion. Zone II is between the distal palmar crease and FDS insertion. Zone III is mid-palm. Zone IV is the carpal tunnel. Zone V is the distal forearm.

4. Nerves **(Figs. 9.19, 9.20, 9.21)**
   - Median nerve **(Figs. 9.22** and **9.23)**
     a. Travels between FDS and flexor pollicis longus (FPL) within the carpal tunnel to enter the wrist
     b. Supplies sensation to the thumb, the index and middle fingers, and the radial half of the ring finger
     c. Significant terminal branches
        - In forearm, motor branches to pronator teres, flexor carpi radialis, palmaris longus, flexor digitorum superficialis
        - Palmar cutaneous nerve
          ♦ Travels between palmaris longus and flexor carpi radialis

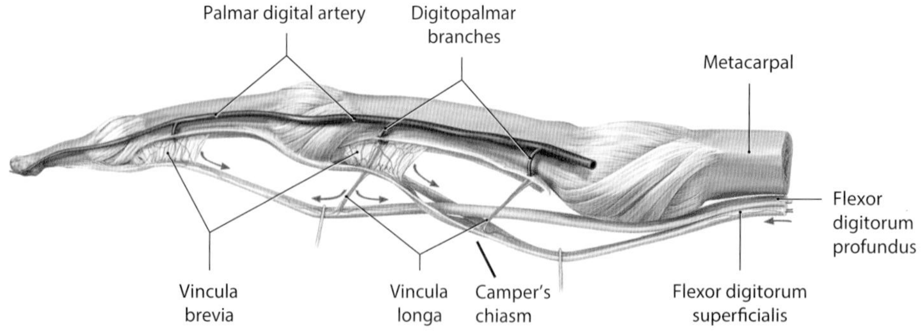

Fig. 9.18 Vascular supply to the flexor tendons. Flexor tendons are supplied within their sheath by branches of the palmar digital arteries via the vincula longa and brevia. Note the flexor digitorum profundus (FDP) traveling through Camper's chiasm to insert on the distal phalanx. (From Schuenke M, Schulte E. General Anatomy and the Musculoskeletal System: Thieme Atlas of Anatomy. New York: Thieme; 2005. Illustration by Karl Wesker.)

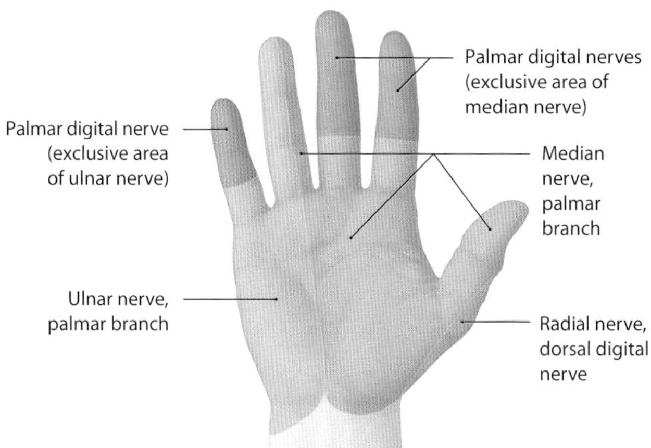

Fig. 9.19 Sensory innervations of palm of the hand. (From Schuenke M, Schulte E. General Anatomy and the Musculoskeletal System: Thieme Atlas of Anatomy. New York: Thieme; 2005. Illustration by Karl Wesker.)

- **Palmar cutaneous nerve branches from median nerve 4 to 6 cm proximal to wrist crease, and injury may result from retraction during volar Henry approach to distal radius, causing sensory change over thenar eminence**
- Supplies sensation to the central palm

- Recurrent motor branch innervates opponens pollicis, abductor pollicis brevis, flexor pollicis brevis
- Anterior interosseus nerve innervates index and middle finger flexor digitorum profundus, FPL, pronator quadrates
- First and second lumbricals innervated by median nerve via branches of digital nerves

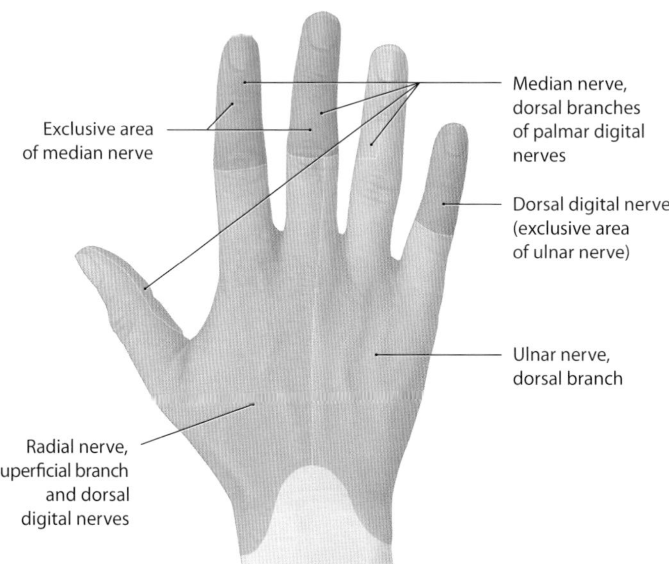

Fig. 9.20 Sensory innervations of dorsum of the hand. (From Schuenke M, Schulte E. General Anatomy and the Musculoskeletal System: Thieme Atlas of Anatomy. New York: Thieme; 2005. Illustration by Karl Wesker.)

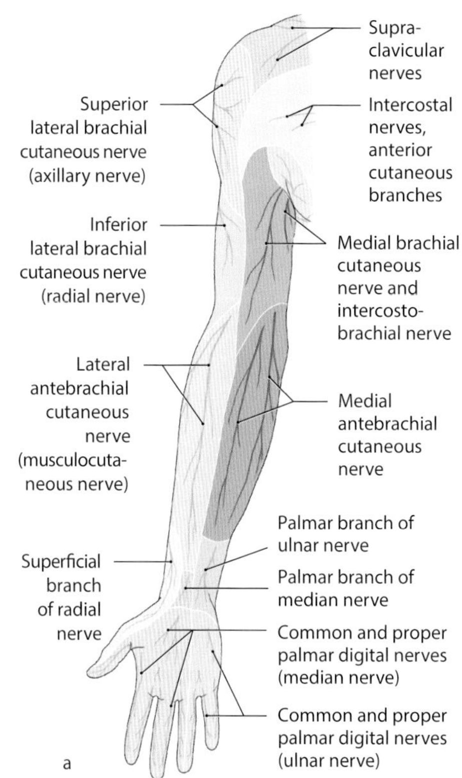

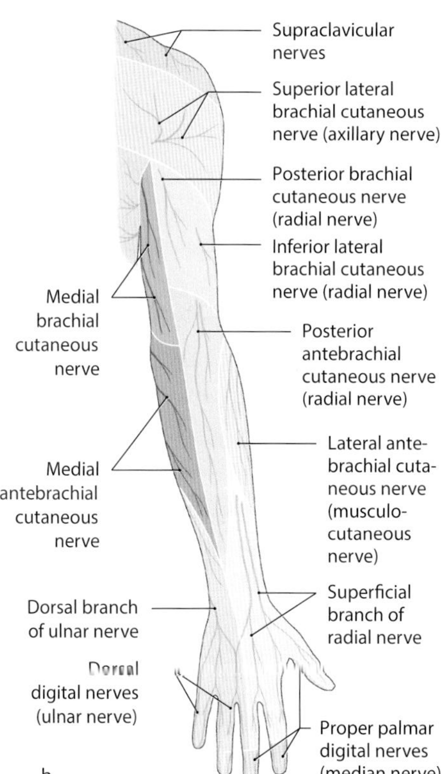

Fig. 9.21 Sensory innervations of **(a)** anterior and **(b)** posterior arm and forearm. (From Schuenke M, Schulte E. General Anatomy and the Musculoskeletal System: Thieme Atlas of Anatomy. New York: Thieme; 2005. Illustration by Karl Wesker.)

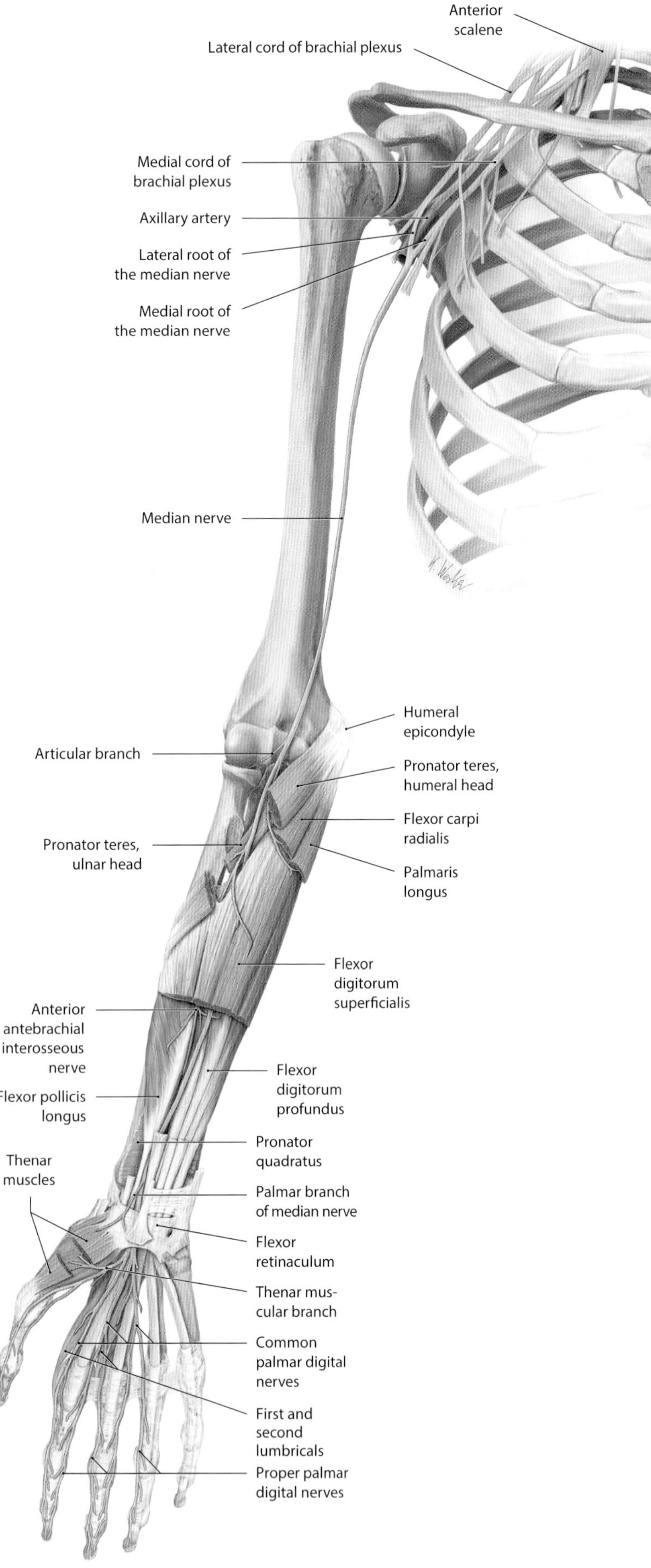

Fig. 9.22 Course of the median nerve. The median nerve is composed of the medial and lateral cords of the brachial plexus. The median nerve runs in the medial bicipital groove and then passes under the bicipital aponeurosis and between the two heads of the pronator teres to the forearm. After giving off the anterior interosseus nerve distal to the pronator teres, the median nerve runs between the flexor digitorum superficialis and the profundus to the wrist. The medial nerve then passes through the carpal tunnel and gives off its terminal branches. (From Schuenke M, Schulte E. General Anatomy and the Musculoskeletal System: Thieme Atlas of Anatomy. New York: Thieme; 2005. Illustration by Karl Wesker.)

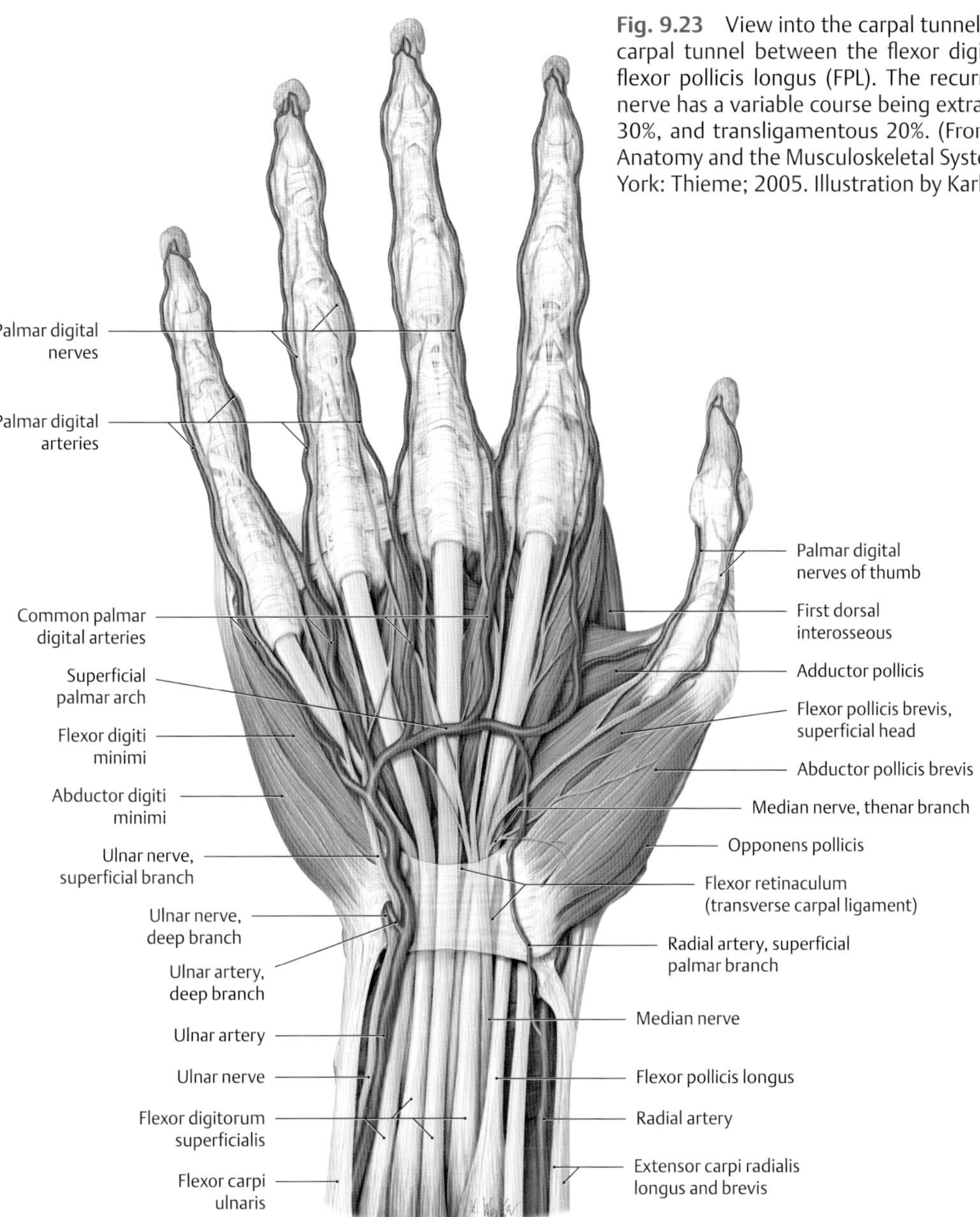

Fig. 9.23 View into the carpal tunnel. Median nerve travels through the carpal tunnel between the flexor digitorum superficialis (FDS) and the flexor pollicis longus (FPL). The recurrent motor branch of the median nerve has a variable course being extraligamentous 50%, subligamentous 30%, and transligamentous 20%. (From Schuenke M, Schulte E. General Anatomy and the Musculoskeletal System: Thieme Atlas of Anatomy. New York: Thieme; 2005. Illustration by Karl Wesker.)

- Ulnar nerve **(Fig. 9.24)**
  a. Enters anterior compartment of forearm through cubital tunnel and enters wrist via Guyon's canal **(Fig. 9.25)**
  b. Supplies sensation to the ulnar half of ring and small fingers
  c. Significant terminal branches
    - In forearm, motor branches to FCU and ring and small finger FDP
    - Dorsal cutaneous branch, 5–7 cm proximal to wrist
    - Within Guyon's canal, ulnar nerve bifurcates into two branches:
      - ♦ Superficial branch is sensory branch and also innervates palmaris brevis
      - ♦ Deep branch innervates all interossei, third and fourth lumbricals, abductor digiti minimi, opponens digiti minimi, flexor digiti minimi, adductor pollicis, and deep head of flexor pollicis brevis
- Radial nerve **(Fig. 9.26)**
  a. Branches into deep and superficial branch in proximal forearm
  b. Supplies sensation to the dorsal first webspace

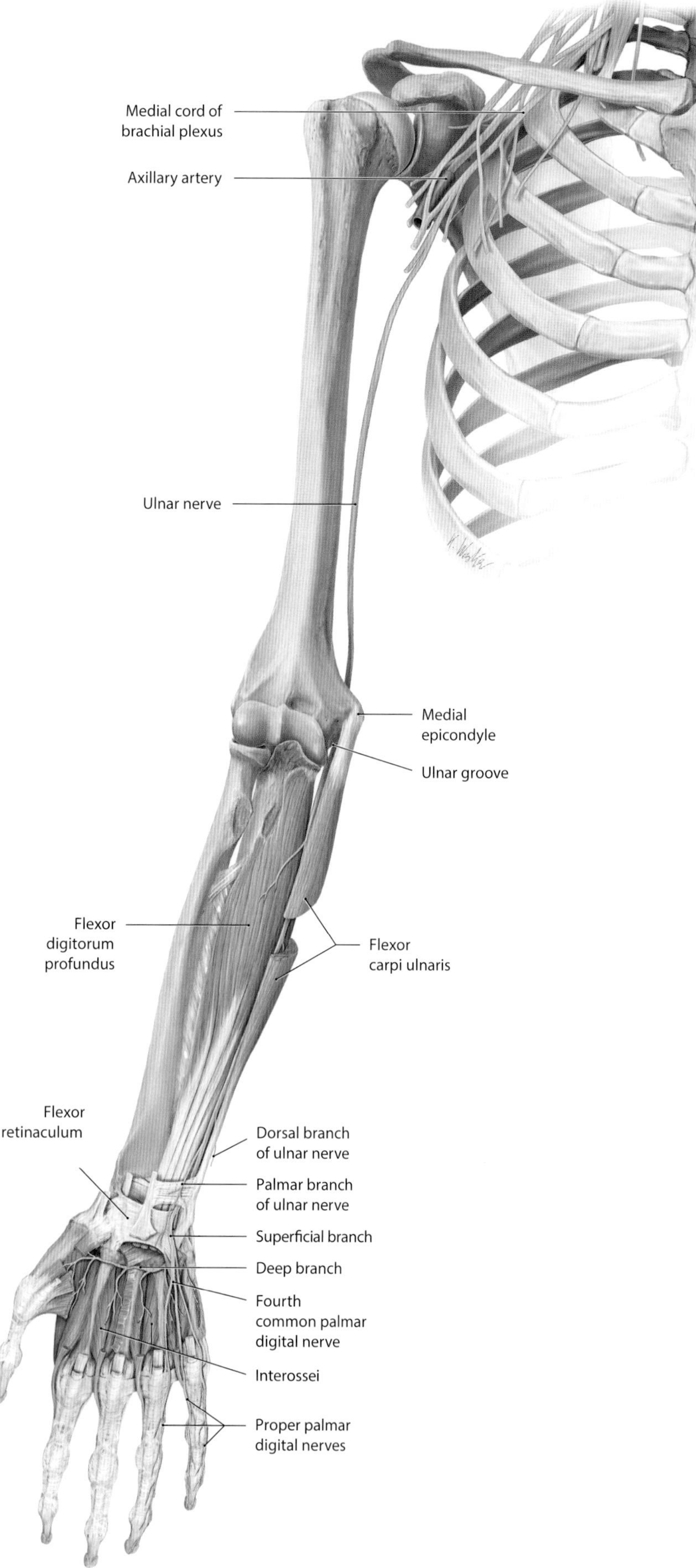

Fig. 9.24 Course of the ulnar nerve. The ulnar nerve is a continuation of the medial cord of the brachial plexus. The ulnar nerve pierces the medial intermuscular septum halfway down the arm. It reaches the elbow joint between the septum and the medial head of the triceps and crosses over the joint just distal to the medial epicondyle. The ulnar nerve then travels between the two heads of the flexor carpi ulnaris (FCU) and then travels beneath the FCU to the wrist. The nerve enters the hand through the ulnar tunnel, where it divides into its superficial sensory and deep motor branch. (From Schuenke M, Schulte E. General Anatomy and the Musculoskeletal System: Thieme Atlas of Anatomy. New York: Thieme; 2005. Illustration by Karl Wesker.)

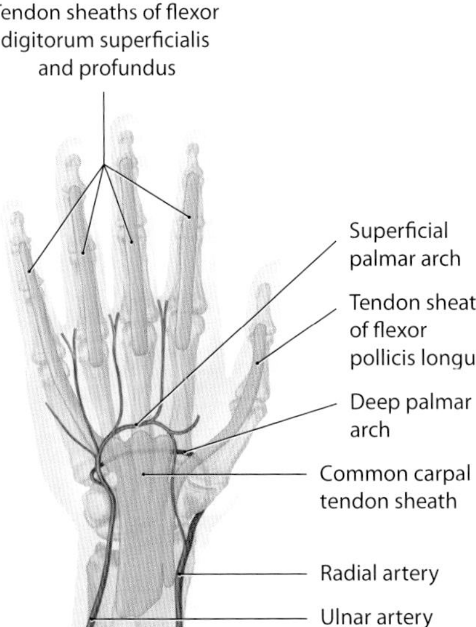

Fig. 9.25 Bony landmarks of the ulnar tunnel (Guyon's canal). The pisiform (ulnar) and the hook of the hamate (distal and radial) provide the bony landmarks that the ulnar artery and nerve travel. The transverse carpal ligament serves as the floor, and the volar carpal ligament the roof of Guyon's canal. (From Schuenke M, Schulte E. General Anatomy and the Musculoskeletal System: Thieme Atlas of Anatomy. New York: Thieme; 2005. Illustration by Karl Wesker.)

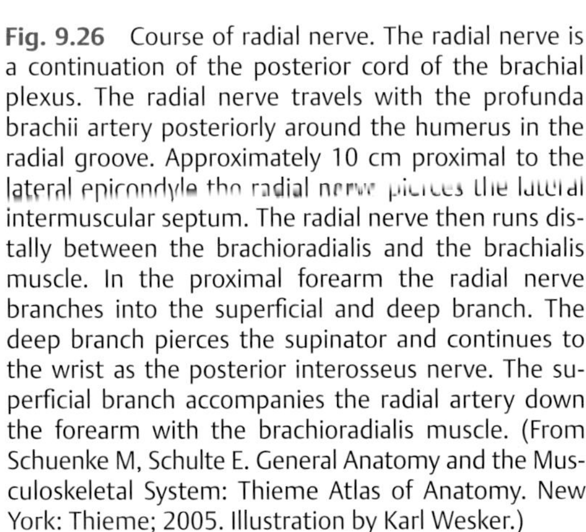

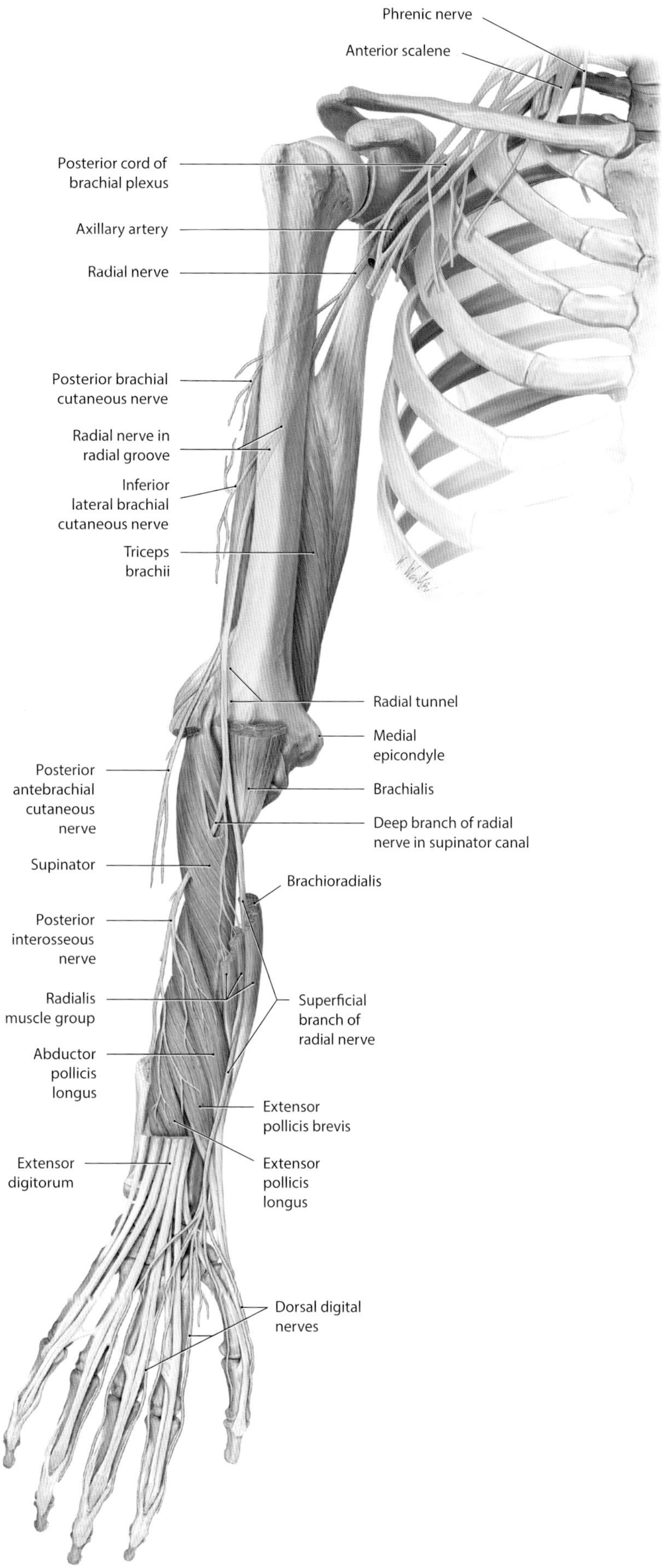

Fig. 9.26 Course of radial nerve. The radial nerve is a continuation of the posterior cord of the brachial plexus. The radial nerve travels with the profunda brachii artery posteriorly around the humerus in the radial groove. Approximately 10 cm proximal to the lateral epicondyle the radial nerve pierces the lateral intermuscular septum. The radial nerve then runs distally between the brachioradialis and the brachialis muscle. In the proximal forearm the radial nerve branches into the superficial and deep branch. The deep branch pierces the supinator and continues to the wrist as the posterior interosseus nerve. The superficial branch accompanies the radial artery down the forearm with the brachioradialis muscle. (From Schuenke M, Schulte E. General Anatomy and the Musculoskeletal System: Thieme Atlas of Anatomy. New York: Thieme; 2005. Illustration by Karl Wesker.)

c. Significant branches

- Muscular branches to triceps, anconeus, extensor carpi radialis longus, brachioradialis [sometimes extensor carpi radialis brevis (ECRB)]
- Posterior interosseous nerve (PIN): continuation of radial nerve; innervates ECRB, supinator, extensor digitorum communis, extensor digiti minimi, extensor carpi ulnaris, extensor indicis, abductor pollicis longus, extensor pollicis longus, extensor pollicis brevis
- Superficial branch radial nerve: branches from radial nerve; emerges between brachioradialis and extensor carpi radialis longus tendon 7 cm from radial styloid to become superficial

5. Vascular

- Ulnar artery: travels radial to ulnar nerve in forearm and is primary supply to superficial palmar arch **(Fig. 9.27)**

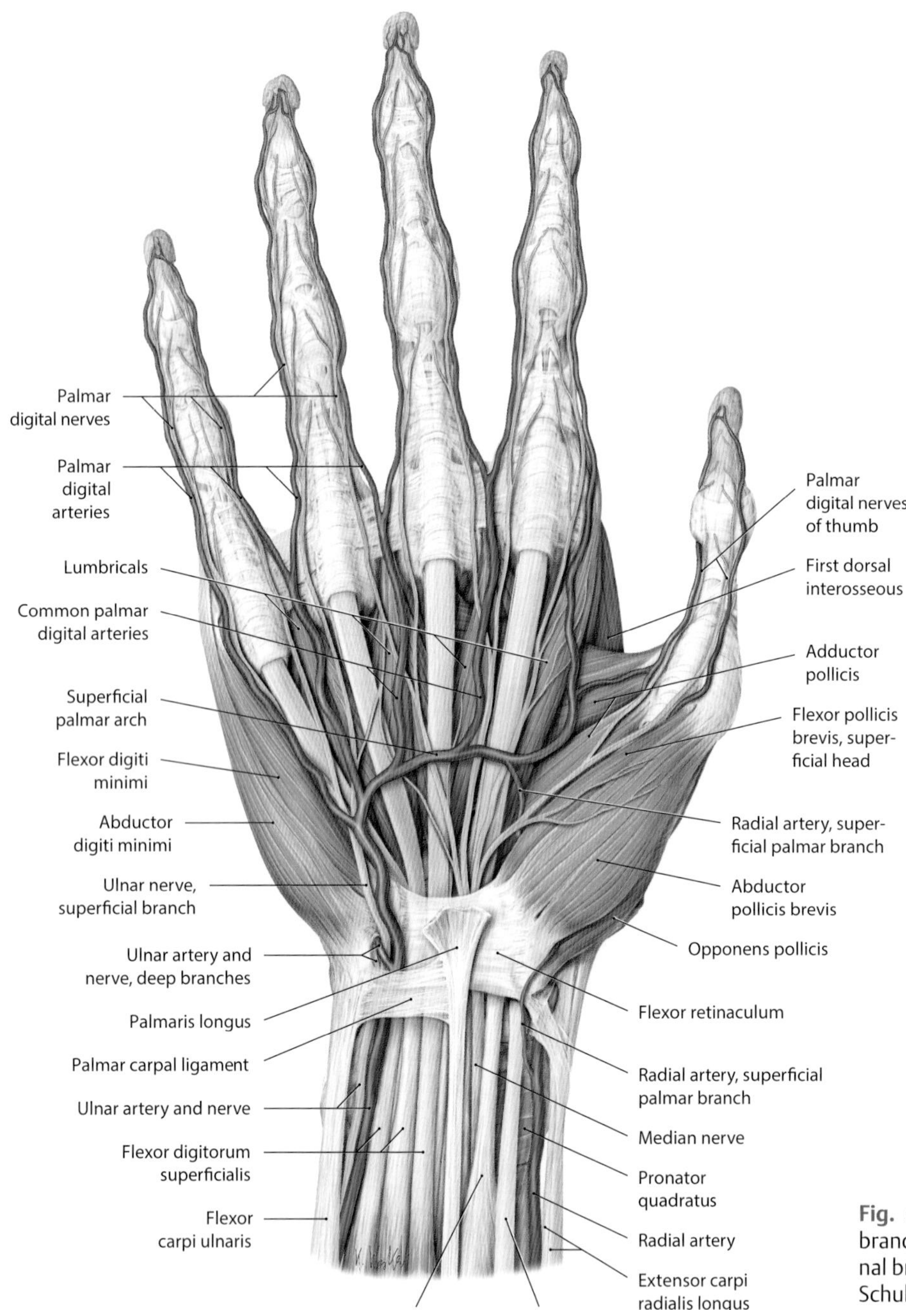

Fig. 9.27 The superficial palmar arch and its branches. The superficial palmar arch is the terminal branch of the ulnar artery. (From Schuenke M, Schulte E. General Anatomy and the Musculoskeletal System: Thieme Atlas of Anatomy. New York: Thieme; 2005. Illustration by Karl Wesker.)

- **Travels with median nerve but goes deep to deep head of pronator teres in the proximal forearm; median nerve splits the two heads of the pronator teres**
- Radial artery: travels between brachioradialis and flexor carpi radialis in the forearm and is primary supply to deep palmar arch (**Figs. 9.28** and **9.29**)
- **Digital neurovascular bundle: nerve lies volar to artery in the finger**

6. Muscles
   - Muscles of the hand (**Figs. 9.30, 9.31, 9.32, 9.33, 9.34** and **Table 9.1**)
   - Muscles of the forearm (**Figs. 9.35, 9.36, 9.37, 9.38, 9.39, 9.40** and **Tables 9.2** and **9.3**)
7. Physical exam of the upper extremity
   - Elbow
     a. Inspection
        - Gross deformity or swelling may indicate fracture
        - Carrying angle: average 11 degrees in men, 13 degrees in women; cubitus varus < 5 degrees and cubitus valgus > 15 degrees

     b. Palpation
        - Tender at medial epicondyle: golfer's elbow or medial collateral ligament (MCL) pathology

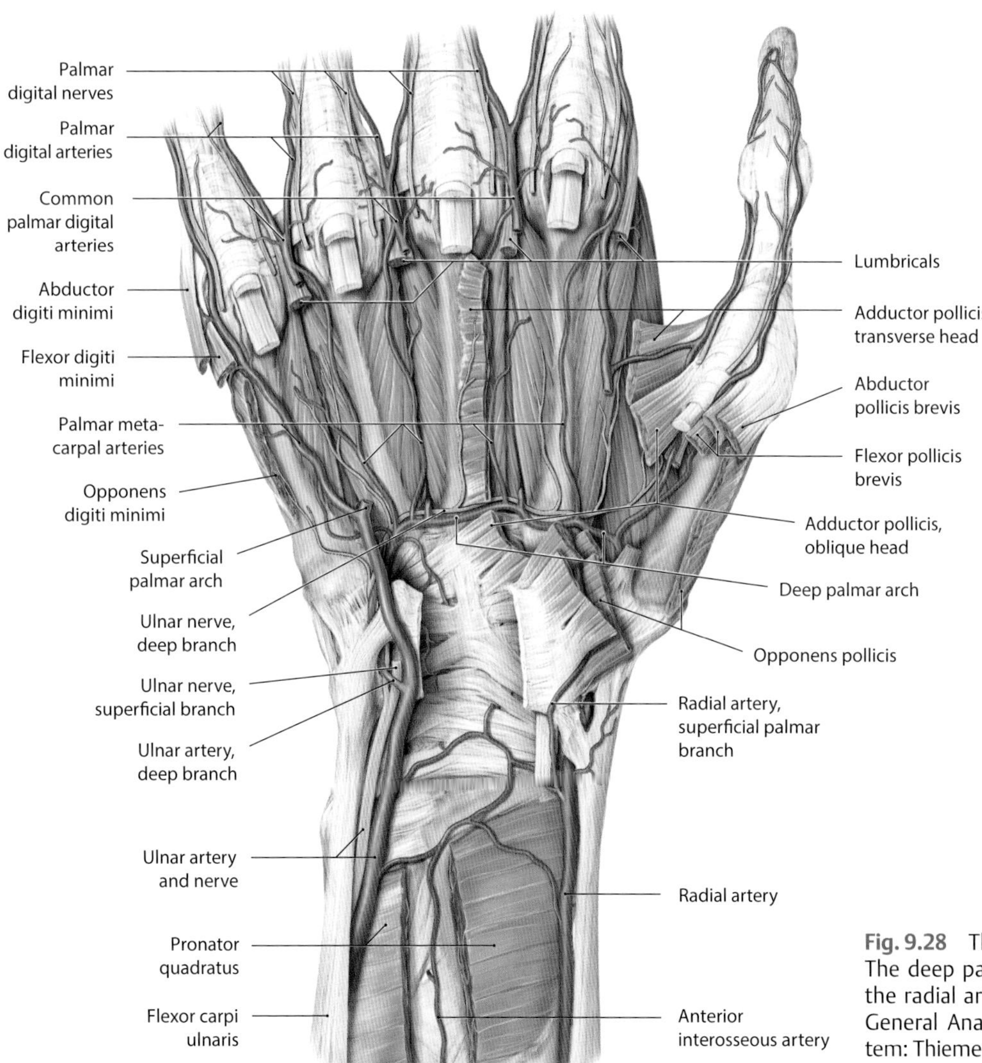

Fig. 9.28 The deep palmar arch and its branches. The deep palmar arch is the terminal branch of the radial artery. (From Schuenke M, Schulte E. General Anatomy and the Musculoskeletal System: Thieme Atlas of Anatomy. New York: Thieme; 2005. Illustration by Karl Wesker.)

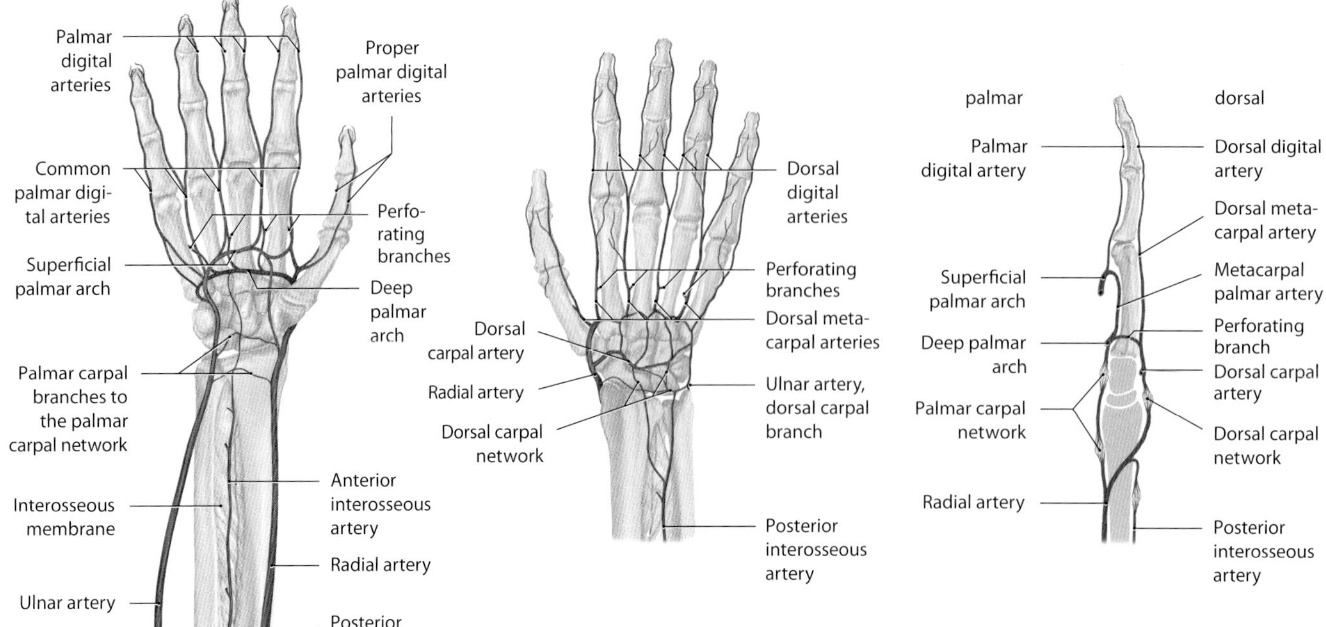

Fig. 9.29 Arterial anastomoses in the hand. The ulnar and radial artery are connected by the superficial and deep palmar arch, the perforating branches, and the dorsal carpal network. (From Schuenke M, Schulte E. General Anatomy and the Musculoskeletal System: Thieme Atlas of Anatomy. New York: Thieme; 2005. Illustration by Karl Wesker.)

- Tender at lateral epicondyle: tennis elbow
- Tender at radial head: fracture, arthritis
- Palpate biceps tendon, absence may be due to biceps tendon rupture

c. ROM
- Extend/flex ROM: 0 to 140–150 degrees
- Supinate 80–90 degrees, pronate 75–90 degrees

d. Neurologic
- Test motor and sensory
- Reflexes: biceps C5, brachioradialis C6, triceps C7; absence or hypoactive indicates a radiculopathy

e. Special tests
- Tennis elbow (lateral epicondylitis): provocative tests include resisted wrist extension
- **Pathology is angiofibroblastic hyperplasia of ECRB tendon**
- Golfer's elbow (medial epicondylitis): provocative tests include resisted flexion and pronation; also pain at medial epicondyle with supination and extension of elbow and wrist
- Radial tunnel: resisted extension of long finger
- Pivot shift: The patient lies supine with arm overhead and elbow extended. The forearm is then supinated with a valgus stress applied while the elbow is flexed. If the patient exhibits apprehension or palpable subluxation of the radial head, then the test is positive for posterolateral rotatory instability.
- Bicep hook test: inability to "hook" biceps due to biceps tendon rupture
- Tinel's sign: percussion of ulnar groove sends tingling or shooting pain in ulnar nerve distribution

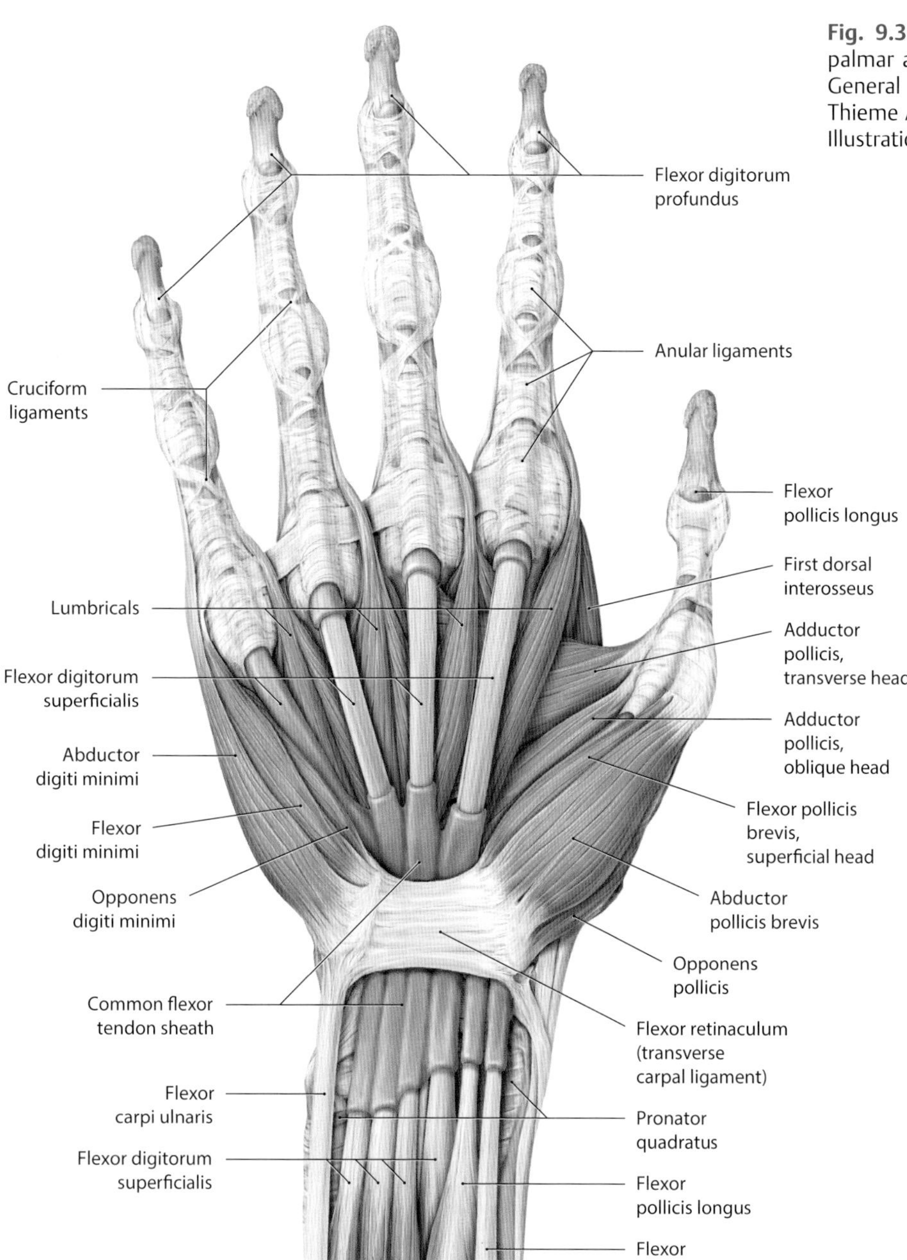

Fig. 9.30 Superficial muscles after removal of a palmar aponeurosis. (From Schuenke M, Schulte E. General Anatomy and the Musculoskeletal System: Thieme Atlas of Anatomy. New York: Thieme; 2005. Illustration by Karl Wesker.)

- Wrist
  a. Inspection
    - Gross deformity or swelling may indicate a fracture
    - Swelling or palpable mass at dorsal or volar aspect of wrist may indicate a ganglion cyst
    - Muscle wasting: thenar atrophy indicative of median nerve pathology
  b. Palpation
    - Snuffbox tenderness may indicate a scaphoid fracture.
    - Tenderness at the radial or ulnar styloid or the carpal row may indicate fracture. Tenderness over the lunate may indicate Kienböck's disease.
    - Tenderness distal to the ulnar styloid may indicate a TFCC tear.
    - Palpate extensor tendons. Tenderness over the first dorsal compartment is de Quervain's synovitis.

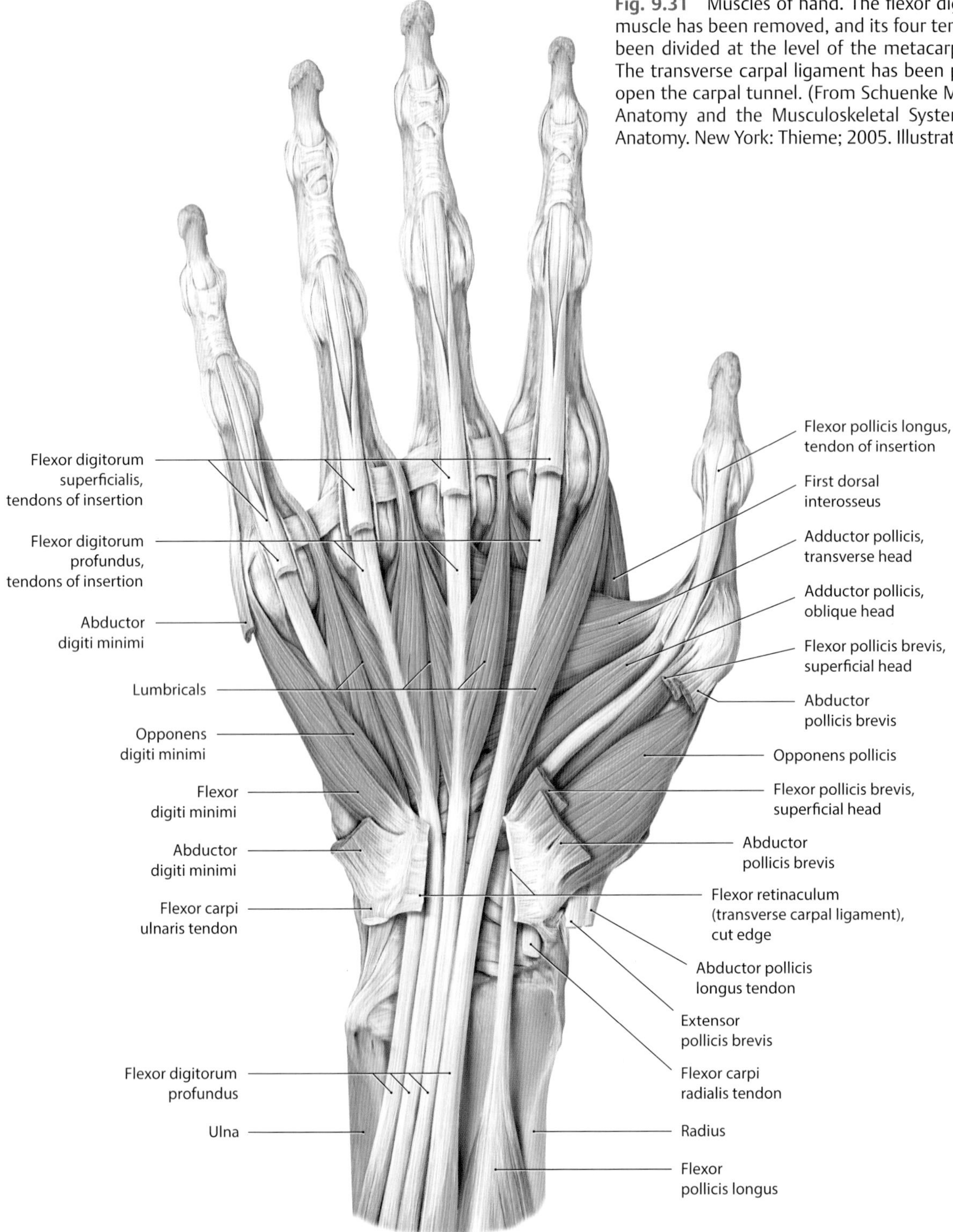

Fig. 9.31 Muscles of hand. The flexor digitorum superficialis muscle has been removed, and its four tendon insertions have been divided at the level of the metacarpophalangeal joints. The transverse carpal ligament has been partially removed to open the carpal tunnel. (From Schuenke M, Schulte E. General Anatomy and the Musculoskeletal System: Thieme Atlas of Anatomy. New York: Thieme; 2005. Illustration by Karl Wesker.)

c. ROM
   - Extend ROM 75 degrees, flexion 80 degrees
   - Radial deviation 15–25 degrees, ulnar 30–45 degrees
   - Only 10 to 15 degrees of pronation and supination from wrist

d. Neurologic
   - Test motor and sensory

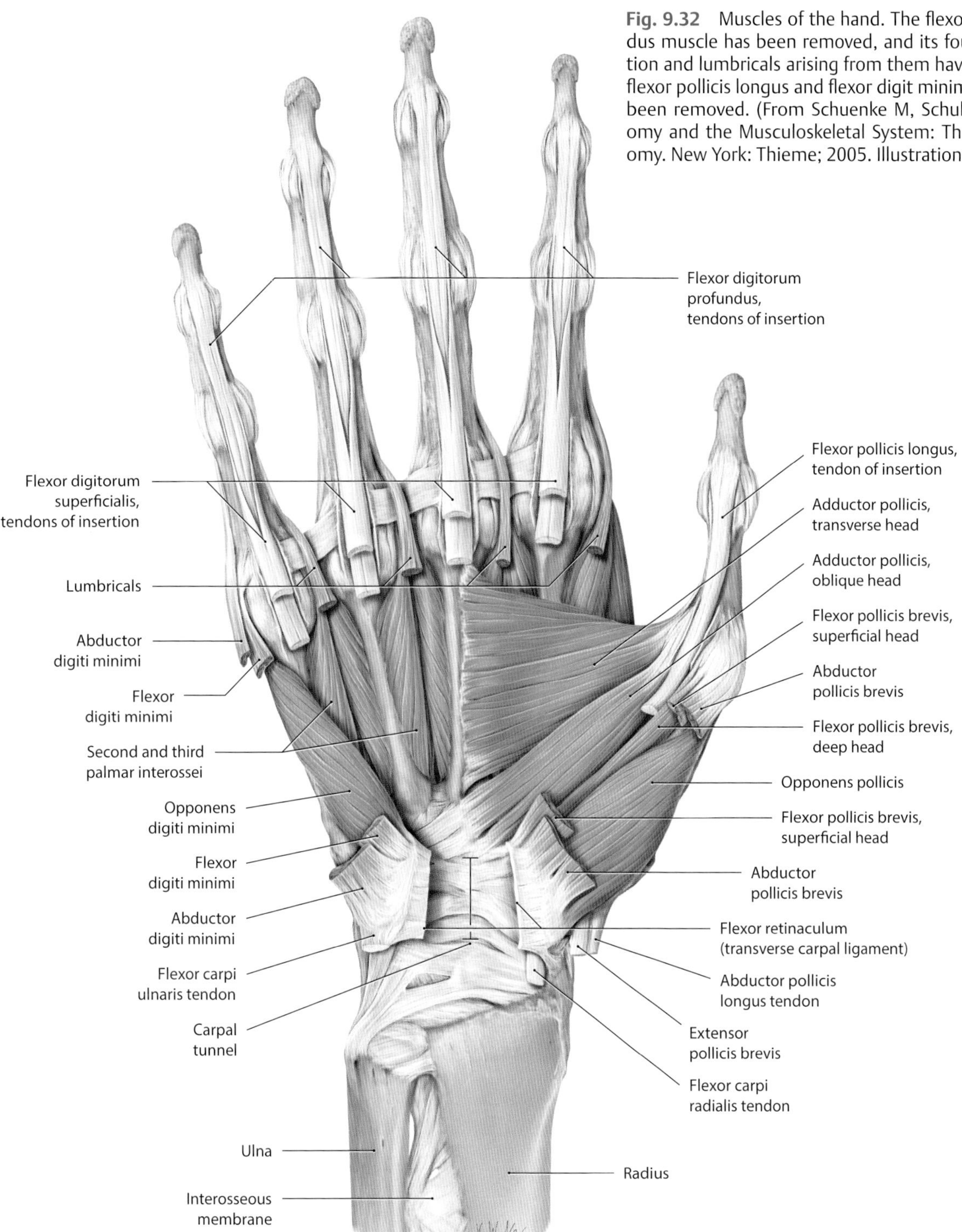

Fig. 9.32 Muscles of the hand. The flexor digitorum profundus muscle has been removed, and its four tendons of insertion and lumbricals arising from them have been divided. The flexor pollicis longus and flexor digit minimi muscles have also been removed. (From Schuenke M, Schulte E. General Anatomy and the Musculoskeletal System: Thieme Atlas of Anatomy. New York: Thieme; 2005. Illustration by Karl Wesker.)

e. Special tests
   - Durkan carpal compression test: manual pressure on carpal tunnel reproduces symptoms of carpal tunnel.
     - **♦ Most sensitive test for carpal tunnel syndrome**
   - Phalen test: wrist flexion reproduces symptoms of carpal tunnel.
   - Tinel's sign: percussion of carpal tunnel sends tingling or shooting pain in median nerve distribution.

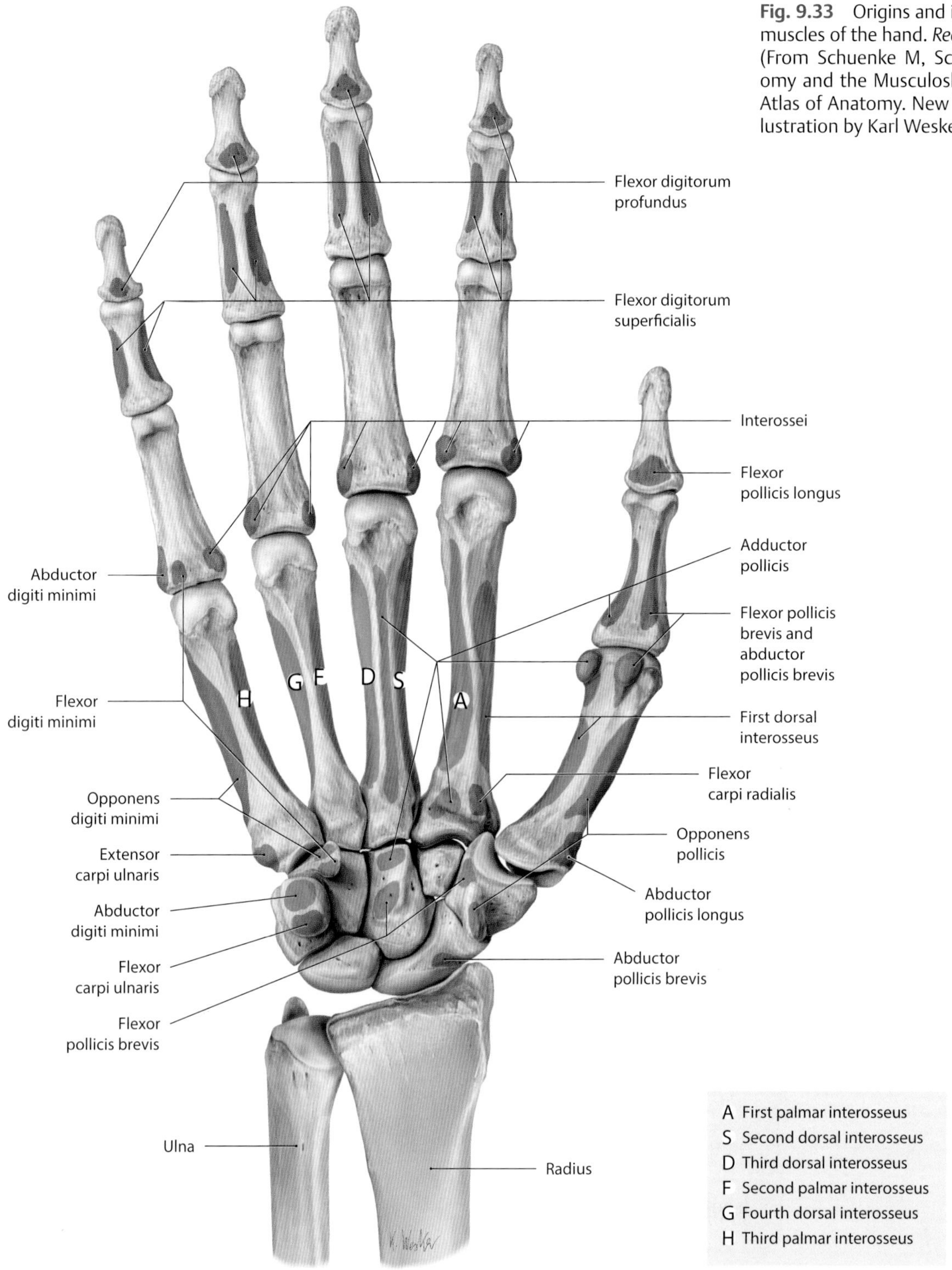

Fig. 9.33 Origins and insertions of the palmar muscles of the hand. *Red,* origin; *blue,* insertion. (From Schuenke M, Schulte E. General Anatomy and the Musculoskeletal System: Thieme Atlas of Anatomy. New York: Thieme; 2005. Illustration by Karl Wesker.)

- Finkelstein test: flex thumb into palm and ulnarly deviate wrist. Pain in first dorsal compartment is suggestive of de Quervain's synovitis.
- Watson scaphoid shift: pain or a clunk with pressure applied to volar scaphoid tubercle and wrist brought from ulnar to radial deviation; compare with contralateral side; tests carpal instability due to scapholunate ligament injury
- Piano key test: stabilize ulna and shuck radius dorsal/volar; subluxation or laxity indicates injury to distal radioulnar joint (DRUJ)

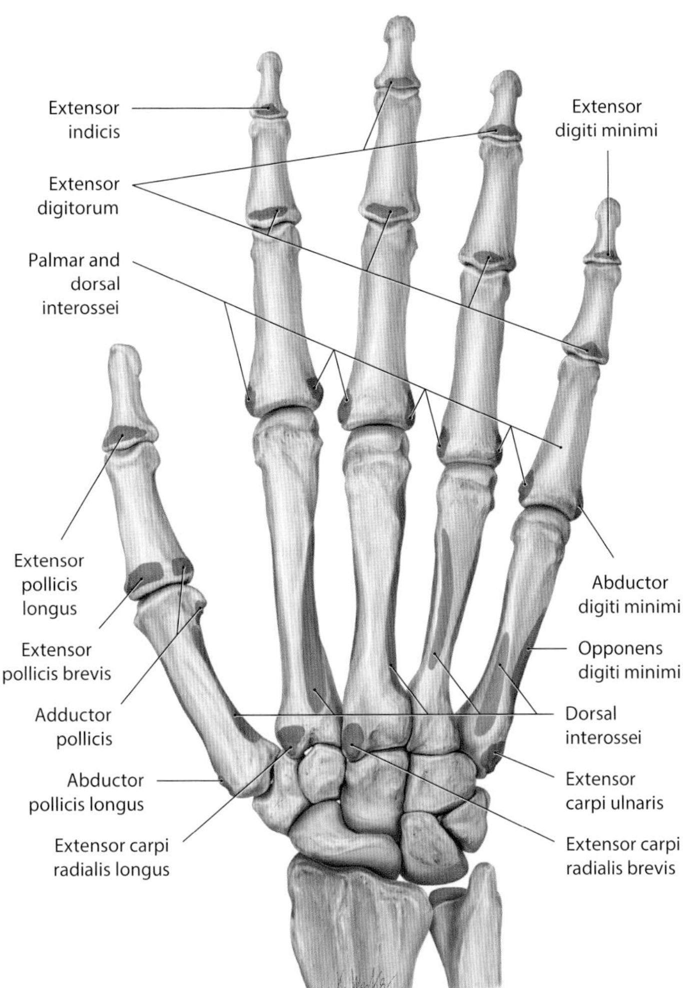

Fig. 9.34 Origins and insertions of the dorsal muscles of the hand. *Red,* origin; *blue,* insertion. (From Schuenke M, Schulte E. General Anatomy and the Musculoskeletal System: Thieme Atlas of Anatomy. New York: Thieme; 2005. Illustration by Karl Wesker.)

- Hand
  a. Inspection
    - Gross deformity or swelling may indicate fracture.
    - Rotational or angular deformity of fingers may indicate facture. Rotation is assessed by having the patient make a fist; all fingers should point toward the scaphoid with no overlap of digits.
    - Finger position: flexed finger may be secondary to flexor tenosynovitis, tendon rupture, or Dupuytren's contracture
    - Fusiform swelling of digit seen in acute infection such as flexor tenosynovitis
    - Swelling of DIP joint due to osteoarthritis; Heberden's nodes
    - Swelling of PIP joint due to osteoarthritis; Bouchard's nodes
    - Swelling of MCP joint seen in rheumatoid arthritis (RA)
    - **Rheumatoid arthritis primarily affects the wrist and MCP joints.**
    - Ulnar drift or boutonniere deformity seen in RA
      - Wasting of hypothenar eminence or first dorsal webspace indicates ulnar nerve injury. Thenar wasting indicates median nerve injury.

Table 9.1 Muscles of the Hand

Muscle	Action	Nerve	Origin	Insertion	Compartment
Abductor pollicis brevis (APB)	Palmar pronation	Median	Scaphoid, trapezium	Proximal phalanx of thumb	Thenar compartment
Flexor pollicis brevis (superficial and deep head)	Thumb MCP flexion	Median/ulnar dual innervation	Transverse carpal ligament, trapezium	Proximal phalanx of thumb (base)	Thenar compartment
Opponens pollicis	Opposes thumb	Median	Trapezium	Thumb metacarpal (lateral)	Thenar compartment
Palmaris brevis	Tenses skin of palm during grip	Ulnar	TCL	Palmar aponeurosis	Hypothenar compartment
Flexor digiti minimi brevis	Small finger MCP flexion	Ulnar	TCL and hamate	Proximal phalanx of small finger (base)	Hypothenar compartment
Opponens digiti minimi	Oppose small finger	Ulnar	TCL and hamate	5th metacarpal (ulnar border)	Hypothenar compartment
Abductor digit minimi (ADM)	Small finger abduction	Ulnar	Pisiform	Proximal phalanx of small finger (ulnar base)	Hypothenar compartment
Adductor pollicis (oblique and transverse head)	Thumb adduction and MCP flexion	Ulnar	Capitate, 2nd and 3rd metacarpal (oblique head), 3rd metacarpal (transverse head)	Proximal phalanx of thumb (ulnar base)	Adductor compartment
Lumbricals: 1st and 2nd	Extend PIP, flex MCP	Median	FDP tendons (radial 1–2)	Radial lateral bands	Intrinsics, not considered a compartment
Lumbricals: 3rd and 4th	Extend PIP, flex MCP	Ulnar	FDP tendon (3–5)	Radial lateral bands	Intrinsics, not considered a compartment
Dorsal interossei Dorsal and Palmar Interossei DAB = Dorsal Abduct PAD = Palmar Adduct	Digit abduction, MCP flexion	Ulnar	Metacarpals	Extensor expansion and proximal phalanx	Dorsal interossei (four)
Palmar interossei	Digit adduction, MCP flexion	Ulnar	Metacarpals	Extensor expansion and proximal phalanx	Palmar interossei (three)

Abbreviations: FDP, flexor digitorum profundus; MCP, metacarpophalangeal; PIP, proximal interphalangeal; TCL, transverse carpal ligament.

b. Palpation
   - Nodules: Dupuytren's disease, cyst, giant cell tumor of tendon sheath
   - Garrod's pads: pads at dorsal PIP joint seen in Dupuytren's disease
   - Tender at A1 pulley: trigger finger
   - Tender on volar aspect of finger at flexor tendons: flexor tenosynovitis

c. ROM
   - MCP: extend/flex 0–90 degrees, adduct/abduct 0–20 degrees
   - PIP: extend/flex 0–110 degrees
   - DIP: extend/flex 0–80 degrees

d. Neurovascular
   - Palpate brachial, radial, and ulnar artery.
   - Allen test (see section IX, Vascular Disorders, below, for an explanation of how to perform this test)
   - Assess perfusion of digits with Doppler; evaluate capillary refill < 2 seconds

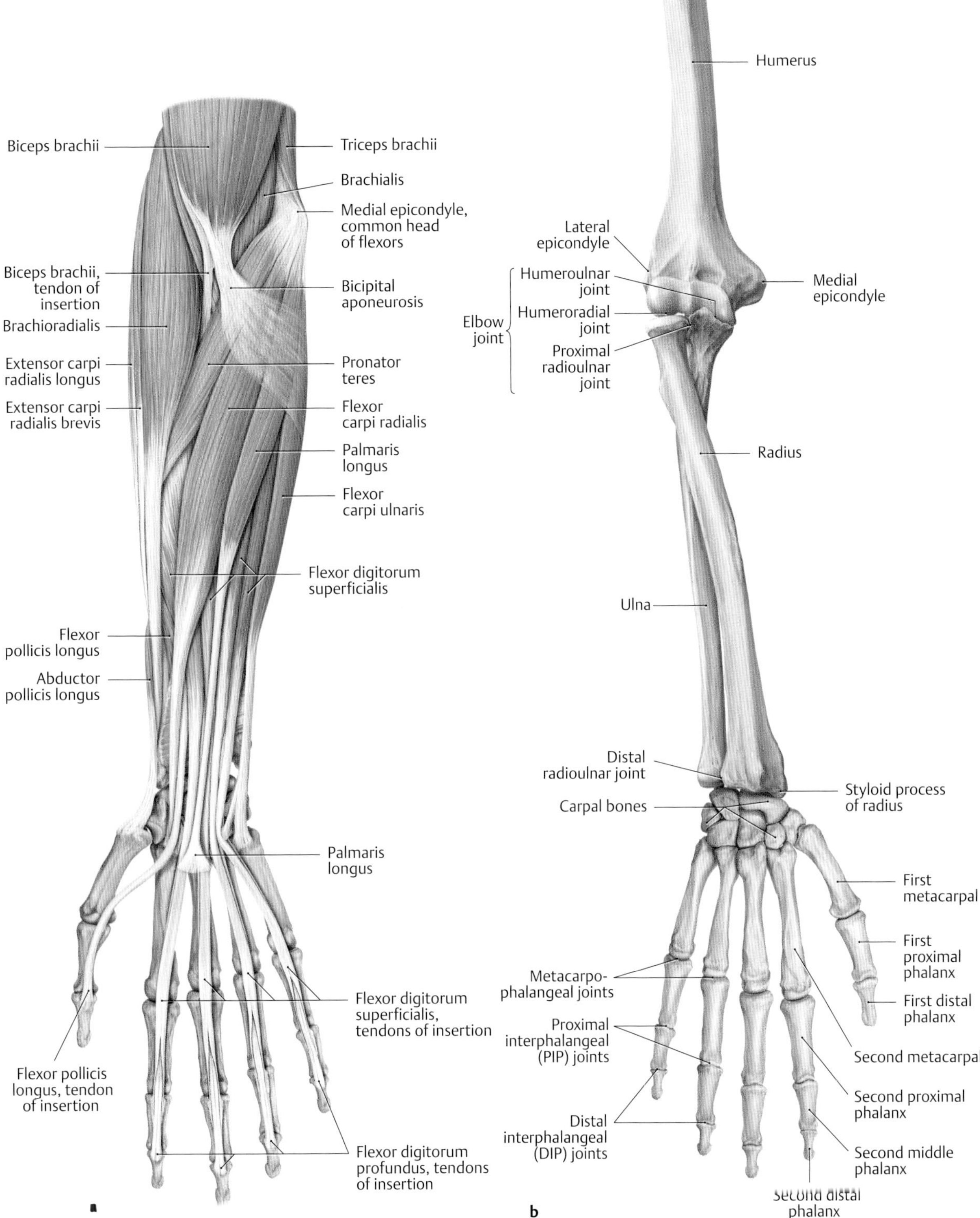

Fig. 9.35 Anterior muscles of the forearm. **(a)** The superficial flexors and mobile wad are shown. **(b)** The mobile wad is removed along with flexor carpi radialis, flexor carpi ulnaris, abductor pollicis longus, palmaris longus, and biceps brachii. (From Schuenke M, Schulte E. General Anatomy and the Musculoskeletal System: Thieme Atlas of Anatomy. New York: Thieme; 2005. Illustration by Karl Wesker.)

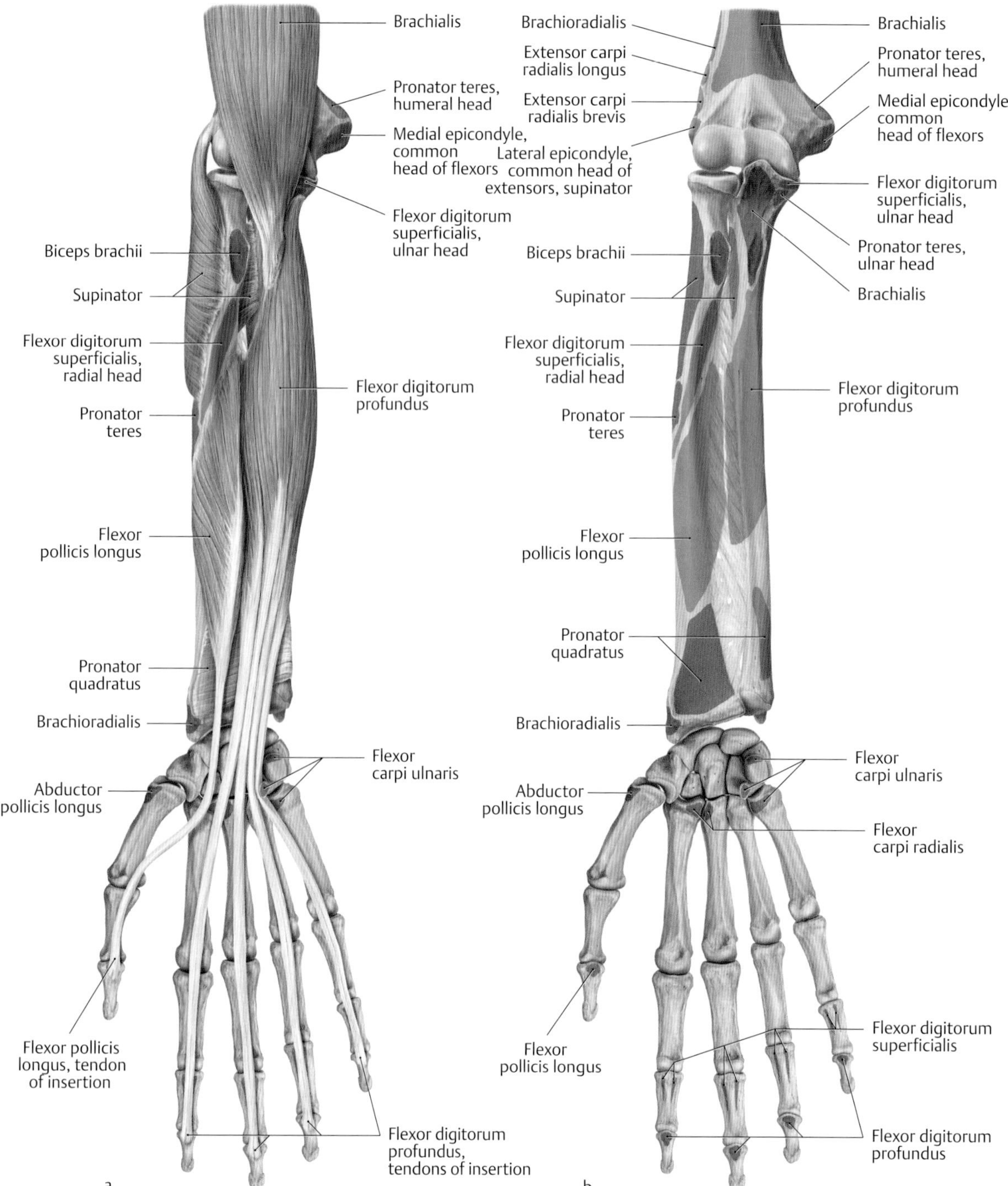

Fig. 9.36 Anterior muscles of the forearm. **(a)** Pronator teres and flexor digitorum superficialis have been removed. **(b)** All the muscles have been removed. *Red,* origin; *blue,* insertion. (From Schuenke M, Schulte E. General Anatomy and the Musculoskeletal System: Thieme Atlas of Anatomy. New York: Thieme; 2005. Illustration by Karl Wesker.)

- Test motor and sensory

e. Special tests

- **Froment sign, Wartenberg sign, intrinsic atrophy, and clawing are all signs of ulnar nerve injury.**
- Elson test: Bend the patient's finger 90 degrees over a table and actively extend it against resistance at the PIP joint. If the DIP joint remains supple and the middle phalanx extends, then the central slip is intact. If the

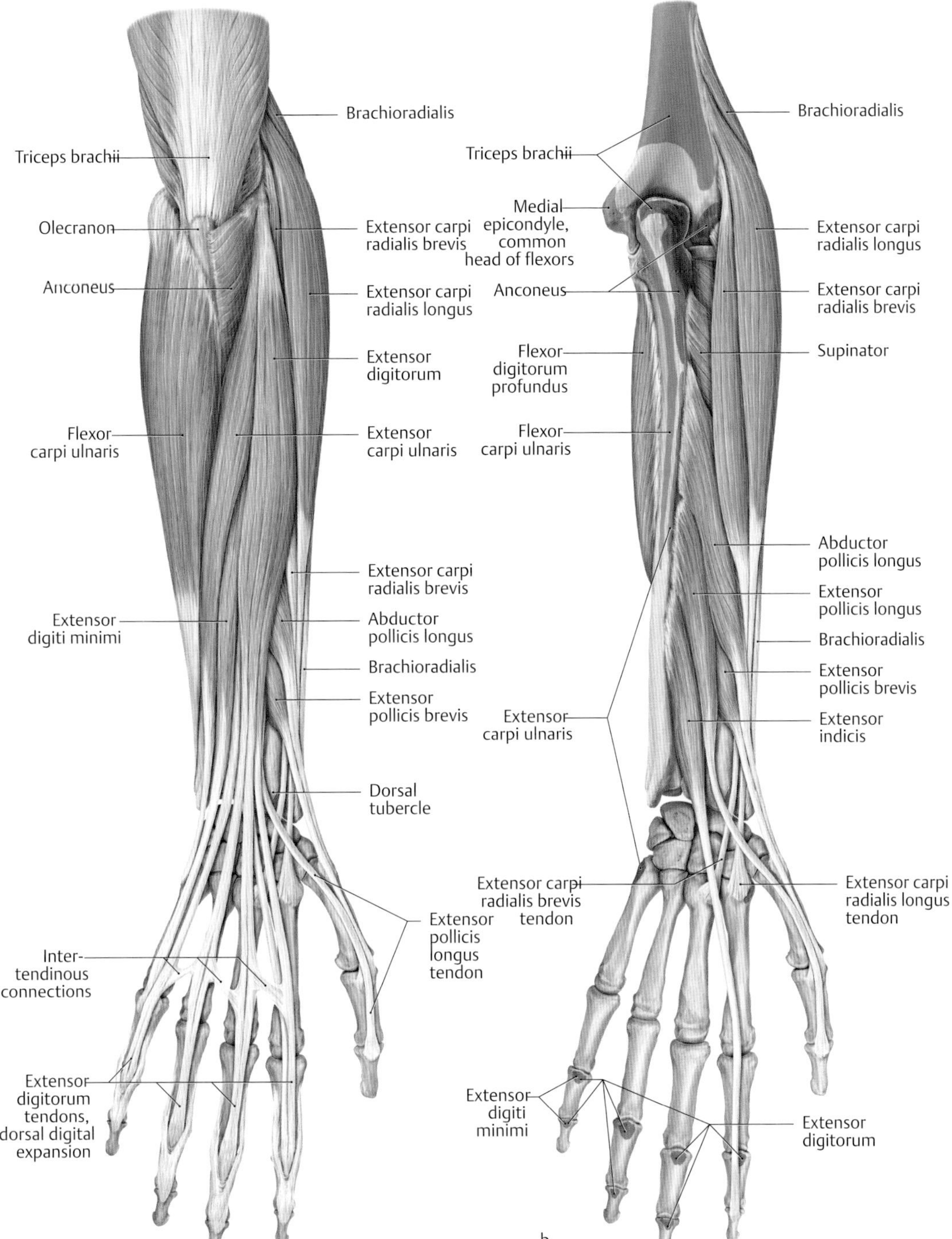

Fig. 9.37 Posterior muscles of the forearm. **(a)** The superficial extensors and mobile wad are shown. **(b)** The triceps brachii, anconeus, flexor carpi ulnaris, extensor carpi ulnaris, and extensor digitorum have been removed. (From Schuenke M, Schulte E. General Anatomy and the Musculoskeletal System: Thieme Atlas of Anatomy. New York: Thieme; 2005. Illustration by Karl Wesker.)

DIP joint is rigid with the absence of PIP extension, then the central slip is ruptured and the lateral bands are extending the DIP.

- Froment sign: IP flexion while attempting to pinch between thumb and index finger due to weak adductor pollicis (ulnar nerve); seen in cubital tunnel and ulnar nerve injuries
- Wartenberg sign: abducted small finger secondary to unopposed pull of EDM and weakness of third palmar interossei (ulnar nerve); seen in cubital tunnel and ulnar nerve injuries

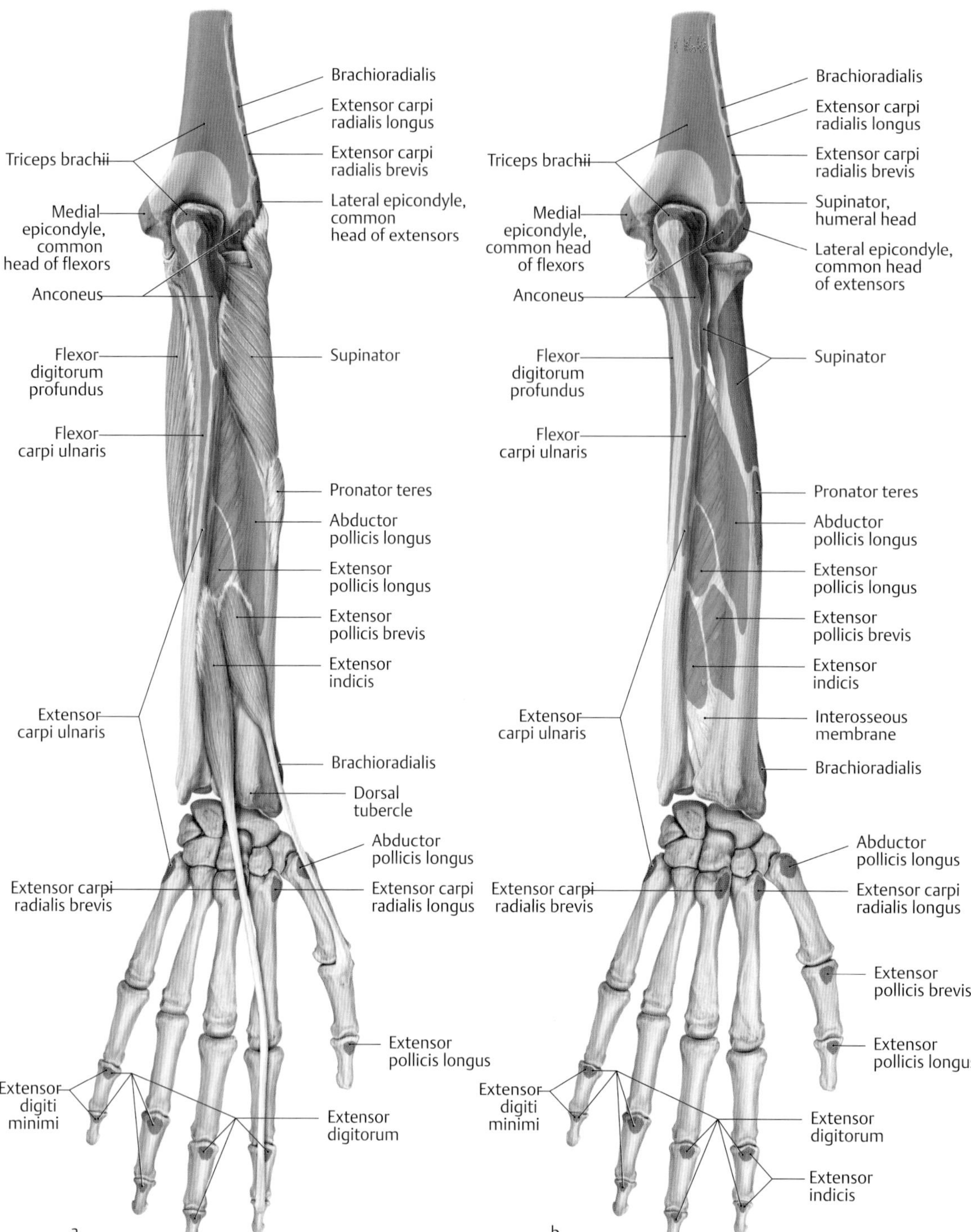

Fig. 9.38 Posterior muscles of the forearm. **(a)** Abductor pollicis longus, extensor pollicis longus, and mobile wad have been removed. **(b)** All the muscles have been removed. *Red,* origin; *blue,* insertion. (From Schuenke M, Schulte E. General Anatomy and the Musculoskeletal System: Thieme Atlas of Anatomy. New York: Thieme; 2005. Illustration by Karl Wesker.)

- Jeanne sign: hyperextension of thumb MCP with key pinch by EPL (radial nerve) due to weak adductor pollicis (ulnar nerve); seen in cubital tunnel and ulnar nerve injuries
- Thumb instability test: radially deviate thumb with the thumb in extension and 30 degrees of flexion to test proper and accessory ulnar collateral ligaments (UCLs), respectively.

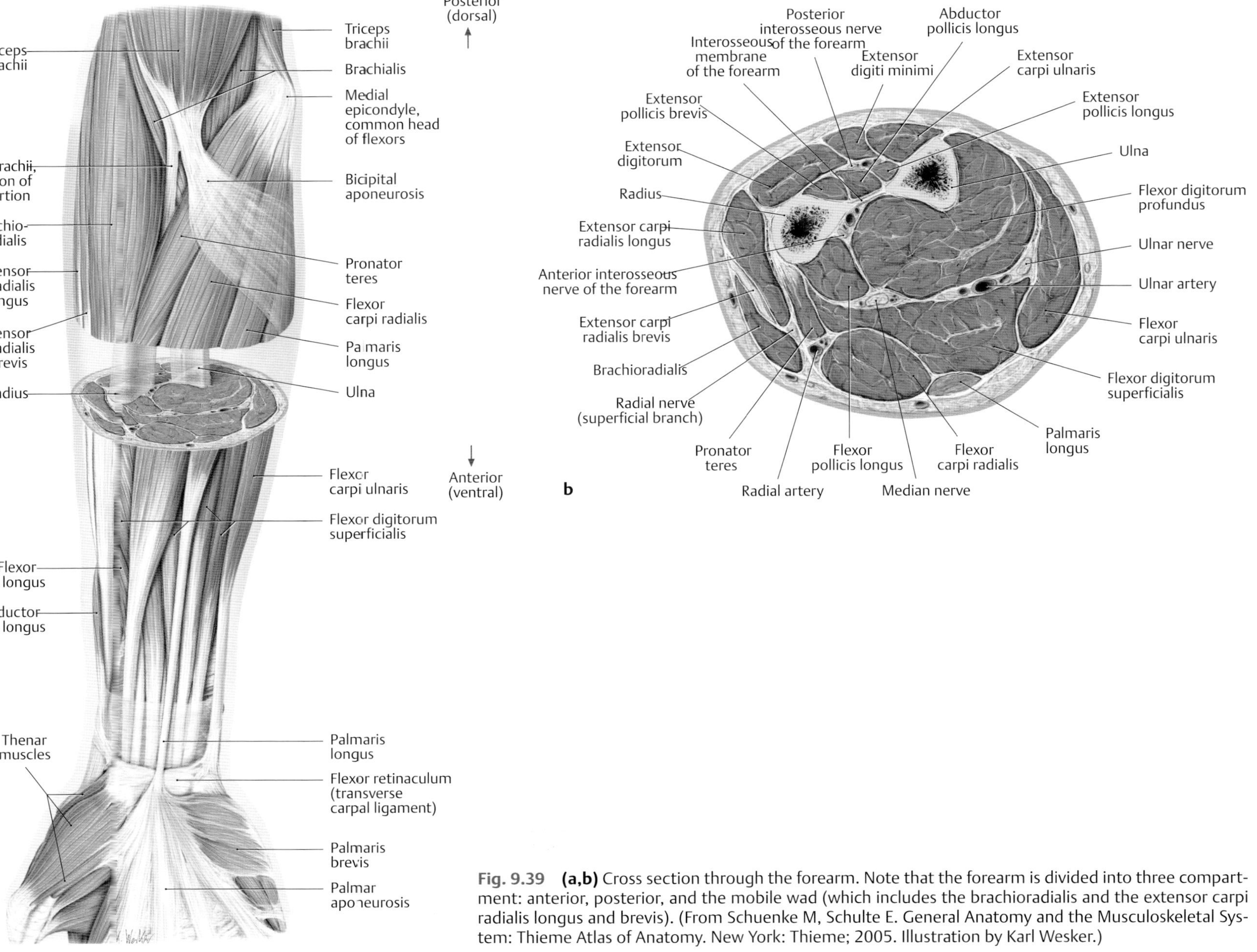

Fig. 9.39 **(a,b)** Cross section through the forearm. Note that the forearm is divided into three compartment: anterior, posterior, and the mobile wad (which includes the brachioradialis and the extensor carpi radialis longus and brevis). (From Schuenke M, Schulte E. General Anatomy and the Musculoskeletal System: Thieme Atlas of Anatomy. New York: Thieme; 2005. Illustration by Karl Wesker.)

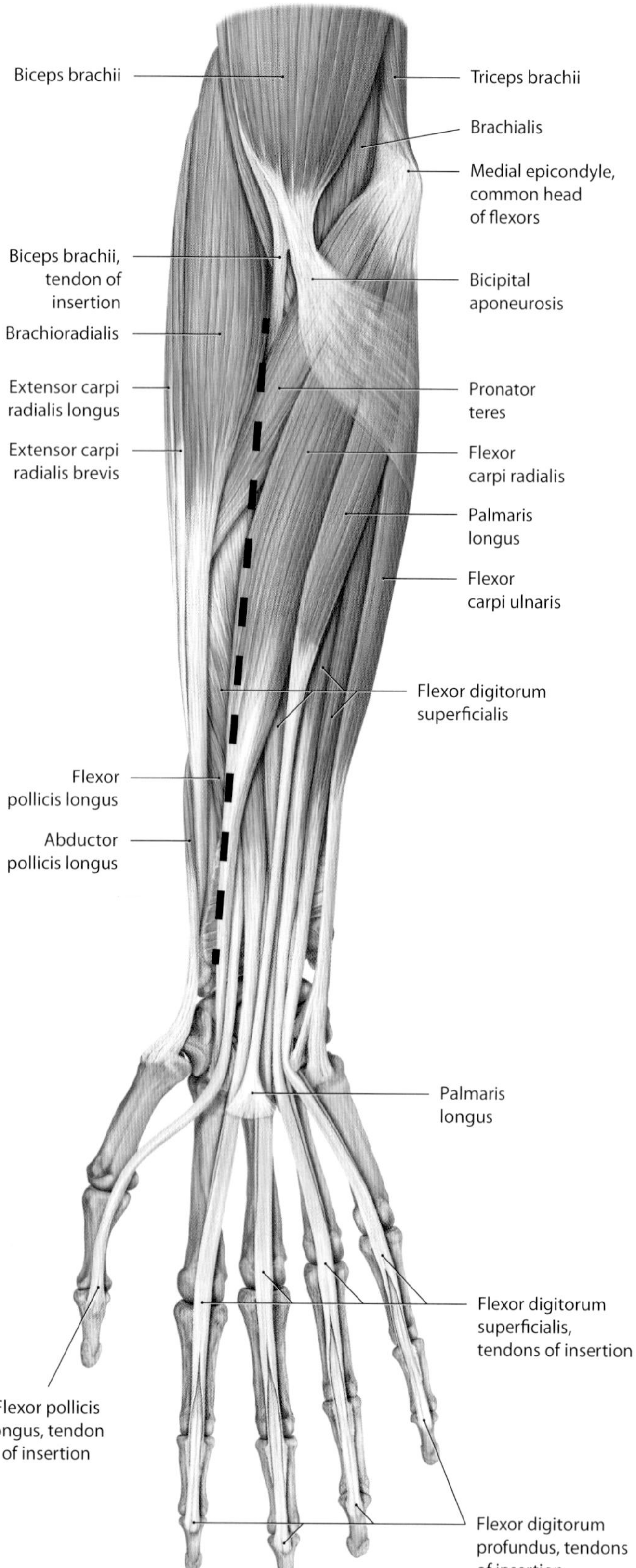

Fig. 9.40 Anterior approach of Henry. Proximally between brachioradialis and pronator teres and distally between flexor carpi radialis and radial artery. (From Schuenke M, Schulte E. General Anatomy and the Musculoskeletal System: Thieme Atlas of Anatomy. New York: Thieme; 2005. Illustration by Karl Wesker.)

Table 9.2 Muscles of the Forearm

Muscle	Action	Nerve	Origin	Insertion	Compartment
Flexor carpi radialis (FCR)	Flex wrist, radial deviation	Median	Medial epicondyle	Base of 2nd/3rd metacarpal	Anterior compartment (superficial)
Palmaris longus	Flex wrist	Median	Medial epicondyle	Flexor retinaculum and palmar aponeurosis	Anterior compartment (superficial)
Pronator teres (humeral and ulnar head)	Pronate and flex forearm	Median	Medial epicondyle, proximal ulna	Lateral mid- radius	Anterior compartment (superficial)
Flexor carpi ulnaris (FCU)	Flex wrist, ulnar deviation	Ulnar	Medial epicondyle, olecranon and proximal ulna	5th metacarpal, pisiform, hook of hamate	Anterior compartment (superficial)
Flexor digitorum superficialis (FDS)	Flex PIP joint	Median	Medial epicondyle, proximal ulna/radius	Middle phalanx	Anterior compartment (superficial)
Flexor digitorum profundus (FDP)	Flex DIP joint	AIN; ulnar (RF, SF, occasionally MF)	Anterior ulna, interosseus membrane	Distal phalanx	Anterior compartment (deep)
Flexor pollicis longus (FPL)	Flex thumb IP joint	AIN	Anterior radius/ proximal ulnar	Distal phalanx of thumb	Anterior compartment (deep)
Pronator quadratus (PQ)	Pronate forearm	AIN	Distal ulna	Anterior radius	Anterior compartment (deep)
Extensor digitorum communis (EDC)	Extend digits	PIN	Lateral epicondyle	Extensor expansion	Posterior compartment (superficial)
Extensor digitorum minimi (EDM)	Small finger extension	PIN	Lateral epicondyle	Extensor expansion 5th digit	Posterior compartment (superficial)
Extensor carpi ulnaris (ECU)	Extend/adduct hand	PIN	Lateral epicondyle	5th metacarpal base	Posterior compartment (superficial)
Anconeus	Extend forearm	Radial	Lateral epicondyle	Dorsal proximal ulna	Posterior compartment (superficial)
Abductor pollicis longus (APL)	Extend and abduct CMC joint	PIN	Proximal dorsal radius/ ulna	1st metacarpal base	Posterior compartment (deep)
Supinator	Supinate forearm	PIN	Posteromedial ulna	Dorsolateral radius	Posterior compartment (deep)
Extensor pollicis brevis (EPB)	Extend thumb at MCP joint	PIN	Proximal dorsal radius	Proximal phalanx of thumb (base)	Posterior compartment (deep)
Extensor pollicis longus (EPL)	Extend thumb at IP joint	PIN	Proximal dorsal ulna	Distal phalanx of thumb (base)	Posterior compartment (deep)
Extensor indicis proprius (EIP)	Extend index finger	PIN	Proximal dorsal ulna	Extensor expansion of index finger	Posterior compartment (deep)
Brachioradialis	Flex forearm	Radial	Lateral condyle	Distal radius	Mobile wad
Extensor carpi radialis longus (ECRL)	Extend wrist	Radial	Lateral condyle	2nd metacarpal base	Mobile wad
Extensor carpi radialis brevis (ECRB)	Extend wrist	Radial/PIN	Lateral condyle	3rd metacarpal base	Mobile wad

Abbreviations: AIN, anterior interosseus nerve; CMC, carpometacarpal, DIP, distal interphalangeal; IP, interphalangeal; MCP, metacarpophalangeal; MF, middle finger; PIN, posterior interosseus nerve; PIP, proximal interphalangeal; RF, ring finger; SF, small finger.

- **More than 30 degrees of laxity indicates an unstable tear. In extension, stress is testing accessory collateral ligament and volar plate. In 30 degrees of flexion, stress is testing collateral ligament.**

- CMC grind test: axial compression and rotation of CMC joint; pain indicates CMC arthritis
- Profundus test: stabilize PIP joint and flex DIP joint; inability to flex DIP joint indicates FDP injury

Table 9.3 Muscles of the Arm

Muscle	Action	Nerve	Origin	Insertion	Compartment
Coracobrachialis	Flex, adduct arm	Musculocutaneous	Coracoid	Humeral midshaft	Anterior
Biceps brachii (long and short head)	Supinate, flex arm	Musculocutaneous	Supraglenoid tubercle (long head), coracoid (short head)	Radial tuberosity	Anterior
Brachialis	Flex forearm	Musculocutaneous (medial), radial (lateral)	Anterior humerus	Ulnar tuberosity	Posterior
Triceps brachii (long, lateral, and medial head)	Extend forearm	Radial	Infraglenoid (long head), posterior humerus (lateral and medial head)	Olecranon	Posterior

Note: also see Chapter 7.

- Sublimis test: extend all fingers and flex a finger at PIP joint; inability to flex PIP joint indicates FDS injury
- Kanavel signs for flexor tenosynovitis: (1) resting flexed posture, (2) pain with passive extension, (3) fusiform swelling, and (4) tenderness volarly over tendon sheath

8. Imaging
   - Elbow
     a. Standard anteroposterior (AP), lateral, and oblique views
     b. Traction radiographs may help delineate distal humerus fractures
     c. Greenspan view evaluates radiocapitellar articulation; useful for radial head fractures; shot with forearm in neutral rotation and radiographic beam angled 45 degrees cephalad
   - Forearm
     a. Standard AP and lateral radiographs; oblique views useful to further evaluate fractures
   - Wrist
     a. Standard PA, lateral, and obliques views
     b. Scaphoid view to evaluate scaphoid fractures; wrist supinated 30 degrees and in ulnar deviation
        - **Clenched fist posteroanterior (PA) view to evaluate scapholunate ligament injury; scapholunate gap of > 3 mm indicates injury**
     c. Carpal tunnel view to evaluate hook of hamate fracture; shot with wrist fully extended, palm placed on cassette, and radiographic beam angled 15 degrees toward palm
     d. Dorsal horizon view: wrist is hyperflexed and the beam of the image intensifier is aimed along the long axis of the radius; to search for a prominent dorsal screw from the volar plate
   - Hand
     a. Standard PA, lateral, and obliques views
     b. Robert's view to evaluate CMC and scaphotrapeziotrapezoid (STT) joints; pronated AP view of thumb
     c. Pronated 30 degree radiographs: look for dorsal fourth/fifth CMC dislocations
9. Surgical approaches
   - Forearm
     a. Anterior (Henry): interval between brachioradialis (radial nerve) and pronator teres (median nerve) proximally; between flexor carpi radialis (median nerve) and radial artery distally **(Fig. 9.40)**
     b. Posterior (Thompson): interval between extensor carpi radialis brevis (radial nerve) and extensor digitorum communis (PIN) **(Fig. 9.41)**
     c. Ulnar: interval between ECU (PIN) and FCU (ulnar nerve)

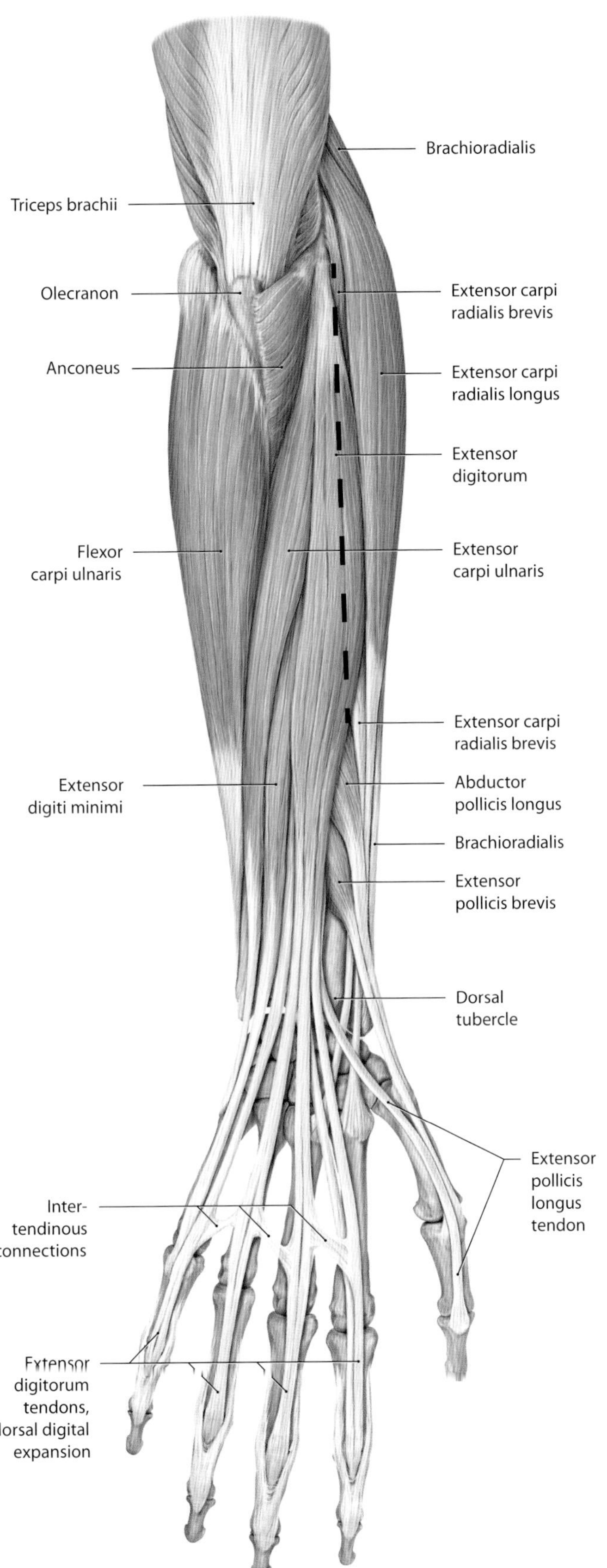

Fig. 9.41 Posterior approach to the radius. Provides exposure to the proximal third of the radius and the interval between the extensor carpi radialis brevis (radial nerve) and the extensor digitorum communis (posterior interosseus nerve). Modified from THIEME Atlas of Anatomy, General Anatomy and Musculoskeltal System, © Thieme 2005, Illustration by [Karl Wesker]

- Wrist
  a. Dorsal: interval between third (extensor pollicis longus) and fourth (extensor digitorum communis); PIN at base of fourth compartment; excise to denervate the carpus **(Fig. 9.42)**
  b. Volar scaphoid: between flexor carpi radialis and radial artery
- Digits
  a. Bruner: zigzag volar incisions across flexor crease to allow access to flexor tendons and prevent transverse scarring at flexion crease **(Fig. 9.43)**
  b. Midlateral: lateral incision dorsal to neurovascular bundle at dorsal extent of interphalangeal crease
  c. Midaxial: lateral incision centered on osseous phalanges

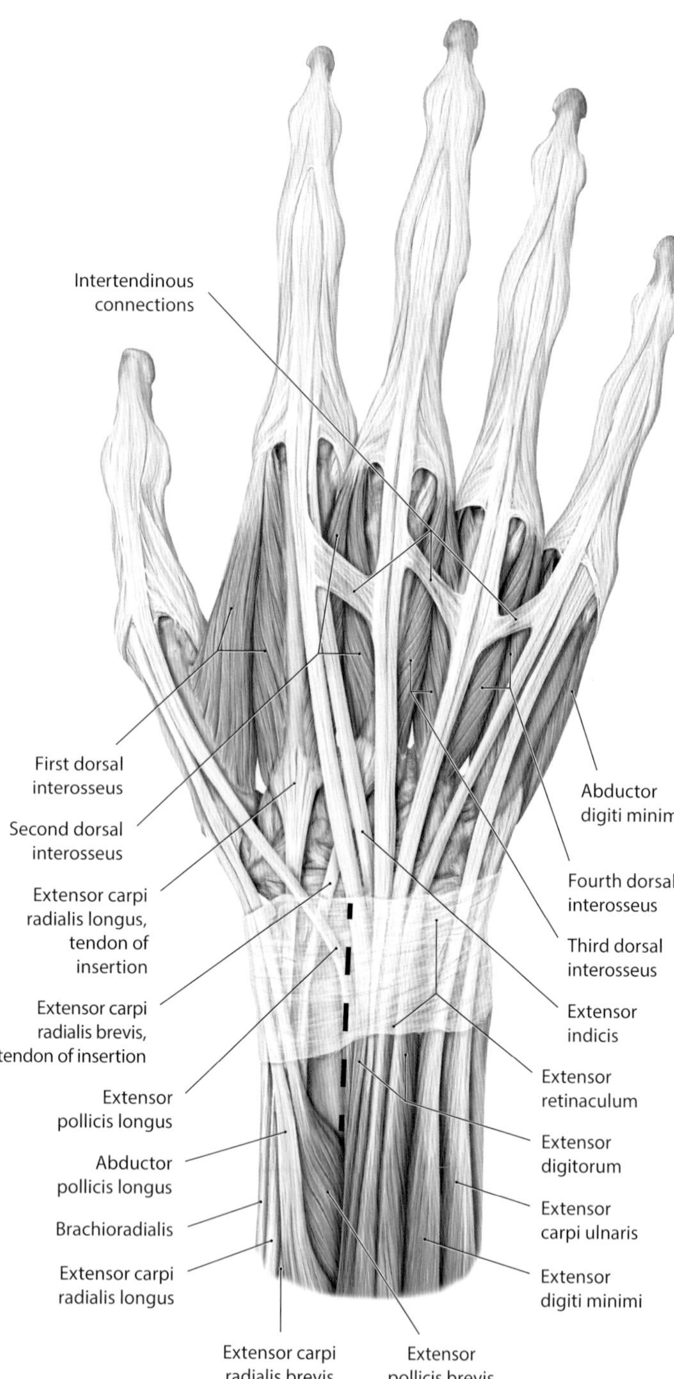

Fig. 9.42 Dorsal approach to wrist. Interval between the third (extensor pollicis longus) and fourth (*extensor digitorum communis*) dorsal compartment of the wrist. Indicated for open reduction and internal fixation (ORIF) of the distal radius or carpal fracture, proximal row carpectomy, wrist fusion, posterior interosseous nerve (PIN) neurectomy, or extensor tendon repair or synovectomy. (From Schuenke M, Schulte E. General Anatomy and the Musculoskeletal System: Thieme Atlas of Anatomy. New York: Thieme; 2005. Illustration by Karl Wesker.)

- Arthroscopy **(Fig. 9.44)**
  a. Indications: TFCC tear, suspected scapholunate or lunotriquetral tear, scaphoid fracture, ulnocarpal impaction, synovitis debridement, wrist ganglion, distal radius fractures to assess joint congruency, removal of loose bodies, septic wrist irrigation and debridement
  b. Portals (named for relationship to extensor compartments):
     - 1–2 portal: risk of injury to superficial radial sensory nerve
     - 3–4 portal: located 1 cm distal to Lister tubercle
     - 4–5: just ulnar to the fourth compartment; should be proximal to the 3–4 portal due to radial inclination
     - 6R: radial to ECU tendon
     - 6U: ulnar to ECU tendon; risk of injury to dorsal sensory branch of ulnar nerve
     - Radial and ulnar midcarpal portals
  c. Complications: nerve injury (superficial radial sensory or dorsal branch of ulnar nerve most common), MCP joint pain secondary to traction, iatrogenic tendon injury (EPL or EDM most common), infection
     - **ECU tendon cannot be visualized arthroscopically.**

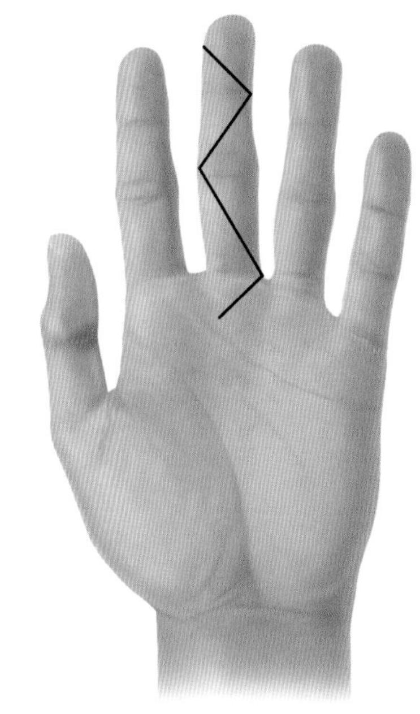

Fig. 9.43 Bruner incision.

II. Trauma

1. Distal radius fracture
   - In elderly, distal radius and vertebral compression fractures are predictive of future hip fracture.
   - Obtain dual-energy X-ray absorptiometry (DEXA) scan in women with distal radius fracture and age > 50 years.
   - Associated injuries: ulnar styloid fracture, DRUJ disruption
     a. Higher degree of initial fracture displacement
     b. Fracture at base associated with TFCC tear
     c. Open reduction and internal fixation (ORIF) of ulnar styloid only if there is associated instability of the DRUJ
   - Imaging
     a. Normal **(Fig. 9.45)**
        - PA radiograph: radial height, 12 mm; inclination, 23 degrees
        - Lateral radiograph volar tilt: 11 degrees
        - Comparative radiographs of contralateral wrist
     b. Ulnar variance: neutral, positive, negative
     c. Assess DRUJ with lateral radiograph
     d. Acceptable reduction criteria: see American Academy of Orthopaedic Surgeons (AAOS) guidelines
   - Classification
     a. Multiple classification schemes: AO, Frykman, Fernandez, Mayo, etc.
     b. Common eponyms
        - Smith: extra-articular volarly displaced fracture
        - Barton: coronal shear fracture/dislocation of radiocarpal joint
        - Colles: low-energy extra-articular dorsally displaced
        - Chauffer's: radial styloid fracture
        - Die punch: depressed articular fracture of lunate fossa

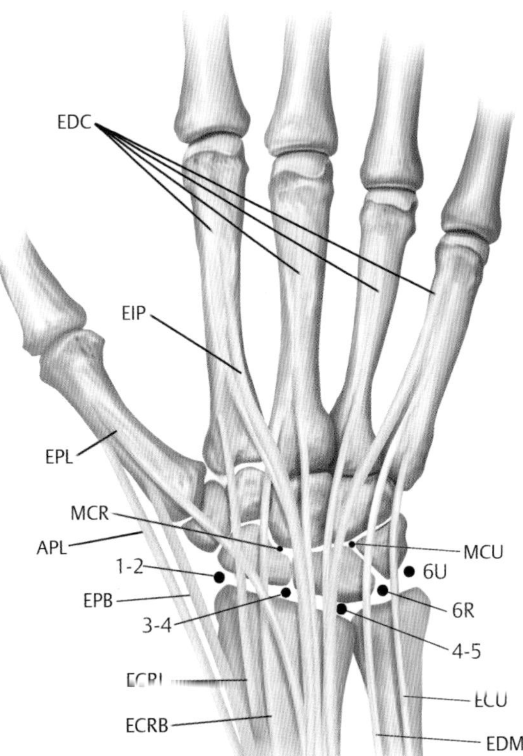

Fig. 9.44 Wrist arthroscopic portals. APL, abductor pollicis longus; ECRB, extensor carpi radialis brevis; ECRL, extensor carpi radialis longus; ECU, extensor carpi ulnaris; EDC, *extensor digitorum communis;* EDM, *extensor digiti minimi;* EIP, extensor indicis proprius; EPB, extensor pollicis brevis; EPL, extensor pollicis longus; MCR, midcarpal joint radial; MCU, midcarpal joint ulnar.

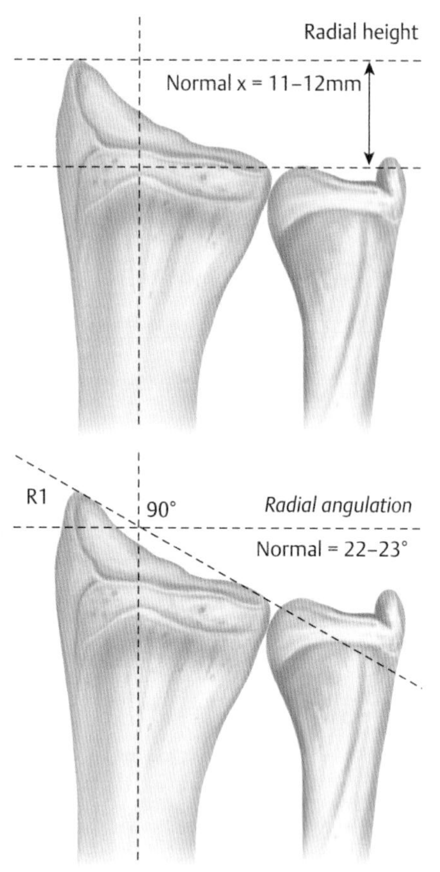

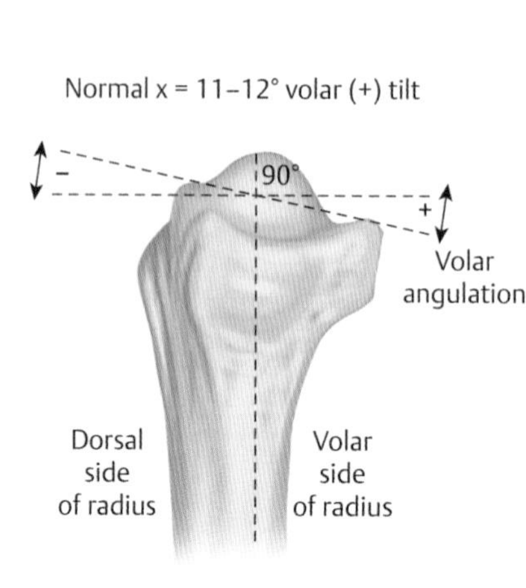

Fig. 9.45 Distal radius radiographic parameters.

- Treatment
  a. Conservative management: closed reduction and immobilization
    - For most extra-articular distal radius fractures
    - Follow with serial radiographs (once a week for 3 weeks)
    - Total length of immobilization: ~6 weeks
    - Conservative management for unstable distal radius fractures in the elderly (age > 65 years) shown to have equivalent outcomes to fixation
  b. Operative treatment
    - Indications for surgery
      - **AAOS Clinical Practice Guidelines: operative fixation of distal radius fractures postreduction (moderate evidence); postreduction radial shortening > 3 mm, dorsal tilt > 10 degrees, intra-articular displacement or stepoff > 2 mm; early active wrist range of motion is not required with stable fixation (moderate evidence); adjuvant treatment with vitamin C (moderate evidence)**
      - Open fractures
      - > 2 mm intra-articular displacement
      - Volar oblique fractures
      - Intra-articular volar shear fractures
      - Die-punch fractures
      - Significant dorsal comminution
    - Methods of fixation
      - Closed reduction and percutaneous pinning
        - Indicated for extra-articular unstable distal radius fractures

- Isolated percutaneous pinning contraindicated in fractures with volar comminution
- ♦ Open reduction and internal fixation
  - Volar distal radius locking plates resist radial shortening and dorsal angulation; buttress the distal radius (biomechanically stronger than dorsal plating)
  - Most common site of flexor tendon rupture with volar plating is the FPL; most common site of extensor tendon injury after volar plating is the EPL due to prominent screws
  - **Dorsal horizon view ensures no dorsal prominent screw**
- ♦ External fixation
  - Works by ligamentotaxis
  - Can injure sensory branch radial nerve
  - Overdistraction can lead to complex regional pain syndrome, stiffness, and limited finger range of motion
  - Bridge plating works as an internal external fixator with greater biomechanical advantage and similar clinical outcomes to volar plating

- Rehabilitation
  a. Physical therapy compared with home exercise shows no significant difference in outcomes.
- Complications
  b. Acute carpal tunnel syndrome
    - Most common neurologic complication; 1–12% in low-energy fracture, 30% in high-energy fracture
    - Decompress nerve if paresthesias are progressive or do not respond to reduction and last > 24–48 hours.

  c. Ulnar nerve neuropathy with DRUJ injuries
  d. Compartment syndrome
  e. EPL rupture
    - Most common tendon rupture thought to be secondary to attrition versus local ischemia secondary to mechanical impingement
    - Treat with transfer of EIP to EPL

  f. ECU or EDM entrapment with DRUJ injuries
  g. Tenosynovitis: first and third dorsal compartments most common
  h. Malunion
    - Revision with osteotomy, ORIF, and bone grafting at > 6 weeks
    - Radial shortening malunion treated with ulnar shortening osteotomy

  i. Reflex sympathetic dystrophy/chronic regional pain syndrome
    - **Vitamin C (500 mg/day) reduces risk of complex regional pain syndrome type I in patients with distal radius fractures.**

2. Carpal fractures
- Scaphoid
  a. Blood supply: dorsal carpal branch of radial artery enters scaphoid tubercle at dorsal tubercle (80% blood supply proximal scaphoid via retrograde flow); superficial palmar branch of radial artery enters distal tubercle and supplies 20% distal scaphoid
  b. Mechanism: fall on outstretched hand with hyperextension and radial deviation of wrist
  c. Presentation: snuffbox tenderness, tenderness to palpation at scaphoid tubercle (volar), pain with axial load of first metacarpal
  d. Imaging

- Obtain PA, lateral, and scaphoid views (30 degrees of wrist extension and 20 degree ulnar deviation)
  - Plain radiographs may initially appear negative.
  - If high clinical suspicion, treat with thumb spica splint and repeat X-rays in 2 weeks
- **MRI: most sensitive test to diagnose occult fractures within 24 hours**
- MRI: can evaluate location of fracture, associated ligament injuries, and vascularity
- Bone scan: effective in diagnosing occult scaphoid fractures if performed within 72 hours
- Computed tomography (CT) scan: best at evaluating fracture characteristics and amount of displacement; less effective at diagnosing occult fractures compared with MRI and bone scan

e. Classification
- Location: waist (most common), tubercle, distal pole, proximal pole
- **Pediatric scaphoid fractures most commonly in distal third because distal pole ossifies before proximal pole, although recent data suggest they occur at other locations as well.**
- Stability: stable (transverse) versus unstable (oblique, comminuted or displaced)

f. Treatment
- Nonoperative
- **Only nondisplaced scaphoid waist, tubercle, or distal plate fractures should be treated conservatively (not proximal pole).**
  - Thumb spica cast immobilization indicated for nondisplaced fractures. (One study has suggested that the thumb does not need to be included in conservative management of nondisplaced waist fractures.)
  - Longer duration of casting the more proximal the fracture; distal waist for 3 months, mid-waist for 4 months, proximal third for 5 months
  - No proven added benefit of short-arm versus long-arm casting
- Operative
  - Indications: > 1 mm displacement, intrascaphoid angle > 35 degrees, unstable vertical or oblique fractures, associated scaphoid fractures with perilunate dislocation, proximal pole fractures, high-demand occupations/sports
  - Percutaneous fixation performed for minimally displaced scaphoid fractures
    - Percutaneous fixation: entails an increased risk of screw prominence of subchondral bone compared with open approach
    - Percutaneous fixation of nondisplaced waist fractures: decreases the time to union and allows early return to work or sports; cost similar to that of casting
  - Open reduction and internal fixation
    - Optimal fixation obtained with long central screw placement
    - **Centrally placed screw is biomechanically strongest**
    - Proximal pole scaphoid fracture best treated with dorsal headless compression screw
    - Nonunion of proximal pole treated with vascularized bone graft ± intraosseous headless screw
    - **Vascularized graft indicated for proximal pole nonunion or nonunion after previously grafted fracture**

        ▪ Nonunion of waist treated with corticocancellous graft or cancellous graft with headless screw

    g. Complications
        ◦ Avascular necrosis: increased incidence with proximal fracture
        ◦ Nonunion: delay in treatment > 28 days greatly increases risk of nonunion; may lead to development of scaphoid nonunion advanced collapse (see Posttraumatic entries in the Arthritis section, below)
        ◦ **Time to treatment > 1 month increases risk of nonunion.**

- Pisiform fracture: uncommon; treat with cast immobilization; if painful nonunion occurs, then excise
- Hook of hamate fracture
    a. Mechanism: blunt trauma to palm; commonly seen in baseball, hockey, racquet sports
    b. Presentation: pain over hook of hamate; may cause ulnar nerve compression or flexor tendon irritation
    c. Imaging: carpal tunnel view or CT scan (note: bipartite hamate has smooth cortical borders)
    d. Treatment: cast immobilization for 4–6 weeks; failure of union with persistent pain is treated with excision of fragment

3. Carpal instability
- Dorsal intercalated segmental instability (DISI): lunate extension
    a. Mechanism: fall on hyperextended and ulnar deviated wrist
    b. Biomechanics: force transmission through scaphoid fossa greater in wrist extension than neutral; force transmission through lunate fossa greater in neutral than extension
    c. Caused by scapholunate rupture; dorsal scapholunate ligament is stronger than volar
    d. Leads to scaphoid hyperflexion and lunate hyperextension
    e. Presentation
        ◦ Snuffbox tenderness, dorsal wrist pain, decreased grip strength
        ◦ Watson test: pain or a clunk with pressure applied to volar scaphoid tubercle and wrist brought from ulnar to radial deviation; compare with contralateral side
    f. Imaging: AP X-ray: scapholunate gap > 3 mm with clenched fist view (Terry Thomas sign), cortical ring sign; lateral X-ray: scapholunate angle > 60 degrees
    g. Arthroscopy: gold standard for diagnosis
    h. Treatment: scapholunate ligament repair (early) or reconstruction (late)
- VISI: lunate flexion
    a. Mechanism: fall on hyperextended and radial deviated wrist
    b. Caused by lunotriquetral rupture; volar lunotriquetral ligament stronger than dorsal
    c. Imaging: lateral X-ray: decreased scapholunate angle (< 30 degrees)
    d. Treatment: closed reduction and percutaneous pinning (CRPP) or ligament repair in acute setting; chronic instability treated with lunotriquetral (LT) fusion
- Perilunate dislocation
    a. Mechanism: high energy, fall on extended arm, ulnar deviated wrist
    b. Presentation: swelling, ecchymosis and painful wrist; acute carpal tunnel syndrome in 25% secondary to volar dislocation of lunate; commonly missed diagnosis; frequently also with scaphoid fracture
    c. Imaging: PA X-ray: break in Gilula's lines, overlapping carpal bones; lateral X-ray: dislocation of lunate or midcarpal joint

- **First look at PA view of the wrist; if Gilula's lines are disrupted, then the carpus is malaligned.**
- **Mayfield classification: counterclockwise direction of ligament disruption**
  - **Stage I: scapholunate**
  - **Stage II: scaphocapitate**
  - **Stage III: lunotriquetral**
  - **Stage IV: lunate dislocation**

d. Sequence of progressive instability: scaphoid extension, opening of space of Poirier, scaphoid failure, distal row dissociation, hyperextension of triquetrum, LT ligament failure, dorsal dislocation of carpus

e. Treatment: emergent closed reduction leads to decreased median nerve symptoms and cartilage cell death; prompt ORIF, ligament repair, and possible acute carpal tunnel release

4. DRUJ injury (see DRUJ section, below)
5. Fracture/dislocation of CMC joints
   - Imaging: pronated 30-degree radiographs to look for dorsal fourth/fifth CMC dislocations; may obtain CT scan for better detail
   - Thumb CMC fracture: deforming forces of Rolando/Bennett fracture: abductor pollicis longus (PIN) and adductor pollicis (ulnar nerve)
   - Small-finger CMC fracture (baby Bennett): deforming force ECU
   - Treatment: attempt closed reduction. These injuries are usually unstable and require CRPP or ORIF.
6. Metacarpal fractures
   - Boxer's fracture: metacarpal neck fracture of small finger
   - Intrinsic muscles lead to apex dorsal angulation
   - Treatment: closed reduction (Jahss maneuver) and immobilized for 3–4 weeks or CRPP/ORIF. Operative indications: intra-articular fracture, rotational malalignment, multiple metacarpal shaft fractures, significant angulation **(Table 9.4)**
   - **Multiple metacarpal shaft fractures should be treated with ORIF to allow immediate motion.**
   - Extensor lag of 7 degrees for every 2 mm of shortening **(Table 9.4)**
7. Gamekeeper's/skier's thumb
   - Valgus instability of thumb MCP due to disruption of ulnar collateral ligament
   - Skier's thumb (acute) versus gamekeeper's (chronic)
   - Two components of UCL: proper (confers stability in MCP flexion) and accessory (confers stability in MCP extension)
   - Physical examination: radially deviate thumb with both thumb in extension and 30 degrees of flexion to test proper and accessory UCL laxity; < 20 degrees indicates partial tear
   - **Stener lesion: occurs when adductor aponeurosis becomes interposed between avulsed UCL**

Table 9.4 Acceptable Angulation of Metacarpal Fractures

	Index/Long	Ring	Small
Metacarpal shaft (degrees)	10–20	30	40
Metacarpal neck (degrees)	10/20	30–40	50–60

- Almost always present if avulsion fracture is significantly displaced on X-ray; requires both proper and accessory ligaments be disrupted; indication for operative repair
- Treatment: immobilization for 4–6 weeks with partial tears. Operative indications for ligament repair: > 30 degrees of laxity compared with contralateral side or Stener lesion

8. Phalanx fractures
   - **Any finger fracture that causes malrotation of the digit should be fixed.**
   - Proximal phalanx fracture
     a. Most commonly apex volar: central slip extends distal fragment and interossei flex proximal fragment
     b. Operative indications: unstable fractures, > 10-degree angulation, 2 mm shortening, rotational deformity
     c. Proximal phalanx fracture malunion with bone in subcondylar fossa region blocking PIP flexion; treat with ostectomy of bone fragment blocking motion
   - Middle phalanx fracture
     a. Treatment: operative indications include unstable fractures, > 10-degree angulation, 2 mm shortening, rotational deformity
     b. Middle phalanx base fracture treated with volar plate arthroplasty; must excise or release collateral ligaments to allow gliding of middle phalanx on articular surface of proximal phalanx
   - Distal phalanx fracture
     a. Treatment: associated nail bed injury; must remove nail, irrigate and repair nail bed
        - Nail bed injury: primary repair versus 2-octylcyanoacrylate (Dermabond): equivalent results with faster procedure with Dermabond
     b. Distal phalanx nonunion: may be treated with ORIF but often requires removal of hardware after union
     c. Nonunion or fibrous union of distal phalanx is common; only treat if clinically symptomatic
     d. Seymour fracture: physeal fracture with nail bed injury in distal phalanx (P3). Treatment: irrigation, debridement, fracture reduction, and nail bed repair
9. PIP dislocation
   - Dorsal dislocation: injury to volar plate and collateral ligament
     a. Associated with fracture of middle phalanx (P2) proximal volar lip
     b. Chronic dislocation may lead to swan neck deformity
     c. Volar plate can become interposed and block reduction; do not pull longitudinal traction when reducing
     d. Treatment: closed reduction and dorsal blocking splint; failed closed reduction usually due to interposition of volar plate and necessitates open reduction; PIP fracture/dislocation with > 40% joint involved/unstable require ORIF or CRPP
   - Volar dislocation: injury to central slip of extensor tendon and collateral ligament
     a. Chronic injury may result in boutonniere deformity (PIP flexion with DIP extension)
     b. Treatment: closed reduction and immobilization in extension
10. DIP dislocation
    - Irreducible dorsal dislocation caused by interposed volar plate
    - Treatment: closed reduction and immobilization in slight flexion; failed reduction secondary to volar plate interposition requires open reduction

III. Tendon Pathology

1. Tendon injury
   - Phases of tendon healing
     a. Inflammatory phase (0–1 week): repair strength dependent on sutures; macrophages phagocytose necrotic tissue and fibroblast migrates to site of injury; tendon weakest after repair at 7–10 days
     b. Proliferative phase (1–3 weeks): strength increasing; fibroblast begins laying down type III collagen, later converted to type I collagen
     c. Remodeling phase (3–12 weeks): tendon does not gain tensile strength until start of remodeling phase; patient tolerates active ROM; collagen organizes and becomes linear
   - Extensor tendon perfusion
     a. At the wrist joint the extensor tendons are perfused via diffusion from the mesotenon. Distally, small vessels perfuse the tendon via the paratenon.
   - Flexor tendon perfusion
     a. Small segmental vessels supply perfusion via short and long vincula; proximally in palm, larger longitudinal vessels from muscle belly enter the tendon
     b. Watershed area over proximal phalanx is nourished via diffusion from synovial fluid. Zone II injuries are primarily supplied by diffusion through synovial sheath.
   - Repair of Flexor tendon injuries
     a. Partial laceration of flexor tendon > 60% or evidence of triggering should be repaired.
     b. Small tendon flaps should be trimmed to prevent triggering.
     c. Most important factor in repair strength of flexor tendon is the number of core sutures crossing repair site
     d. Four to six core strands provide strength for early active ROM.
     e. Epitendinous suture decreases gap formation, improves strength and contour (10–50%)
     f. Preserve A2 and A4 pulley; preserve oblique pulley in thumb
     g. Risk of tendon rupture highest until 3 weeks after surgery and occurs at suture knots

IV. Flexor Tendon Zones (Fig. 9.17)

1. Zone I: distal to FDS insertion
   - Jersey finger: avulsion injury of FDP
     a. Mechanism: forced extension of DIP joint during grip
     b. Physical exam: finger is slightly extended at DIP joint compared with others
     c. Classification: Leddy and Packer **(Table 9.5)**
        - **Type 1 injury is worst (tendon in palm), whereas type 3 is best.**

Table 9.5 Leddy and Packer Classification of Zone I Flexor Tendon Rupture and Treatment

Type	Flexor Digitorum Profundus Location	Timing of Repair
I	Retracted to palm	Within 7 days
II	Still within sheath, indicating vincula still intact	Up to 6 weeks after injury
III	Bony avulsion fragment at distal interphalangeal	Up to 6 weeks after injury

d. Treatment: acutely repair direct tendon repair (type I) or ORIF fragment (type III); chronic injuries with full passive ROM can be treated with two-stage graft reconstruction with silicone rod followed by free tendon graft

e. Complications

   - **Overadvancement of FDP by > 1 cm decreases excursion of other FDP tendons because they share the same muscle belly, resulting in DIP flexion contracture or quadrigia.**
   - Up to 20% rerupture rate

2. Zone II: "no-man's land"; FDS insertion to distal palmar crease; FDS/FDP in same tendon sheath and often both injured; neurovascular injury common; direct repair of both tendons; traditionally poor outcomes secondary to adhesion formation but improved due to postoperative rehab protocols (see Rehabilitation, below)
3. Zone III: palm; direct repair recommended; high incidence of neurovascular injuries
4. Zone IV: carpal tunnel; direct tendon repair; transverse carpal ligament should be repaired to prevent bowstringing
5. Zone V: distal forearm, direct tendon repair
6. Thumb TI, TII, TIII: direct repair
   - **Chronic FPL laceration with full passive range of motion can be treated with transfer of FDS of ring finger.**
7. Rehabilitation
   - Early active ROM protocol: may decrease adhesion but entails the risk of rerupture or gap formation
   - Kleinert protocol: low force and tendon excursion; dorsal blocking splint at 45 degrees of flexion and elastic bands attached to digits; patient actively extends and elastic bands passively flex
   - Duran protocol: low force and tendon excursion; dorsal blocking splint with passive flexion with other hand and active extension of digits
   - If patient cannot comply with instructions (e.g., child), treat with cast immobilization.
8. Extensor tendons zones **(Fig. 9.46)**
   - Zones: odd numbers located over joints
   - **Odd number annular pulleys (A1, A3, A5) also located over joints, but in opposite order**
   - Zone I: mallet finger: rupture of terminal extensor tendon

     a. Mechanism: forced flexion of extended fingertip

     b. Treatment:
        - Within 12 weeks: DIP extension splint; operative indication: volar subluxation of distal phalanx (pin the DIP joint to keep reduced)
        - Chronic injury (> 12 weeks): surgical reconstruction of terminal extensor tendon; chronic injury may lead to swan neck deformity requiring repair
        - Painful stiff DIP joint treated with arthrodesis

     c. Complications: injury treated closed often with residual extensor lag
   - Zone II: located over middle phalanx; most commonly secondary to laceration or crush injury
   - Zone III: boutonniere deformity; rupture of central slip and volar subluxation of lateral bands causing PIP flexion and DIP hyperextension

     a. Most common mechanisms: volar PIP dislocation or lacerations

     b. Physical exam: Elson test: bend patient's finger 90 degrees over table and actively extend it against resistance at PIP joint; if DIP joint remains supple and middle phalanx extends, then central slip is intact; if DIP joint is

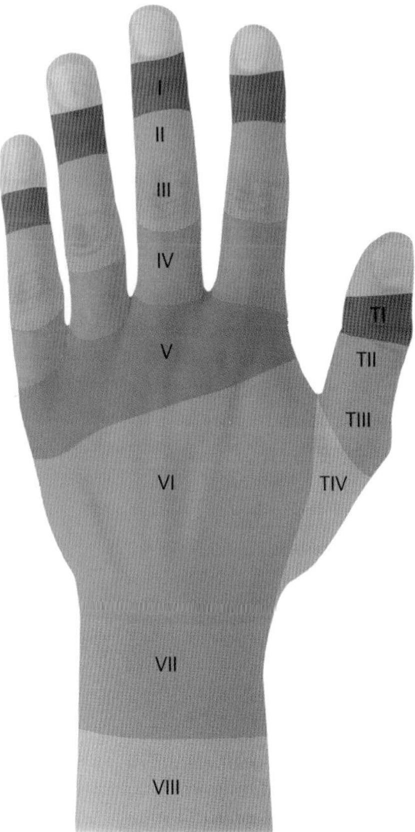

Fig. 9.46 Extensor tendon zones.

rigid with the absence of PIP extension, then central slip is ruptured and lateral bands are extending the DIP

c. Treatment: full-time PIP extension splinting for 4 weeks with MCP and DIP joints free; chronic injuries may require central slip reconstruction or lateral band transferred dorsally

- Zone IV: located over proximal phalanx; common complication of tendon repair in this zone is adhesion formation
- Zone V: located over MCP/CMC joint
  a. Beware of "fight bites," which require irrigation and debridement.
  b. Sagittal band rupture "boxer's knuckle"
    - Most commonly affects long finger
    - Most commonly subluxes ulnarly due to radial sagittal band rupture
    - Physical exam: patient unable to actively extend MCP, but able to maintain MCP extension if passively placed into extension
    - **Sagittal band rupture: patient able to maintain but not attain MCP extension**
    - Treatment: acute injuries (≤ 1 week) treated with MCP extension splint; delay in diagnosis or treatment (> 1 week) require surgical reconstruction of sagittal band
- Zone VI: located over metacarpals
- Zone VII: located over wrist; adhesion formation after repair common

9. Repair
   - Extensor tendon injuries > 60% tendon laceration
10. Reconstruction
    - Chronic EPL rupture reconstruct with EIP to EPL transfer
11. Complications
    - Most common complication is adhesion formation
    - Lumbrical plus finger: paradoxical IP joint extension while attempting to flex digit; lumbricals originate from FDP, so when FDP lacerated, active contraction of FDP pulls on lumbricals, which causes extension of IP joints; causes include excessively long FDP tendon graft, FDP laceration distal to lumbrical insertion, and amputation of distal phalanx distal to central slip insertion; treat with FDP repair (if laceration) or release of lumbrical
12. Stenosing tenosynovitis/trigger digit
    - Pathology: inflammation of flexor tendon sheath
    - Mechanism: catching of flexor tendons at A1 pulley
    - Associated conditions: diabetes, rheumatoid arthritis, amyloidosis
    - Treatment: conservative treatment with night splinting, nonsteroidal anti-inflammatory drugs (NSAIDs), and steroid injections; diabetics less responsive to steroid treatment; if conservative treatment fails, then operative treatment with release of A1 pulley
    - **In children, in addition to A1 pulley, triggering may be due to more proximal decussation of FDS tendon; may need release of single FDS tendon slip**
    - Complications: injury to radial digital nerve in treatment of trigger thumb; crosses surgical field at A1 pulley
13. Retinacular cysts
    - Pathology: firm round cysts arising from pulley system; does not move with tendon motion; may be painful with gripping
    - Treatment: needle aspiration or excision
14. De Quervain's tenosynovitis
    - Pathology: inflammation of first dorsal compartment (APL/EPB)
    - Associated with postpartum state, and with golf and racquet sports

- Physical exam: positive Finkelstein test, radial-sided wrist pain
- Treatment: splinting, first dorsal compartment steroid injection; if conservative treatment fails, then first dorsal compartment release
- Complications

  a. Failure to decompress after release is often due to failure to recognize a distinct EPB sheath.

  b. Injury to radial sensory nerve causing numbness and painful neuroma formation; avoid surgical trauma during dissection

15. Intersection syndrome
    - Overuse injury at junction of first [EPL/abductor pollicis brevis (APB] compartment crossing over second (ECRL/ECRB) compartment
    - Palpable crepitus and pain with resisted wrist extension and thumb extension
    - Associated with rowers
    - Treatment: steroid injection to second compartment; release of first and second dorsal compartments
16. Snapping ECU
    - Pathology: rupture of ECU subsheath causes subluxation of ECU tendon with wrist supination; ECU is only extensor tendon that has its own fibro-osseus tunnel
    - Associated with rowers and tennis players
    - Physical exam: audible snap with wrist supination and ulnar deviation; on pronation, it relocates
    - Treatment: acute (< 6 weeks): immobilization with forearm in pronation and radial deviation; chronic: ECU subsheath reconstruction

V. DRUJ

1. TFCC
   - Mechanism: axial load on pronated wrist
   - Anatomy: TFCC stabilizes DRUJ; composed of ECU subsheath, articular disk, meniscus homologue, dorsal and volar radioulnar ligaments, ulnolunate and ulnotriquetral ligaments **(Fig. 9.47)**
   - Central portion poorly vascularized, periphery well vascularized
   - **As with the meniscus in the knee, only peripheral tears can be repaired.**
   - Symptoms/physical exam: ulnar-sided wrist pain, pain distal to ulnar styloid, pain with resisted ulnar deviation
   - Imaging: radiographs usually negative; MRI detects TFCC tear; arthrography shows active extravasation at ulnar wrist
   - TFCC classification: Palmer type I (traumatic), type II (degenerative) **(Table 9.6)**

   Treatment: treat initially with NSAIDs and immobilization; arthroscopic or open repair indicated if nonoperative treatment fails
2. Instability
   - Acute injury may occur in isolation or in association with Galeazzi (distal radial shaft fracture), Essex-Lopresti, or ulnar styloid injuries
   - Chronic instability due to TFCC injury, ulnar styloid nonunion, or distal radius malunion
   - Imaging: best evaluated on lateral radiograph, which shows dorsal displacement of ulna; AP radiograph may show widening of DRUJ
   - Treatment: acutely in Galeazzi injury, must assess DRUJ stability after radius fixation; if unstable, consider pinning when reduced (typically in supination) with or without TFCC repair

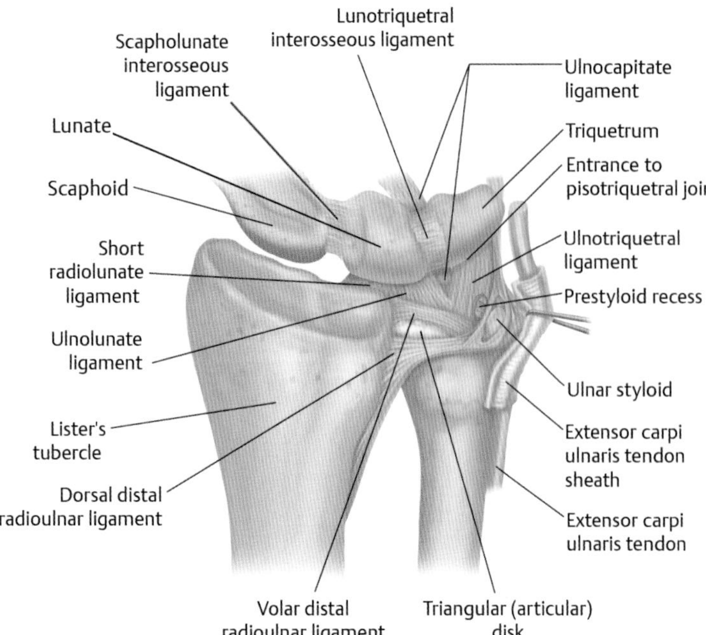

Fig. 9.47 Triangular fibrocartilage complex anatomy. The triangular fibrocartilage complex (TFCC) is composed of an extensor carpi ulnaris (ECU) subsheath, articular disk, meniscus homologue, dorsal and volar radioulnar ligaments, and ulnolunate and ulnotriquetral ligaments.

a. Chronic instability due to distal radius malunion requires corrective osteotomy.
b. Chronic instability due to ligament injury requires ligament repair or reconstruction.

3. DRUJ arthritis
   - Physical exam: pain at dorsum of the wrist, worse with pronation/supination; may perform diagnostic injection of lidocaine into DRUJ, resulting in improved supination/pronation and grip strength
   - Imaging: PA/lateral radiographs for degenerative changes of DRUJ
   - Conservative treatment: NSAIDs, steroid injection, Munster splint limiting forearm rotation
   - Surgical treatment
     a. Ulnar hemiresection arthroplasty: must perform TFCC repair to avoid instability; appropriate for manual laborers
     b. Suave-Kapandji procedure: DRUJ fusion with distal ulnar osteotomy/pseudarthrosis; appropriate for manual laborers
     c. Darrach procedure: excision of distal ulna; may produce distal ulnar instability; appropriate for low-demand elderly patients, such as those with RA
     d. Ulnar head/DRUJ replacement
4. Ulnocarpal impingement syndrome
   - Pathology: impact of ulna on carpal bones due to positive ulnar variance
   - Causes: distal radius fracture with shortening, Galeazzi fracture, Essex-Lopresti injury with shortening, injury to distal radius epiphysis, Madelung deformity or naturally occurring ulnar positive variance
   - Physical exam: pain localized to dorsum at the DRUJ, pain with ulnar deviation, positive ballottement test (dorsal and palmar displacement of ulna while wrist is ulnar deviated)
   - Imaging: PA radiograph to evaluate ulnar variance; positive ulna variance increases with pronation and power grip; may consider obtaining these views; MRI evaluates TFCC, which may be torn secondary to impingement; look for bone edema on proximal ulnar side of lunate
   - Associated injury: TFCC tear

Table 9.6 Palmer Classification of Triangular Fibrocartilage Complex (TFCC) Tears

Type I: traumatic tears	
IA	Central traumatic tear
IB	Ulnar avulsion
IC	Distal avulsion
ID	Radial avulsion from sigmoid notch
Type II: degenerative tears	
IIA	TFCC wear
IIB	IIA + lunate or ulnar chondromalacia
IIC	TFCC perforation + lunate or ulnar chondromalacia
IID	IIC + lunotriquetral ligament perforation
IIE	IID + ulnocarpal and distal radioulnar joint arthritis

- Treatment: ulnar shortening osteotomy for ulnar positive variance and DRUJ incongruity; Darrach procedure is an option for low-demand elderly patients
- Cystic changes of carpal bones resolve after operative treatment

VI. Arthritis

1. Posttraumatic
   - Scaphoid lunate advanced collapse (SLAC) **(Table 9.7)**
     a. Pathology: chronic scapholunate interosseus ligament tear leading to unopposed scaphoid flexion and lunate extension (DISI pattern), resulting in an abnormal wear pattern
     b. Imaging: Watson classification describes the predictable progression of degenerative arthritis from the radial styloscaphoid to radioscaphoid, to capitolunate joint.
        - **The radiolunate joint is spared in a SLAC wrist.**

     c. Lateral radiograph: increased scapholunate angle > 60 degrees
     d. PA radiograph: widening of scapholunate interval > 3 mm
     e. Treatment depends on the stage of SLAC arthritis
        - **Treatment of SLAC/scaphoid nonunion advanced collapse (SNAC) wrists depends on which joints are unaffected. On a PA radiograph of the wrist, determine which joints are spared from arthritis. In SLAC/SNAC stage I and II, the radiolunate joint should be normal, and both proximal row carpectomy (PRC) and four-corner are possible. In SLAC/SNAC stage III, the capitolunate joint is affected. Because the capitate head is no longer normal, stage III can not be treated with a PRC.**
        - **Following PRC, the primary stabilizer of the wrist is the radioscaphocapitate ligament. It prevents the carpus from drifting ulnarly.**
   - Scaphoid nonunion advanced collapse (SNAC)
     a. Pathology: scaphoid nonunion leads to abnormal wear patterns and progressive arthritis similar to a SLAC wrist.
     b. Imaging: radiographic stages of SNAC are similar to those of SLAC. A stage II SNAC wrist has degenerative changes of the scaphocapitate joint.
     c. Radiolunate articulation is generally spared.
     d. Treatment **(Table 9.8)**
2. Distal radioulnar joint arthritis (see DRUJ section, above)

Table 9.7 Radiographic Stages of Scaphoid Lunate Advanced Collapse (SLAC) Wrist

Stage	X-Ray Findings	Treatment
I	Degenerative changes localized to radial styloid	Radial styloidectomy and scaphoid stabilization
II	Degenerative changes of radioscaphoid joint	Proximal row carpectomy or scaphoid excision and four-corner fusion
III	Degenerative changes of capitolunate joint	Scaphoid excision and four-corner fusion; note: proximal row carpectomy is contraindicated in capitolunate arthritis
IV	Pan-carpal arthritis	Total wrist arthrodesis versus total wrist arthroplasty

Table 9.8 Radiographic Stages and Treatment of Scaphoid Nonunion Advanced Collapse (SNAC) Wrist

Stage	X-Ray Findings	Treatment
I	Degenerative changes localized to radial scaphoid and radial styloid	Radial styloidectomy and scaphoid fixation with bone grafting
II	Degenerative changes of radioscaphoid joint plus scaphocapitate joint	Scaphocapitate fusion and distal scaphoid excision or scaphoid excision and four-corner fusion
III	Degenerative changes of periscaphoid (including capitolunate joint)	Scaphoid excision and four-corner fusion
IV	Pan-carpal arthritis	Total wrist arthrodesis versus total wrist arthroplasty

3. Primary osteoarthritis
   - Thumb CMC arthritis
     a. Pathology
        - **Attenuation of anterior oblique ligament (beak) leading to dorsoradial subluxation of metacarpal and degenerative changes**
        - Recent evidence suggests dorsal ligaments may be as important or more important.

     b. Physical exam: tenderness at trapeziometacarpal joint, decreased pinch and grip strength, positive CMC grind test; late findings are metacarpal adduction, compensatory MCP hyperextension, and contracture
        - **"Shoulder sign" and Z deformity with MCP hyperextension are seen.**

     c. Imaging: Robert's view: pronated AP view of thumb **(Table 9.9)**

     d. Treatment
        - Nonoperative treatment with thumb spica splints, NSAIDs and steroid injections
        - Injection with saline, steroid, or hyaluronic acid have equal efficacy.

Table 9.9 Eaton and Littler Classification of Thumb Carpometacarpal (CMC) Arthritis

Stage	Radiographic Findings	Treatment
I	Normal, except slight joint space widening secondary to synovitis	1. Conservative treatment 2. Arthroscopic synovectomy and debridement 3. If excessive joint laxity and pain, then volar ligament reconstruction 4. Osteotomy
II	Joint space narrowing, osteophytes ≤ 2 mm	1. Conservative treatment 2. Trapezial excision ± LRTI (or implant) 3. Young heavy laborers: trapezial metacarpal arthrodesis (an option) or osteotomy
III	Significant joint space narrowing, osteophytes > 2 mm	1. Conservative treatment 2. Trapezial excision ± LRTI (or implant) 3. Young heavy laborers: trapezial metacarpal arthrodesis
IV	Pan-trapezial arthritis	Trapezial excision ± LRTI (or implant)

Abbreviation: LRTI, ligament reconstruction and tendon interposition.

- Many different operative techniques and procedures for trapezium excision and ligament reconstruction and tendon interposition (LRTI). Trapezium excision is the most important step of the procedure, and no technique has been shown to have superior outcomes to trapeziectomy and hematoma distraction arthroplasty.
- If in conjunction with MCP hyperextension (Z deformity), can manage MCP with pinning in flexion (hyperextension 10–20 degrees), capsulodesis of volar plate (hyperextension 20–40 degrees), or MCP fusion (fixed deformity, deformity > 40 degrees, advanced arthritis)

• Thumb MCP arthritis

a. Not commonly involved in primary osteoarthritis

b. Treatment: arthrodesis

• STT arthritis

a. Must differentiate between CMC arthritis and STT arthritis on radiographs of patients with radial-sided wrist pain

b. Idiopathic or caused by SLAC wrist due to rotation of scaphoid or CMC arthritis (stage IV)

c. Treatment: isolated STT arthritis treated with arthrodesis or distal scaphoid excision; pantrapezial arthritis requires trapeziectomy

• Pisotriquetral arthritis

a. Treatment: conservative with steroid injections; operative treatment with pisiform excision or fusion

• MCP arthritis

a. Presentation: loss of motion with pain

b. Treatment:

- NSAIDs or corticosteroid injection
- Arthroplasty: most common in middle finger. Silicone implants are still the gold standard, but pyrocarbon implants have good results as well.
- Arthrodesis: rarely indicated

• PIP arthritis

a. Physical exam: joint contracture, fibrosis of collateral ligaments, Bouchard's nodes caused by marginal osteophytes

b. Treatment

- Collateral ligament excision, volar plate release and osteophyte excision: indicated for predominant contracture with minimal joint involvement
- Arthroplasty: indicated for long and ring finger > index and small fingers with good bone stock and no rotational deformity
- **Index finger should usually not be replaced due to high stresses placed during pinch; fuse instead.**
- Arthrodesis: headless screw fixation has highest fusion rate. Joint should be fused in increasing degree of flexion (radial → ulnar): index finger, 40 degrees; long finger, 45 degrees; ring finger, 50 degrees; small finger, 55 degrees

• DIP arthritis

a. Sustains the highest joint forces in the hand causing arthritis, pain, and deformity

b. Heberden's nodes

c. Nail splitting, deformity or loss of gloss

d. Treatment: arthrodesis with headless screw fixation/wires (0–20 degrees of flexion)

f. Mucous cyst: mass from DIP joint secondary to osteoarthritis

- Treatment: surgical excision with debridement of osteophyte, which decreases risk of recurrence

VII. Autoimmune Disease

1. Rheumatoid arthritis
   - Subcutaneous nodules over extensor surfaces are most common extra-articular manifestation in the upper extremity
   - Tendon problems
     a. Tendon ruptures due to attrition over bony prominences or chronic tenosynovitis
     b. Flexor tendons
        - **Mannerfelt lesion: FPL rupture due to attrition/tendinopathy from synovitis/osteophyte from STT joint; treat with tendon graft reconstruction (palmaris longus), transfer of FDS ring finger or IP fusion**
        - Tenosynovitis of the flexor tendons in the carpal tunnel may present with median nerve symptoms. Treatment is tenosynovectomy in addition to carpal tunnel release.
        - Trigger finger: treatment is A1 pulley release and tenosynovectomy
     c. Extensor tendons
        - Extensor digitorum communis and extensor digit minimi to ring and small finger are the most susceptible to rupture.
        - Sagittal band rupture
        - Vaughan-Jackson syndrome: attritional ruptures of extensor tendons in rheumatoid arthritis; rupture begins with EDM and continues radially
        - **EDM is extensor tendon most prone to rupture due to dorsal prominence of distal ulnar head**
        - Treatment of extensor digitorum communis (EDC) fourth and fifth digit rupture with EIP transfer has no effect on index finger extension
        - Treatment of multiple EDC rupture with FDS middle/ring transfer to EDC: tendons should be passed radially and dorsally around radius to improve ulnar deviation of digits and avoid synovitis of wrist
   - Joints
     a. Elbow
        - Diffuse synovitis causes joint destruction and ligamentous laxity; can cause radial nerve palsy
        - Physical exam: fixed flexion contractures, radial instability due to attenuation of annular ligament, varus or valgus instability, ulnar neuropathy
        - Larsen radiographic staging for RA **(Table 9.10)**
        - Larsen stages I and II best treated with synovectomy, with arthroscopic synovectomy being more effective in patients with flexion arc < 90 degrees
        - Prosthetic arthroplasty for higher grade disease (Larsen stage III), with semiconstrained arthroplasty performing better (than unconstrained) after previous radial head resection

Table 9.10 Larsen Radiographic Staging for Rheumatoid Arthritis

Stage	Radiographic Findings
I	Soft tissue findings only; near-normal radiographs
II	Periarticular erosions; may be soft tissue swelling or evidence of osteopenia
III	Marked joint space narrowing
IV	Extensive erosions with involvement of subchondral bone plate
V	Extensive articular damage and loss of contour

- Semiconstrained preferred to constrained due to high rate of prosthetic loosening in constrained

b. Rheumatoid wrist
   - Chronic extensive synovitis leading to wrist deformity: supination, volar dislocation, radial deviation and ulnar translocation
   - Treatment
     - Early disease: ECRL to ECU transfer to counter deforming forces and synovectomy
     - Midcarpus preserved: radiolunate arthrodesis (Chamay technique)
     - Advanced disease: wrist arthrodesis or wrist arthroplasty (cemented with poor bone stock, uncemented with good bone stock)

c. Caput ulnae syndrome
   - Chronic synovitis results in DRUJ instability, supination of carpal bones away from ulna, and dorsal subluxation and prominence of ulnar head; leads to attritional rupture of extensor tendons
   - Treatment: Darrach procedure, Suave-Kapandji procedure, or arthroplasty options

d. PIP joint
   - Boutonniere deformity: attenuation of central slip results in flexion if PIP joint, volar subluxation of lateral bands
   - **Deformity: PIP flexion and DIP hyperextension**
     - Treatment: full-time PIP extension splinting; chronic injuries may require central slip reconstruction or lateral band transferred dorsally
   - Swan neck deformity: attenuation of volar plate results in hyperextension of PIP, dorsal subluxation of lateral bands
   - **Deformity: PIP hyperextension and DIP flexion**
     - Treatment: flexible deformities should be splinted to prevent PIP hyperextension. Operative treatment includes FDS tenodesis or Fowler's central slip tenotomy. Stiff contracture is treated with arthrodesis.

e. MCP joint
   - Ulnar deviation caused by extensive synovitis, extensor tendon subluxation, and radial deviation of wrist
   - Treatment: Early disease can be treated with soft tissue realignment procedures. Definitive treatment with MCP arthroplasty relieves pain and restores alignment (though ulnar deviation returns eventually). Thumb MCP joint involvement is treated with arthrodesis.

2. Juvenile rheumatoid arthritis (JRA)
   - Autoimmune inflammatory arthropathy lasting > 6 weeks prior to age 16
   - Diagnosis of exclusion; must rule out infection
   - Majority of patients are seronegative for rheumatoid factor
   - Classification of JRA

     a. Polyarticular: > 5 joints involved, symmetric; hand most commonly involved; ulnar deviated wrist and radially deviated digits (opposite of adult RA)

     b. Pauciarticular: most common; < 5 joints involved, asymmetric larger joints
        - **Associated with uveitis or iridocyclitis; ophthalmologic slit-lamp exam mandatory**

     c. Systemic (Still's disease): acute onset with multiple joints involved, fevers, splenomegaly, rash

3. Psoriatic arthritis
   - Rash precedes joint involvement; no tenosynovitis

- Characteristic findings: sausage digits and nail pitting
- Imaging: DIP joint has "pencil in cup" deformity; centripedal erosions differentiate from DIP osteoarthritis (OA)
- Treatment: medical treatment [disease-modifying antirheumatic drugs (DMARDs)]

4. Gout
   - Deposition of monosodium urate crystals in joint leading to inflammatory response causing joint destruction; diagnosis generally made by microscopic analysis of joint fluid
   - Radiographs: periarticular erosions; tophi may be visible
   - Microscopic needle shaped, weakly negative birefringent monosodium urate crystals
   - Treatment: colchicine (inhibits granulocyte migration), indomethacin, corticosteroids for acute flares; allopurinol (xanthine oxidase inhibitor) to prevent flares, probenecid (increases uric acid excretion in urine)
5. Pseudogout
   - Deposition of calcium pyrophosphate crystal
   - Microscopic rod shaped, positively birefringent calcium pyrophosphate crystals
   - Radiographs: chondrocalcinosis of TFCC
   - Treatment: NSAIDs, splints for acute flare

- **Gout: negatively birefringent monosodium urate crystals**
- **Pseudogout: positively birefringent calcium pyrophosphate crystals**

6. Scleroderma
   - Skin is taut, shiny, and edematous with loss of regular skin folds
   - May present with Raynaud's phenomenon, calcinosis cutis, PIP flexion contractures, fingertip atrophy, or digital ulcerations
   - Treatment
     a. Arthrodesis for PIP flexion contractures
     b. Digital sympathectomy for refractory Raynaud's phenomenon
     c. Fingertip ulcerations treated with debridement and possible amputation
7. Pulmonary hypertrophic osteoarthropathy
   - Caused by malignant lung neoplasm, familial inheritance, or pulmonary disease
   - Digital clubbing, morning stiffness, arthralgia, ossifying periostitis
   - Radiographs: Periosteal thickening or elevation
   - Treatment: for pulmonary cause of disorder

VIII. Nerve Disorders

1. Compressive neuropathy
   - Electrophysiology
     a. Electromyogram (EMG): measures electrical potential of muscle cells after they are electrically stimulated, and provides information regarding fibrillations, sharp waves, motor recruitment, and insertional activity of the muscle
     b. Nerve conduction study (NCS): measures both motor and sensory nerve conduction velocity (NCV)
        - Amplitude loss = axonal injury
        - Latency slowing = myelin degeneration
   - Double crush phenomenon

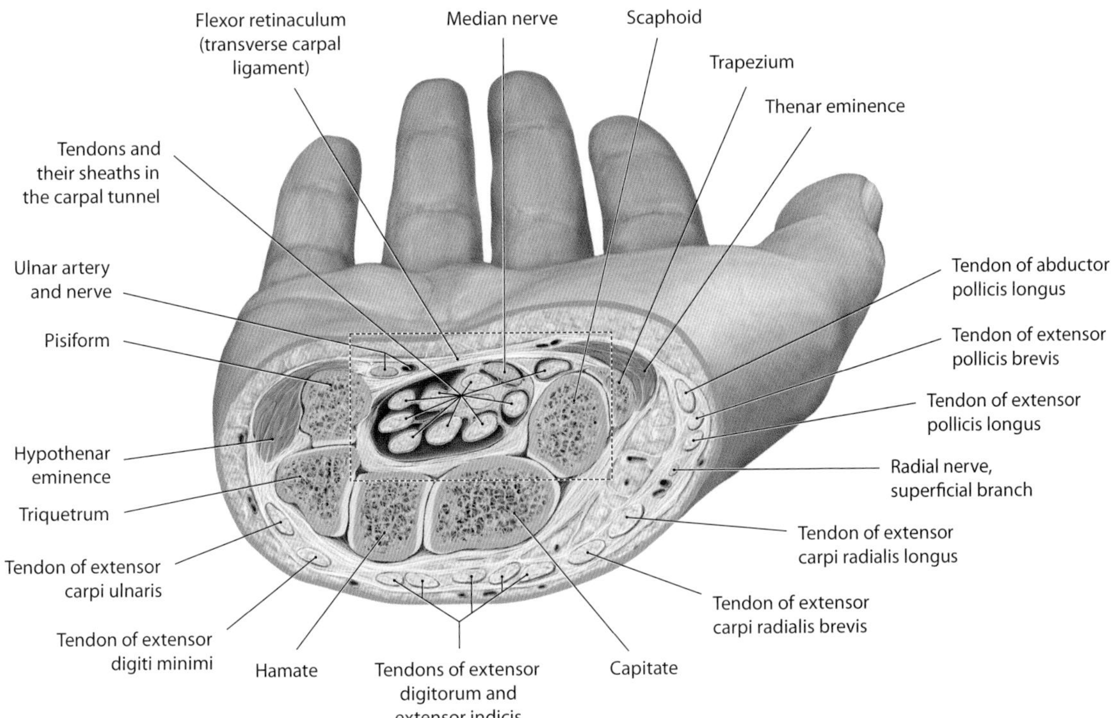

Fig. 9.48 The carpal tunnel. The carpal tunnel contains nine flexor tendons and median nerve. The flexor pollicis longus (most radial structure), four flexor digitorum superficialis and four flexor digitorum profundus tendons. The flexor carpi radialis is not in the carpal tunnel. (From Schuenke M, Schulte E. General Anatomy and the Musculoskeletal System: Thieme Atlas of Anatomy. New York: Thieme; 2005. Illustration by Karl Wesker.)

a. Proximal nerve entrapment (e.g., cervical radiculopathy) may coexist with distal nerve compression. Disruption of axonal transport of nutrients proximally makes the nerve more susceptible to compression distally.
b. Both sites of compression must be decompressed to relieve symptoms.

- Median
  a. Carpal tunnel **(Fig. 9.48)**
    - Anatomy: contains nine flexor tendons and median nerve; flexor pollicis longus (one), flexor digitorum superficialis (four), flexor digitorum profundus (four)
    - **Contents of carpal tunnel: median nerve, flexor pollicis longus, flexor digitorum superficialis, flexor digitorum profundus**
    - Flexor carpi radialis is not in the tunnel
    - Transverse carpal ligament attaches to scaphoid tubercle/trapezium radially and pisiform/hamate ulnarly **(Fig. 9.49)**
    - Associated conditions: diabetes, pregnancy, obesity, inflammatory arthritis, alcoholism, storage diseases, chronic renal failure, hypothyroidism, occupational repetitive tasks
    - Symptoms: night pain, paresthesias, or pain in radial 3½ digits; weakness
    - Physical exam: Durkan compression test (most sensitive test), Self-Administered Hand Diagram (most specific test), Tinel's test, Phalen's test, Semmes-Weinstein filament testing
    - **Semmes-Weinstein testing most sensitive for early diagnosis; tests the threshold of slowly adapting fibers**
    - Paresthesias or pain in radial 3½ digits; thenar atrophy in advanced cases; electrodiagnostic tests are not necessary to confirm diagnosis

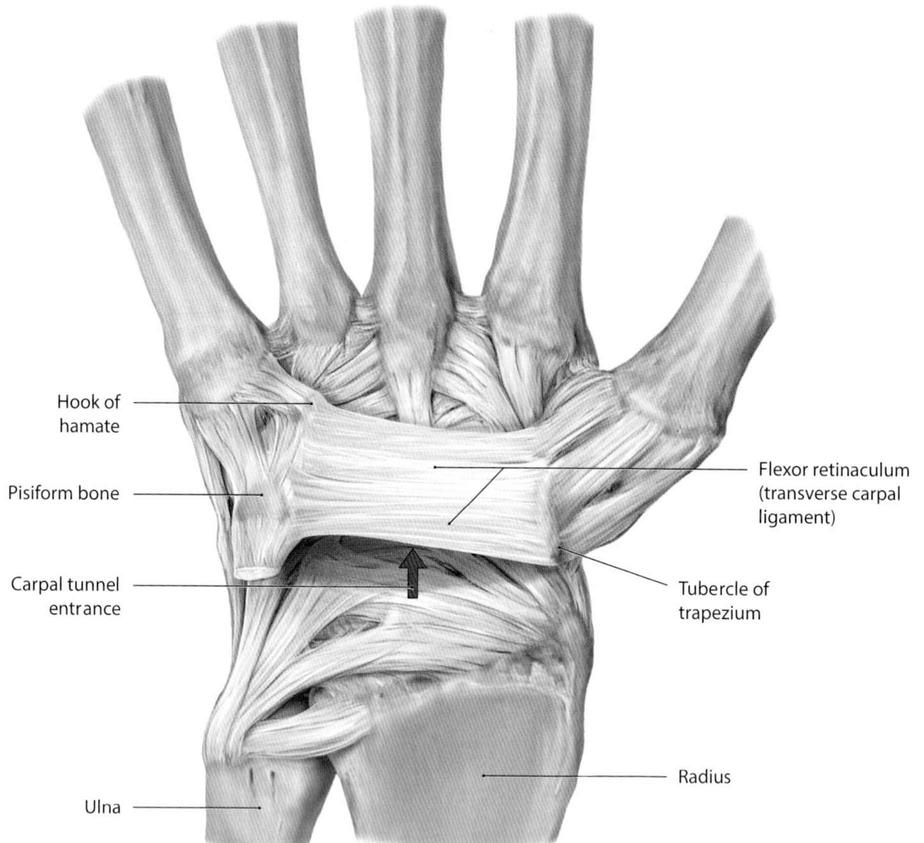

Fig. 9.49 Transverse carpal ligament. The transverse carpal ligament attaches to the scaphoid tubercle and trapezium radially and the pisiform and hamate ulnarly. (From Schuenke M, Schulte E. General Anatomy and the Musculoskeletal System: Thieme Atlas of Anatomy. New York: Thieme; 2005. Illustration by Karl Wesker.)

- Beware: C7 radiculopathy will produce paresthesia in index, middle, and ring fingers; also with triceps and wrist flexion weakness
- Carpal tunnel pressures in neutral: normal, 2.5 mm Hg, and 30 mm Hg in wrist flexion; carpal tunnel wrist in neutral, 30 mm Hg, and with flexion may be 90–110 mm Hg
- Nonoperative treatment: night splint, NSAIDs, and local steroid injection
- Operative treatment: carpal tunnel release
- No added benefit to performing flexor tenosynovectomy in addition to carpal tunnel release
- Achieve preoperative grip and pinch strength 3 months following carpal tunnel release

b. Pronator syndrome **(Figs. 9.50** and **9.51)**
  - Compressive neuropathy at elbow/proximal forearm
  - Symptoms: pain and tenderness at volar aspect of forearm, activity-induced paresthesias; lack of night symptoms compared with carpal tunnel
  - Physical exam: pain or paresthesias in radial 3½ digits, provocative maneuvers include pain with elbow flexion against resistance if Lacertus fibrosis involved, pain with resistive forearm pronation if pronator teres involved, or pain with resisted flexion of middle finger if FDS involved
  - Potential site of entrapment
    - Ligament of Struthers: vestigial band travels from supracondylar process to medial epicondyle **(Fig. 9.52)**
    - Supracondylar process: osseus structure on anterior distal humerus; best seen on lateral radiograph; affects 1% of patients

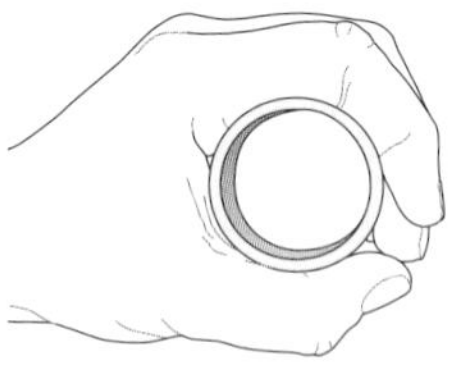

In a healthy hand, the thumb can be abducted to fully grasp a cylindrical object

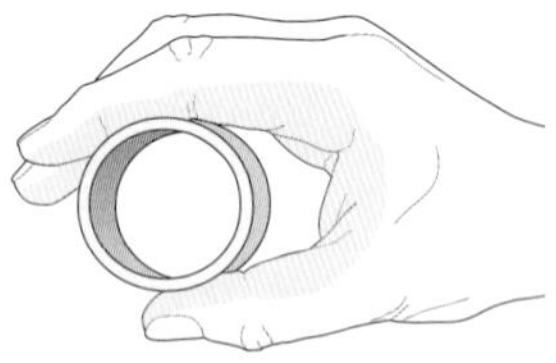

With a proximal median nerve lesion, the thumb cannot be fully abducted

Fig. 9.50 Hand of benediction following a proximal median nerve lesion. When patients try to make a fist, they can flex only the ulnar fingers. There may be associated sensory disturbances in the radial 3½ digits. This is due to the loss of first and second lumbricals and the index and middle FDP. (From Schuenke M, Schulte E. General Anatomy and the Musculoskeletal System: Thieme Atlas of Anatomy. New York: Thieme; 2005. Illustration by Karl Wesker.)

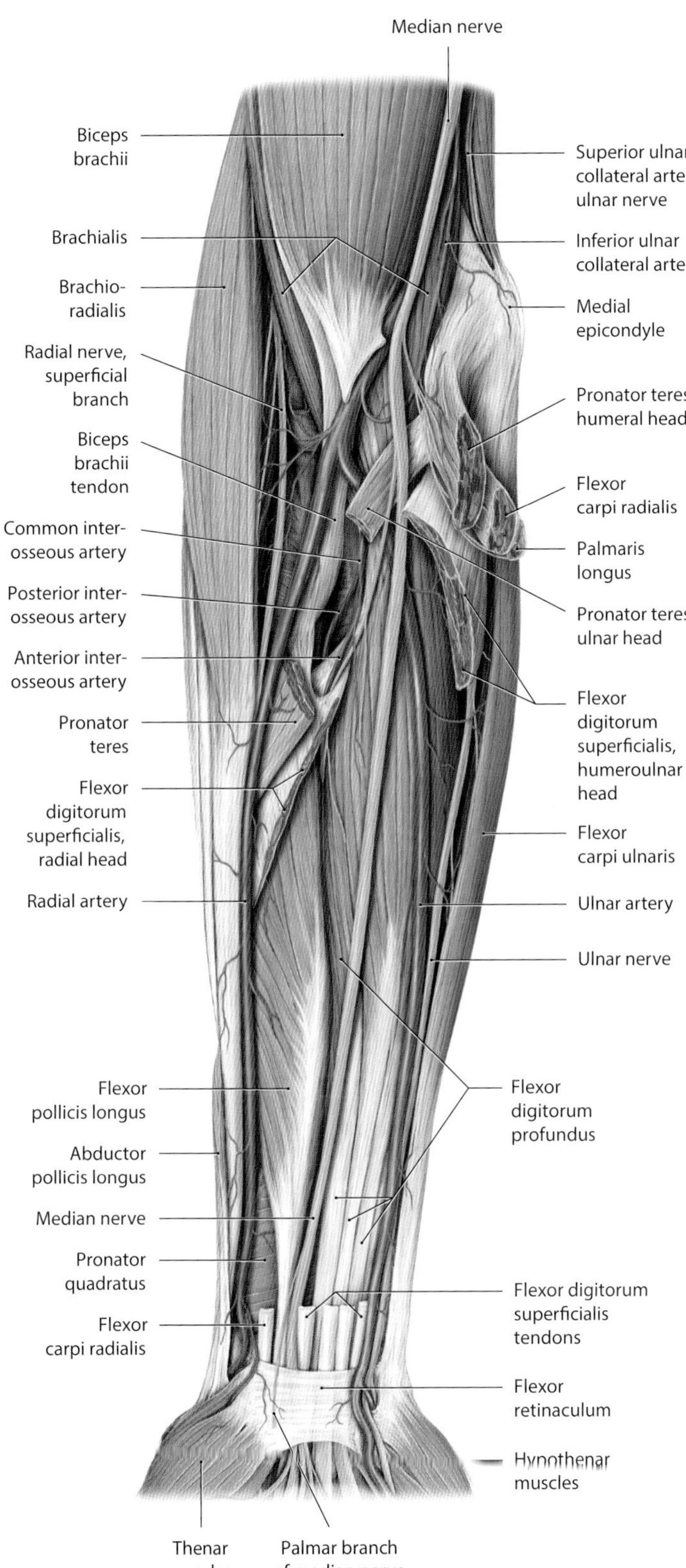

Fig. 9.51 Course of median nerve in the forearm. The pronator teres (humeral head) is reflected. Potential sites of the median nerve entrapment include between the pronator teres, FDS aponeurotic arch, ligament of Struthers, supracondylar process above the medial epicondyle, and lacertus fibrosis. (From Schuenke M, Schulte E. General Anatomy and the Musculoskeletal System: Thieme Atlas of Anatomy. New York: Thieme; 2005. Illustration by Karl Wesker.)

- Lacertus fibrosis (bicep aponeurosis)
- Between two head of pronator teres
- FDS aponeurotic arch

◦ Treatment: nonoperative treatment with splints and NSAIDs; decompression if nonoperative treatment fails

c. Anterior interosseus nerve syndrome

◦ Anatomy: supplies motor to FPL, index and long FDP, and pronator quadratus; no sensory supply; motor branch comes off median nerve 4–6 cm distal to elbow

◦ Sites of compression

- Site of compression of pronator syndrome
- Gantzer muscle: accessory head of FPL
- Enlarged bicipital bursa

◦ Symptoms: motor deficits only; no sensory complaints

◦ Physical exam: tests pronator quadratus by resisted pronation with elbow maximally flexed; test FPL and index FDP by having patient make the “OK” sign; weak pinch and grip

◦ EMG nerve test helpful for diagnosis

◦ **Parsonage-Turner may cause anterior interosseous nerve (AIN) palsy; often palsy preceded by viral illness and shoulder pain; tends to resolve over 4–6 months**

◦ Treatment

- Nonoperative: splinting elbow at 90 degrees for 8–12 weeks and NSAIDs
- Operative: decompression if nonoperative treatment fails

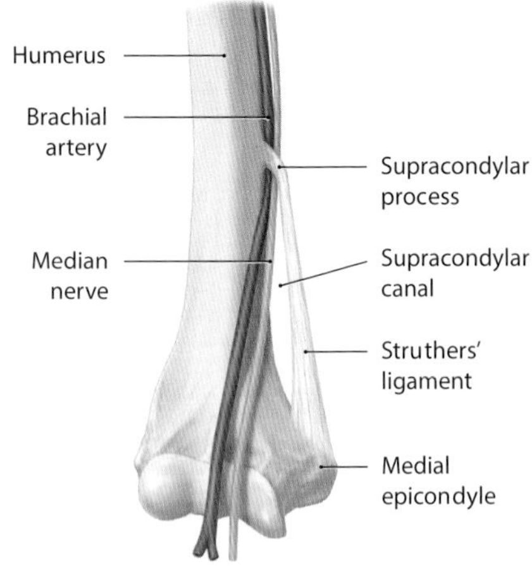

Fig. 9.52 Supracondylar process of the humerus. The supracondylar process is rare (0.7%); a bony outgrowth above the medial epicondyle. When present, it can serve as an attachment for a connective tissue band referred to as the ligament of Struthers, which ends on the medial epicondyle. This fibro-osseus supracondylar canal can entrap and compress the brachial artery and medial nerve. From THIEME Atlas of Anatomy, General Anatomy and Musculoskeltal System, © Thieme 2005, Illustration by [Karl Wesler]

• Ulnar

a. Cubital tunnel

◦ Anatomic sites of compression

- Arcade of Struthers: band of deep fascia covering ulnar nerve 8 cm proximal to medial epicondyle, connecting medial head of triceps to medical intermuscular septum
- Medial intermuscular septum
- Medial epicondyle
- Cubital tunnel: floor is MCL and elbow joint capsule, roof is Osbourne's ligament (aponeurotic attachment of FCU)
- Anconeus epitrochlearis: anomalous muscle found in 10% patients undergoing cubital tunnel release
- Arcuate ligament: FCU aponeurosis between ulnar and humeral heads of FCU in proximal forearm

◦ Associated conditions: cubitus varus/valgus, burns, heterotopic ossification, fracture and nonunions of medial epicondyle, medial epicondylitis, ganglion cysts, tumors

◦ Symptoms: night pain, paresthesias in ulnar 1½ digits; pain exacerbated by elbow flexion or shoulder abduction

◦ Physical exam

- Findings: first web space atrophy, interosseus atrophy, ring or small finger clawing, subluxation of ulnar nerve at medial epicondyle, weak pinch **(Fig. 9.53)**
- Froment sign: IP flexion while attempting to pinch between thumb and index finger due to weak adductor pollicis **(Fig. 9.54)**

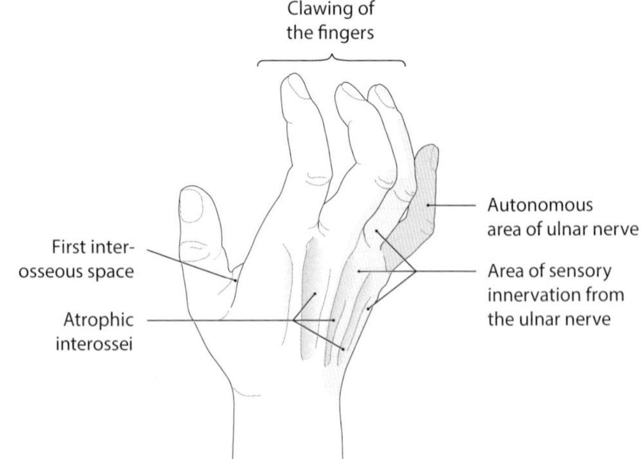

Fig. 9.53 Claw hand due to ulnar nerve lesion. Ulnar nerve lesion may present with claw hand and atrophy of the interossei musculature. Sensory abnormalities are frequently confined to the small finger. (From Schuenke M, Schulte E. General Anatomy and the Musculoskeletal System: Thieme Atlas of Anatomy. New York: Thieme; 2005. Illustration by Karl Wesker.)

- Wartenberg sign: abducted small finger secondary to unopposed pull of EDM and weakness of third palmar interossei
- Jeanne sign: hyperextension of thumb MCP with key pinch by EPL (radial n.) due to weak adductor pollicis (ulnar n.)
- Other physical exam maneuvers that reproduce symptoms: direct compression test, Tinel's, and elbow flexion

∘ Treatment

- Nonoperative treatment with nighttime extension splinting and NSAIDs
- **Operative treatment with decompression; no proven benefit to addition of anterior subcutaneous transposition even if subluxation of nerve present**

∘ Complications

- Persistent posteromedial elbow pain due to iatrogenic injury and neuroma formation of medial antebrachial cutaneous nerve
- Recurrence secondary to scar formation or inadequate release

b. Ulnar tunnel/Guyon's canal **(Fig. 9.55)**

∘ Anatomy

- Boundaries of Guyon's canal:
  - Roof: volar carpal ligament, palmaris brevis, hypothenar fat
  - Floor: transverse carpal ligament, pisohamate and pisometacarpal ligament, and opponens digiti minimi
  - Medial (ulnar) wall: FCU, pisiform, abductor digiti minimi
  - Lateral (radial) wall: hook of hamate
- Zones of injury:
  - Zone 1: proximal to bifurcation of ulnar nerve affecting both motor and sensory fibers

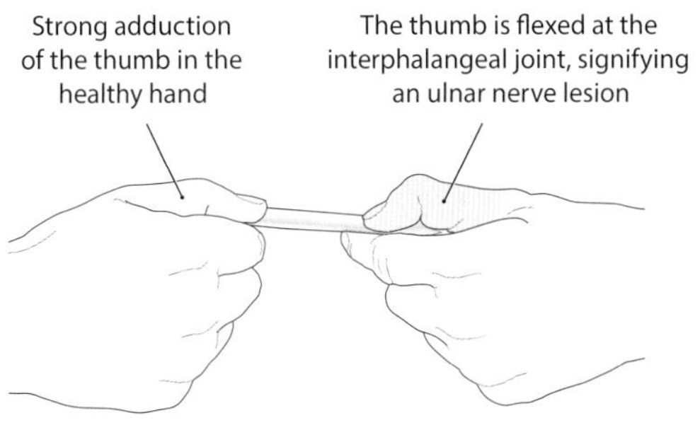

Strong adduction of the thumb in the healthy hand

The thumb is flexed at the interphalangeal joint, signifying an ulnar nerve lesion

Fig. 9.54 Froment sign. The thumb flexes at the interphalangeal joint when attempting to pinch between the thumb and index finger due to a weak adductor pollicis (ulnar nerve lesion). (From Schuenke M, Schulte E. General Anatomy and the Musculoskeletal System: Thieme Atlas of Anatomy. New York: Thieme; 2005. Illustration by Karl Wesker.)

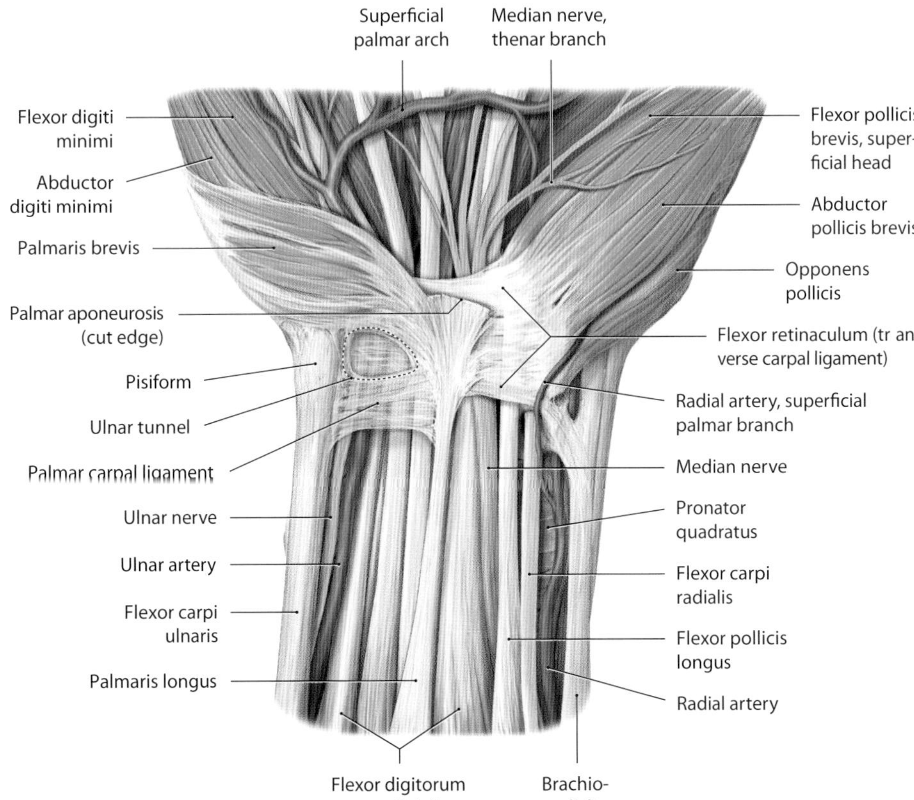

Fig. 9.55 Course of the ulnar artery and nerve in the ulnar tunnel. The borders of the ulnar tunnel (Guyon's canal) is the palmar carpal ligament (roof), transverse carpal ligament (floor), hook of the hamate (radial), and pisiform (ulnar). The ulnar nerve bifurcates within the canal into superficial sensory and deep motor branches (more radial). (From Schuenke M, Schulte E. General Anatomy and the Musculoskeletal System: Thieme Atlas of Anatomy. New York: Thieme; 2005. Illustration by Karl Wesker.)

- Zone 2: distal to bifurcation of ulnar nerve where deep motor branch runs to innervate interossei (affects motor only)
- Zone 3: distal to bifurcation where superficial sensory branch runs (affects sensation only)

◦ Dorsal sensory branch is proximal to Guyon's canal, so compression here will have intact dorsal ulnar sensation

◦ Deep motor nerve innervates intrinsics (except radial two lumbricals), adductor pollicis, and deep head of flexor pollicis brevis (FPB)

◦ Causes include: ganglion (most common) or lipoma (zone I or II), repetitive trauma, hook of hamate fracture, pisiform dislocation, ulnar artery thrombosis or aneurysm (zone III), palmar brevis hypertrophy

◦ Physical exam: depends on site of compression; Froment sign, Wartenberg sign, clawing of ring and small finger

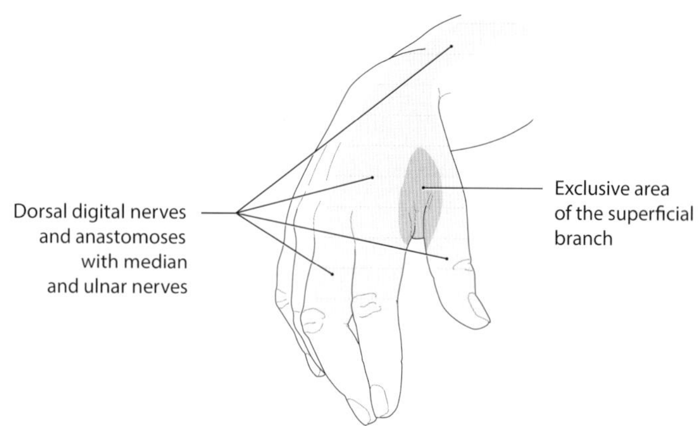

Fig. 9.56 Wrist drop due to a radial nerve lesion. (From Schuenke M, Schulte E. General Anatomy and the Musculoskeletal System: Thieme Atlas of Anatomy. New York: Thieme; 2005. Illustration by Karl Wesker.)

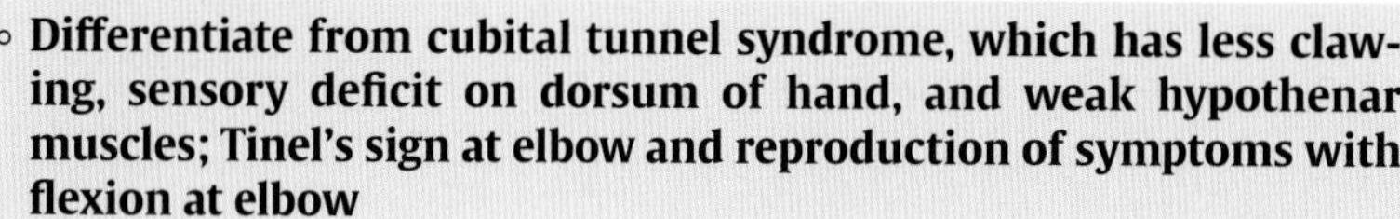
◦ **Differentiate from cubital tunnel syndrome, which has less clawing, sensory deficit on dorsum of hand, and weak hypothenar muscles; Tinel's sign at elbow and reproduction of symptoms with flexion at elbow**

◦ Diagnostic testing: MRI to look for ganglion; CT to look for hook of hamate fracture; Doppler ultrasound (US) to evaluate ulnar artery

◦ Treatment
  - ♦ Nonoperative: splinting and NSAIDs
  - ♦ Operative: decompression when symptoms are severe or nonoperative treatment failed

• Radial **(Fig. 9.56)**

a. Proximal compression/injury
  - ◦ Etiologies: humeral shaft fracture, direct compression ("Saturday night palsy"), prolonged tourniquet
  - ◦ Physical exam: weakness of elbow extension, wrist/finger extension
  - ◦ Treatment: observation; if no recovery by 3 months, then EMG/NCS; possible exploration
  - ◦ **Radial nerve injury after a humerus fracture is treated nonoperatively, with a 85–95% recovery rate.**
  - ◦ **If EMG after 6 weeks shows no recovery, continue to observe and repeat the EMG at 12 weeks.**
  - ◦ **If no recovery at 3–6 months, perform exploratory surgery.**

b. PIN syndrome
  - ◦ Anatomic sites of compression
    - ♦ Arcade of Frohse: proximal edge of supinator
    - ♦ Distal edge supinator
    - ♦ ECRB edge
    - ♦ Fascial band at radial head
    - ♦ Radial artery recurrent leash of Henry
    - ♦ Other causes include Monteggia fracture/dislocation, chronic radial head dislocation, rheumatoid synovitis
  - ◦ Symptoms/physical exam: pain at lateral elbow, pain at wrist capsule due to innervation of dorsal wrist capsule, motor weakness; terminal

branch of PIN lies on the floor of fourth dorsal compartment; radial deviation of wrist with active extension (ECRL intact, ECU out); no sensory complaints

- **Differentiate from extensor tendon injury by wrist tenodesis**
- Diagnostic test: EMG may be helpful
- Treatment: nonoperative, with splinting, activity modification, and NSAIDs; failure to improve after 3 months requires decompression

c. Radial tunnel syndrome

- **Same site of compression as PIN syndrome, presenting with pain only**
- Anatomic site of decompression: same as PIN syndrome
- Symptoms manifest as pain, with tenderness more anterior and distal than lateral epicondylitis; no motor weakness
- Physical exam: no muscle weakness; lateral elbow and dorsoradial forearm pain; pain with resisted long finger extension; diagnosis may be made by diagnostic/therapeutic injection
- May coexist with lateral epicondylitis
- Treatment: nonoperative, with splint, NSAIDs, and activity modification for at least 1 year; surgical decompression if nonoperative therapy fails

d. Radial sensory nerve entrapment

- **Wartenberg syndrome: compression between brachioradialis and ECRL in distal forearm producing sensory changes only (no motor)**
- Etiology: direct trauma, external fixation, handcuffs, tight casts, tight watchband
- Symptoms: pain and numbness over dorsoradial hand
- Physical exam: provocative maneuver includes forearm pronation, which compresses nerve between ECRL and brachioradialis reproducing symptoms; positive Tinel's sign
- Treatment: nonoperative treatment with splint, NSAIDs, and activity modification for 6 months; surgical decompression if nonoperative therapy fails; variable results

• Thoracic outlet syndrome

a. Neurogenic (usually lower trunk of brachial plexus) or vascular (subclavian vessels)
b. Etiology: first cervical rib, vertebral transverse process, scalene muscle abnormalities, fibrous band, clavicle or cervical rib malunion, athletes such as rowers or weight lifters
c. Symptoms: vague upper extremity pain, paresthesias or fatigue
d. Physical exam: provocative maneuver
   - Roos test: have patient hold hand above head and repeatedly open/close hand for 1 minute
   - Adson test: hand at side and neck extended and turned toward hand, resulting in loss of radial pulse or reproduction of symptoms
   - Wright test: abduction of arm with neck extended and turned toward contralateral side
   - Diagnostics: chest X-ray to rule out Pancoast tumor; C-spine X-ray to evaluate cervical rib; duplex ultrasound if suspect vascular compromise; electrodiagnostic tests generally do not aid in diagnosis
   - Treatment: physical therapy focused on shoulder girdle (first line); if persistent pain or neurovascular compromise, then perform surgery directed toward etiology

• Shoulder

a. Suprascapular nerve

- Anatomy: C5-C6 nerve root; suprascapular nerve travels below the transverse scapular ligament; suprascapular artery passes above, nerve below; suprascapular nerve supplies supraspinatus and then travels through spinoglenoid notch to supply infraspinatus
- **Suprascapular artery travels above transverse scapular ligament, nerve travels below; mnemonic: Army over Navy**
- Sites of entrapment
  - Suprascapular notch: supraspinatus and infraspinatus affected
  - Spinoglenoid notch: only infraspinatus affected
- Etiology: ganglion, blunt trauma, fractures
- Physical exam: posterolateral shoulder pain, tenderness at suprascapular notch; weakness with abduction to 90 degrees (supraspinatus), external rotation weakness, posterior scapula atrophy
- Diagnostics test: MRI to look for mass, EMG/NCS
- Treatment: If no compressive mass is seen on MRI, then treat with a shoulder rehabilitation program. A compressive mass or failure of nonoperative treatment requires surgical decompression.

b. Musculocutaneous nerve
- Anatomy: C5-C7; supplies bicep brachii, coracobrachialis, half of brachialis; sensation via lateral antebrachial cutaneous nerve
- Etiology: shoulder dislocation compressing coracobrachialis, iatrogenic injury from retraction intraoperatively
- Symptoms/physical exam: lateral arm paresthesias, elbow flexion weakness
- Treatment: observation, rarely requires surgery

c. Long thoracic nerve palsy
- Anatomy: C5-C7; innervates serratus anterior; maintains scapula position and assists with shoulder elevation
- **Injury causes medial rotation of inferior scapular pole and elevation of scapula**
- Etiology: repetitive stretch injury, direct trauma, iatrogenic (e.g., axillary node dissection)
- Treatment
  - Nonoperative: observation, bracing, and scapula strengthening for at least 6 months
  - Operative: Split pectoralis major transfer

d. Spinal accessory nerve palsy
- Anatomy: cranial nerve XI; innervates trapezius and sternocleidomastoid

e. Injury causes trapezius palsy and resultant lateral rotation of inferior scapular pole and depression of scapula
- Etiology: direct blow, acromioclavicular (AC) dislocations, iatrogenic injury (e.g., neck dissections)
- Treatment
  - Nonoperative: observation and trapezius strengthening
  - Operative: modified Eden-Lange procedure, which entails transfer of rhomboid major/minor and levator scapulae

f. Axillary nerve compression (quadrilateral space syndrome)
- Anatomy
  - **Quadrilateral space boundaries: medial, long head of triceps; lateral, humeral shaft; superior, teres major; inferior, teres minor**
  - Axillary nerve runs through quadrilateral space with posterior humeral circumflex artery

Table 9.11 Seddon and Sunderland Classifications

Seddon	Sunderland	Pathology	Prognosis
Neurapraxia	Type 1	Myelin injury	Usually full recovery
Axonotmesis	Type 2	Axonal injury with intact endoneurium, perineurium, and epineurium	Usually complete recovery but may take weeks to months
	Type 3	Axonal and endoneurium injury with intact perineurium and epineurium	Partial recovery
	Type 4	Axonal, endoneurium, and perineurium injury with intact epineurium	Poor recovery
Neurotmesis	Type 5	Complete nerve disruption	No spontaneous regeneration

- Etiology: anterior glenohumeral dislocations, trauma, throwing athletes
- Physical exam: provocative pain with shoulder abduction, elevation, and external rotation; tenderness over quadrilateral space
- Diagnostic: angiography shows compression with shoulder abduction
- Treatment
  - ♦ Nonoperative: activity modification
  - ♦ Operative: fibrous band release or teres minor release

- Brachial neuritis/Parsonage-Turner syndrome
  a. Rare disorder of unknown etiology that causes pain or weakness of upper extremity
  b. Often presents following viral illness; 1–2 weeks of intense shoulder pain that subsides, then onset of weakness; commonly involves AIN
  c. Treatment: observation

2. Nerve injury
- Peripheral nerve injuries
  a. Classification: Seddon and Sunderland **(Table 9.11)**
  b. Nerve regenerates ~1 mm/day
  c. Most effective repair is primary epineural repair
  d. Repair of segmental nerve loss with conduits, decellularized allograft, or autograft
    - **Nerve repair with autograft has the best outcomes compared with conduits and decellularized allograft.**
    - Autograft sources: sural, medial, and lateral antebrachial cutaneous nerves
    - **Age is the leading prognostic factor for nerve recovery; age > 30 years yields worse prognosis**
    - **Location is second prognostic factor; proximal worse than distal**
  e. Chronic injuries may be treated with tendon or nerve transfers
    - Classic tendon transfers (see Tendon transfers, below, for full description)
      - ♦ Radial nerve palsy: flexor carpi radialis to extensor digitorum communis (restore digital extension); palmaris longus to extensor pollicis longus (restore thumb extension); pronator teres to extensor carpi radialis brevis (restore wrist extension)

- Brachial plexus **(Fig. 9.57)**
  a. Brachial plexus is divided into roots, trunks, divisions, cords, and branches. Mnemonic: Randy Travis Drinks Cold Beer.

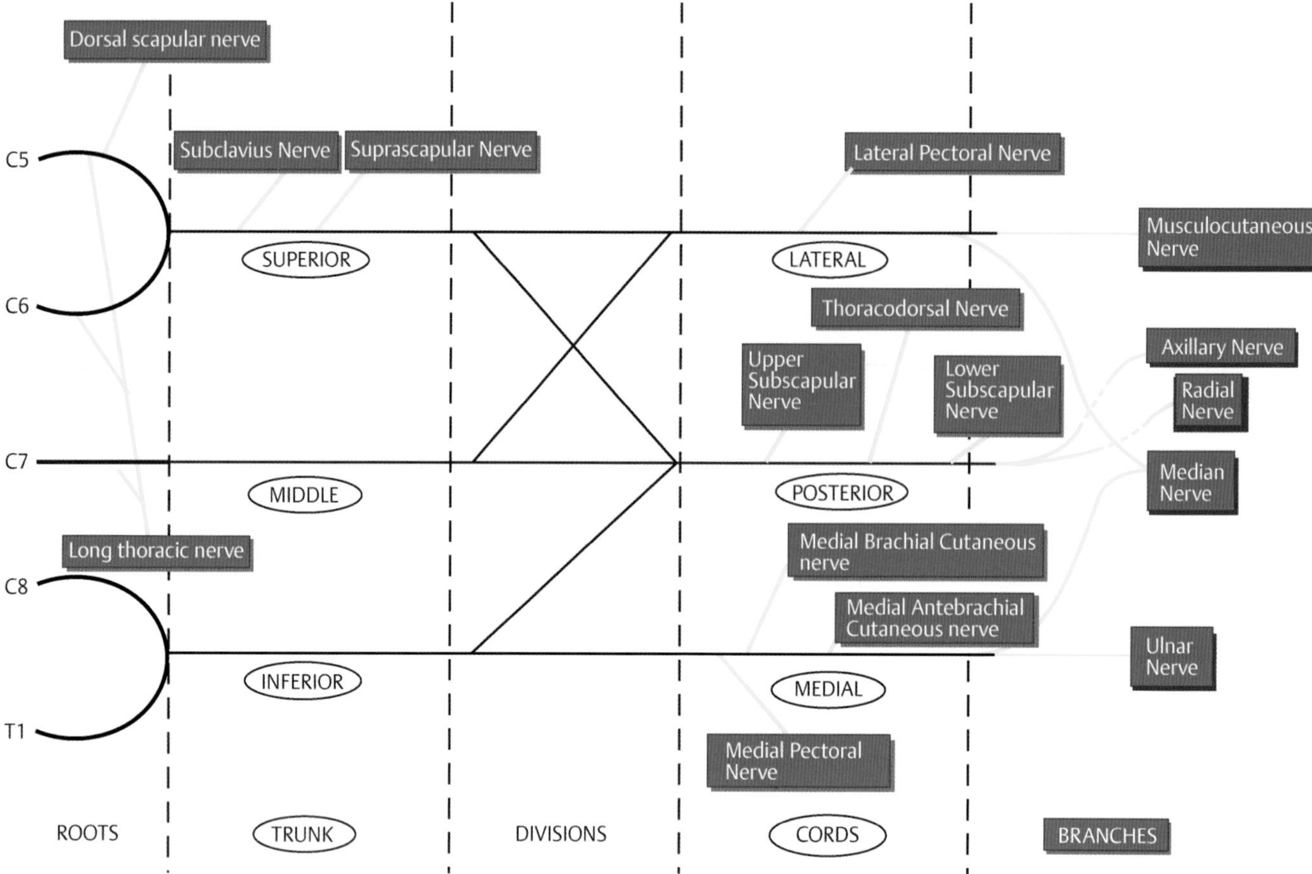

Fig. 9.57 Brachial plexus diagram.

- Anatomy
  a. Proximal to distal: roots, trunks, divisions, cords, terminal branches
  b. Classic from C5-T1
  c. Anatomic variants of brachial plexus:
     - Prefixed C4-C8
     - Postfixed C6-T2
  d. Terminal nerve branches that arise from roots can help delineate the level of the lesion. If muscles work, then the injury is distal to the roots.
     - **Horner's syndrome is indicative of a preganglionic lower trunk injury (C8-T1).**
     - Phrenic nerve (C3-C5)
     - Long thoracic nerve (C5–7)
     - Dorsal scapular nerve (C5)
     - Paraspinal muscles
  a. Terminal nerve branch that arises from a trunk is the suprascapular and subclavius nerve
     - **The C5 and C6 nerve roots join to make the superior trunk (at Erb's point). The suprascapular nerve branches from the superior trunk at Erb's point.**
  b. There are no terminal branches off of the divisions.
  c. Terminal branches of lateral cord: musculocutaneous and median nerves
  d. Terminal branches of posterior cord: axillary and radial nerves

e. Terminal branch of medial cord: ulnar and median nerves

- Classification
  a. Preganglionic versus postganglionic
  b. Preganglionic lesions (nerve root avulsions) have worst prognosis; not repairable
  c. Postganglionic lesions are either stretched or torn. If a focal nerve lesion is present, it can be directly repaired or nerve grafted (sural cable grafts).
  d. Anatomic description of level of injury: supraclavicular, retroclavicular, infraclavicular. Infraclavicular injuries have a better prognosis than supraclavicular injuries.
- Mechanism: motorcycle or motor vehicle accidents; shoulder forced caudad (favors injury of upper plexus); forced abduction of shoulder (favors injury of lower plexus)
- Obstetric brachial plexus palsy: see Chapter 4
- Acute evaluation
  a. Physical exam including motor strength and sensory exam; test rhomboids (dorsal scapular nerve) and serratus anterior (long thoracic nerve); if functioning, then C5 injury is postganglionic
  b. Examine eyes for evidence of Horner's syndrome: ptosis, miosis, and anhidrosis indicating a preganglionic T1 avulsion
  c. Complete vascular exam
  d. Radiographs
    - Chest X-ray to look for scapulothoracic dissociation, clavicle fracture, or first/second rib fractures, which may indicate brachial plexus injury; if phrenic nerve injured, hemidiaphragm will be elevated
    - CT of cervical spine to look for multiple transverse process fractures, which may indicate root avulsion injury or cervical fracture/spinal cord injury
    - Shoulder X-rays
    - CT myelography is gold standard in evaluation; obtain 3–4 weeks after injury
    - **Look for pseudomeningoceles in preganglionic ruptures.**
    - MRI largely replacing CT myelography in evaluation of plexus injuries
- Long-term workup
  a. EMG between 2–6 weeks; can determine difference between pre- and postganglionic injuries; must allow wallerian degeneration to occur before EMG is useful
  b. NCS
    - **Sensory nerve action potentials (SNAPs) are normal in patients with preganglionic lesions because the sensory cell bodies are intact within the dorsal root ganglion.**
- Treatment
  a. Priorities (in decreasing order of importance): elbow flexion, shoulder abduction, wrist extension/finger flexion, wrist flexion/finger extension, and intrinsic function
  b. Indications
    - Penetrating trauma of the brachial plexus treated with immediate exploration and repair
    - Gunshot wounds: nerve injury usually due to neurapraxia
    - Blunt trauma causing preganglionic injury: early tendon transfers (3–6 weeks)
    - Blunt trauma causing postganglionic injuries: treatment is delayed to allow regeneration of nerves (3–6 months)

- Late identification and treatment (1 year after initial injury): patients typically do poorly with nerve grafting and best treated with tendon transfers

c. Nerve grafting: better for upper and middle trunk because innervated muscle is more proximal; poor results for lower trunk lesions due to distal nature of muscles and increased time required for reinnervation

- **Lose ~ 1% a day of the motor end plate of a denervated muscle, or ~ 50% of the motor end plates at 1 year, so nerve injuries left unaddressed for more than 12–18 months, or nerve injures far from their motor end plate (high ulnar nerve injuries, for example) have poor likelihood of functional motor recovery**
- Sources: sural nerval, ipsilateral cutaneous nerve, ipsilateral vascularized ulnar nerve

d. Neurotization (nerve transfer): transfer of functional but less important motor nerve to nonfunctioning nerve innervating a more important muscle

- Extraplexal sources: spinal accessory nerve, intercostal nerve, contralateral C7, and hypoglossal nerve
- Intraplexal sources: phrenic nerve, ulnar nerve, triceps motor branch
- Common transfers
  - Ulnar nerve branch from FCU to musculocutaneous nerve to restore elbow flexion (biceps): Oberlin transfer
  - Triceps motor branch to axillary nerve to restore shoulder abduction (deltoid)
  - **Oberlin transfer: ulnar nerve branch to musculocutaneous nerve to restore elbow flexion**

e. Free muscle transfer: gracilis most commonly used

- Tendon transfers

a. Indicated for late presentation or early transfer for lower root injuries (due to time to innervation of distal muscles and loss of motor end plates)

b. Lose one motor grade with transfer; transfer muscle with 5/5 motor grade

c. Common tendon transfers

- Musculocutaneous nerve palsy
  - Lose elbow flexion
    - Free gracilis transfer
    - Transfer pectoralis major/latissimus dorsi to biceps
    - Or transfer common flexor mass more proximal on humerus (Steindler flexorplasty)
- Radial nerve/PIN palsy
  - Lose elbow extension
    - Transfer deltoid, latissimus, or biceps to triceps
  - Lose wrist extension
    - Transfer pronator teres to ECRB
  - Lose finger extension
    - Transfer flexor carpi radialis (FCR) to extensor digitorum communis (EDC) (FDS and FCU also described)
  - Lose thumb extension
    - Transfer palmaris longus (PL) to EPL
    - Or transfer FDS to radial lateral band
- Ulnar nerve palsy
  - Lose thumb adduction

- Transfer FDS, ECRB, or BR (brachioradialis) to adductor pollicis
  - Lose finger abduction
    - Transfer APL, ECRL or EIP to first dorsal interosseus
- Low median nerve palsy
  - Lose thumb opposition and abduction
    - Transfer ring FDS through a pulley created by FCU to base of proximal phalanx or APB (Bunnell opponensplasty)
    - Or EIP (directed around ulna) to base of proximal phalanx
    - Abductor digiti quinti (ADQ) to APB (Huber)
    - PL to APB (Camitz)
- High median nerve palsy
  - Lose thumb IP flexion
    - Transfer BR to FPL
  - Lose index and long finger flexion
    - Side-to-side transfer FDP ring and small fingers to FDP index and middle fingers

IX. Vascular Disorders

1. Anatomy
   - **Ulnar artery is dominant in 88% of patients; it contributes to the superficial palmar arch.**
   - Radial artery contributes to deep palmar arch and princeps pollicis
   - 80% of individuals have complete arches; if either ulnar or radial artery is injured, there are enough collaterals to complete arch and supply digits; presence of an incomplete arch (20%) can be detected by Allen test
2. Diagnostics
   - Allen test: Manually compress both radial and ulnar arteries proximal to wrist and ask patient to open and close hand several times. Then release radial artery and continue to compress the ulnar artery and evaluate digital reperfusion. Repeat the test, releasing the ulnar artery and compressing the radial artery.
   - Duplex ultrasound: evaluates true and false aneurysms; evaluates perfusion.
   - Three-phase bone scan:
     a. Phase I (2 minutes): similar to arteriogram; evaluates perfusion
     b. Phase II (5–10 minutes): evaluates soft tissue and inflammation
     c. Phase III (2–3 hours): not helpful in evaluating vascular disorder of hand; positive phase III that does not correlate with phase I-II diagnosis: reflex sympathetic dystrophy
   - Arteriography: gold standard for thrombotic and embolic sources
3. Occlusive
   - Hypothenar hammer syndrome
     a. Most common vascular occlusive disease of hand
     b. Hypothenar hammer syndrome: posttraumatic ulnar artery thrombosis at Guyon's canal caused by blunt trauma to hypothenar eminence
     c. Common in carpenters or anyone who uses palm as a "hammer" during work
     d. Diagnostic studies: Doppler or arteriogram
     e. Treatment: resection of thrombosed segment, sympathectomy

- Embolic
  a. Most commonly cardiac origin; other origins: subclavian vessels due to thoracic outlet syndrome
  b. Treatment: emergent embolectomy and anticoagulation
- Thromboangiitis obliterans (Buerger disease)
  a. Inflammation of small and medium vessels of hand and feet with subsequent thrombosis
  b. Most commonly occurs in young male smokers
  c. Symptoms: Raynaud's phenomenon, severe rest pain, cold intolerance, digital ulceration or ischemia
  d. Treatment: smoking cessation (most important); avoidance of cold and medications that cause vasoconstriction; amputation
- Vasospastic disease
  a. Raynaud's phenomenon: vasospastic disease with known cause
     - Causes: scleroderma, systemic lupus erythematosus (SLE), RA, dermatomyositis, CREST syndrome (calcinosis, Raynaud's phenomenon, esophageal dysmotility, sclerodactyly, and telangiectasia), thoracic outlet syndrome, polycythemia, cryoproteinemia, ergot pharmaceuticals, beta blockers, reflex sympathetic dystrophy
     - Symptoms: unilateral, peripheral pulses absent
     - Treatment: directed at underlying cause; avoid smoking and cold
  b. Raynaud's disease: idiopathic
     - Most commonly affects premenopausal women
     - Symptoms: bilateral, peripheral pulses present
     - Treatment: calcium channel blockers, smoking cessation and avoidance of cold; if conservative treatment fails, then digital sympathectomy

4. Aneurysm/pseudoaneurysm
   - Presentation: pulsatile mass, caused by blunt or penetrating trauma
   - Diagnostic: Doppler ultrasound or arteriography; order MRI if diagnosis unclear
   - Treatment: surgical exploration with ligation, repair, or excision of lesion
5. Compartment syndrome
   - Increased intracompartmental pressure leading to decrease capillary blood flow restricting tissue perfusion/oxygenation
   - Causes: high-energy trauma, supracondylar humerus fractures (most common cause in children), burns
   - Clinical diagnosis: pain with passive stretch (most sensitive), pain out of proportion, tense compartment; late findings include paresthesias, pallor, pulselessness, and paralysis
   - Equivocal physical exam findings with high index of suspicion or unresponsive patients must have compartment monitoring
   - Treatment: emergent fasciotomies
     a. Three forearm compartments: mobile wad, dorsal, and volar
     b. Ten hand compartments: thenar, hypothenar, four dorsal interossei, three volar interossei, adductor pollicis; note: carpal tunnel release done in same setting
   - Volkmann ischemic contracture
     a. Sequelae of compartment syndrome with muscle fibrosis and contracture
     b. Most common physical exam finding of untreated compartment syndrome of hand: intrinsic minus posture before MCP extension and after flexion from imbalance of relatively strong extrinsic muscles to weak intrinsic muscles

X. Osteonecrosis

(Note: osteonecrosis is most common in the lunate, followed by the scaphoid and capitate head.)

1. Preiser's disease
   - Avascular necrosis of scaphoid
   - Uncommon; average age at onset, 45 years
   - Symptoms: insidious onset of dorsoradial wrist pain; decreased grip strength; snuffbox tenderness; no history of trauma or prior fracture
   - Imaging
     a. Radiographs: may show sclerosis or fragmentation
     b. MRI: to evaluate early disease and vascularity; enables classification of complete involvement (type I) or partial involvement (type II)
   - Treatment: no consensus or algorithm; may try period of immobilization but has had limited success; other procedures include core decompression, microfracture, revascularization procedures, allograft replacement, or salvage procedures such as proximal row carpectomy or scaphoid excision and four-corner fusion
2. Kienböck's disease
   - Avascular necrosis of lunate
   - Most common in males of ages 20–40 years
   - Etiology: multiple factors including ulnar negative variance, singular vacular supply to lunate (I pattern [single vessel] blood supply thought to be highest risk), altered geometry of lunate, repetitive trauma
   - Symptoms: dorsal wrist pain, mild swelling, limited wrist range of motion or grip strength
   - Imaging: X-rays of wrist, PA view of wrist evaluates ulnar variance; MRI detects early disease, decreased T1 signal
   - Treatment based on Lichtman classification **(Table 9.12)**

Table 9.12 Lichtman Classification

Stage	Radiographic Findings	Treatment
I	No changes on X-ray; MRI finding, decreased T1 signal of lunate	Cast immobilization
II	Lunate sclerosis	▪ Joint leveling procedure for ulnar negative patients with radial shortening osteotomy ▪ Ulnar positive variance; undergo capitate shortening with capitohamate fusion ▪ Distal radius core decompression to stimulate vascular response ▪ Revascularization with pedicle grafts ▪ Adolescents should undergo temporary STT pinning
IIIA	Lunate collapse, no scaphoid rotation or carpus	Same as stage II
IIIB	Lunate collapse, fixed scaphoid rotation (ring sign), capitates migrates proximally; load shifted over lunate further progressing collapse	Address carpal instability with proximal row carpectomy or STT fusion; can consider radial shortening osteotomy
IV	Lunate collapse with degenerative changes of midcarpal or radiocarpal	Proximal row carpectomy or wrist fusion or total wrist arthroplasty

Abbreviation: STT, scaphotrapeziotrapezoid.

XI. Dupuytren's Contracture

1. Anatomy/pathoanatomy
   - Dupuytren's contracture manifests as the result of pathological transformation of normal palmar fascial structures, leading to formation of cords (highly organized collagen structures) and nodules (dense collections of myofibroblasts).
   - Normal anatomic structures are generally referred to as bands, whereas pathological structures are referred to as cords.
   - Normal structures: pretendinous bands, spiral band, natatory ligament, lateral digital sheet, retrovascular band, Grayson's ligament
     a. Grayson's and Cleland's ligaments run volar and dorsal, respectively, to neurovascular bundle in digit.
     b. Grayson's is volar, toward the ground.
     c. Grayson's ligament can become part of spiral cord, whereas Cleland's ligament is generally not involved in Dupuytren's contracture, although it can be.
     d. Spiral bands pass deep into the palm around the metacarpal head and deep (dorsal) to the neurovascular bundle and merge with the lateral digital sheet.
   - Pathological cords: spiral cord, central cord, lateral cord, retrovascular cord, intercommissural cord of first web space, abductor digiti minimi cord, natatory cord
     a. Spiral cord has contributions from pretendinous band, spiral band, lateral digital sheet, and Grayson's ligament.
     b. Spiral cord displaces neurovascular bundle volarly (superficial) and midline as cord thickens and straightens
2. Pathophysiology
   - **Myofibroblasts are fibroblasts with contractile actin microfilaments that are the pathological cellular entity in Dupuytren's contracture.**
   - Phases
     a. Proliferative: high concentration of disorganized fibroblasts and myofibroblasts
     b. Involutional: fibroblasts align themselves longitudinally
     c. Residual: relatively acellular with high collagen content
   - Higher levels of type III collagen found in Dupuytren's fascia
   - Associated with basic fibroblast growth factor, platelet-derived growth factor, transforming growth factor-β, which may play roles in mediating pathological cellular proliferation
3. Epidemiology
   - More prevalent in people of Northern European ancestry
   - Associated with diabetes, smoking, alcoholism, HIV, epilepsy (although this may represent relationship with antiseizure medication)
   - Dupuytren's diathesis: a form of the disease that is more aggressive in nature and associated with a higher rate of recurrence; associated with younger age at onset, strong family history, bilateral disease, and ectopic disease
     a. Ectopic sites include dorsal knuckle pads (Garrod's nodes), penile fibromatosis (Peyronie's disease), and plantar fibromatosis (Ledderhose disease)
4. Treatment
   - Nonoperative
     a. Collagenase: injectable *Clostridium histolyticum*–derived collagenase used to produce lysis and rupture of cords; Food and Drug Administration (FDA) approved in 2010

- Operative
  a. Indications: MCP contracture > 30 degrees, PIP flexion contractures
  b. Percutaneous needle aponeurotomy: small-gauge needle used to rupture cords; higher risk of recurrence than with open surgery
  c. Limited fasciectomy: removal of macroscopically pathological fascial tissue via multiple 1- to 1.5-cm transverse incisions
  d. Total palmar fasciectomy: removal of all palmar fascia, including normal-appearing tissue; high complication rate
  e. Dermofasciectomy: removal of fascia as well as overlying skin
     - Some studies have demonstrated no advantage in recurrence rate or motion with dermofasciectomy compared with standard fasciectomy, but this technique may be considered for recurrent or diathesis cases.
  f. Skin incisions and deficits may be managed in several different ways, including V-Y advancement, skin grafting, secondary intention, and Z-plasty.
     - Open-palm McCash technique may control edema, reduce hematoma formation, and allow early motion.
  g. Arthrodesis or amputation may be required in advanced cases.

5. Complications
   - Recurrence is most common complication
   - Hematoma
   - Neurovascular injury, hematoma, complex regional pain syndrome (CRPS), infection

XII. Infection

1. Felon
   - Infection of volar pulp of fingertip; pulp is composed of multiple small compartments of subcutaneous fat separated by septa; abscess forms, increasing the intracompartmental pressure and swelling of digit, causing pain
   - Most common organism: *Staphylococcus aureus*
   - Etiology: penetrating energy (finger-stick glucose) or spread from paronychia
   - Treatment: incision and drainage (I&D) with midlateral incision; break up septa to decompress fingertip of infection; leave incision open
2. Paronychia
   - Infection of the nail fold
   - Acute
     a. Etiology: nail biting, thumb sucking, or other minor trauma
     b. Most common hand infection
     c. Most common organism: *S. aureus*
     d. Early paronychia present with pain, swelling and erythema around nail folds; no fluctuance present; treat with warm soaks, antibiotics, and avoid offending behavior (nail biting)
     e. Paronychia progressing with fluctuance should undergo treatment with I&D, partial/total nail removal, and antibiotics.
   - Chronic
     a. Occurs in individuals with prolonged exposure to water (dishwasher, florists, etc.)
     b. Symptoms: recurrent bouts of inflammation of the nail fold; as a result, nail fold becomes blunted and retracted; nail may hypertrophy
     c. Common organism found: *Candida albicans*
     d. Treatment

- Nonoperative: warm soaks, topical antifungals, and avoidance of offending agents
- Operative: marsupialization

3. Bite
   - Human: "fight bite" involving MCP joint
     a. Common organisms: *Streptococcus, Staphylococcus, Eikenella corrodens*
     b. Treatment: I&D and intravenous (IV) antibiotics
   - Animal
     a. Most common organisms: *Pasteurella*, from dog *(Pasteurella canis)* and cat *(Pasteurella multocida)* bites
4. Flexor tenosynovitis
   - Most common organism: *S. aureus*
   - **Kanavel signs: (1) resting flexed posture, (2) pain with passive extension, (3) fusiform swelling, and (4) tenderness volarly over tendon sheath**
   - Horseshoe abscess: thumb and small finger sheaths communicate at the wrist; infection of one finger can lead to infection of the other
   - Treatment: If recognized early, treat with IV antibiotics. Failure to improve after 24 hours necessitates operative intervention. In general, the treatment is I&D of the flexor tendon sheath.
5. Deep space infection
   - Deep palmar spaces: thenar, hypothenar, midpalmar
   - Collar-button abscess: webspace between digits
   - Treatment: I&D, IV antibiotics
6. Septic arthritis
   - Commonly penetrating injuries or "fight bite"
   - Most common organism: *S. aureus*
   - In sexually active, consider gonococcal infection
   - Treatment: I&D, IV antibiotics
7. Herpetic whitlow
   - Most common in dental workers, respiratory therapists, and children
   - Symptoms/physical exam: fingertip pain, swelling, erythema, burning pain, and clear vesicles; vesicles will coalesce over a 2-week period and form bullae (virus-shedding active).
   - Treatment: oral acyclovir lessens symptoms; I&D contraindicated because of increasing risk of bacterial superinfection
8. Fungal
   - Onychomycosis: common organisms *Trichophyton rubrum* and *Candida*. Treatment with oral antifungal and nail removal has greater success.
   - Sporothrix schenckii: spores implanted from penetrating injury while gardening, classically rose bush thorns. Presentation: subcutaneous infection with ulceration and proximal lymph node swelling. Treatment: oral itraconazole preferred over potassium iodide due to a lower side-effects profile.
   - Histoplasmosis: endemic to Ohio–Mississippi River Valley. Presentation: tenosynovitis, pulmonary complaints, chest X-ray findings. Diagnosed by urinary antigen. Treatment: tenosynovectomy and IV amphotericin B
   - Coccidiomycosis: endemic to southwestern US. Presentation: synovitis, arthritis, osteomyelitis, and pulmonary complaints. Treatment: surgical debridement and IV amphotericin B
9. Gas gangrene
   - Common organism: *Clostridium* species
   - Occurs in grossly contaminated wounds
   - Treatment: extensive irrigation and debridement

10. High-pressure injection injury

- **High-pressure injection injuries entail an extensive amount of tissue damage/necrosis and require emergent and aggressive debridement, with amputation rates as high as 50–80%.**

- High rate of amputation of digit
- Treatment: immediate operative irrigation and debridement

11. Miscellaneous
   - Mycobacterial
      a. Symptoms of chronic papules or ulcers that may progress to tenosynovitis, arthritis, or osteomyelitis
      b. *Mycobacterium tuberculosis:* caseating granuloma; cultured on Lowenstein-Jensen medium
      c. *Mycobacterium marinum:* common in marine environments. Treatment: irrigation and debridement; ethambutol, rifampin, or clarithromycin
   - Anthrax
      a. Gram-negative anaerobe *Bacillus anthracis*
      b. Cutaneous manifestations are small painless macule that ulcerates and progresses to black eschar; may progress with lymphadenopathy and fevers
      c. Treatment: IV penicillin, doxycycline, quinolones; then transition to oral antibiotics
   - Diabetes: increased amputation rate associated with renal failure and deep polymicrobial or gram-negative infection; antibiotics

12. Differential
   - Brown recluse spider bite, pyogenic granuloma, pyogenic gangrenosum, acute gout, rheumatoid arthritis

XIII. Microvascular

1. Amputation
   - Indications for replantation
      a. Thumb
      b. Multiple digits
      c. Amputation in child
      d. Amputation at hand/wrist or proximal
      e. Single digit in zone I
   - Contraindications
      a. Zone II amputation (proximal to FDS insertion)
      b. Crushed or mangled amputation with multisystem injury
      c. Prolonged ischemia
         - Cold ischemia > 12 hours if amputation proximal to carpus or > 24 hours for amputated digit
         - Warm ischemia > 6 hours if amputation proximal to carpus or > 12 hours for amputated digit
      d. Segmental amputation
   - Operative technique
      a. Amputated tissue should be stored in moist gauze in plastic bag and then placed in ice-water bath.
      b. Sequence: bone stabilization (usually with shortening to allow resection of damaged vessels and subsequent end-to-end repair) → extensor tendon repair → flexor tendon repair → arterial repair → nerve repair → venous repair → loose closure

- **Replant structure by structure is faster than digit by digit in multiple digit replantation.**

- Postoperative care
  a. Warm environment
  b. Hydration with monitoring of blood pressure and urine output
  c. Vasoconstrictive agents such as caffeine and nicotine prohibited
  d. Monitoring of digital temperature, capillary refill, and finger pulp turgor; decrease in temperature > 2°C in 1 hour or temperature of < 30°C suggests diminished perfusion of digit
- Outcome
  a. Complications
    - Most common cause of early failure (< 12 hours) is arterial insufficiency from thrombosis due to persistent vasospasm; manifested by decrease in temperature, loss of capillary refill, loss of Doppler signal, pale color
      - Manage with heparin infusion, release of potentially tight bandage, dependent positioning, ganglion blockade, or early exploration
    - Late failure more commonly due to venous congestion marked by dark red skin color, slowed capillary refill, engorgement of tissue
      - Treat with release of dressing, elevation, application of heparin-soaked sponge to nail bed, leeches, or, if unsuccessful, exploration and revision
      - Leeches: *Hirudo medicinalis* produce anticoagulant hirudin
        - Must watch for potential *Aeromonas hydrophila* infection associated with leeches; can treat with prophylactic antibiotics
  b. Most important factor influencing outcome is mechanism of injury (crush mechanism has worst outcome); male gender and cigarette smoking also negative risk factors

    - **Most important factor influencing outcome is mechanism of injury (crush mechanism has worst outcome)**

  c. Tenolysis is most common secondary procedure
  d. Most common complication is infection; cold intolerance can also occur
- Pharmacology
  a. Baby aspirin (81 mg/d) and dextran 40 (20 mL/h) may be used for anticoagulation.
  b. IV heparin (1,000 U/h) may be used for crush injuries.
  c. Allopurinol: xanthine oxidase inhibitor: inhibition of conversion of hypoxanthine to xanthine may reduce reperfusion injury.

2. Soft tissue coverage
- Graft: tissue transferred from donor to recipient site without its own vascular supply
  a. Split-thickness skin graft (STSG): preferred for dorsal hand wounds
  b. Full-thickness skin graft (FTSG): preferred for volar hand and fingertip wounds; more durable, better sensibility, and contracts less than STSG
- Flap: tissue transferred from donor site to recipient site with its own vascular supply; can be classified by donor site, tissue type, vascular supply, and method of transfer
  a. Donor site: local versus distant
  b. Tissue type
    - Single tissue: fascia, muscle, or bone
    - Composite: e.g., cutaneous, fasciocutaneous, musculocutaneous, osteocutaneous
  c. Vascular supply

- Random pattern: no named arteriovenous pedicle; depends on microcirculation, so length/width ratio should not exceed 2:1; e.g., cross-finger and thenar flaps
- Axial pattern: named arteriovenous pedicle, thus more predictable blood supply; e.g., radial forearm flap

d. Method of transfer
- Advancement: along a linear axis
- Rotation: pivoted around a fixed point
- Transposition: flap rotated over incomplete skin bridge into recipient site.
- **Z-plasty with 30-, 45-, and 60-degree limbs allow 25%, 50%, and 75% lengthening, respectively.**
- Interpolated: cross over or under intact skin; may require second-stage division of flap if over intact skin; e.g., cross-finger flap
- Free flap: flap with known arteriovenous supply is removed from donor site (including division of blood supply) and revascularized at recipient site by microsurgical reanastomosis

- Reconstructive ladder: hierarchy of wound management used to describe coverage procedures of increasing complexity
- **Reconstructive ladder:**

a. Healing by secondary intention
b. Primary closure
c. Delayed primary closure
d. Split-thickness skin graft
e. Full-thickness skin graft
f. Random-pattern local flap
g. Axial-pattern local flap
h. Random-pattern distant flap
i. Axial-pattern distant flap
j. Free flap

- Common sites/coverage

a. Volar digit: cross-finger flap for more proximal defect than tip
b. Finger tip
- Young children with fingertip amputation can be treated with dressing changes even if bone exposed; also may attempt composite flap in young children (reattachment of amputated tissue without vascular repair)
- V-Y advancement can be used for finger tip injuries with more dorsal than volar soft tissue loss.
- Thenar flap may be used for tip injuries of index or middle fingers; stiffness is a potential complication.
- Cross-finger flap for volar oblique injuries with dorsal skin of adjacent digit used to cover wound and STSG used to cover donor site

c. Thumb tip
- Moberg flap: volar advancement flap that may be used for small (< 2 cm) volar thumb defect; IP or MCP contracture is common complication

d. Dorsal thumb
- Kite flap: first dorsal metacarpal artery–based flap

e. Dorsal hand
- Radial forearm flap: supplied by radial artery and can include part of radial diaphysis, forearm fascia, brachioradialis, and palmaris longus

- Lateral arm flap: supplied by posterior radial collateral artery
- Groin flap: supplied by superficial circumflex iliac artery

f. Thumb index web
- Z-plasty

- Flap coverage of lower extremity wounds

a. Proximal third tibia
- Medial: medial gastrocnemius rotational flap; supplied by medial branch of sural artery
- Lateral: lateral gastrocnemius rotational flap; supplied by lateral branch of sural artery
- Middle third tibia: soleus flap; supplied by perforating branches of posterior tibial and peroneal arteries
- Distal third tibia: fasciocutaneous perforator flaps or free flaps (gracilis, latissimus dorsi, or rectus abdominis)

- Bone flaps
- Tissue expansion

XIV. Hand Tumors (see Chapter 2)

XV. Congenital

1. Embryology
   - Limb bud appears at 4th week of gestation and develops into a paddle (34–38 days), which is followed by separation of the digits (onset 38–40 days).
   - The limb bud induces formation of the apical ectodermal ridge (AER), which is a major signaling center for proper development.
   - The zone of polarizing activity (ZPA) is another major signaling center essential for maintaining development along the anterior-posterior (radial-ulnar) axis.
   - Dorsoventral axis (extensor-flexor) mediated by Wnt7a protein
2. Types
   - Failure formation

a. Congenital amputation: thought to be due to vascular insult to AER and usually occurs at level of proximal forearm
- Treat with early prosthetic fitting.

b. Radial longitudinal deficiency (RLD): longitudinal failure of formation of radial forearm, wrist, and hand structures
- Bayne and Klug classification **(Table 9.13)**; type IV aplastic radius most common
- Often associated with other congenital malformations
  - ♦ Thrombocytopenia and absent radius (TAR): anemia and thrombocytopenia at birth that improves in first year of life; autosomal recessive; thumb is present
  - ♦ **Thumb is present in TAR**
  - ♦ Fanconi's anemia: pancytopenia; autosomal recessive
  - ♦ Holt-Oram syndrome: atrial septal defects and arrhythmias; autosomal dominant
  - ♦ VATER (*v*ertebral anomalies, *a*nal atresia, *t*racheoesophageal fistula, *e*sophageal atresia, and *r*enal agenesis) syndrome: sporadic

Table 9.13 Bayne and Klug Classification of Radial Longitudinal Deficiency

Type	Deficiency
I	Short radius due to delayed appearance of distal radial epiphysis
II	Deficient growth of proximal and distal radial epiphysis
III	Partial radial aplasia; most commonly proximal radius still present
IV	Absent radius

- Workup should include echocardiogram, complete blood count (CBC), and renal ultrasound
- **Syndromes associated with radial longitudinal deficiency include TAR, Fanconi's anemia, Holt-Oran syndrome, and VATER. Workup should include echocardiogram, CBC, and renal ultrasound.**
- Treatment
  - Early stretching and casting to stretch tight radial structures and maintain passive motion
  - Surgical options include centralization [align ulna to third metacarpal (MC)] and radialization (align ulna to second MC)
  - Avoid surgery in setting of significant elbow stiffness.

c. Ulnar longitudinal deficiency (ULD): longitudinal failure of formation of ulnar forearm, wrist, and hand structures
- Less common than RLD and less frequently associated with syndromes
- Usually sporadic in nature but occasionally autosomal dominant inheritance patterns
- Wrist is usually stable but elbow dysfunction more common (elbow instability, radial head dislocation, radiohumeral synostosis)
- Surgical options include excision of ulnar anlage, corrective osteotomy of radius or humerus, or single bone forearm

d. Cleft hand
- Usually bilateral, involves feet, familial and involves missing metacarpals (as opposed to symbrachydactyly)
- Treatment goals include cleft closure and thumb web reconstruction.

• Failure differentiation

a. Radioulnar synostosis: can treat with observation unless bilateral involvement for which osteotomy with fusion in pronation for one arm and supination for other arm may be done

b. Symphalangism: congenital digital stiffness, which can range from fibrous symphalangism to bony fusion
- Hereditary form is autosomal dominant and associated with correctable hearing loss
- Nonhereditary form seen with syndactyly, Apert syndrome, and Poland syndrome
- Treatment: usually observation, but can perform angular osteotomy at end of adolescent growth for cosmesis or function

c. Camptodactyly: congenital digital flexion deformity usually occurs in PIP of fifth digit
- Type I: seen in infancy and treated with stretching and splinting
- Type II: due to abnormal lumbrical insertion or abnormal FDS origin/insertion; may be treated surgically with exploration and transfer of abnormal tendon; more commonly seen in adolescent girls
- Type III: severe flexion contractures with multiple digit involvement usually associated with a syndrome
- Treatment: generally nonoperative management, but if functional deficit remains, realignment through osteotomy may be performed at skeletal maturity

d. Clinodactyly: congenital curvature of digit in radioulnar plane; most commonly seen in small finger
- When seen in association with Down syndrome, often entails short second phalanx
- Treatment: generally conservative but if there is significant angulation with delta phalanx, treat with early excision if delta phalanx is separate bone and digit is too long; otherwise, osteotomy to correct deformity

e. Flexed thumb: may be due to either pediatric trigger thumb or congenital clasped thumb

f. Pediatric trigger thumb: mechanical triggering of thumb may lead to interphalangeal flexion contracture if untreated

  - Treatment: may respond to splinting or may be treated with surgical release of A1 pulley; radial digital nerve of thumb at risk during surgical release of A1 pulley
  - **Radial digital nerve of thumb at risk during surgical release of A1 pulley**
  - Congenital clasped thumb: flexion/adduction deformity of thumb MCP joint due to hypoplastic or absent extensor pollicis brevis; rigid deformities may involve hypoplastic extensors, thenar muscle hypoplasia, first web skin deficiency, and UCL deficiency
    - Treatment: supple deformities treated with splinting or long/ring FDS transfer to EPB; rigid deformities may require MCP, FPB, AddP release, transfer of extensor or opponens tendons, and/or first web space deepening

g. Arthrogryposis: manifests in hand with weakness, flexed/ulnar deviated wrist, (MCP)/IP stiffness and adducted thumb

  - Treatment: can perform tendon transfers if passive motion can be achieved, but fusion may be more functional in some cases

h. Syndactyly: congenital webbing or fusion of digits due to failure of apoptosis between digits

  - Classified as incomplete versus complete (involvement of entire length of nail)
  - Classified as simple or complex based on absence or presence of bony connection, respectively
  - Most commonly involves long and ring fingers
  - Severe syndactyly seen in Apert syndrome due to defect in fibroblast growth factor receptor 2 *(FGFR2)* gene
    - Also associated with Poland's syndrome, Holt-Oram syndrome, and Carpenter syndrome
  - Treatment: usually perform surgical release at 9–12 months, earlier if tethering of digits; in case of multiple syndactyly, only one digit should be released at a time to avoid vascular compromise
    - Most common complication after surgery is web creep

- Duplication

a. Preaxial polydactyly: thumb duplication **(Table 9.14)**

  - **Type VII associated with Holt-Oram syndrome, Fanconi anemia, Blackfan-Diamond anemia, hypoplastic anemia, imperforate anus, cleft palata, and tibial defects**
  - Type IV most common (43%)
  - Treatment: usually with ablation of lesser digit; if digits of equal size, then generally preserve ulnar thumb to preserve ulnar collateral ligament for pinch
    - Bilhaut-Cloquet procedure: removal of central portions of duplicated thumbs with repair of radial half of radial thumb to ulnar half of ulnar thumb; can be used for symmetric Wassel I, II, or III

b. Postaxial polydactyly: small finger duplication

  - Ten times more common in African Americans; autosomal dominant
  - If present in Caucasians, then may be associated with syndrome
  - Type A: well-formed extra digit; treated with ablation of ulnar digit
  - Type B: rudimentary skin tag, which may be tied off in nursery

Table 9.14 Wassel Preaxial Polydactyly Classification

Type	Description
I	Bifid distal phalanx
II	Duplicated distal phalanx
III	Bifid proximal phalanx
IV	Duplicated proximal phalanx (most common)
V	Bifid metacarpal
VI	Duplicated metacarpal
VII	Triphalangism

c. Central polydactyly: extra ring, middle, or index finger
   - Less common than other forms of polydactyly and commonly associated with syndactyly
   - Treatment: early surgery with osteotomy and ligament reconstructions to prevent angular growth deformities

- Overgrowth

  a. Macrodactyly: nonhereditary digital enlargement
   - 90% unilateral and 70% involve multiple digits
   - Classification
     - ♦ Static: present at birth with linear growth with age
     - ♦ Progressive: not apparent at birth but disproportionate growth with age
   - Treatment: epiphysiodesis when digit reaches size of same-sex parent
     - ♦ Also angular or shortening osteotomy, debulking, nerve stripping, narrowing osteotomy

- Undergrowth

  a. Thumb hypoplasia
   - Blauth classification **(Table 9.15)**
   - Thumb function dependent largely on CMC stability
   - Treatment
     - ♦ Type I: no treatment
     - ♦ Type II-IIIA (stable CMC): stabilization of MCP ULC, web deepening, and extrinsic extensor reconstruction
     - ♦ Type IIIB-V (unstable CMC): index pollicization
     - ♦ **Decision to perform pollicization for thumb hypoplasia largely dependent on CMC stability (difference between Blauth types IIIA and IIIB)**

- Constriction ring syndrome: malformation due to intrauterine rings or bands that constrict fetal tissue

  a. Four categories
   - Simple constriction rings
   - Deformity of distal part with or without lymphedema
   - Acrosyndactyly
   - Amputation

  b. Treatment: with lymphatic or vascular compromise, treat with band excision

Table 9.15 Blauth Thumb Hypoplasia Classification

Type	Description
I	Minor shortening and narrowing
II	Thenar hypoplasia, MCP instability, adduction contracture
IIIA	Type II plus hypoplastic metacarpal, extrinsic tendon abnormalities, and stable CMC joint
IIIB	Type II plus partial metacarpal aplasia, extrinsic tendon abnormalities, and unstable CMC joint
IV	Pouce flottant (floating thumb): absent thenar muscles and functioning tendons with connection to hand by skin bridge
V	Absent thumb

Abbreviations: CMC, carpometacarpal; MCP, metacarpophalangeal.

- Generalized
  a. Congenital dislocation radial head
     - Dome-shaped radial head often associated with other congenital anomalies, hypoplastic capitellum, and bilateral involvement
     - Most common presenting complaint is cosmetic deformity of painless mass over posterior elbow; forearm rotation and flexion/extension affected
     - Treatment: observation unless significant pain and motion restriction; can perform radial head excision at skeletal maturity
     - **Poland's syndrome: symbrachydactyly of fingers, hypoplasia of hand and forearm, and chest wall hypoplasia affecting one side of the body**
     - Extent of hand and chest involvement varies
     - Symbrachydactyly: due to absence or shortening of middle phalanx
     - Chest wall hypoplasia: due to absence of the sternocostal head of pectoralis major
     - Other associated conditions: scoliosis, Sprengel's deformity, dextrocardia, asymmetric breasts, radioulnar synostosis, absent flexor/extensor tendons, absent nails
     - Unilateral, right > left side
  b. Apert syndrome: complex syndactyl of bilateral hands/feet, craniosynostosis and dysmorphic facial features (high prominent forehead with flat posterior skull and broad-spaced eyes)
     - Autosomal dominant, mutation in *FGFR2* gene
     - First brachial arch syndrome
     - Syndrome includes bilateral complex syndactyl of hands and feet, symphalangism (ankylosis of IP joints), craniosynostosis, hypertelorism, glenoid hypoplasia, radial synostosis, and cognitive dysfunction
  c. Madelung's deformity
     - **Wrist deformity caused by growth disturbance of volar/ulnar distal radius physis; often caused by Vickers' ligament (abnormal ligament between lunate and radius)**
     - Bilateral Madelung's deformity associated with Leri-Weill dyschondrosteosis, which is caused by mutation or deletion of the *SHOX* gene on X or Y chromosome
     - Often asymptomatic but may manifest symptoms of decreased forearm rotation, median nerve compression, or ulnocarpal impaction
     - Treatment: may perform early release of Vickers' ligament or osteotomy of radius with or without distal ulna resection

10

Foot and Ankle

Craig R. Lareau, Jason T. Bariteau, and Christopher W. DiGiovanni

I. Foot and Ankle Anatomy

1. Bones
   - Twenty-six non-sesamoid bones of the foot: seven tarsals, five metatarsals, and 14 phalanges **(Figs. 10.1, 10.2, 10.3, 10.4)**
   - Divided into hindfoot (calcaneus and talus), midfoot (navicular, three cuneiforms, and cuboid) and forefoot (metatarsals and phalanges) **(Fig. 10.5)**
     a. Tarsal bones include all bones in the hindfoot and midfoot
   - Calcaneus **(Figs. 10.6** and **10.7)**
     a. Sustentaculum tali (the "constant fragment") is the eminence on the anteromedial calcaneus that supports the medial talar body and forms part of the anterior and middle facets of the subtalar joint; also creates inferior groove for the flexor hallucis longus (FHL)
        - Constant fragment rarely moves with hindfoot pathology (e.g., calcaneal fracture) due to its strong ligamentous attachments to the talus
        - **Reconstruct fracture fragments to the constant fragment in calcaneus fractures.**
   - Talus **(Figs. 10.8** and **10.9)**
     a. Talar dome wider anteriorly; ankle more stable in dorsiflexion (DF)
     b. No muscular attachments or tendon insertions; two thirds covered with cartilage
     c. Primary blood supply to the talar body: artery of the tarsal canal (from the posterior tibial artery)
     d. Secondary blood supply to the talar body: deltoid branch of the posterior tibial artery
     e. The talar head and neck are supplied by the dorsalis pedis and peroneal arteries, which anastomose to form the artery of the tarsal sinus.
   - Navicular
     a. Medial plantar projection: attachment for the posterior tibial tendon
     b. Tenuous centripetal blood supply
   - Cuneiforms: medial, intermediate (middle), and lateral
   - Cuboid: grooved on its plantar surface by the peroneus longus
   - Metatarsals (MTs)
     a. First MT has plantar cristae for articulation with the sesamoids contained within the flexor hallucis brevis (FHB)
     b. Deep transverse intermetatarsal ligaments connect the MT heads
        - First interspace: ligament connects second MT head to fibular sesamoid
     c. Phalanges (great toe has two phalanges, remaining toes have three)
   - Accessory bones: os trigonum, os peroneum, accessory navicular, etc.
     a. Os trigonum syndrome commonly occurs in dancers with symptoms at the "en-pointe" position and is treated with arthroscopic or open excision if conservative management fails.

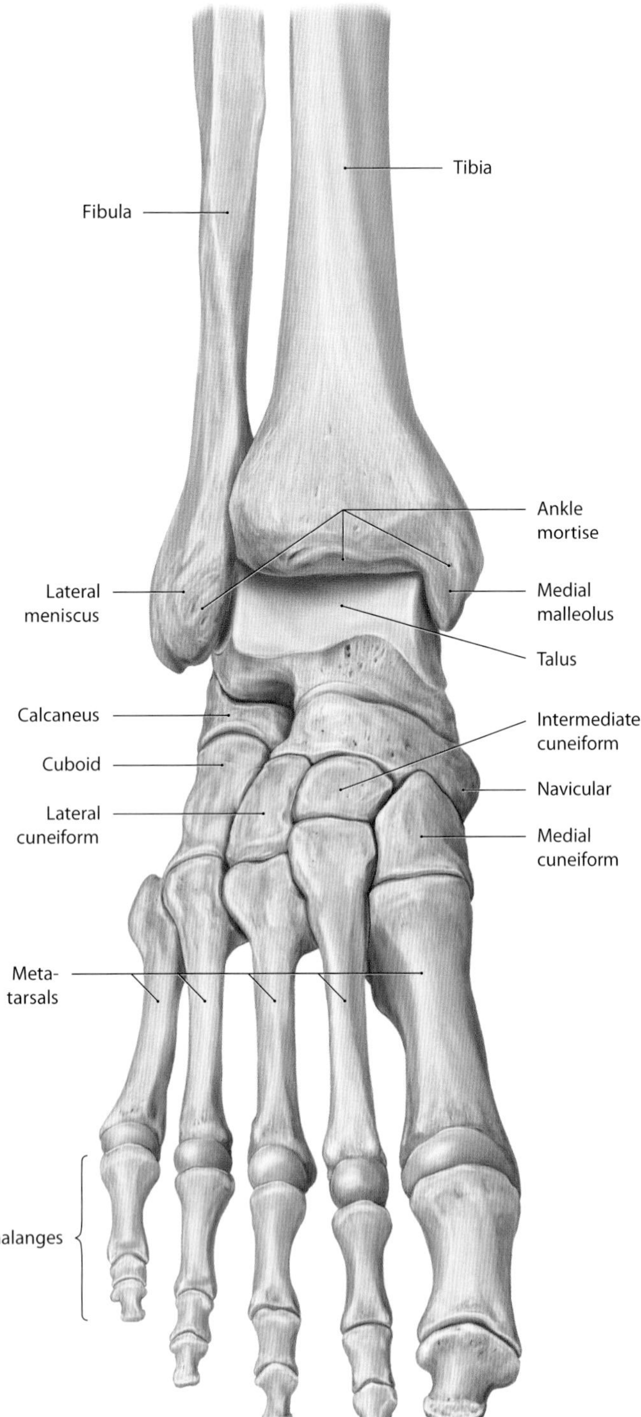

Fig. 10.1 The articulating bones in different joints of the right foot. Anterior view with the talocrural joint in plantar flexion. (From Schuenke M, Schulte E. General Anatomy and the Musculoskeletal System: Thieme Atlas of Anatomy. New York: Thieme; 2005. Illustration by Karl Wesker.)

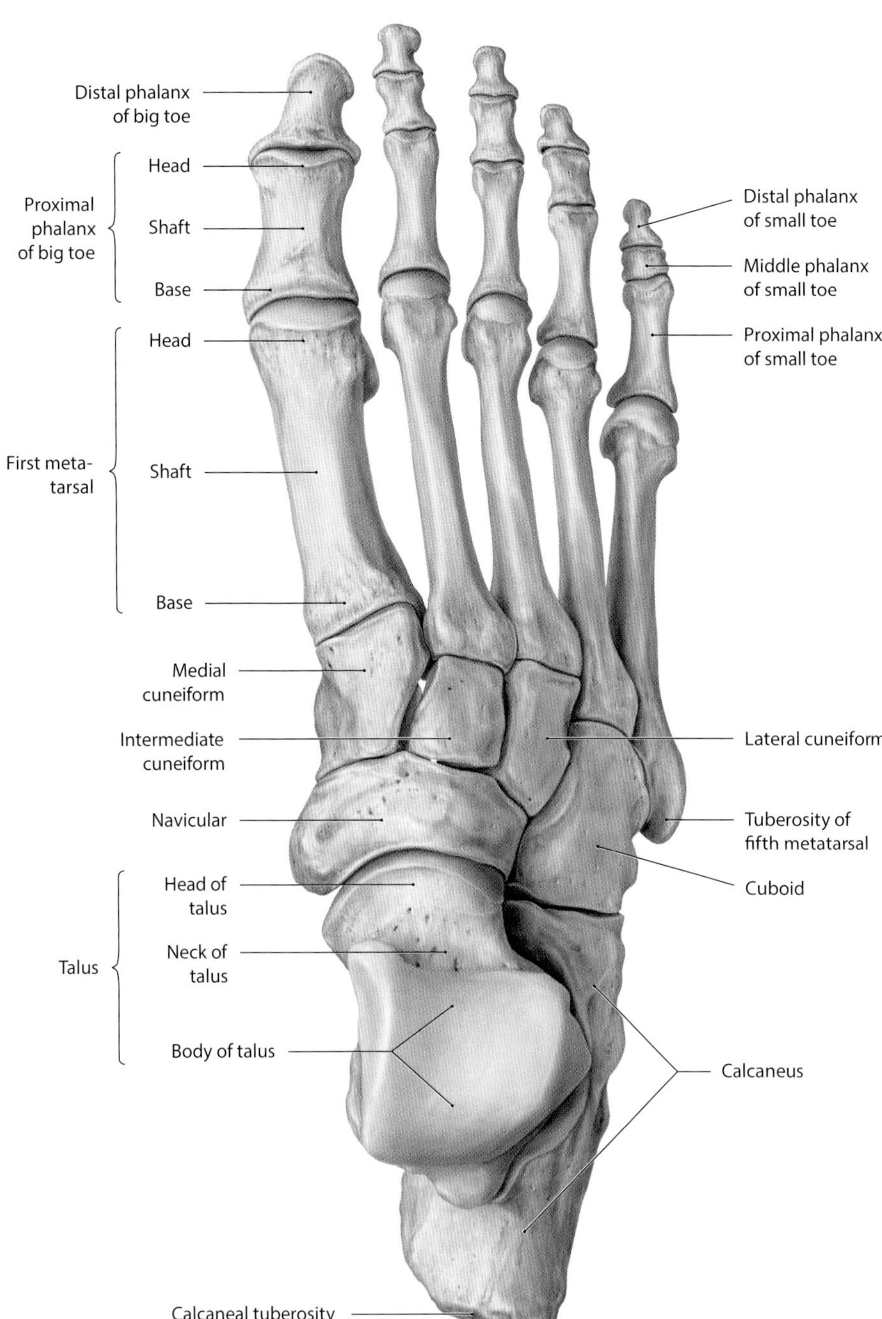

Fig. 10.2 The bones of the right foot. Dorsal view. (From Schuenke M, Schulte E. General Anatomy and the Musculoskeletal System: Thieme Atlas of Anatomy. New York: Thieme; 2005. Illustration by Karl Wesker.)

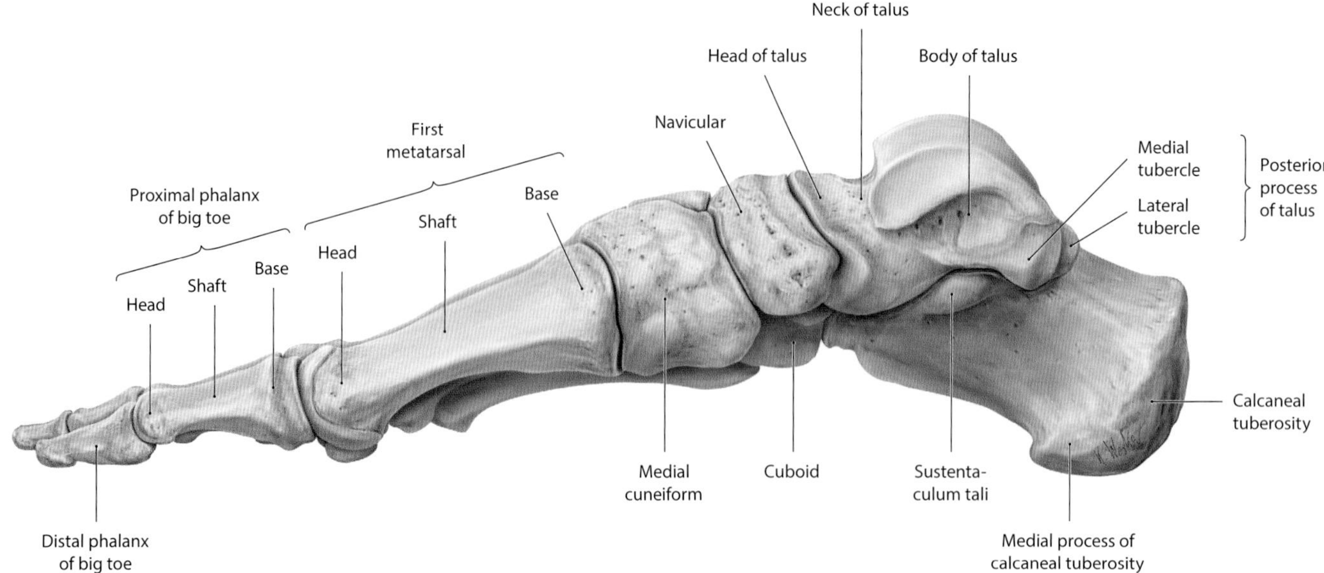

Fig. 10.3 The bones of the right foot. Medial view. (From Schuenke M, Schulte E. General Anatomy and the Musculoskeletal System: Thieme Atlas of Anatomy. New York: Thieme; 2005. Illustration by Karl Wesker.)

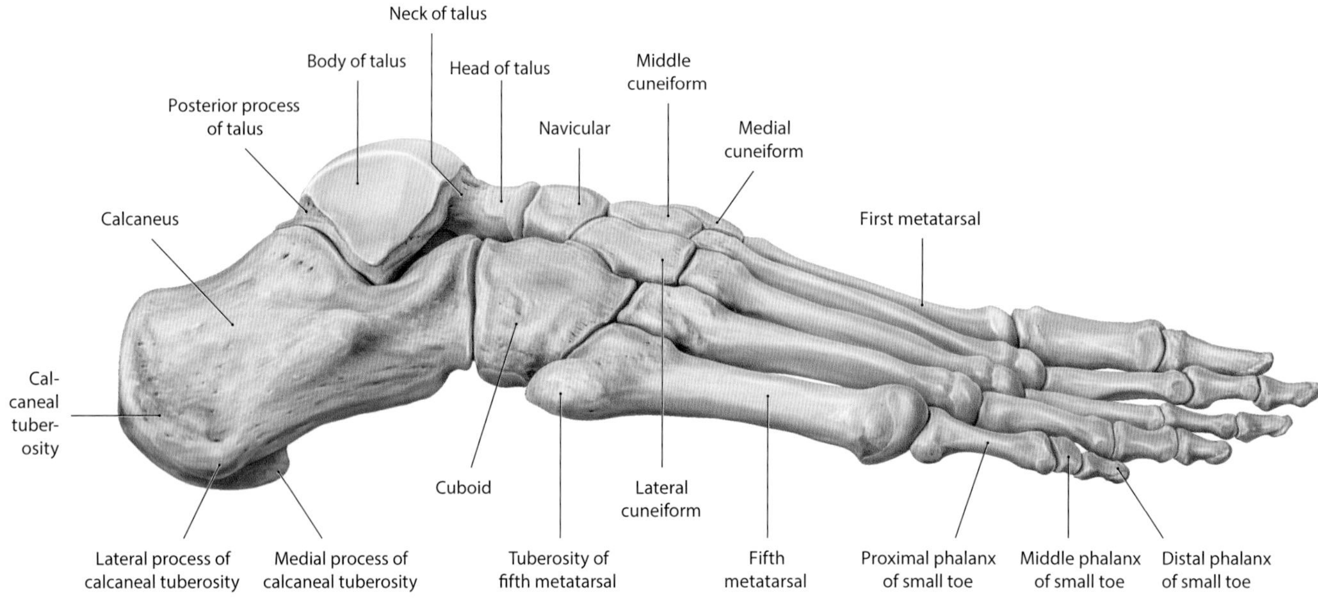

Fig. 10.4 The bones of the right foot. Lateral view. (From Schuenke M, Schulte E. General Anatomy and the Musculoskeletal System: Thieme Atlas of Anatomy. New York: Thieme; 2005. Illustration by Karl Wesker.)

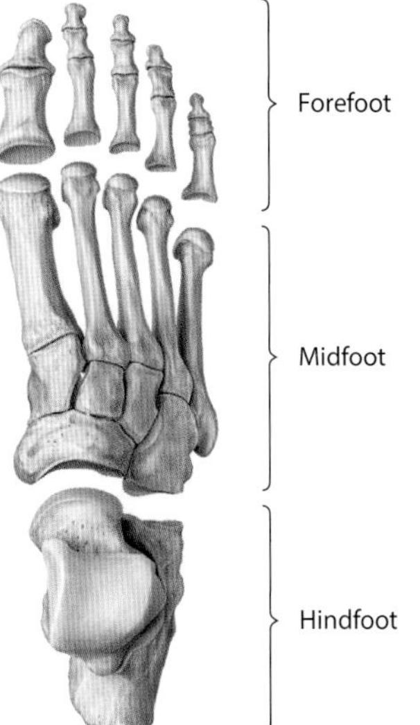

Fig. 10.5 Functional subdivision of the pedal skeleton. Right foot, dorsal view. The skeleton of the foot is often subdivided, based on functional and clinical criteria, as follows: hindfoot (calcaneus and talus); midfoot (cuboid, navicular, cuneiforms, and metatarsals); forefoot (the proximal, middle, and distal phalanges). (From Schuenke M, Schulte E. General Anatomy and the Musculoskeletal System: Thieme Atlas of Anatomy. New York: Thieme; 2005. Illustration by Karl Wesker.)

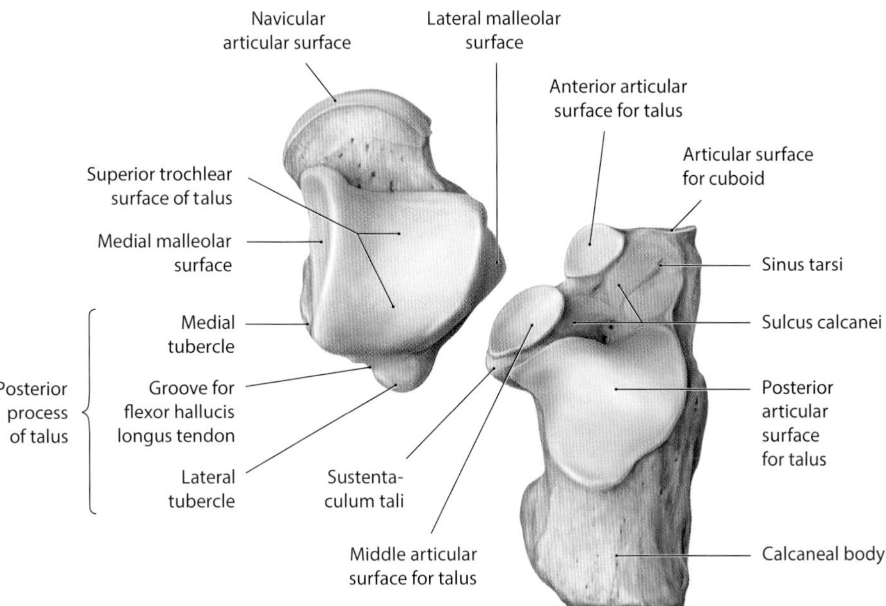

Fig. 10.6 The right talus and calcaneus. Dorsal view. The two tarsal bones have been separated at the subtalar joint to demonstrate their articular surfaces. (From Schuenke M, Schulte E. General Anatomy and the Musculoskeletal System: Thieme Atlas of Anatomy. New York: Thieme; 2005. Illustration by Karl Wesker.)

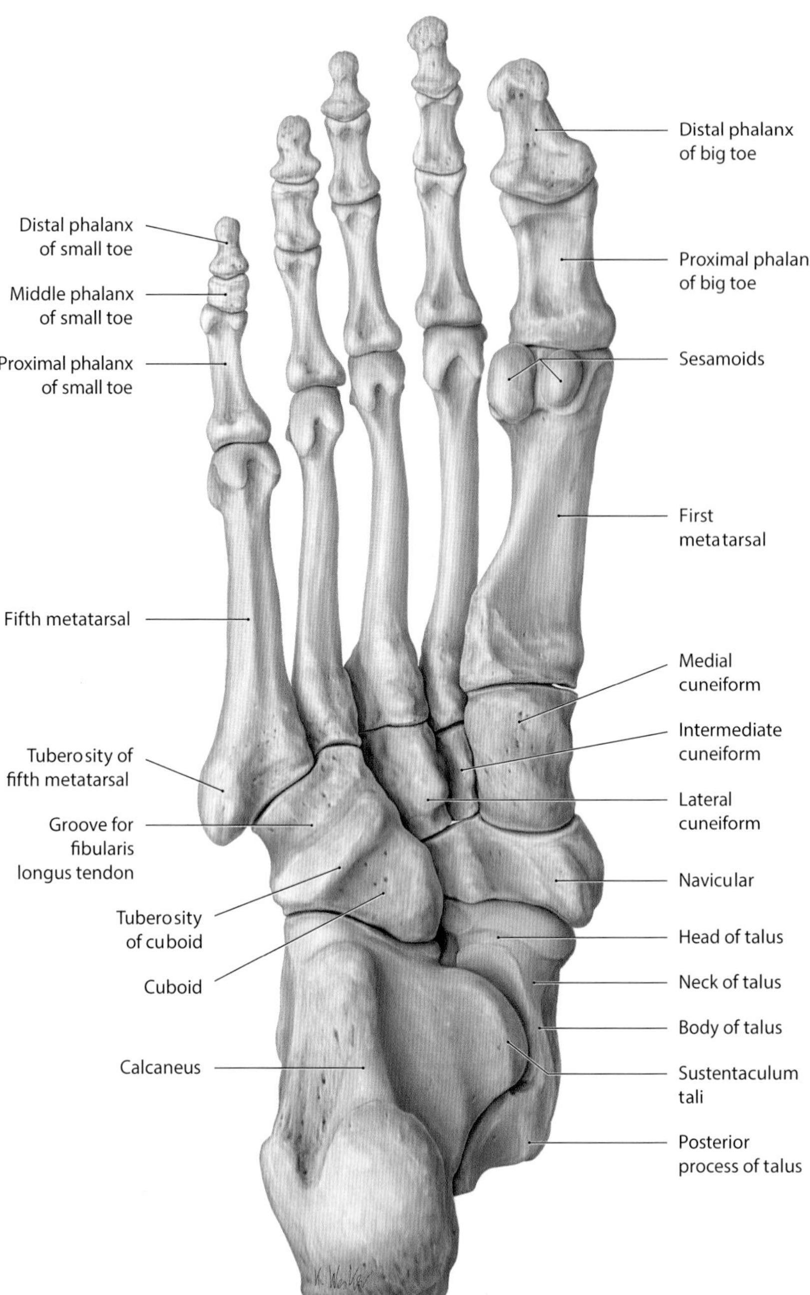

Fig. 10.7 The right talus and calcaneus. Plantar view. The two tarsal bones have been separated at the subtalar joint to demonstrate their articular surfaces. (From Schuenke M, Schulte E. General Anatomy and the Musculoskeletal System: Thieme Atlas of Anatomy. New York: Thieme; 2005. Illustration by Karl Wesker.)

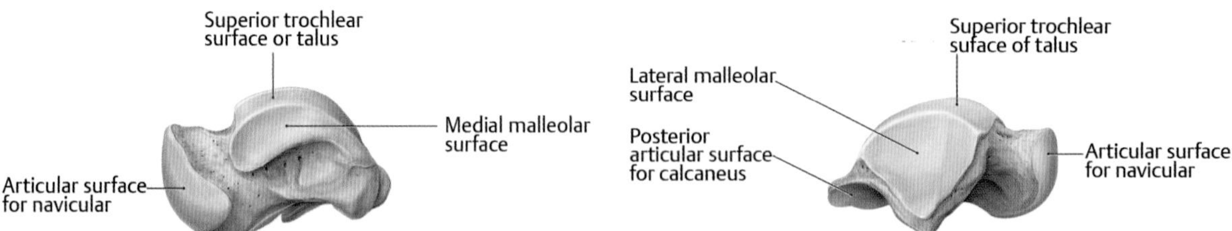

Fig. 10.8 The right talus and calcaneus. Medial view. The two tarsal bones have been separated at the subtaler joint to demonstrate their articular surfaces. (From Schuenke M, Schulte E. General Anatomy and the Musculoskeletal System: Thieme Atlas of Anatomy. New York: Thieme; 2005. Illustration by Karl Wesker.)

Fig. 10.9 The right talus and calcaneus. Lateral view. The two tarsal bones have been separated at the subtalar joint to demonstrate their articular surfaces. (From Schuenke M, Schulte E. General Anatomy and the Musculoskeletal System: Thieme Atlas of Anatomy. New York: Thieme; 2005. Illustration by Karl Wesker.)

2. Joints
   - Tibiotalar (ankle) joint
     a. The mortise, which articulates with the talus, is composed of the tibial plafond, medial malleolus, and lateral malleolus (**Figs. 10.10, 10.11, 10.12**).
     b. Deltoid ligament: main stabilizer of the ankle during stance
        - Superficial deltoid: tibionavicular, anterior tibiotalar, and tibiocalcaneal ligaments

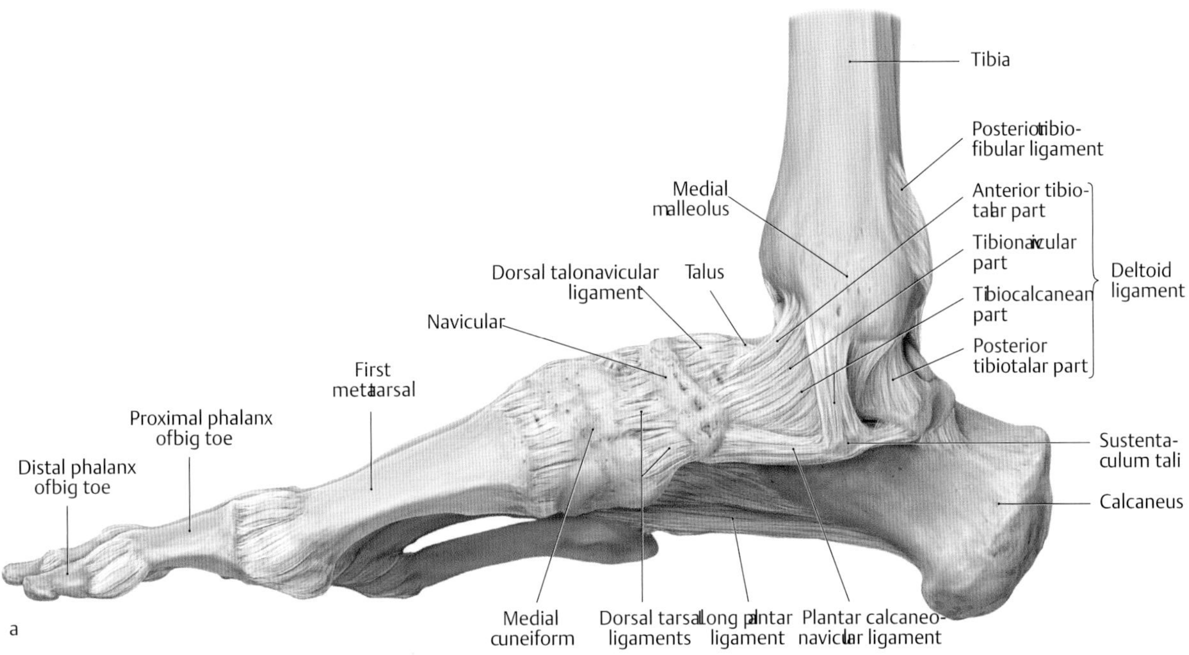

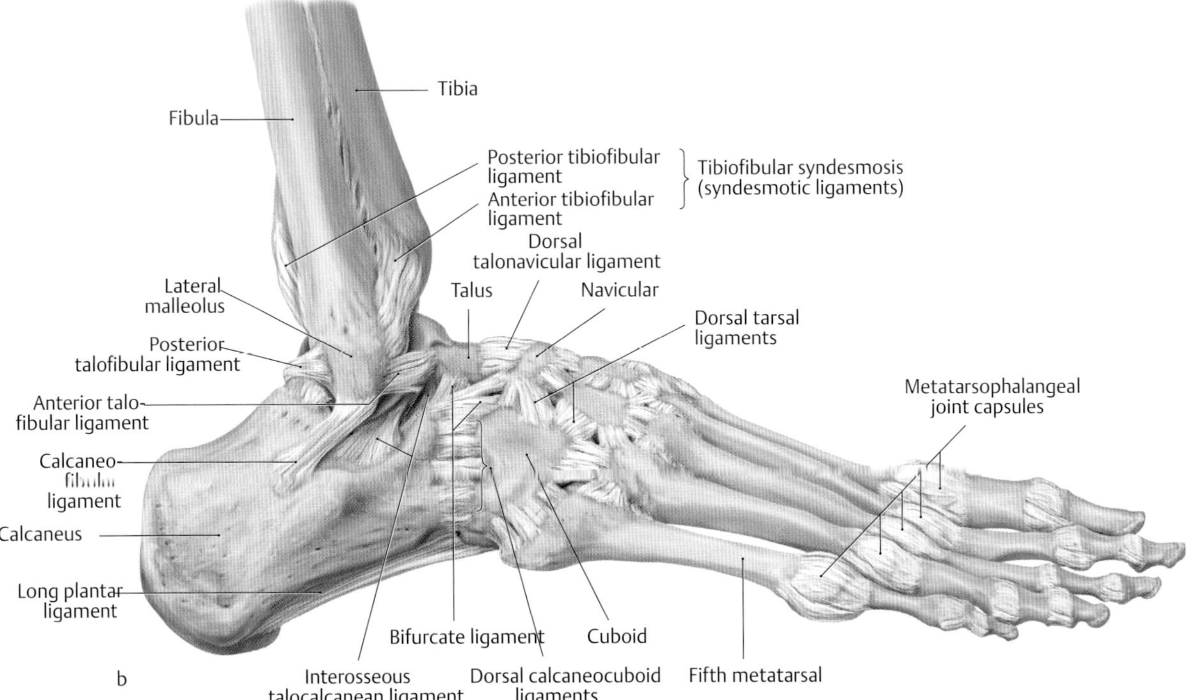

Fig. 10.10 **(a)** The ligaments of the right foot, medial view. **(b)** The ligaments of the right foot, lateral view. (From Schuenke M, Schulte E. General Anatomy and the Musculoskeletal System: Thieme Atlas of Anatomy. New York: Thieme; 2005. Illustration by Karl Wesker.)

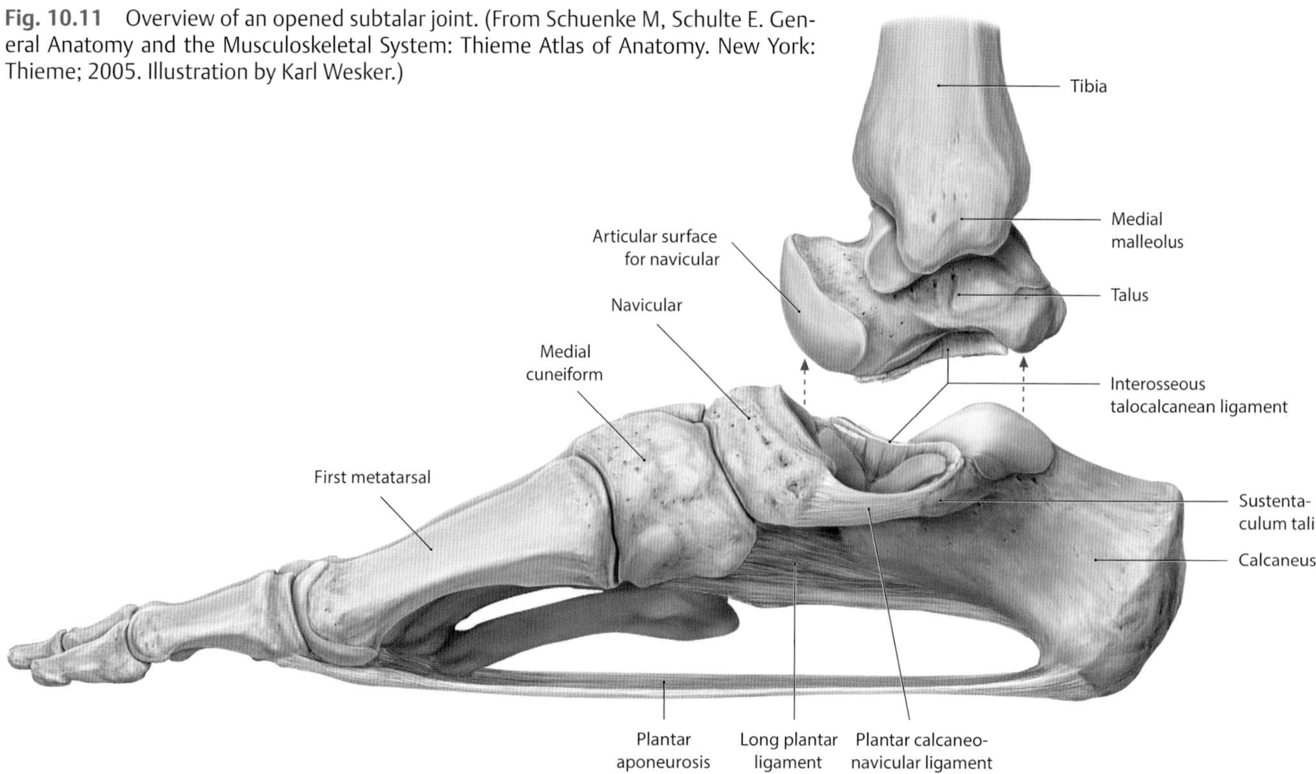

Fig. 10.11 Overview of an opened subtalar joint. (From Schuenke M, Schulte E. General Anatomy and the Musculoskeletal System: Thieme Atlas of Anatomy. New York: Thieme; 2005. Illustration by Karl Wesker.)

- Origin: anterior colliculus; resists valgus ankle force
- Crosses tibiotalar, subtalar, and talonavicular (TN) joints

- Deep deltoid = anterior and posterior tibiotalar ligaments
  - Origin = posterior colliculus
  - Resists lateral talar translation and external rotation

c. Lateral ankle ligaments resist varus forces
- Anterior talofibular ligament (ATFL): resists inversion with the ankle in plantarflexion (PF)
  - Intracapsular, weakest of three ligaments
- Calcaneofibular ligament (CFL): resists inversion with the ankle in neutral/DF
- Posterior talofibular ligament (PTFL): strongest of three ligaments, rarely torn

- Inferior tibiofibular joint (syndesmosis): resists lateral talar translation

a. Convex medial distal fibula articulates with concave incisura fibularis

b. Composed of four ligaments: anterior inferior tibiofibular ligament (AITFL), posterior inferior tibiofibular ligament (PITFL), transverse tibiofibular, and interosseous
- PITFL is strongest, and often injured last

- Hindfoot joints include the subtalar (ST) and transverse tarsal (Chopart) joints

a. The ST joint is stabilized by medial, lateral, interosseous talocalcaneal, and cervical ligaments.

b. Transverse tarsal (midtarsal or Chopart) joints: TN and calcaneocuboid (CC) joints

c. The spring (plantar calcaneonavicular) ligament, which originates at the sustentaculum tali, is critical in maintaining the arch.
- Rupture of this ligament can occur with or contribute to severe pes planovalgus deformity; seen on coronal magnetic resonance imaging (MRI)

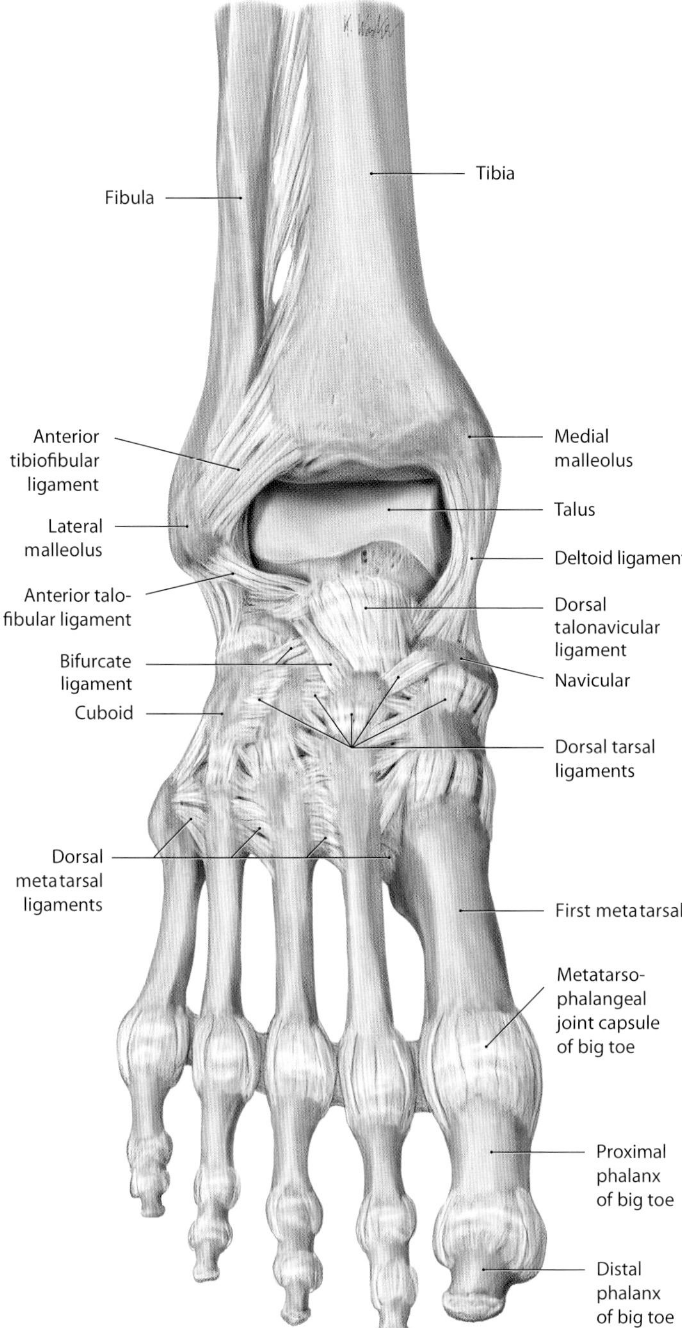

Fig. 10.12 The ligaments of the right foot. Anterior view (talocrural joint in plantar flexion). (From Schuenke M, Schulte E. General Anatomy and the Musculoskeletal System: Thieme Atlas of Anatomy. New York: Thieme; 2005. Illustration by Karl Wesker.)

- Midfoot joints include the naviculocuneiform (NC), intercuneiform, and tarsometatarsal (TMT; a.k.a. Lisfranc) joints
  a. Lisfranc joints
    - No ligamentous connection between the bases of the first and second MT.
    - So-called Lisfranc ligament connects the medial cuneiform to the second MT.
- Metatarsophalangeal (MTP) joints: primary stabilizer is the plantar plate
  a. Also supported by the collaterals and plantar ligaments

3. Muscles **(Figs. 10.13, 10.14, 10.15,** and **Table 10.1)**
   - Major tendons crossing the ankle joint into the foot (extrinsic muscles):
     a. Anterior: tibialis anterior (TA), extensor hallucis longus (EHL), extensor digitorum longus (EDL), peroneus tertius

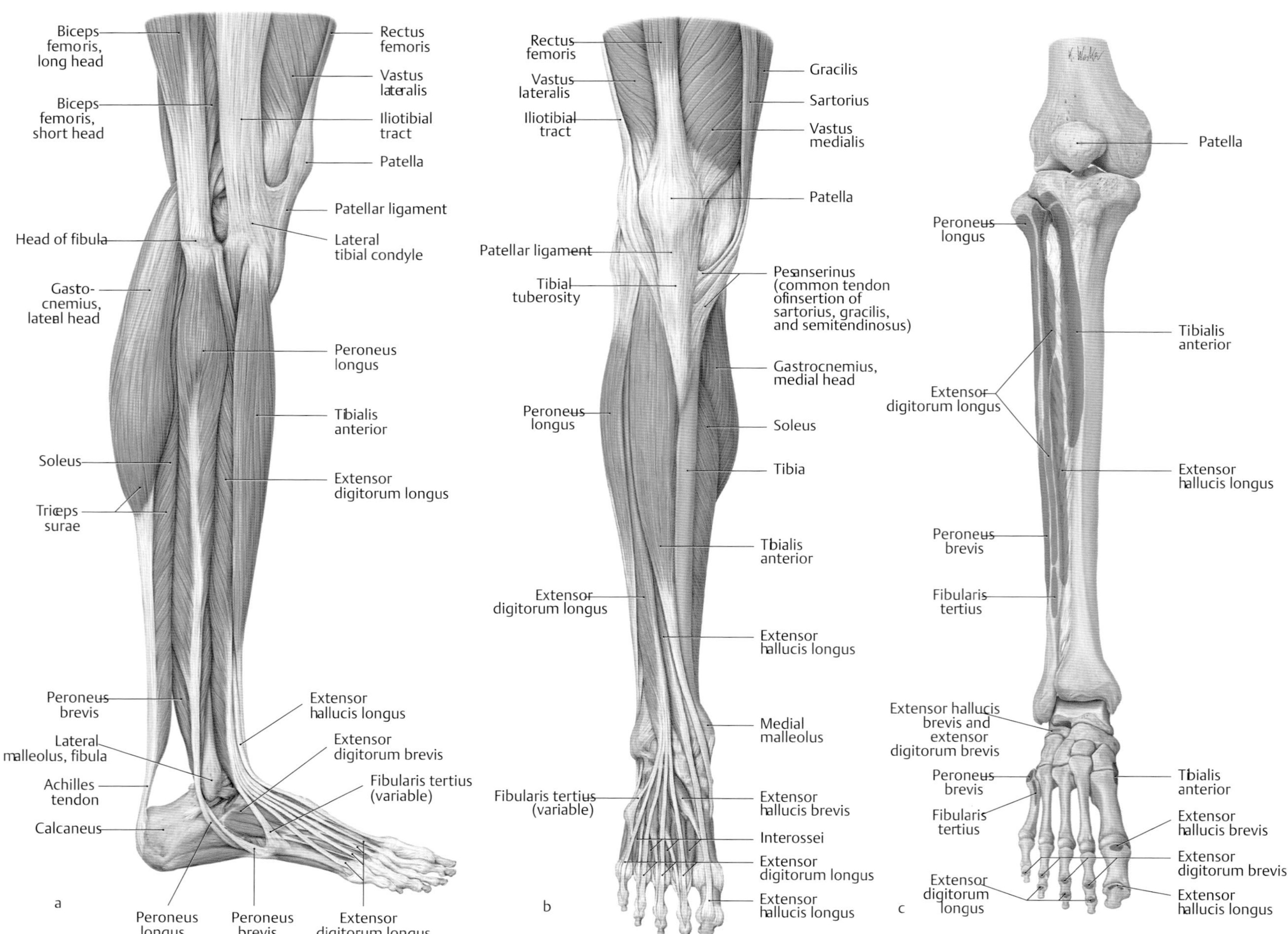

Fig. 10.13 The muscles of the right leg. **(a)** Lateral view. **(b)** Anterior view. **(c)** All the muscles have been removed. (From Schuenke M, Schulte E. General Anatomy and the Musculoskeletal System: Thieme Atlas of Anatomy. New York: Thieme; 2005. Illustration by Karl Wesker.)

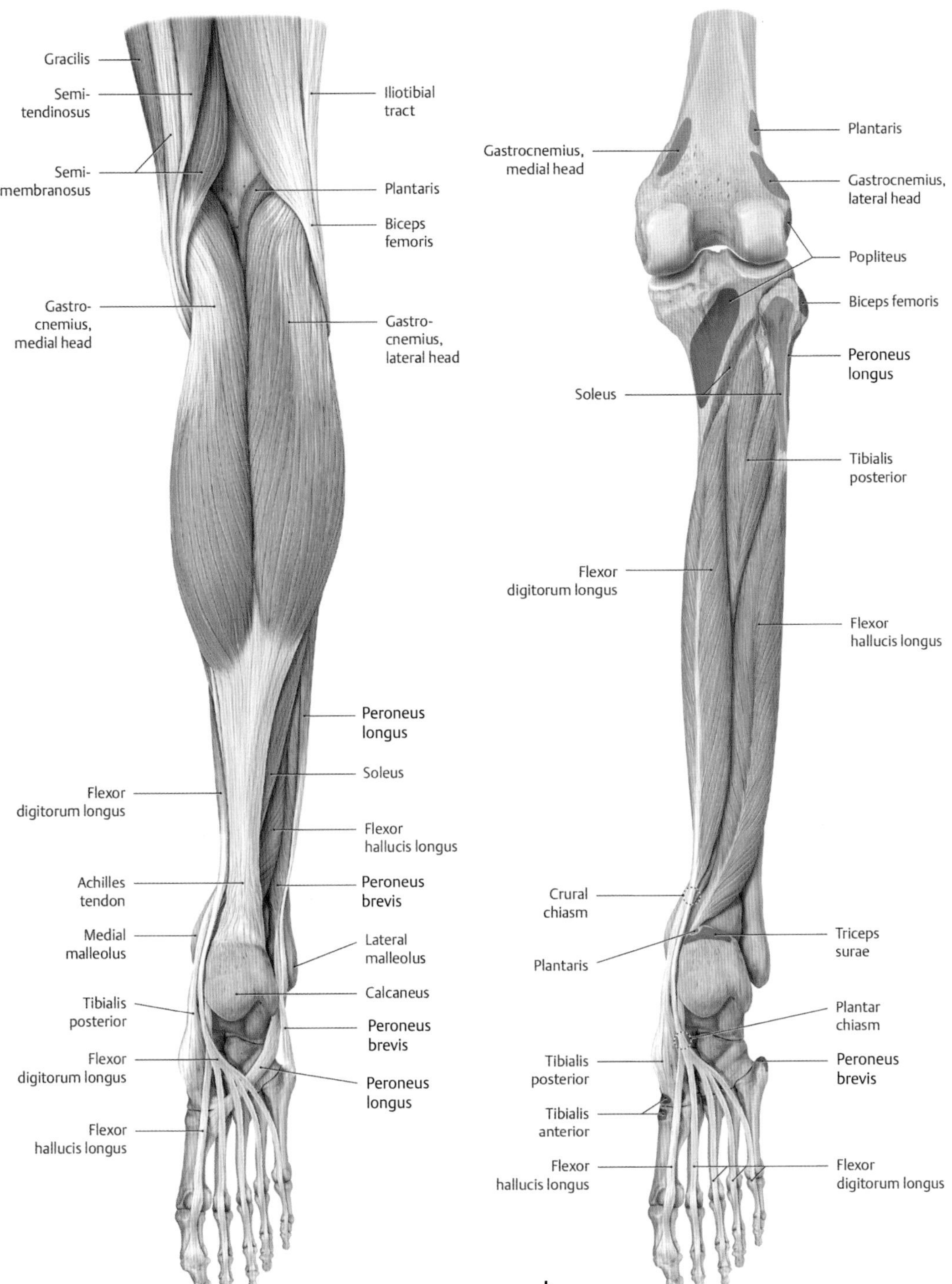

Fig. 10.14 The muscles of the right leg from the posterior view. **(a)** The bulge of the calf is produced mainly by the triceps surae muscle (the soleus plus the two heads of the gastrocnemius). **(b)** Both heads of the gastrocnemius have been removed. (*continued on page 442*)

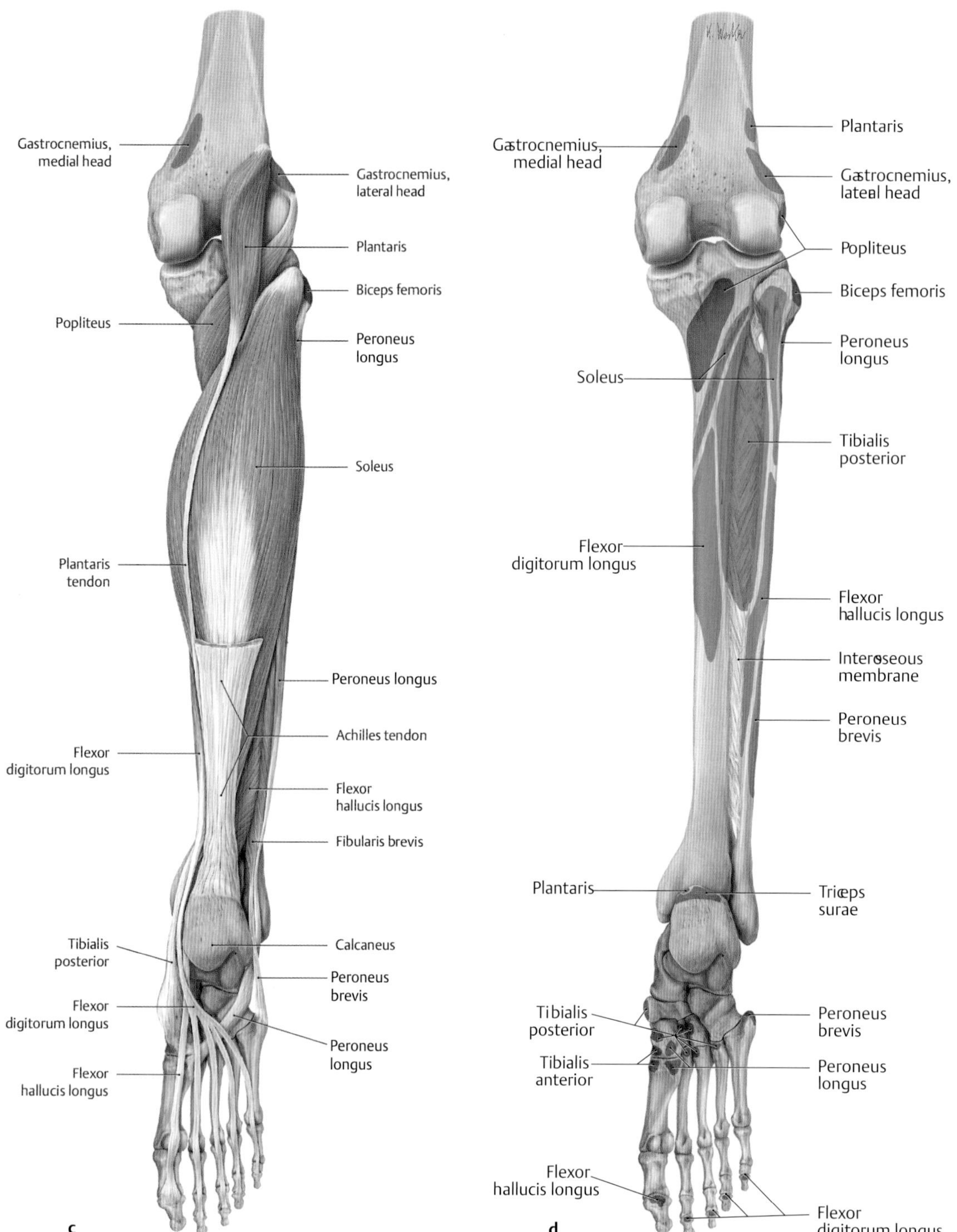

Fig. 10.14 (*continued*) **(c)** The triceps, surae, plantaris, and popliteus muscles have been removed. **(d)** All of the muscles have been removed. (From Schuenke M, Schulte E. General Anatomy and the Musculoskeletal System: Thieme Atlas of Anatomy. New York: Thieme; 2005. Illustration by Karl Wesker.)

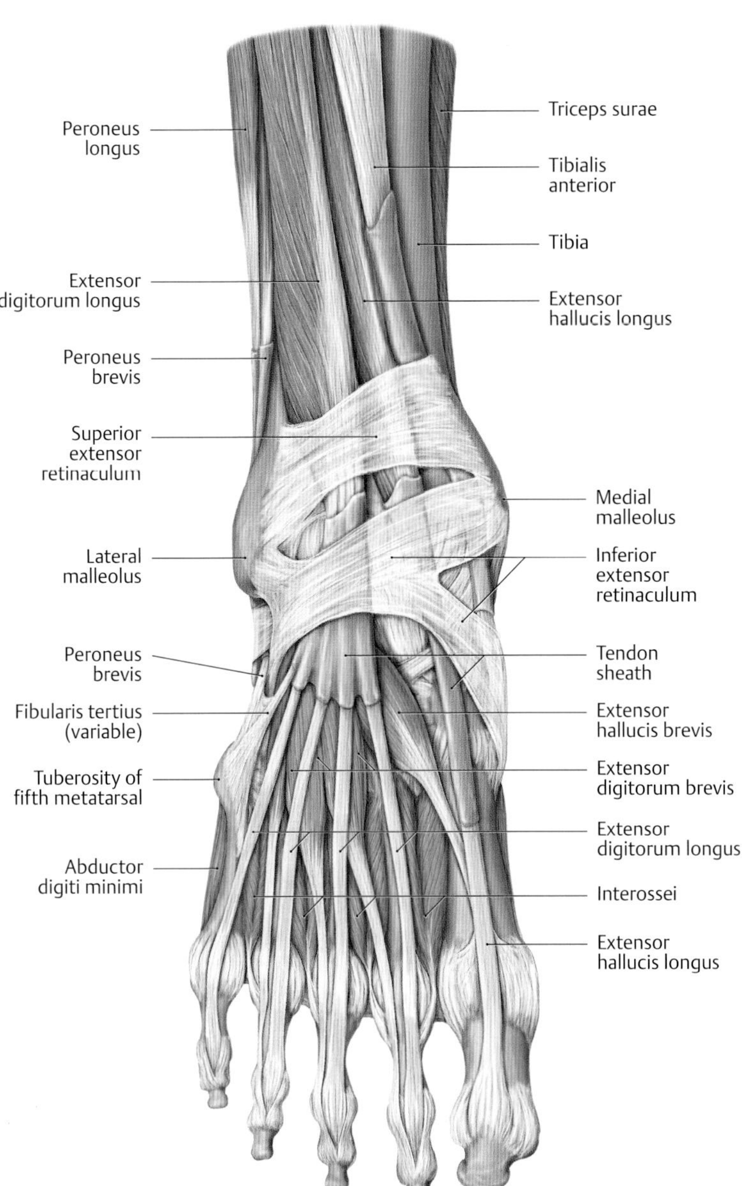

Fig. 10.15 The tendon sheaths and retinacula of the right foot. **(a)** Anterior view. (*continued on page 444*)

Fig. 10.15 (*continued*) **(b)** Medial view. **(c)** Lateral view. (From Schuenke M, Schulte E. General Anatomy and the Musculoskeletal System: Thieme Atlas of Anatomy. New York: Thieme; 2005. Illustration by Karl Wesker.)

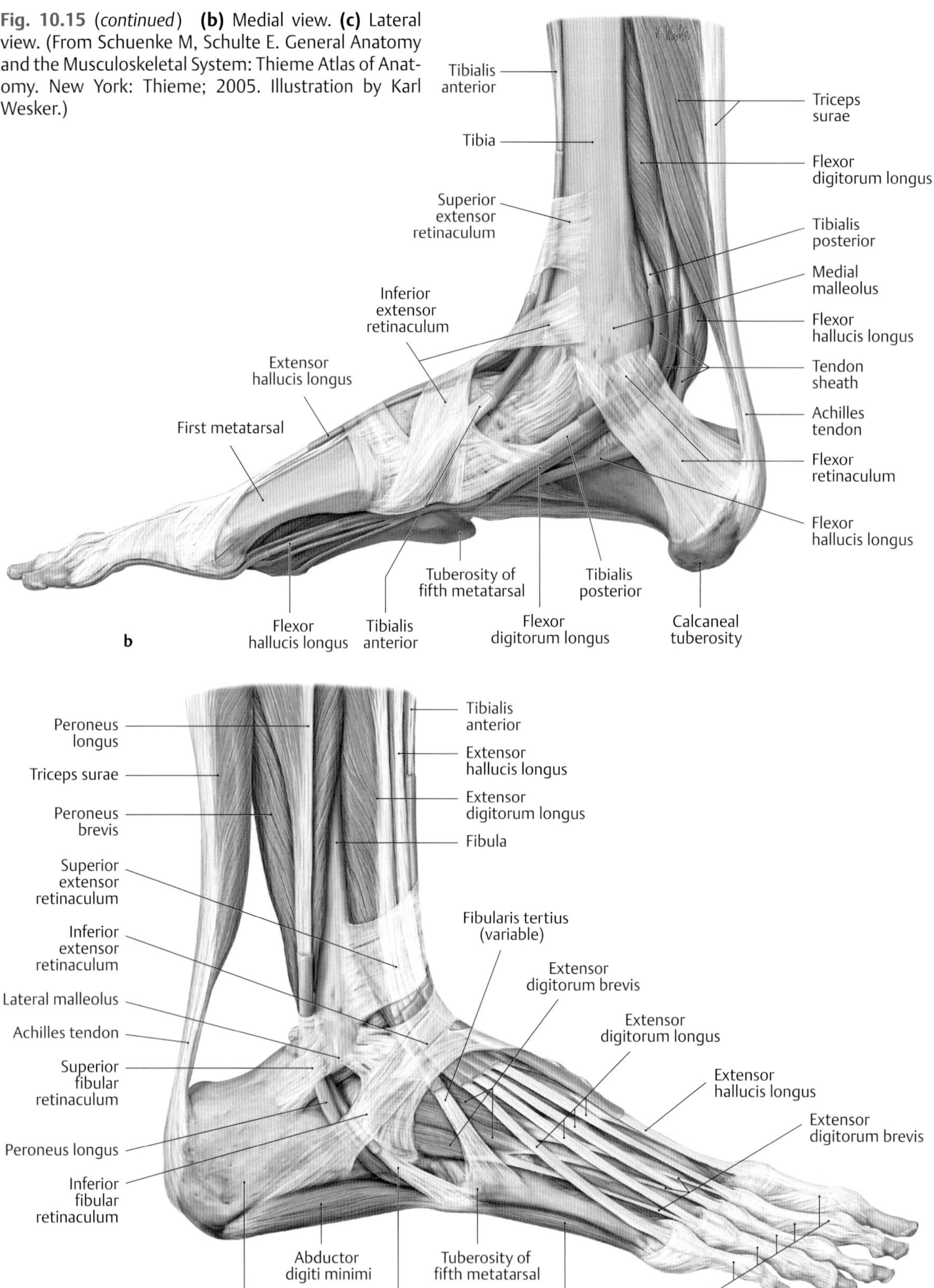

Table 10.1 Anatomy: Muscle Origins, Insertions, Nerve Supply, Action, and Compartment

Muscle	Origin	Insertion	Nerve Supply	Action	Compartment
TA	Lateral condyle of tibia, IO membrane	First cuneiform and base of first MT	DP	Dorsiflexes ankle, inverts foot	Anterior
EDL	Proximal fibula	Dorsum of middle and distal phalanges	DP	Extends toes 2–5, dorsiflexes ankle	Anterior
EHL	Anterior surface of fibula	Base of distal phalanx of great toe	DP	Dorsiflexes great toe	Anterior
Peroneus tertius	EDL and medial fibular shaft	Dorsal base of fifth MT	DP	Dorsiflexes, everts and abducts foot	Anterior
PL	Head of fibula, upper fibular shaft	Plantar aspect of medial cuneiform and first MT base	SP	Everts foot, plantarflexes ankle	Lateral
PB	Inferior two thirds of lateral fibular surface	Fifth MT base	SP	Everts foot, plantarflexes ankle	Lateral
Gastrocnemius	Posterior femoral condyles	Calcaneal tuber (via Achilles tendon)	Tibial	Plantarflexes ankle, flexes knee	Superficial posterior
Soleus	Posterior fibular head, middle third of medial tibial shaft	Calcaneal tuber (via Achilles tendon)	Tibial	Plantarflexes ankle	Superficial posterior
Plantaris	Lateral supracondylar line of distal femur	Middle third of posterior calcaneus (just medial to Achilles)	Tibial	Plantarflexes ankle, flexes knee	Superficial posterior
PT	Posterosuperior aspects of tibia and fibula, IO membrane	Navicular tuberosity, medial cuneiform, plantar MTs 2–4	Tibial	Inverts foot, plantarflexes ankle	Deep posterior
FDL	Posterior surface of tibia	Plantar surfaces of bases of second to fifth distal phalanges	Tibial	Flexes toes 2–5, plantarflexes ankle	Deep posterior
FHL	Inferior two thirds of posterior surface of fibula	Base of distal phalanx of great toe	Tibial	Flexes great toe, plantarflexes ankle	Deep posterior

Abbreviations: DP, deep peroneal; EDL, extensor digitorum longus; EHL, extensor hallucis longus; FDL, flexor digitorum longus; FHL, flexor hallucis longus; IO, intraosseous; MT, metatarsal; PB, peroneus brevis; PL, peroneus longus; PT, posterior tibialis; SP, superficial peroneal; TA, tibialis anterior.

b. Lateral: peroneus longus (PL) and peroneus brevis (PB)
   - PB lies anterior and medial to the PL in the retromalleolar groove

c. Posterior: Achilles (confluence of the gastrocnemius and soleus muscles, strongest and largest tendon in the body)
   - Rotates ~ 90 degrees: soleus fibers insert on the medial aspect of the Achilles tendon footprint; gastrocnemius fibers insert on the lateral aspect (due to embryological limb bud rotation)

d. Medial: posterior tibialis (PT), flexor digitorum longus (FDL), and flexor hallucis longus (FHL)
   - **From anterior to posterior: PT, FDL, Vein, Artery, Nerve, FHL; use mnemonic "Tom, Dick, and a Very Angry Nervous Harry"**
     - ♦ Posterior tibial vein and artery and tibial nerve
   - PT initiates hindfoot inversion during gait
   - In the ankle, the FDL is medial/anterior to the FHL; crosses in midfoot (knot of Henry) where FHL goes deep (dorsal) to FDL

e. Plantar foot muscles layers (**Figs. 10.16, 10.17, 10.18** and **Table 10.2**)
   - Intrinsic muscles dominate the first and third layers
   - Extrinsic muscles contribute more to the second and fourth layers
   - Medial and lateral plantar nerves travel in the second layer

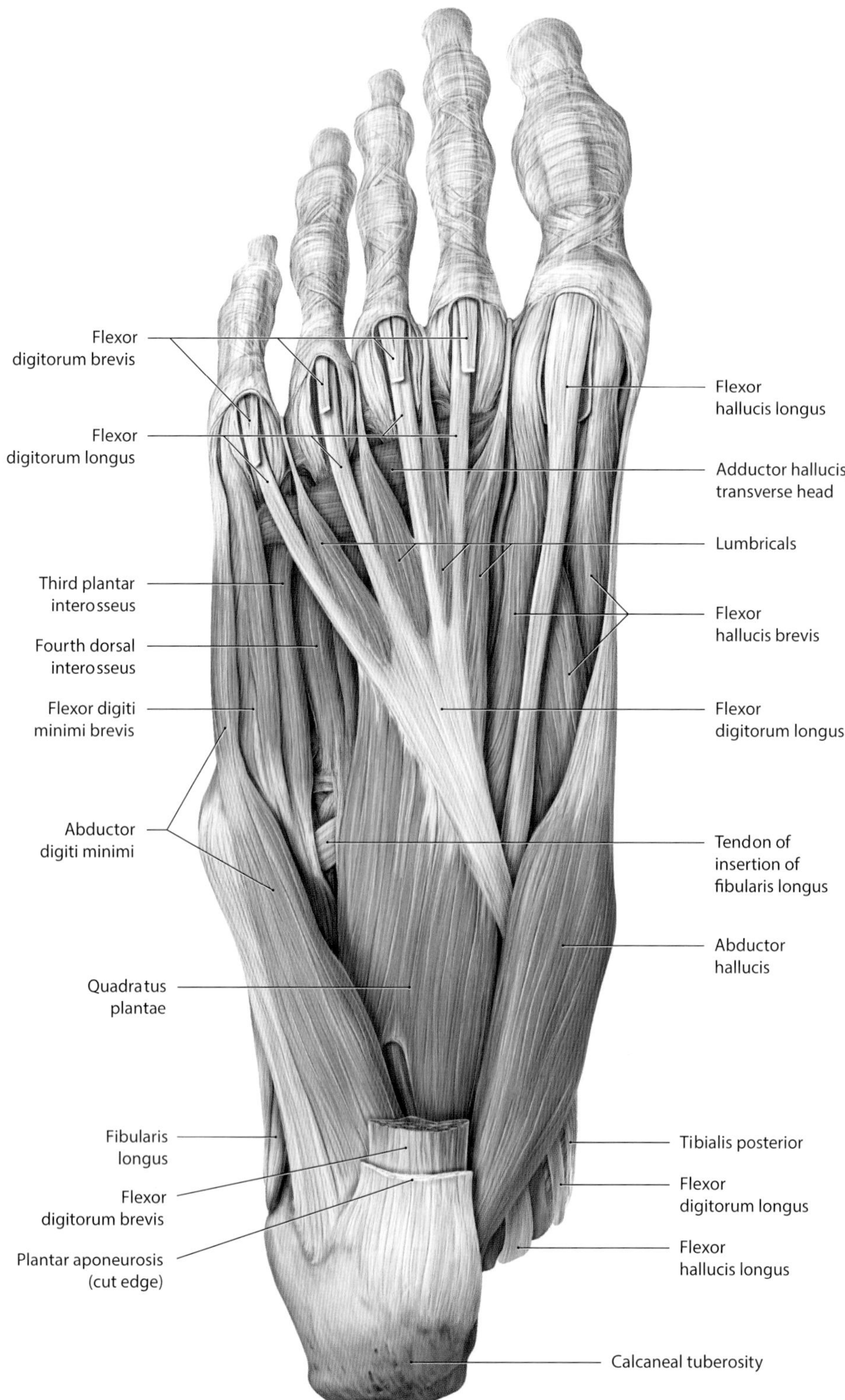

Fig. 10.16 The short muscles of the right foot from the plantar view. (From Schuenke M, Schulte E. General Anatomy and the Musculoskeletal System: Thieme Atlas of Anatomy. New York: Thieme; 2005. Illustration by Karl Wesker.)

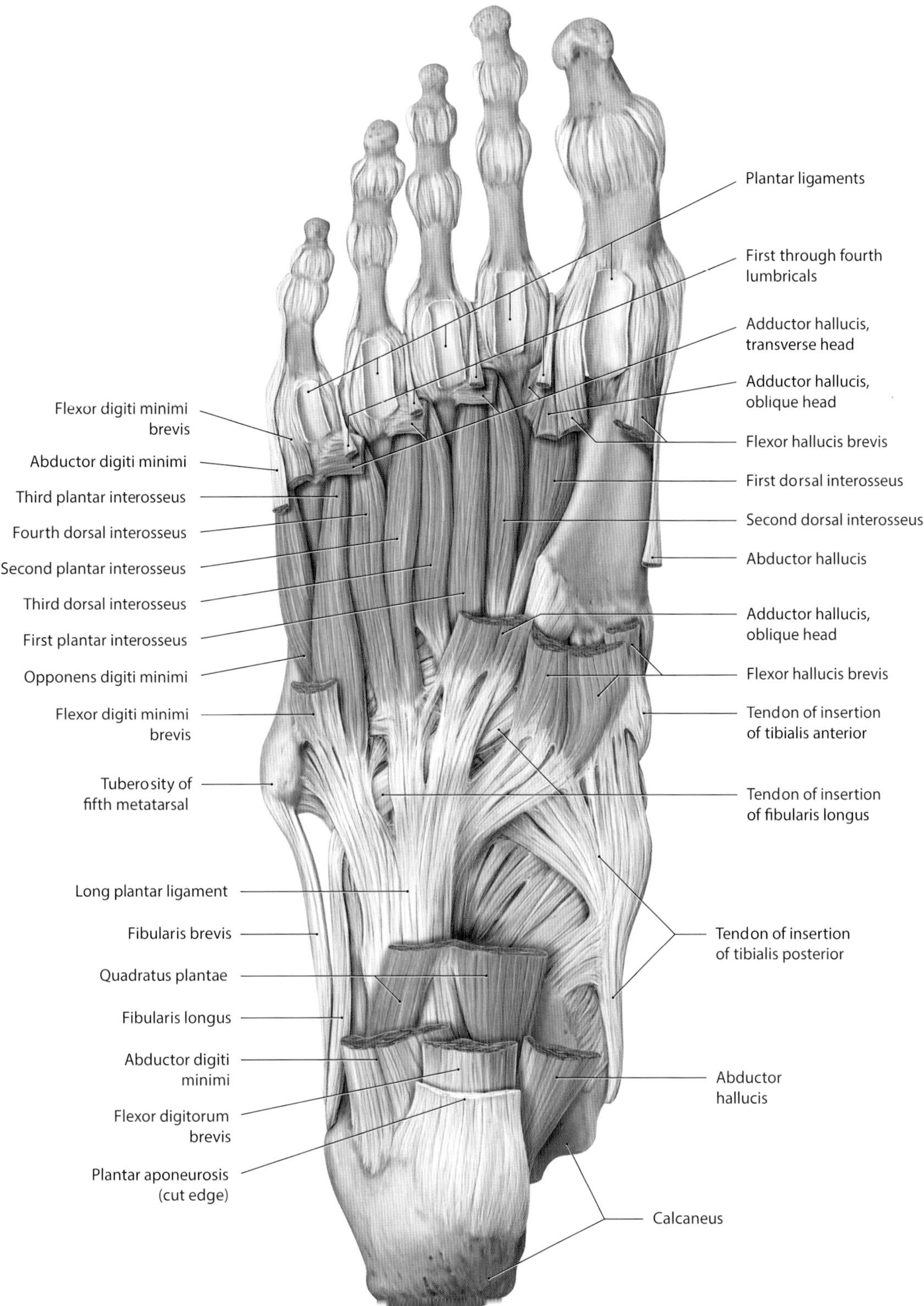

Fig. 10.17 The short muscles of the right foot from the plantar view. (From Schuenke M, Schulte E. General Anatomy and the Musculoskeletal System: Thieme Atlas of Anatomy. New York: Thieme; 2005. Illustration by Karl Wesker.)

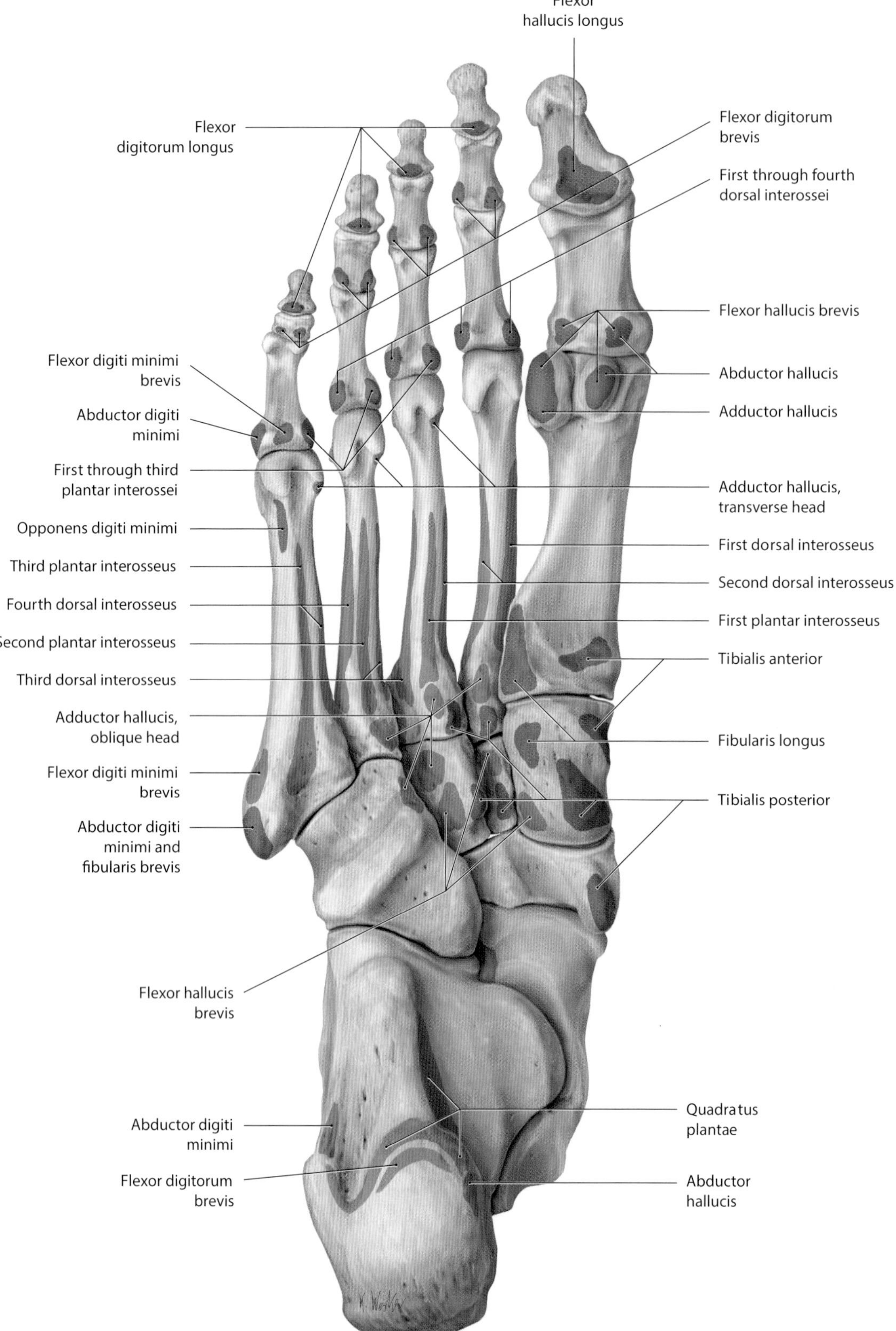

Fig. 10.18 Muscle origins and insertions on the plantar view of the right foot. Muscle originas are in red; muscle/tendon unit insertions are in blue. (From Schuenke M, Schulte E. General Anatomy and the Musculoskeletal System: Thieme Atlas of Anatomy. New York: Thieme; 2005. Illustration by Karl Wesker.)

- Deep plantar arch exists in the fourth layer
- The lumbrical muscles are plantar to the transverse MT ligament, while the interossei are dorsal.

f. Extensor digitorum brevis (EDB): single dorsal intrinsic foot muscle
- Originates from the superolateral calcaneus
- Inserts at base of the proximal phalanges [except hallux: extensor hallucis brevis (EHB)]
- Located lateral to EDL of each toe

g. Plantar calcaneal (heel) spurs occur in the flexor digitorum brevis (FDB) origin.

4. Nerves **(Figs. 10.19, 10.20, 10.21)**
- Tibial nerve **(Fig. 10.22)**

a. Supplies all the intrinsic muscles of the foot except for the EDB (deep peroneal [DP] nerve)

b. Travels in tarsal tunnel beneath flexor retinaculum and splits into medial plantar nerve (MPN), lateral plantar nerve (LPN), and calcaneal sensory branch
- MPN innervates the FHB, abductor hallucis (AbH), FDB, and first lumbrical muscle, and supplies sensation to the plantar medial 3½ digits.
- LPN innervates the remaining intrinsics, and supplies sensation to the plantar lateral 1½ digits.

c. MPN runs deep to the AbH; LPN runs under the quadratus plantae (QP).

d. First branch of the LPN (Baxter's nerve) supplies the abductor digiti quinti.

- Superficial peroneal (SP) nerve

a. The medial and intermediate dorsal cutaneous nerves of the SP nerve supply sensation to the dorsum of the foot except for the first web space.

b. The dorsal medial cutaneous nerve (branch of the SP nerve) supplies sensation to the dorsomedial aspect of the great toe and is at risk during hallux valgus correction surgery

Table 10.2 Plantar Foot Muscles Layers

Layer	Muscles
First (most plantar)	AbH, FDB, ADM
Second	QP, Lumbricals, FDL, FHL
Third	FHB, AdH, FDMB
Fourth (most dorsal)	Dorsal and plantar interossei, PL, PT

Abbreviations: AbH, abductor hallucis; AdH, adductor hallucis; ADM, abductor digiti minimi; FDB, flexor digitorum brevis; FDL, flexor digitorum longus; FDMB, flexor digiti minimi brevis; FHB, flexor hallucis brevis; FHL, flexor hallucis longus; QP, quadratus plantae; PL, peroneus longus; PT, posterior tibialis.

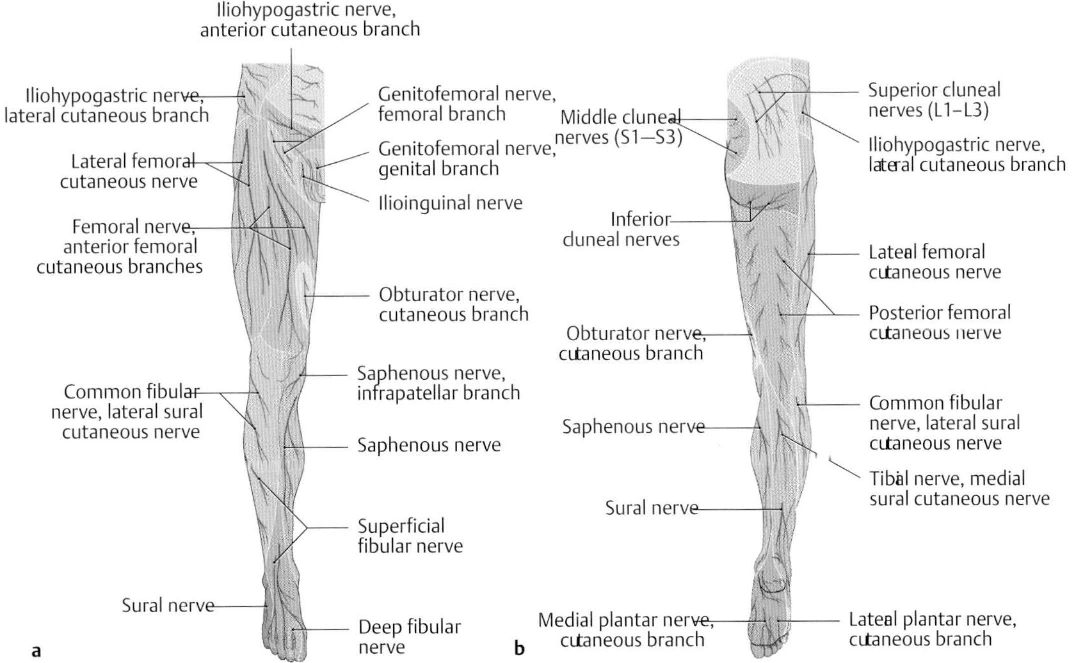

Fig. 10.19 (a) Pattern of peripheral sensory innervation in the right lower limb. **(b)** Pattern of peripheral sensory innervation in the left lower limb. (From Schuenke M, Schulte E. General Anatomy and the Musculoskeletal System: Thieme Atlas of Anatomy. New York: Thieme; 2005. Illustration by Karl Wesker.)

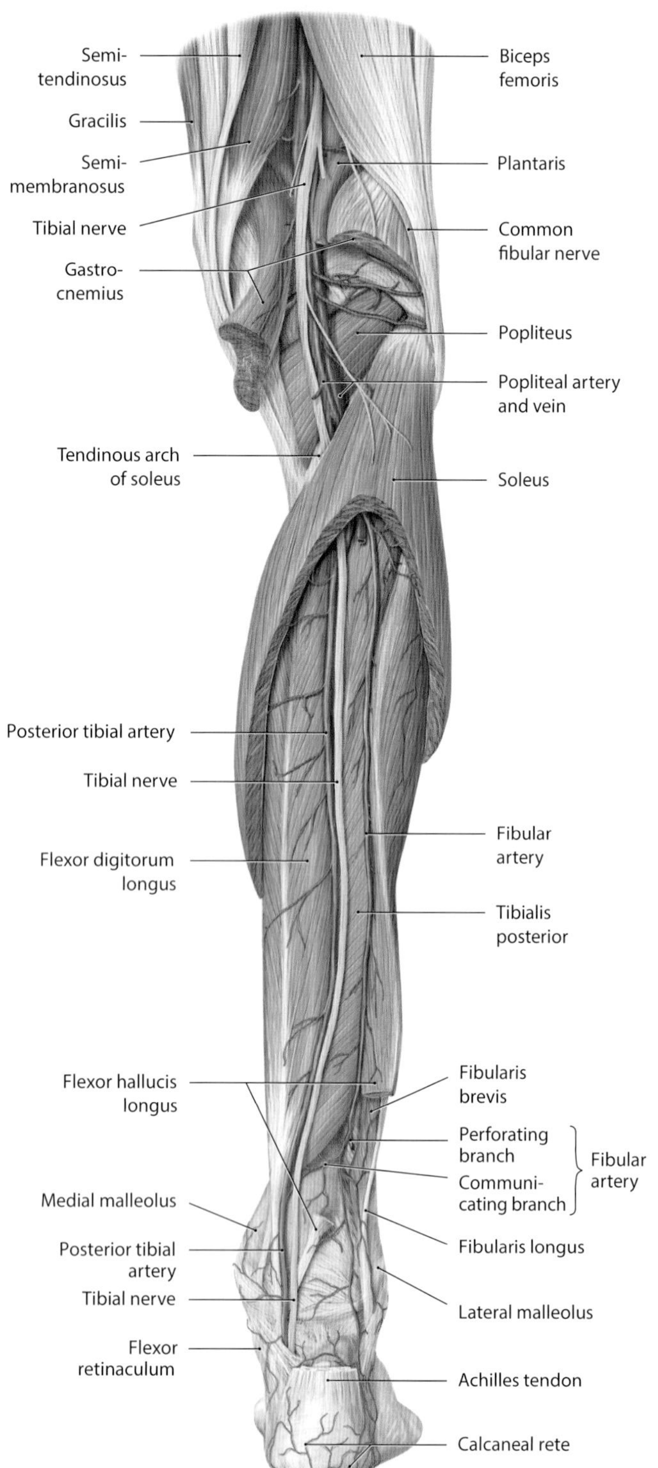

Fig. 10.20 The neurovascular structures in the superficial and deep posterior compartments. Right leg, posterior view. Neurovascular structures in the deep posterior compartment after partial removal of the triceps surae and the deep layer of the fascia of the leg. The popliteal artery divides into the anterior and posterior tibial arteries at the distal border of the popliteus. The anterior tibial artery pierces the interosseous membrane (not shown here) and passes to the anterior side of the leg, entering the anterior compartment. The posterior tibial artery, accompanied by the tibial nerve, passes below the tendinous arch of the soleus into the deep posterior compartment, almost immediately gives off the fibular artery, and then continues distally behind the medial malleolus to the plantar side of the foot. The deep posterior compartment is one of four poorly distensible muscle compartments in the leg ("fibro-osseous canals"), which are potential sites for the development of a compartment syndrome following a vascular injury (see p. 445). (From Schuenke M, Schulte E. General Anatomy and the Musculoskeletal System: Thieme Atlas of Anatomy. New York: Thieme; 2005. Illustration by Karl Wesker.)

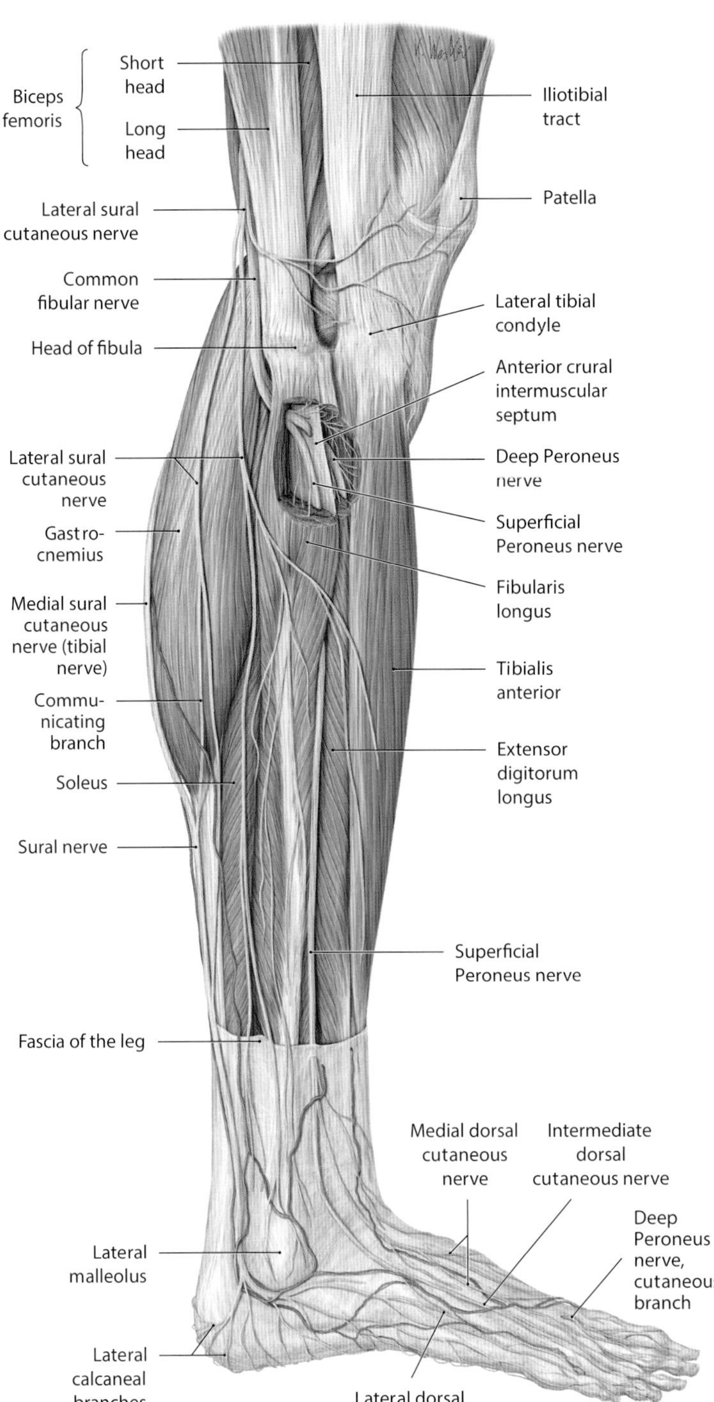

Fig. 10.21 Division of the common fibular nerve into the deep and superficial fibular nerves. (From Schuenke M, Schulte E. General Anatomy and the Musculoskeletal System: Thieme Atlas of Anatomy. New York: Thieme; 2005. Illustration by Karl Wesker.)

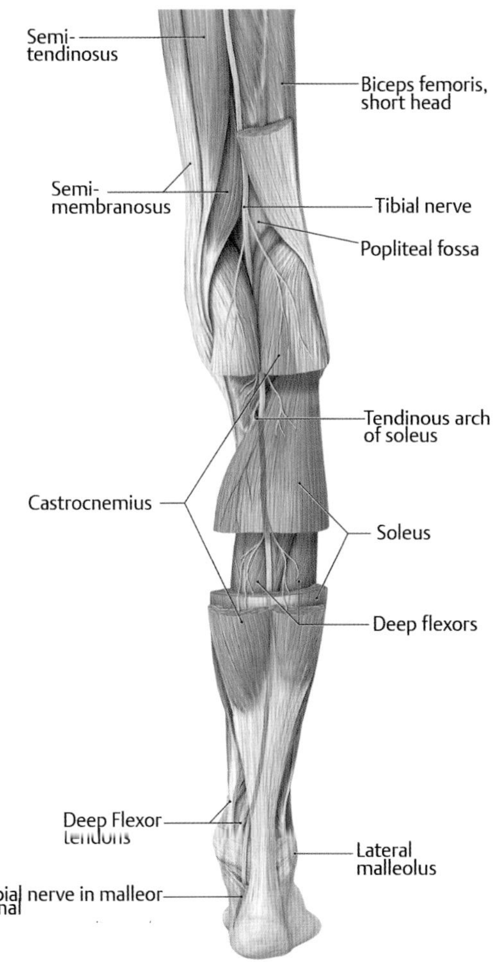

Fig. 10.22 Course and motor distribution of the sciatic nerve: the tibial part (tibial nerve). Right lower limb, posterior view. (From Schuenke M, Schulte E. General Anatomy and the Musculoskeletal System: Thieme Atlas of Anatomy. New York: Thieme; 2005. Illustration by Karl Wesker.)

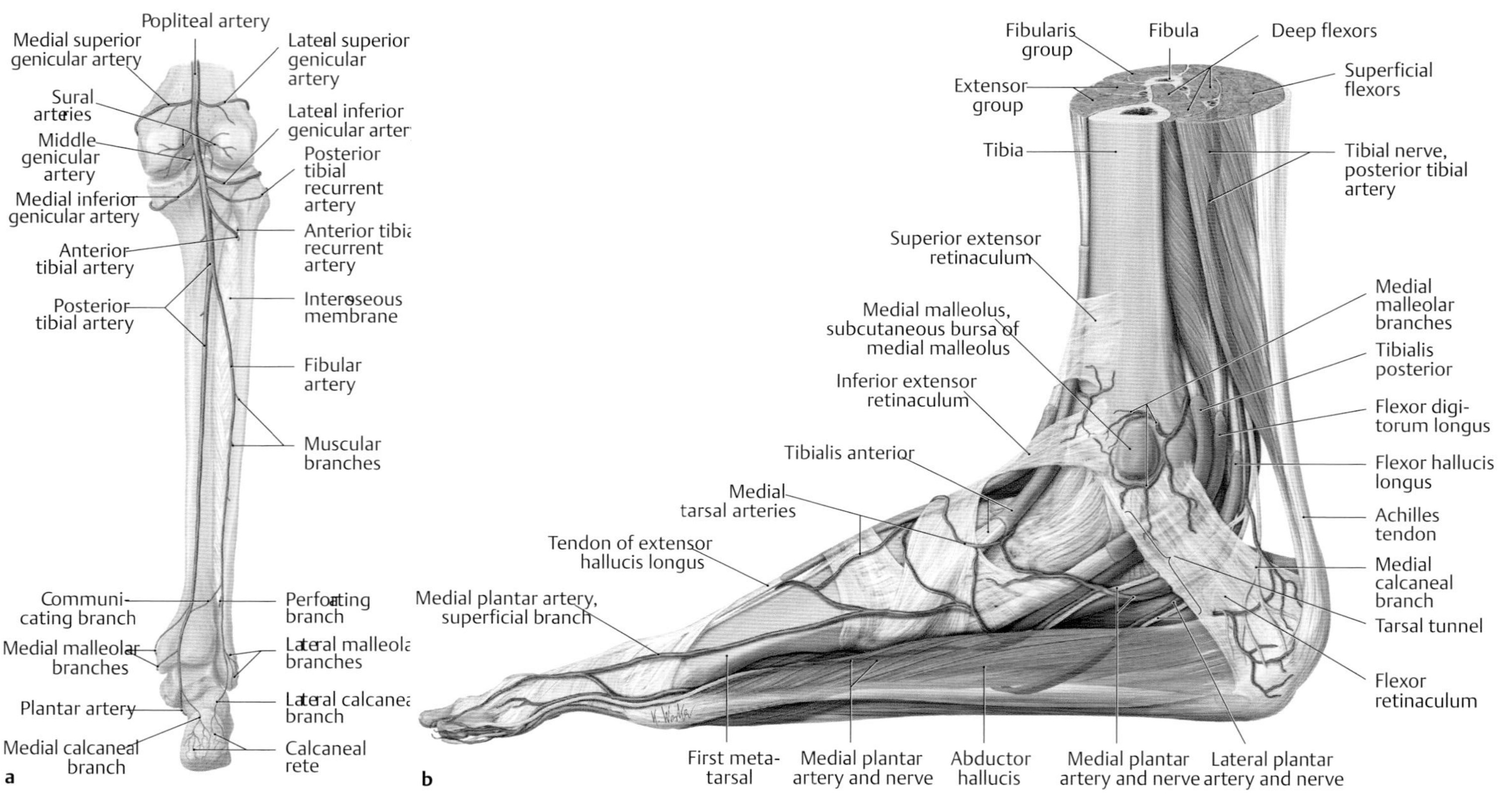

Fig. 10.23 **(a)** The arteries of the leg. Posterior view. **(b)** The neurovascular structures of the medial malleolar region. (From Schuenke M, Schulte E. General Anatomy and the Musculoskeletal System: Thieme Atlas of Anatomy. New York: Thieme; 2005. Illustration by Karl Wesker.)

- Deep peroneal (DP) nerve
  a. Lateral terminal recurrent branch of DP nerve supplies the EDB
  b. Medial terminal branch of DP nerve supplies sensation to first web space
- Saphenous nerve (posterior to greater saphenous vein)
  a. All sensation to the foot is supplied by the sciatic nerve except for the medial foot (saphenous nerve is the termination of the femoral nerve).
- Sural nerve: supplies sensation to the lateral aspect of the foot
- Digital nerves course plantar to the transverse MT ligaments (interdigital).
- **Morton's neuromas develop here, most commonly in second or third interspace**

5. Vessels **(Figs. 10.20** and **10.23)**
   - Dorsalis pedis artery: continuation of the anterior tibial artery of the leg **(Fig. 10.24)**
     a. Largest branch, the deep plantar artery, runs between the first and second MTs and contributes to the plantar arch (implicated in foot compartment syndrome)
   - PT artery **(Fig. 10.25)**
     a. Divides into medial and lateral plantar branches beneath the AbH muscle
     b. The larger lateral branch receives the deep plantar artery and forms the plantar arch in the fourth layer of the plantar foot.
6. Surgical approaches **(Figs. 10.26, 10.27, 10.28** and **Table 10.3)**
7. Arthroscopy **(Table 10.4)**

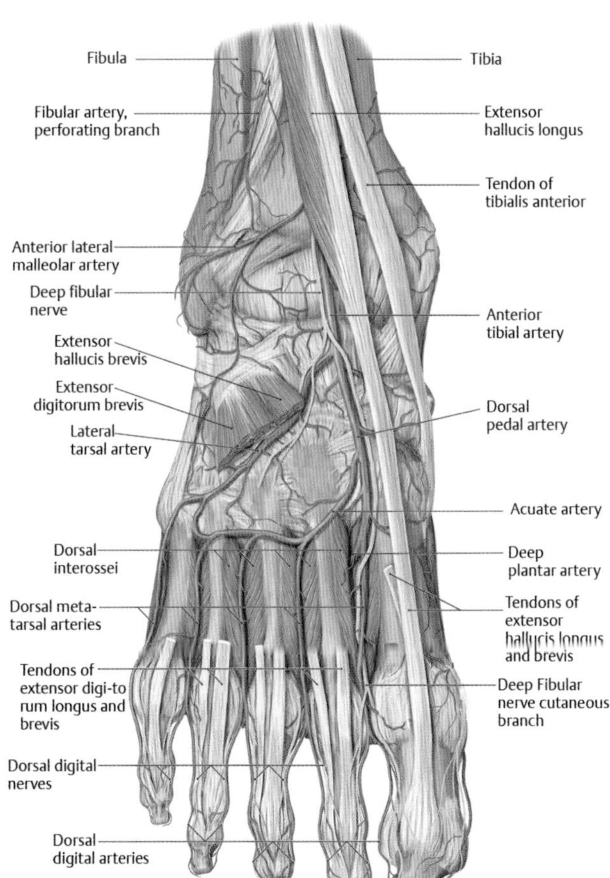

Fig. 10.24 The dorsal arteries and nerves of the foot. (From Schuenke M, Schulte E. General Anatomy and the Musculoskeletal System: Thieme Atlas of Anatomy. New York: Thieme; 2005. Illustration by Karl Wesker.)

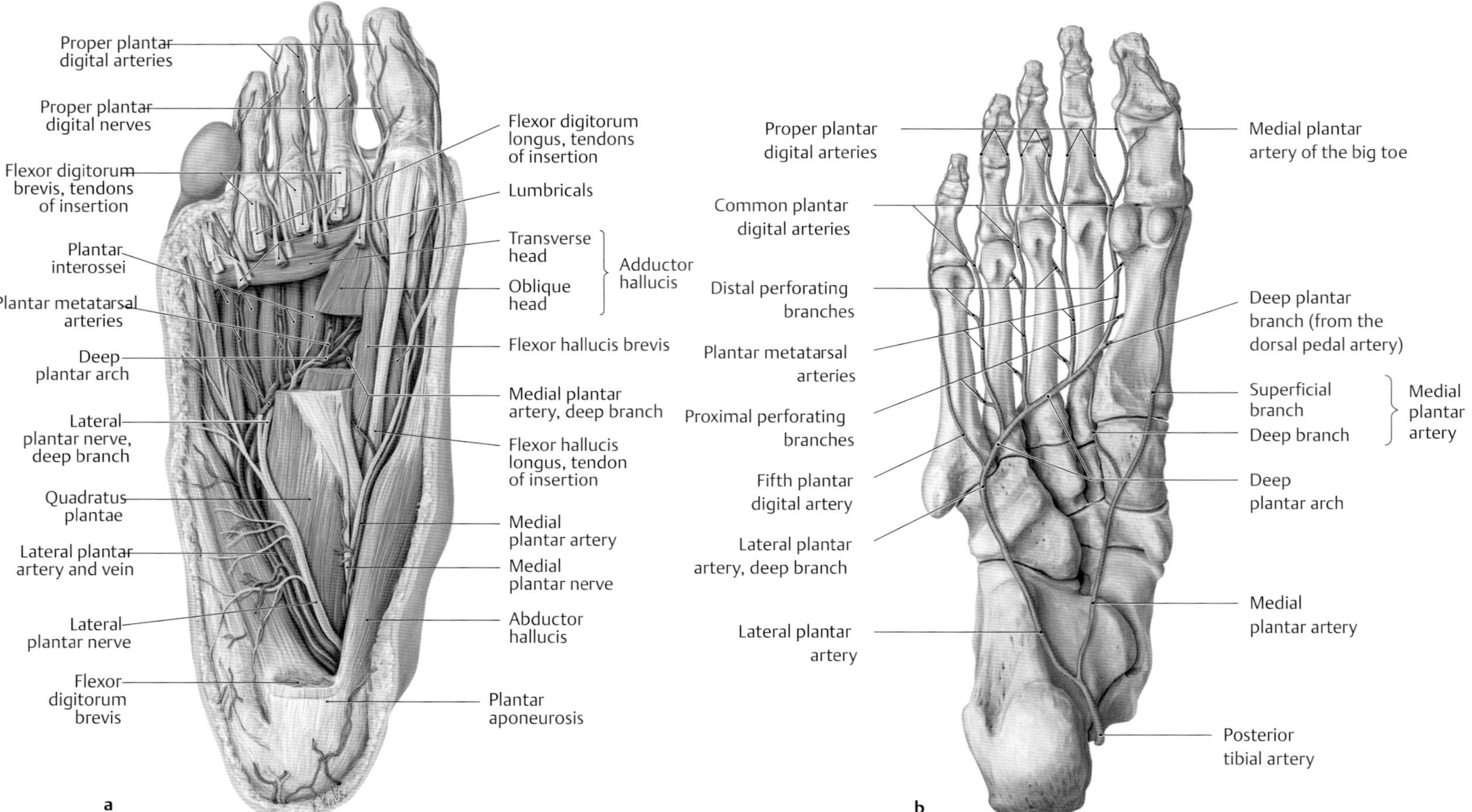

Fig. 10.25 **(a)** The plantar arteries and nerves of the foot (deep layer). **(b)** Overview of the plantar arteries of the foot. (From Schuenke M, Schulte E. General Anatomy and the Musculoskeletal System: Thieme Atlas of Anatomy. New York: Thieme; 2005. Illustration by Karl Wesker.)

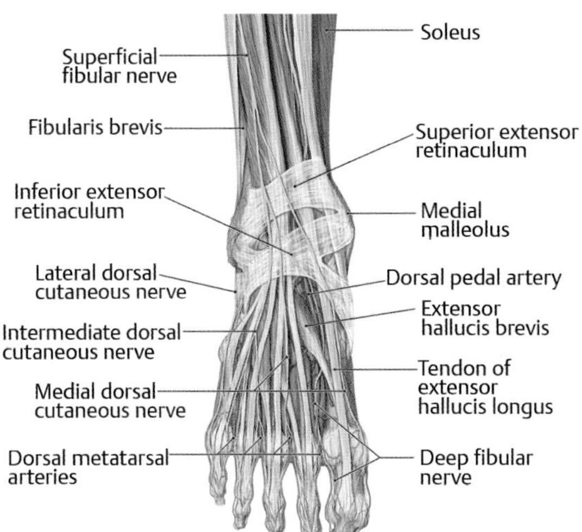

Fig. 10.26 The neurovascular structures of the anterior compartment and dorsum of the foot. (From Schuenke M, Schulte E. General Anatomy and the Musculoskeletal System: Thieme Atlas of Anatomy. New York: Thieme; 2005. Illustration by Karl Wesker.)

Fig. 10.27 Right leg, posterior view. Neurovascular structures in the deep posterior compartment after partial removal of the triceps surae and the deep layer of the fascia of the leg. The posterior tibial artery, accompanied by the tibial nerve, passes below the tendinous arch of the soleus into the deep posterior compartment, almost immediately gives off the fibular artery, and then continues distally behind the medial malleolus to the plantar side of the foot. (Modified from Schuenke M, Schulte E. General Anatomy and the Musculoskeletal System: Thieme Atlas of Anatomy. New York: Thieme; 2005. Illustration by Karl Wesker.)

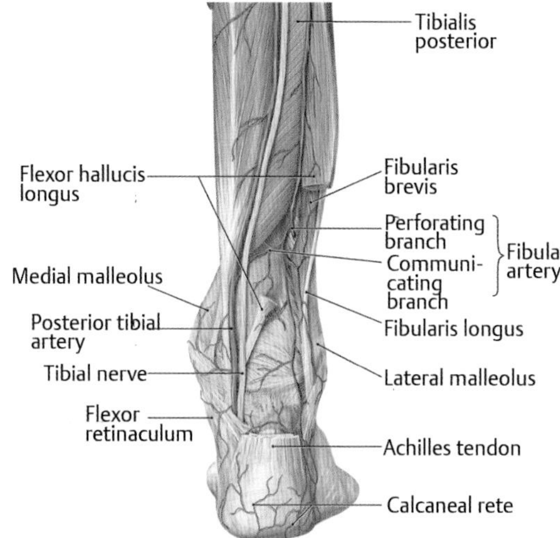

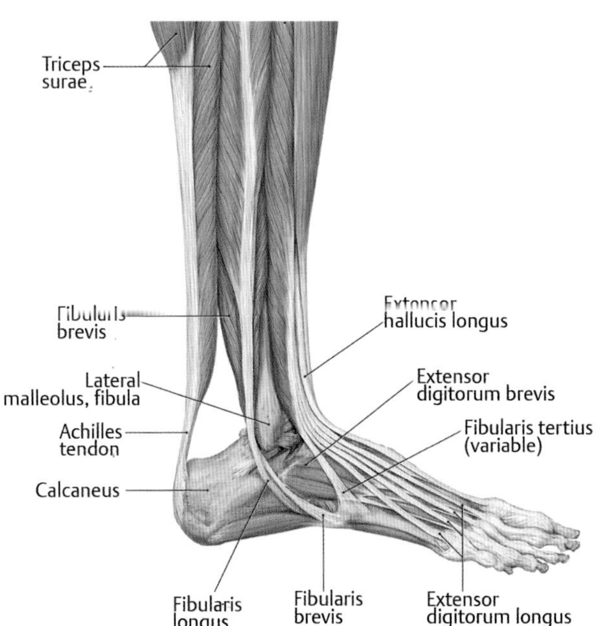

Fig. 10.28 The muscles of the right leg. Lateral view. (From Schuenke M, Schulte E. General Anatomy and the Musculoskeletal System: Thieme Atlas of Anatomy. New York: Thieme; 2005. Illustration by Karl Wesker.)

Table 10.3 Surgical Approaches

Approach	Interval	Risks
Anterior approach to the ankle **(Fig. 10.29)**	Between EHL (DP nerve) and EDL (DP nerve)	Anterior NV bundle (retract medially)
Anteromedial approach to the ankle **(Fig. 10.29)**	Medial to tibialis anterior (DP nerve)	Saphenous nerve
Anterolateral approach to the ankle **(Fig. 10.29)**	Lateral to EDL (DP nerve)	SP nerve (anterior)
Approach to the medial malleolus **(Fig. 10.30)**	No internervous plane	Saphenous nerve Long saphenous vein
Posteromedial approach to the ankle **(Fig. 10.31)**	Achilles and posteromedial aspect of tibia	Posterior tibial artery Tibial nerve
Posterolateral approach to the ankle **(Fig. 10.29)**	Between peroneals (SP nerve) and FHL (tibial nerve)	Peroneal artery Sural nerve
Lateral approach to the lateral malleolus **(Fig. 10.29)**	Subcutaneous	Sural nerve (posterior) SP nerve (anterior)
Extensile lateral approach to the calcaneus **(Fig. 10.32)**	Between peroneals (SP nerve) and Achilles (tibial nerve)	Sural nerve
Lateral approach to the hindfoot (sinus tarsi approach) **(Fig. 10.32)**	Between peroneus tertius (DP nerve) and peroneals (SP nerve)	Lesser saphenous vein Sural nerve
Medial utility incision (approach to talus and talonavicular joint) **(Fig. 10.31)**	Between tibialis anterior (DP nerve) and tibialis posterior (tibial nerve)	Saphenous vein and its branches
Lisfranc (midfoot) approach (centered dorsally over first TMT joint) **(Fig. 10.30)**	EHL (DP nerve) tendon sheath incised and tendon retracted laterally	Dorsalis pedis artery and DP nerve lie lateral to the EHL

Abbreviations: DP, deep peroneal; EDL, extensor digitorum longus; EHL, extensor hallucis longus; FHL, flexor hallucis longus; NV, neurovascular; SP, superficial peroneal; TMT, tarsometatarsal.

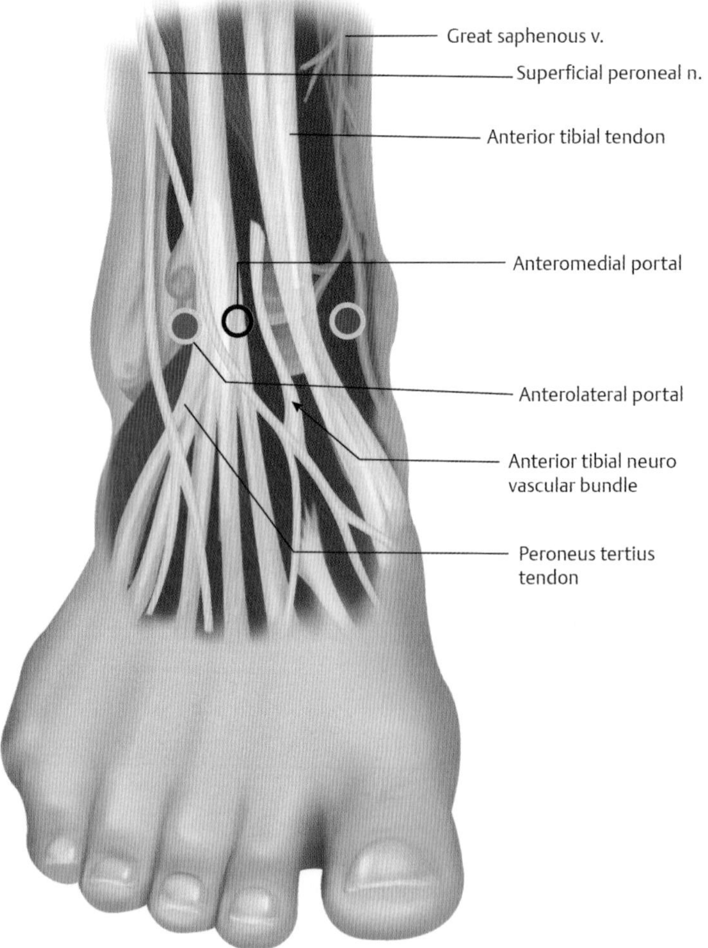

Fig. 10.29 Ankle arthroscopic portals and relevant anatomy and the most commonly used anteromedial and anterolateral portals.

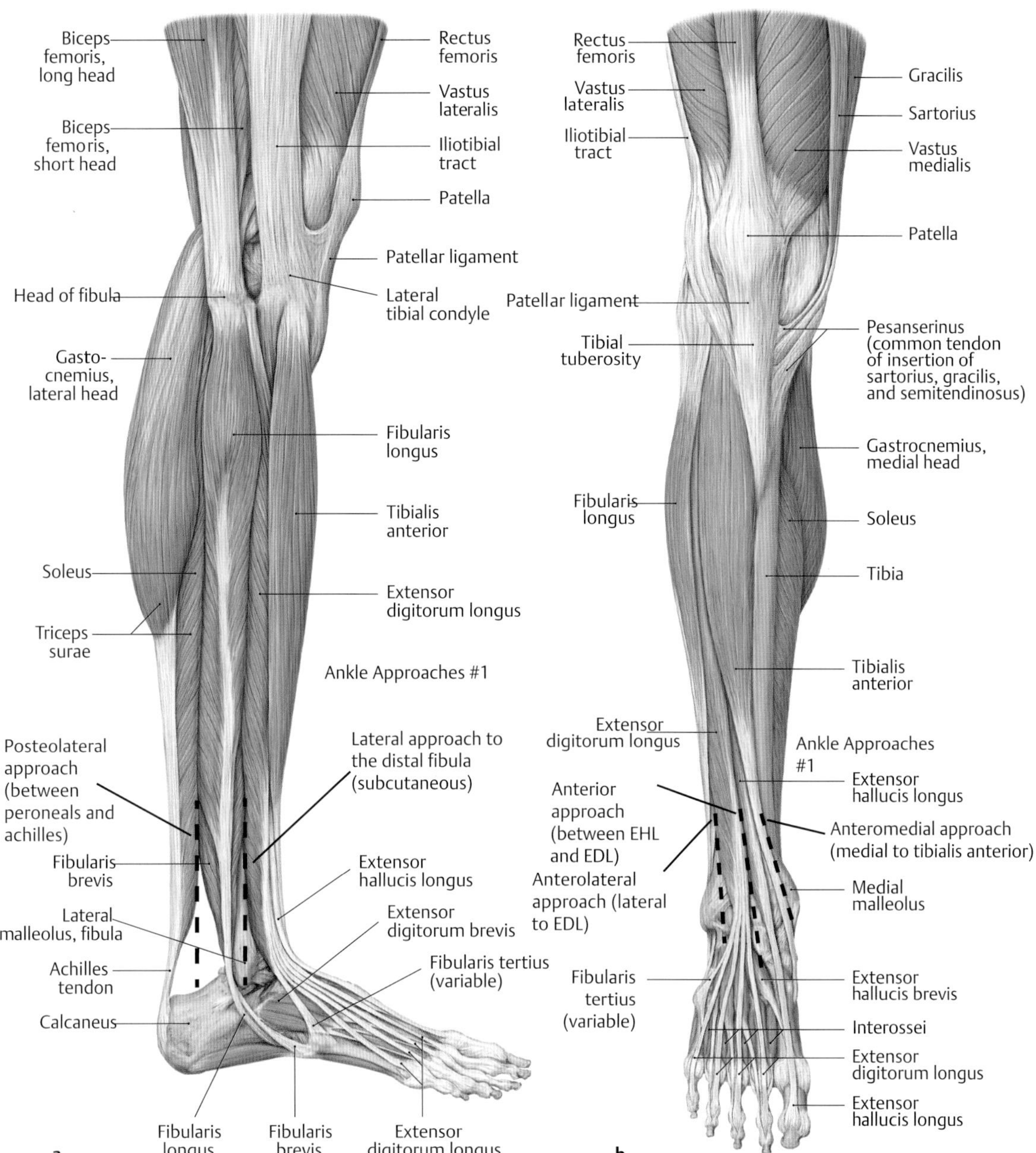

Fig. 10.30 Ankle approaches. **(a)** lateral view; **(b)** frontal view. (Modified from Schuenke M, Schulte E. General Anatomy and the Musculoskeletal System: Thieme Atlas of Anatomy. New York: Thieme; 2005. Illustration by Karl Wesker.)

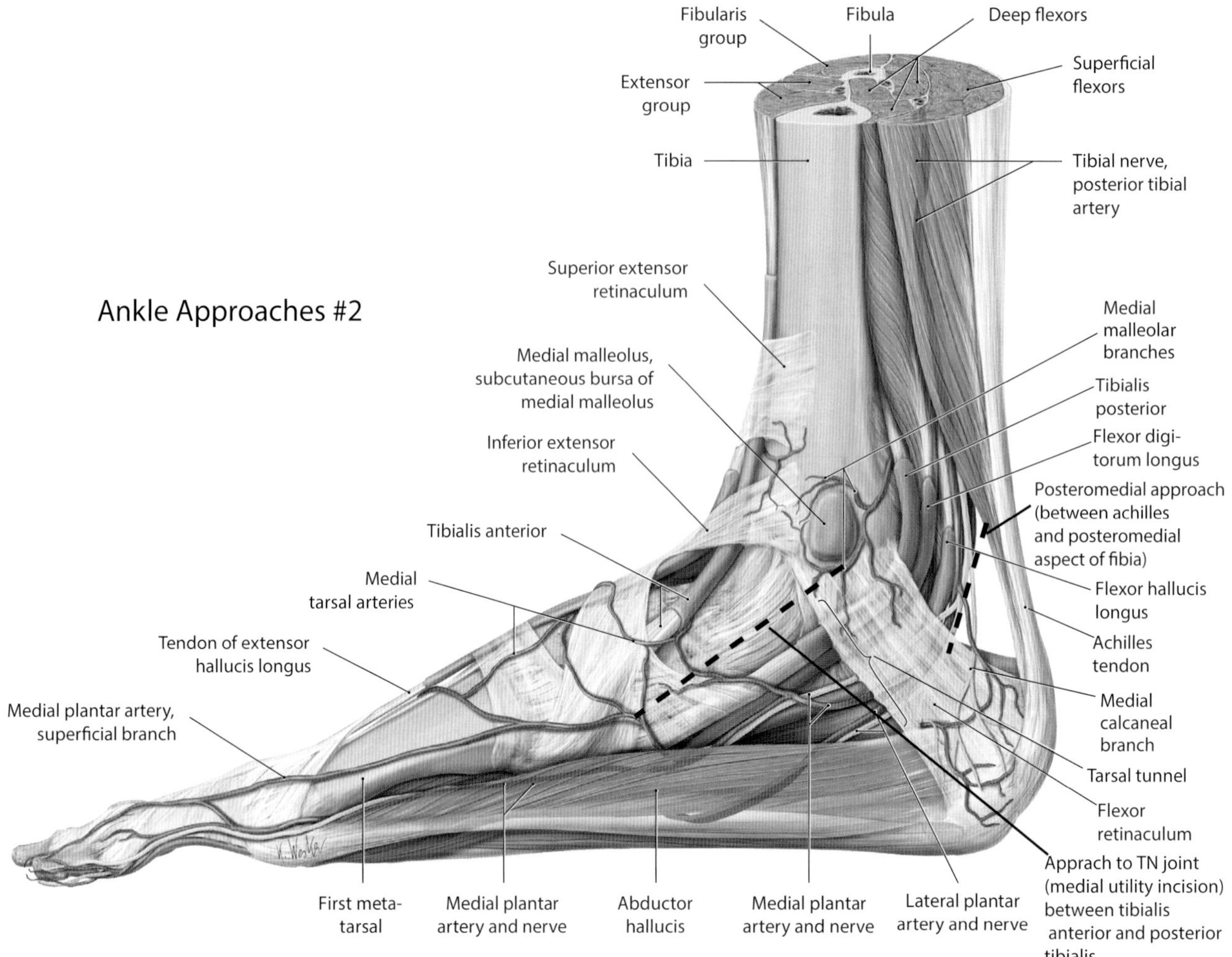

Fig. 10.31 Ankle Approaches 2. TN, talonavicular. (Modified from Schuenke M, Schulte E. General Anatomy and the Musculoskeletal System: Thieme Atlas of Anatomy. New York: Thieme; 2005. Illustration by Karl Wesker.)

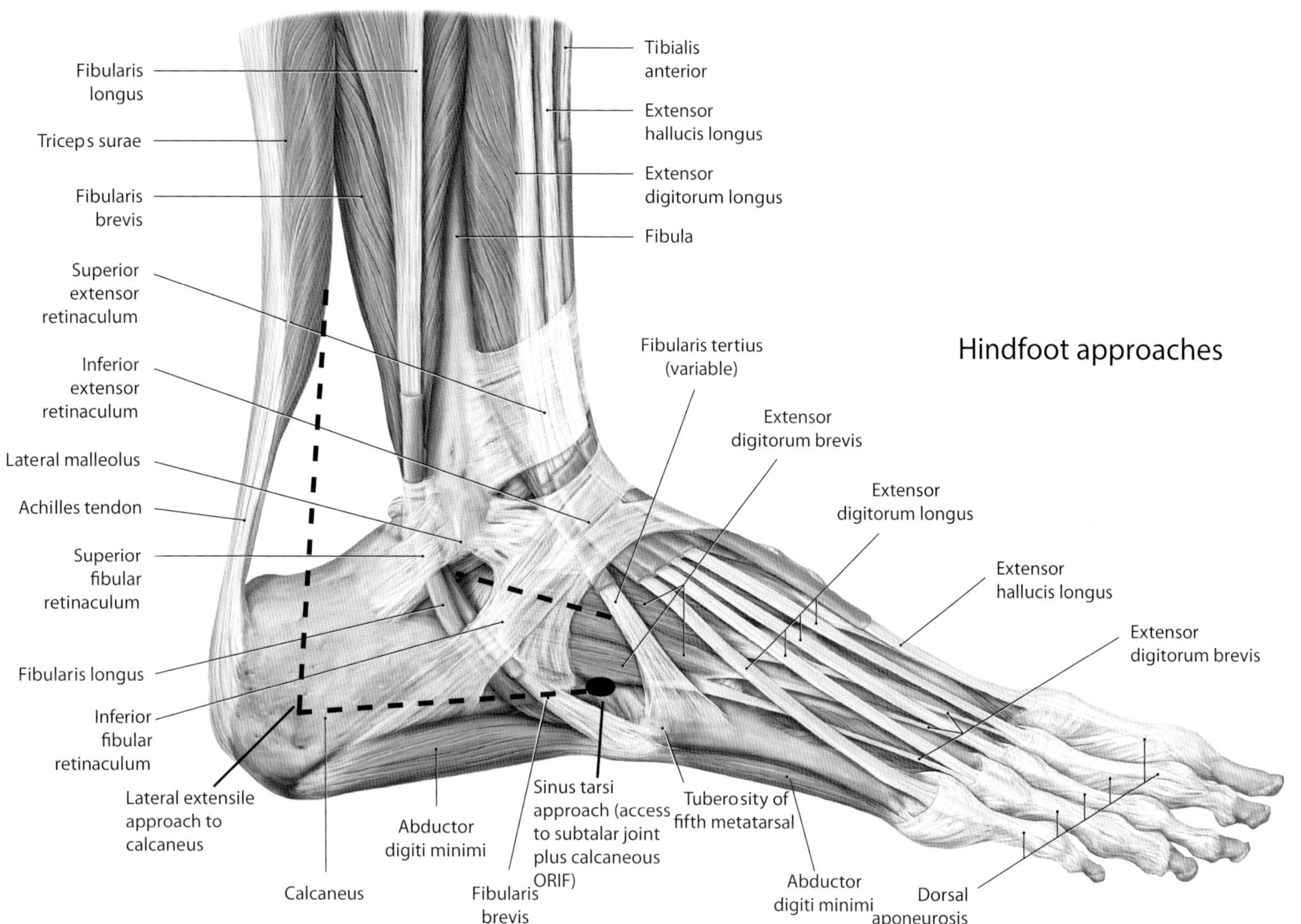

Fig. 10.32 Hindfoot approaches. ORIF, open reduction and internal fixation. (Modified from Schuenke M, Schulte E. General Anatomy and the Musculoskeletal System: Thieme Atlas of Anatomy. New York: Thieme; 2005. Illustration by Karl Wesker.)

Table 10.4 Arthroscopy **(Fig. 10.33)**

Portal Location	Risks
Anterolateral **(Figs. 10.33** and **10.34)**	Dorsal intermediate cutaneous branch of SP nerve
Anteromedial **(Figs 10.33** and **10.35)**	Saphenous nerve and greater saphenous vein
Anterocentral (not recommended) **(Fig. 10.33)**	Dorsalis pedis artery
Posteromedial **(Figs. 10.35** and **10.36)**	Posterior tibial artery and tibial nerve
Posterolateral **(Fig. 10.36)**	Sural nerve

Abbreviation: SP, superficial peroneal.

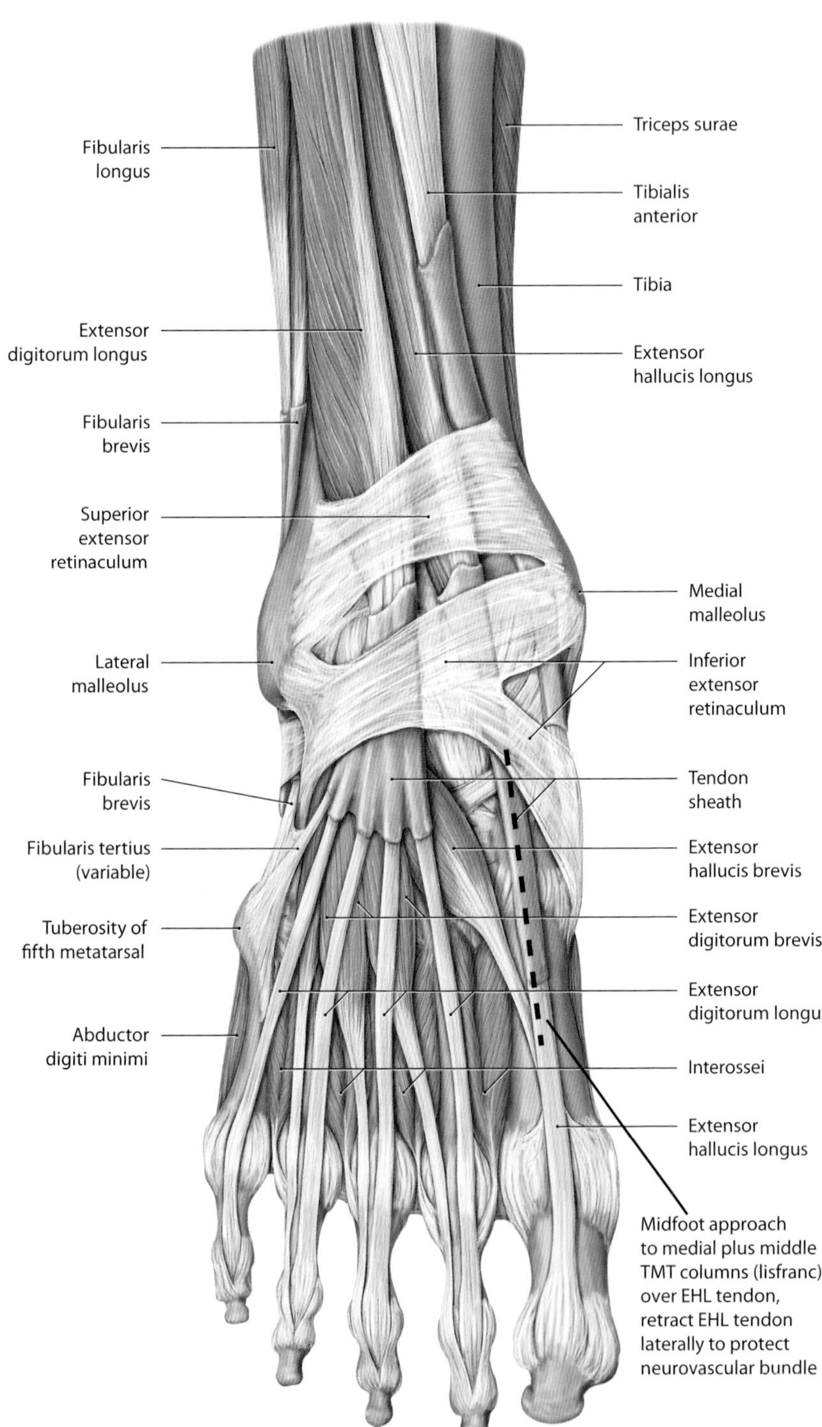

Fig. 10.33 Midfoot approaches. EHL, extensor hallucis longus; TMT, tarsometatarsal. Modified (From Schuenke M, Schulte E. General Anatomy and the Musculoskeletal System: Thieme Atlas of Anatomy. New York: Thieme; 2005. Illustration by Karl Wesker.)

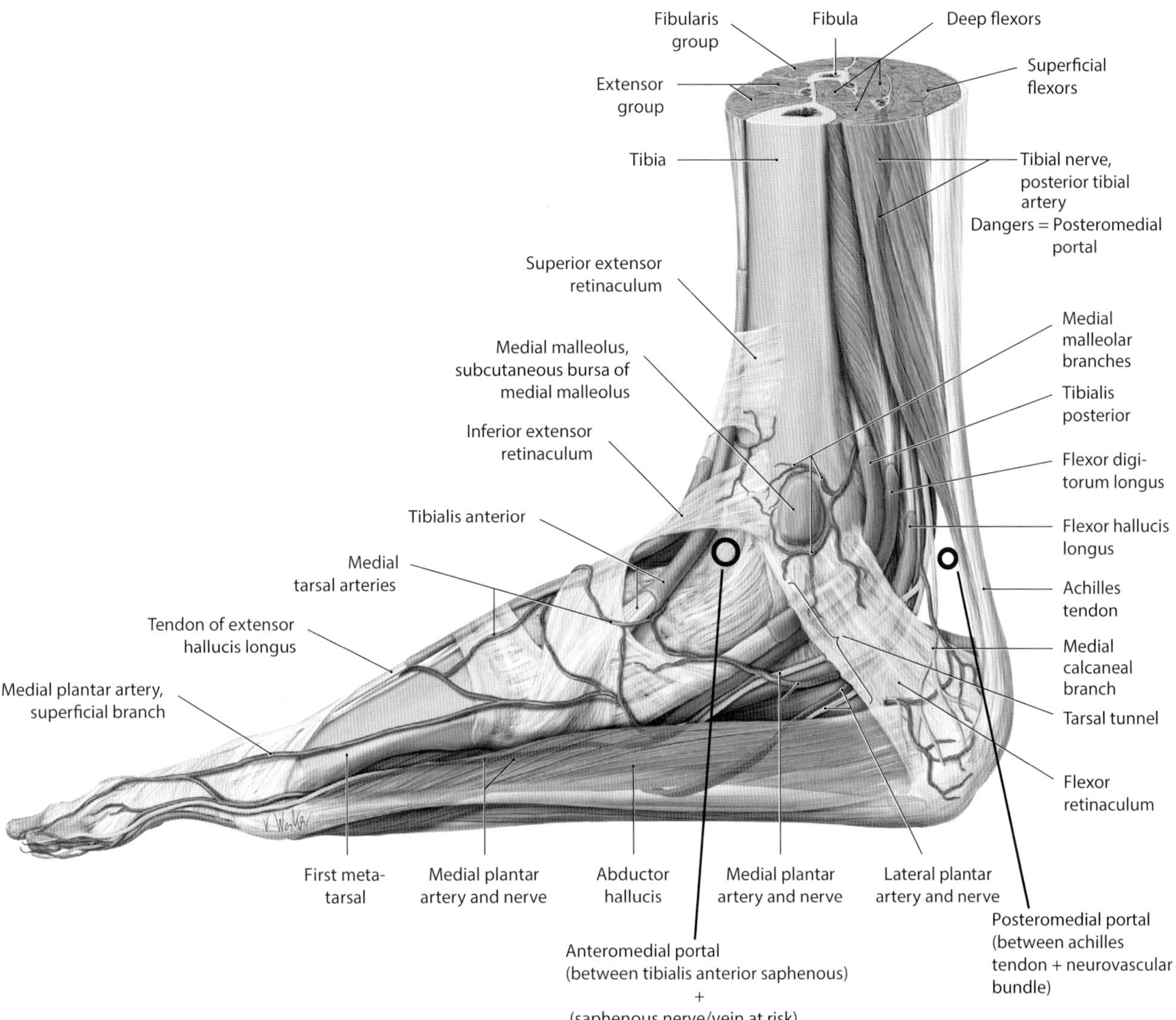

Fig. 10.34 Antroscopy portals/dangers 1. (Modified from Schuenke M, Schulte E. General Anatomy and the Musculoskeletal System: Thieme Atlas of Anatomy. New York: Thieme; 2005. Illustration by Karl Wesker.)

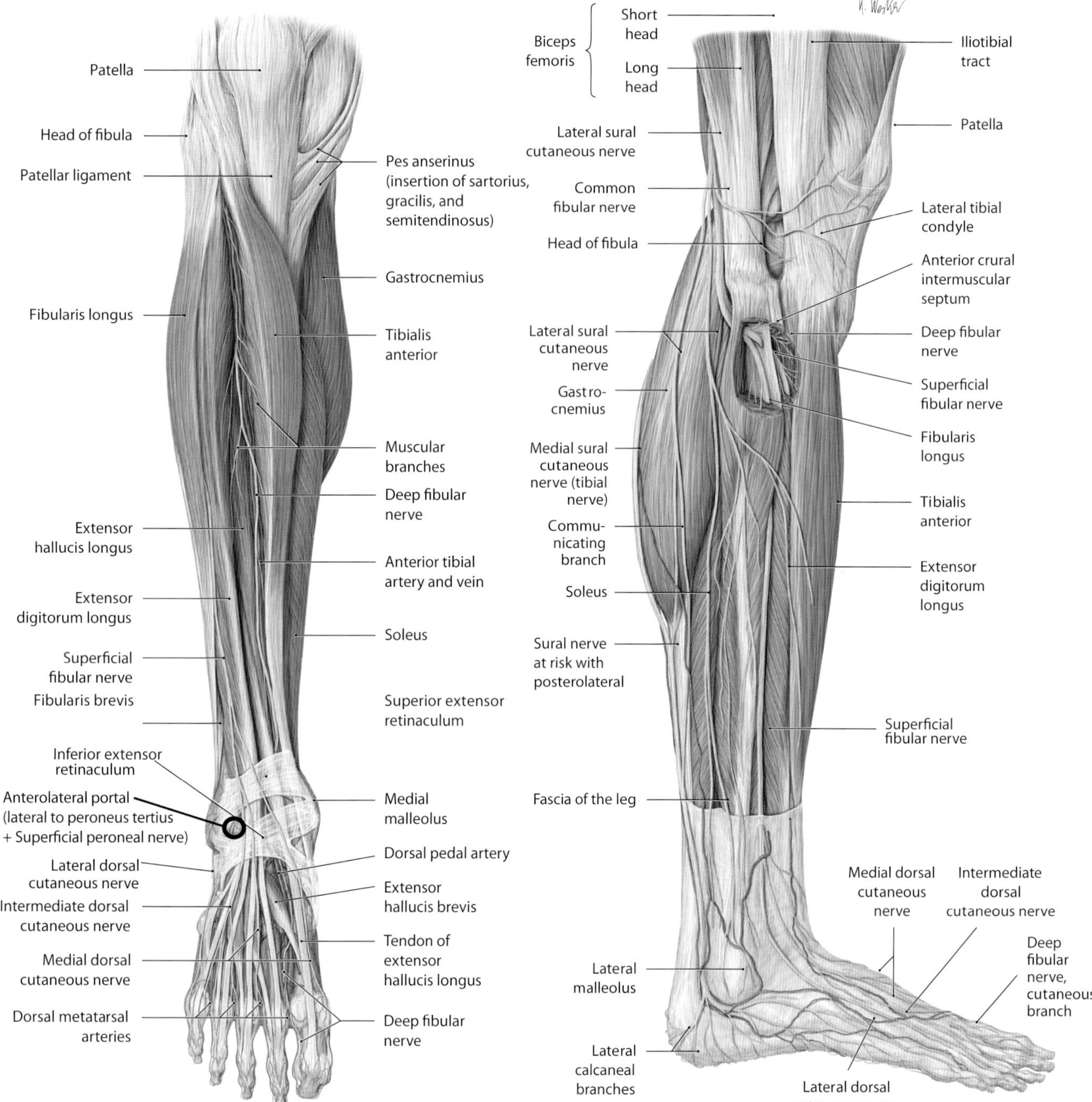

Fig. 10.35 Antroscopy portals/dangers 2. (Modified from Schuenke M, Schulte E. General Anatomy and the Musculoskeletal System: Thieme Atlas of Anatomy. New York: Thieme; 2005. Illustration by Karl Wesker.)

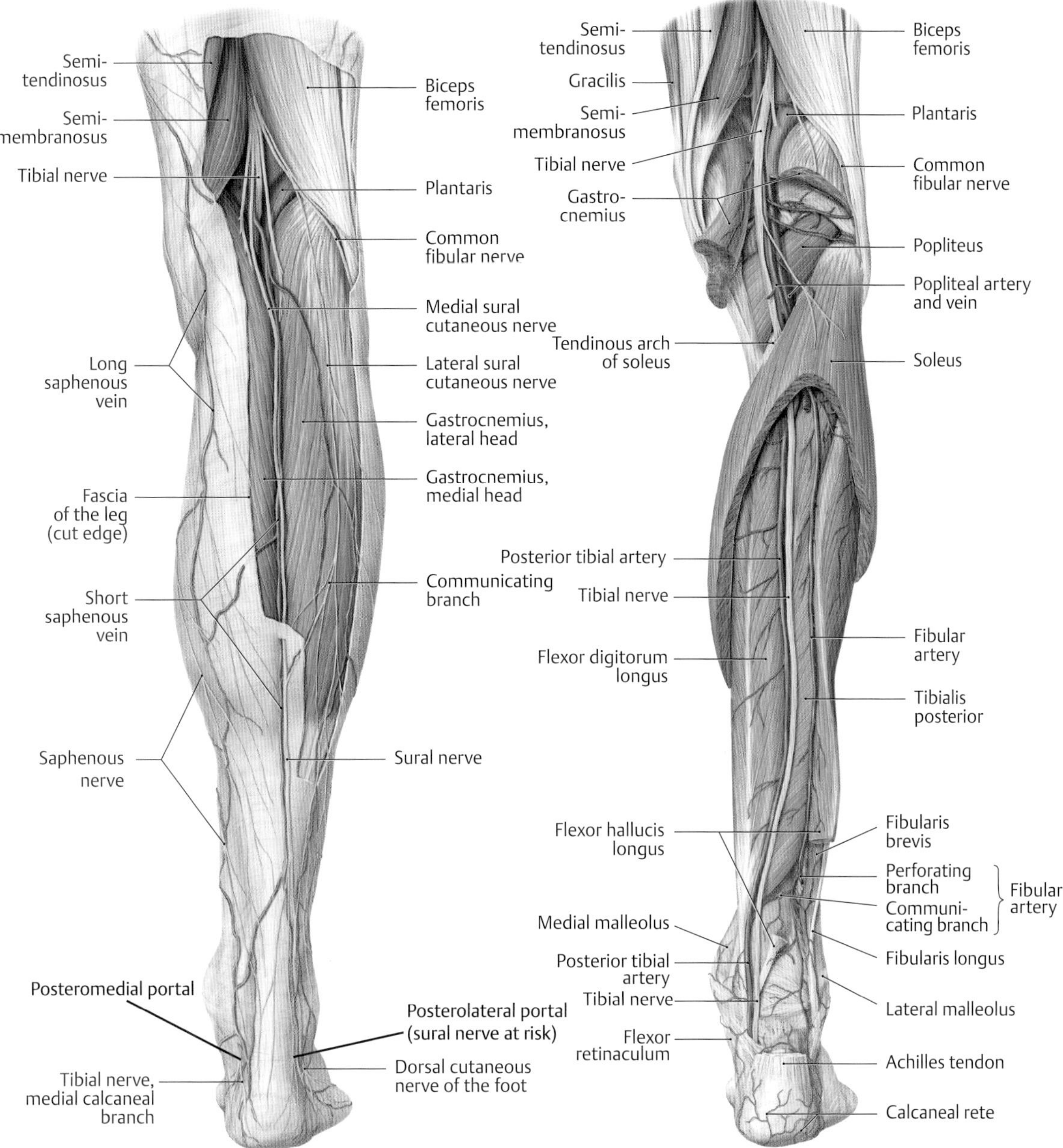

Fig. 10.36 Antroscopy portals/dangers 3. (Modified from Schuenke M, Schulte E. General Anatomy and the Musculoskeletal System: Thieme Atlas of Anatomy. New York: Thieme; 2005. Illustration by Karl Wesker.)

II. Foot and Ankle Biomechanics

1. Ankle
   - Responsible for most sagittal plane motion of the foot and ankle
   - Some contribution to inversion/eversion and rotation
2. Syndesmosis
   - Fibula rotates ~ 2 degrees in the incisura during gait
   - With DF, the distal fibula externally rotates and translates proximally.
3. Hindfoot and midfoot
   - Transverse tarsal joints
     a. Provide stability of the hindfoot/midfoot; rigid lever at heel-rise
     b. During heel-strike (hindfoot valgus, forefoot abduction, and ankle DF), the axes of the transverse tarsal joints are parallel and supple, allowing them to adapt to uneven ground **(Fig. 10.37)**.
     c. During toe-off (hindfoot varus, forefoot adduction, and ankle PF), the axes of these joints diverge. This causes these joints to lock, creating a rigid lever arm during push-off.
        - Failure of the PT tendon to lock the transverse tarsal joints in patients with posterior tibial tendon insufficiency (PTTI) results in an inability to perform single-limb heel-rise.
   - The foot is divided into three columns:
     a. Medial column: first MT, medial cuneiform, navicular
        - Least sagittal plane motion, rigid lever-arm during push-off
     b. Intermediate column: second and third MTs, middle and lateral cuneiforms
     c. Lateral column: fourth and fifth MTs and cuboid
        - Most sagittal plane motion; helps foot adapt to uneven ground
   - Ligamentous stability of the midfoot is provided by the longitudinal and transverse ligaments on the plantar and dorsal surfaces of each joint.
     a. Plantar ligaments are thicker and stronger than dorsal ligaments.
     b. Primary stabilizer of the longitudinal arch: interosseous ligaments
     c. Secondary stabilizer of the longitudinal arch: plantar fascia
   - Lisfranc joint complex is stable due to bony and ligamentous architecture
     a. Middle cuneiform ends more proximally so that the second MT is recessed proximally ("keystone" providing bony stability) **(Fig. 10.38)**
     b. The cuneiforms and medial three MT bases are trapezoidal (wider dorsally than plantarly), allowing for sagittal plane stability with weight bearing.
     c. Dorsal and plantar ligaments extend from the second MT to cuneiforms
        - Largest/strongest of these ligaments is the Lisfranc ligament, which connects the base of the second MT to the medial cuneiform.
        - **Injury to the Lisfranc ligament leads to Lisfranc joint instability.**

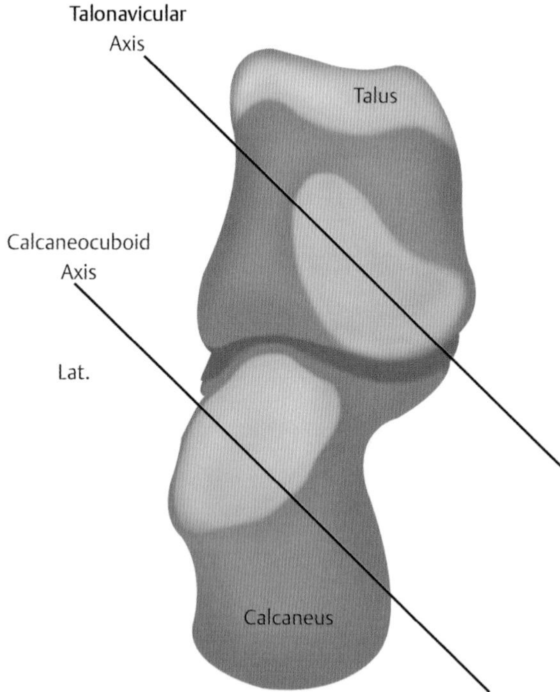

Fig. 10.37 During heel-strike (hindfoot valgus, forefoot abduction, and ankle dorsiflexion), the axes of the transverse tarsal joints are parallel and supple, allowing them to adapt to uneven ground.

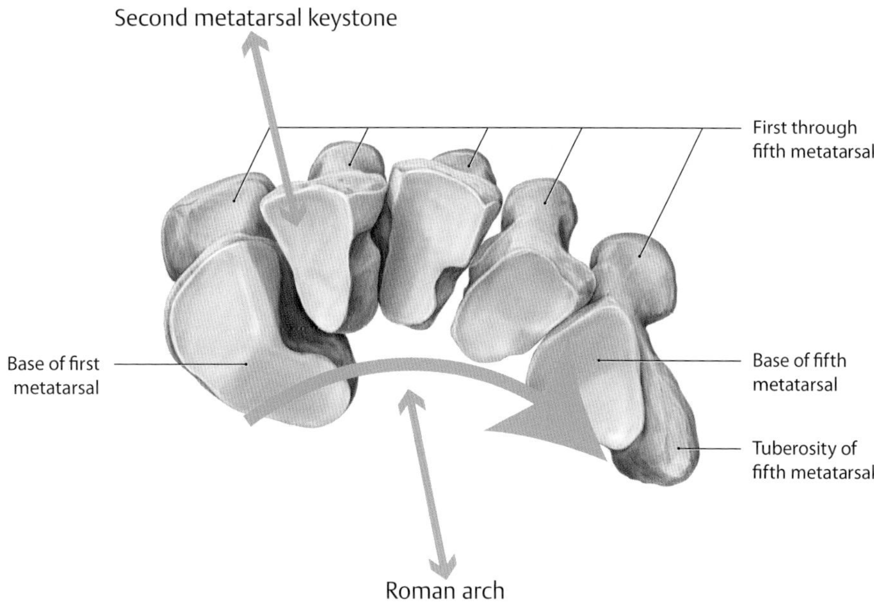

Fig. 10.38 Proximal articular surfaces. Right foot, proximal view. Tarsometatarsal joints: bases of the first through fifth metatarsals. (From Schuenke M, Schulte E. General Anatomy and the Musculoskeletal System: Thieme Atlas of Anatomy. New York: Thieme; 2005. Illustration by Karl Wesker.)

4. Forefoot
   - All structures distal to the TMT joints
   - First MT bears 50% of the weight during gait.
   - The second MT is usually the longest and experiences more stress than the other lesser metatarsals by virtue of its length and stability (constraint).
   - Intrinsic tendons pass plantar to the MTP joint axis proximally (flexion force) and dorsal to the axis distally (extension force).
     a. Weil osteotomy can lead to plantar migration of this center of rotation, and cause a "cock-up" ("floating toe") toe deformity (tendons become dorsal to the MTP axis and hence extend).
   - Loss of intrinsic function from hereditary motor sensory neuropathy (HMSN) [e.g., Charcot-Marie-Tooth (CMT) disease] leads to claw toes.
5. Foot positions versus foot motions
   - Foot positions: varus/valgus (hindfoot), abduction/adduction (midfoot), equinus/calcaneus (ankle)
   - Foot motions (defined in three axes of rotation) **(Fig. 10.39)**
     a. Sagittal plane motion: DF/PF
     b. Coronal plane motion: inversion/eversion
     c. Transverse plane motion: forefoot/midfoot adduction/abduction, ankle/hindfoot internal/external rotation
     d. Triplanar motion
        - Supination: adduction, inversion, PF
        - Pronation: abduction, eversion, DF
     e. If the heel is in a subtalar neutral position, the forefoot should be parallel with the floor to meet the ground flush (plantigrade).
        - If the first ray is elevated, the forefoot is in varus (supination); if the first ray is flexed, the forefoot is in valgus (pronation).
        - In a long-term flatfoot deformity, the forefoot compensates by supinating to attempt to achieve a plantigrade foot.

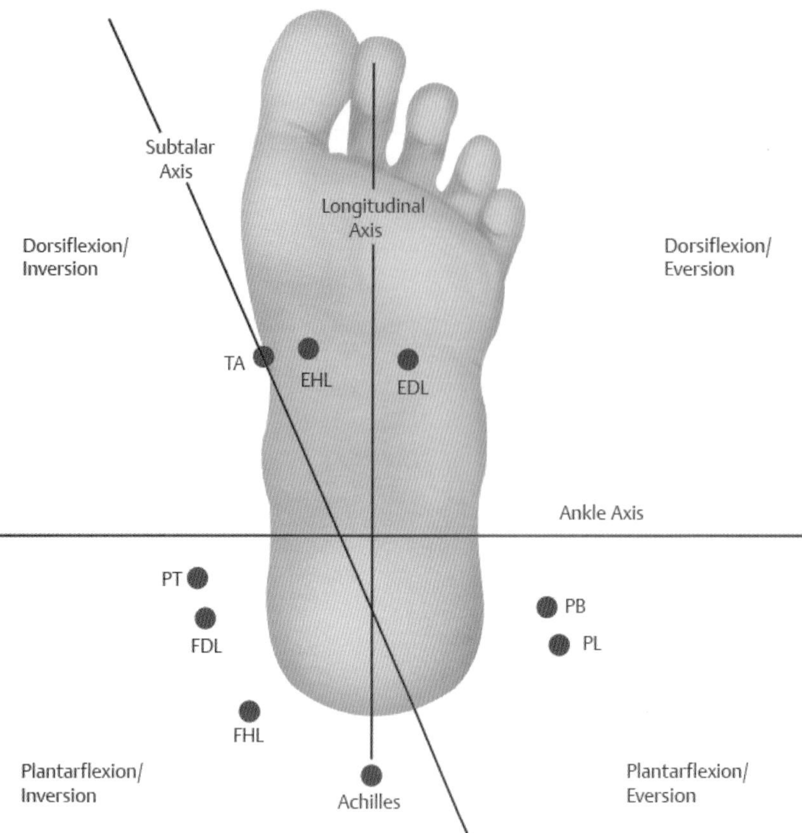

Fig. 10.39 Foot axes and muscles acting in those planes. EDL, extensor digitorum longus; EHL, extensor hallucis longus; FDL, flexor digitorum longus; FHL, flexor hallucis longus; PB, peroneus brevis; PL, peroneus longus; PT, posterior tibialis; TA, tibialis anterior.

III. Physical Examination of the Foot and Ankle

1. Inspection
   - Alignment
     a. Cavovarus: elevated longitudinal arch with hindfoot varus and plantarflexed first ray **(Fig. 10.40)**
     b. Pes planus: flat longitudinal arch with hindfoot valgus **(Fig. 10.41)**
2. Vascular examination
   - If DP and PT pulses are not palpable, consider noninvasive studies
   - Predictive for healing:
     a. Ankle-brachial index (ABI) > 0.5 (normal range, 0.9 to 1.3)
     b. Toe pressure > 40 mm Hg
     c. Transcutaneous oxygen pressure (Tc_{PO_2}) > 40 mm Hg
3. Neurologic examination
   - Sensory examination
     a. Assess all five cutaneous nerves supplying the foot **(Fig. 10.42)**.
     b. Inability to sense a Semmes-Weinstein 5.07 monofilament is most predictive of development of foot ulceration in patients with neuropathy (tests for protective sensation).
   - Motor examination
     a. Keep in mind the location of the tendon in relation to the axis of the ankle.
     b. The following muscles should be tested:
        - Tibialis anterior (L3–4): ankle DF
        - Extensor hallucis longus (L4–5): great toe DF

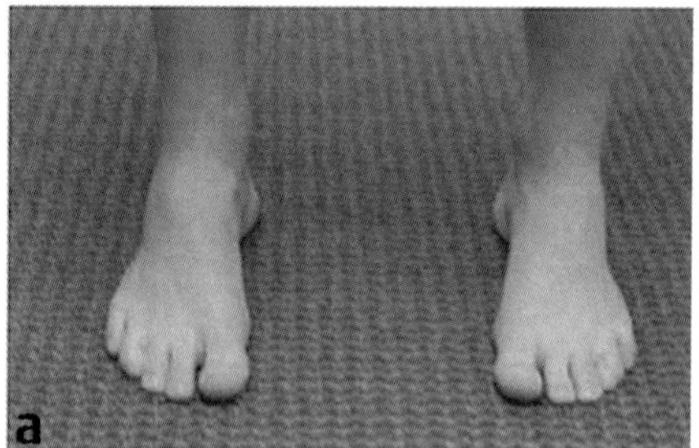

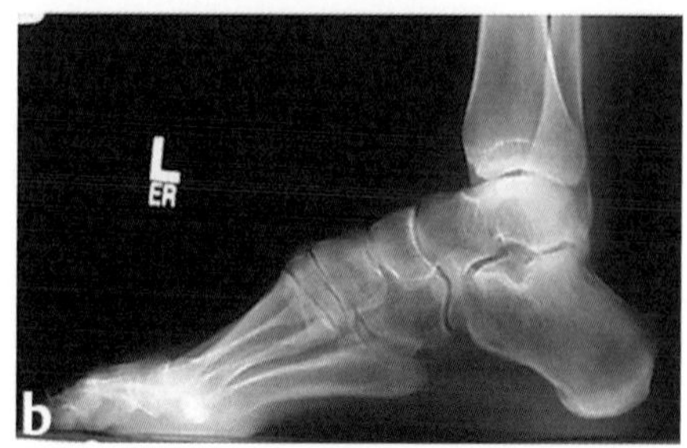

Fig. 10.40 Cavovarus foot. **(a)** Clinical photo. **(b)** Radiograph.

- PL and PB (L5-S1): hindfoot eversion
    - Posterior tibialis (L4–5): hindfoot inversion
    - Gastrocnemius-soleus (S1): ankle PF
  c. Neurologic deficits can be secondary to more proximal etiology
4. Palpation and stability
  - Palpate tendons for swelling, nodules, and subluxation.
  - Tinel's signs can be checked at the following locations:
    a. Tarsal tunnel (tibial nerve)
    b. Anterolateral leg (SP nerve)
    c. Anterior ankle and dorsal hindfoot at inferior extensor retinaculum (DP nerve): anterior tarsal tunnel syndrome
    d. Inferior margin of the abductor hallucis (Baxter's nerve)
  - The web spaces should be palpated for interdigital (Morton's) neuromas and an associated Mulder's sign (palpable click with reproduction of radiating pain when dorsally directed pressure is applied to the plantar web space while compressing the MT heads).
  - Stability of the lateral ankle ligaments can be assessed as follows:
    a. Anterior drawer test:
      - Anteriorly directed pressure on the hindfoot with the ankle in 20 degrees of PF evaluates the ATFL.
      - Test with ankle in neutral/DF evaluates the CFL.
    b. Talar tilt test: > 15 degrees of tilt signifies rupture of both the ATFL and CFL.
      - **Most common acute musculoskeletal injury in dancers: an inversion sprain of the ankle due to relative peroneal muscle weakness**
  - Resisted eversion can reproduce peroneal subluxation/dislocation if the superior peroneal retinaculum has been acutely disrupted.

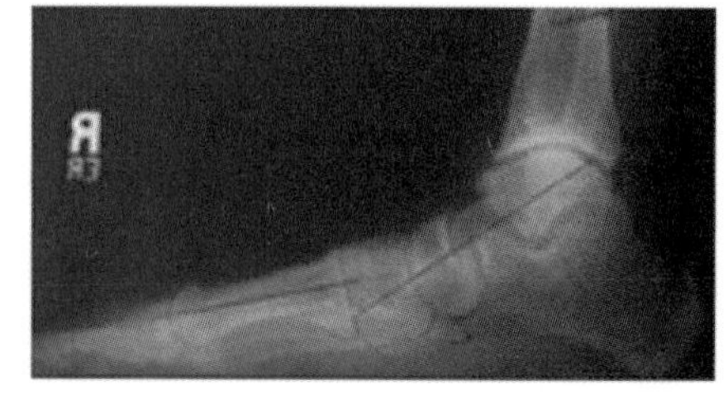

Fig. 10.41 Pes planus radiograph.

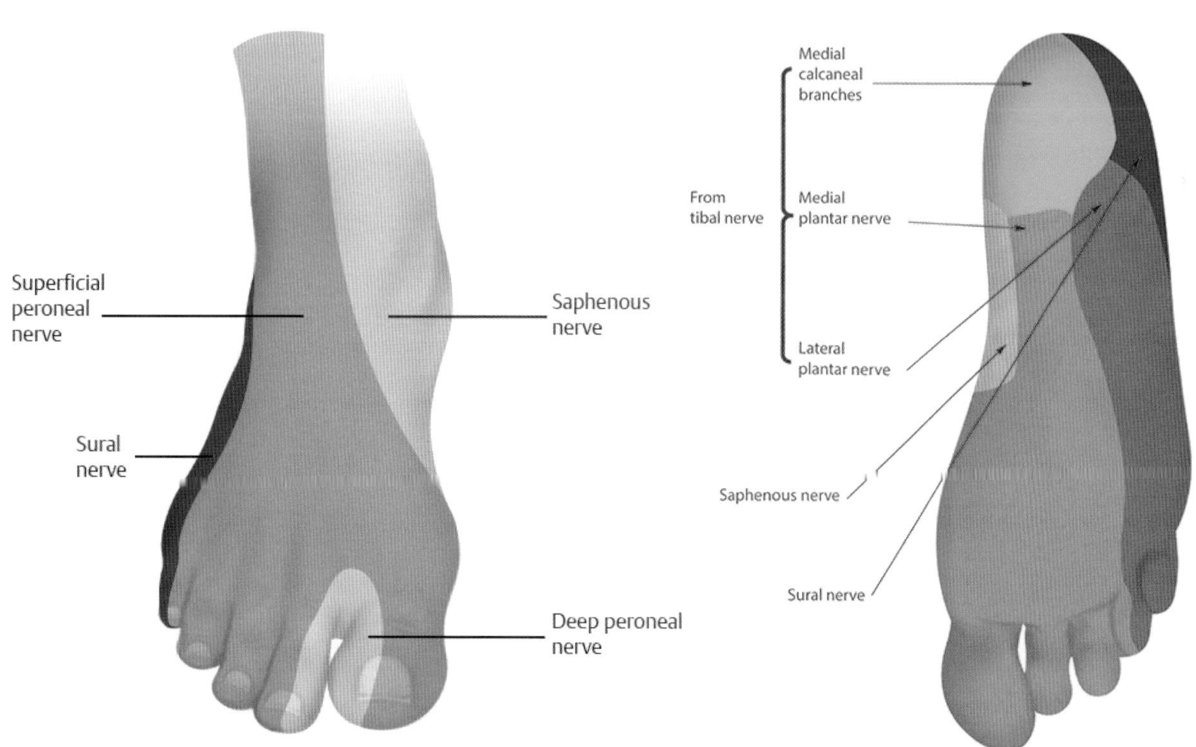

Fig. 10.42 The cutaneous nerves supplying the foot. All the nerves should be assessed.

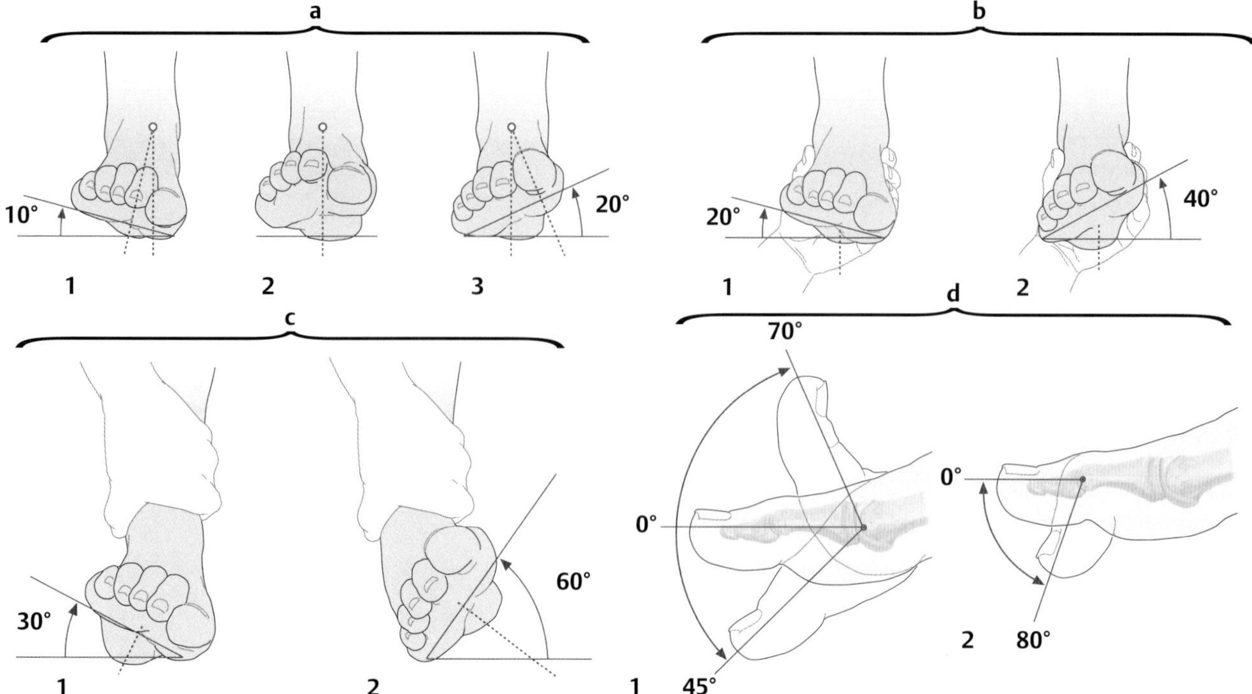

Fig. 10.43 **(a)** Range of motion of the subtalar joint. Right foot, anterior view. 1, everted by 10 degrees; 2, neutral (0-degree) position; 3, inverted by 20 degrees. **(b)** Range of pronation/supination of the transverse tarsal and tarsometatarsal joints. 1, range of pronation of the forefoot: 20 degrees; 2, range of the supination of the forefoot: 40 degrees. **(c)** Total range of motion of the forefoot and hindfoot. Right foot, anterior view. 1, eversion and pronation of the forefoot: 30 degrees; 2, inversion and supination of the forefoot: 60 degrees. **(d)** Range of motion of the joints of the big toe. Lateral view. 1, flexion/extension of the first metatarsophalangeal joint; 2, flexion of the first interphalangeal joint. (From Schuenke M, Schulte E. General Anatomy and the Musculoskeletal System: Thieme Atlas of Anatomy. New York: Thieme; 2005. Illustration by Karl Wesker.)

5. Range of Motion **(Fig. 10.43)**
   - Assess active/passive ROM and compare with the contralateral side.
   - Increased ankle DF can be indicative of an Achilles tendon rupture.
   - Silfverskiöld test: assessment of ankle DF with the hindfoot inverted in positions of full knee flexion and then full knee extension, to differentiate isolated gastrocnemius from combined gastrocnemius and soleus (Achilles) contracture; predicated on the fact that the gastrocnemius takes its origin above the knee
     a. Normally, there should be ~ 10 degrees of DF with the knee extended
     b. With the knee flexed, ankle DF should increase by 10 degrees
        - Increased DF with knee flexion: gastrocnemius contracture
        - Unchanged DF with knee flexion: Achilles contracture

IV. Radiographic Evaluation of the Foot and Ankle

1. Ankle
   - Standard weight-bearing views: anteroposterior (AP), mortise (15 degrees internally rotated), lateral
     a. Normal talocrural angle: 83 ± 4 degrees
     b. Medial clear space = superior clear space ≤ 4 mm
     c. Tibiofibular clear space (between medial wall of fibula and incisural surface of tibia) < 6 mm
   - Gravity or manual external rotation stress can be used to diagnose suspected deltoid ligament and syndesmotic injuries.
   - Anterior drawer and talar tilt views are helpful to diagnose ankle instability.

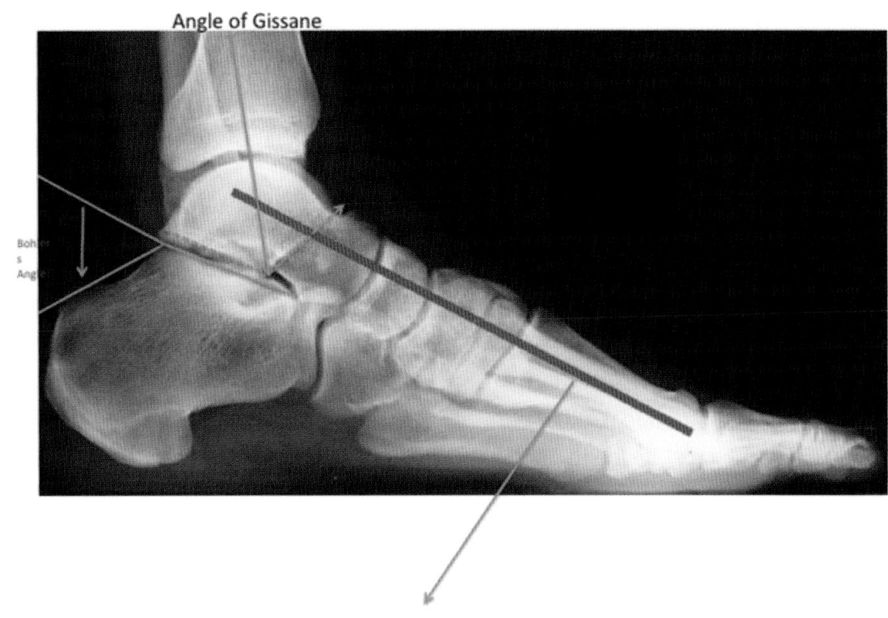

Fig. 10.44 Meary's line (lateral talo–first metatarsal angle).

2. Foot
   - Standard weight-bearing views of the foot: AP (medial and middle column visualized), oblique (middle and lateral column visualized), lateral
     a. On lateral view, sagittal alignment of the foot is assessed using Meary's line (talus-first MT angle) (normal: 0–4 degrees) **(Fig. 10.44)** to diagnose pes planus or cavus.
     b. Angle of Gissane (normal: 95–105 degrees): angle between the lateral margin of the posterior facet and the anterior beak of the calcaneus
     c. Böhler's angle (normal: 20–40 degrees): angle between a line drawn from the highest point of the anterior process to the highest point of the posterior facet and a line drawn tangential to the superior edge of the tuberosity
3. Special views
   - Canale view (maximum equinus, 15 degrees' pronation, X-ray beam directed 75 degrees cephalad from horizontal): optimal talar neck view
   - Harris (axial) view (foot maximally dorsiflexed, beam angled at 45 degrees): assess calcaneal comminution, subtalar joint involvement, heel alignment, loss of height, widening, impingement on peroneal space
   - Broden views (ankle internally rotated 40 degrees, neutral flexion, views taken at 10, 20, 30, and 40 degrees from vertical): primarily allows visualization of the posterior facet of the ST joint (and medial/anterior facets to a lesser degree)
   - Sesamoid view: assess sesamoids and MT–sesamoid articulations
4. Comparison contralateral views, or stress views, should be used in cases of suspected ligamentous injury (Lisfranc, syndesmotic, plantar plate)
5. Imaging procedures
   - Computed tomography (CT): helpful in evaluating complex fractures (pilon, talus, calcaneus, Lisfranc, midfoot) and tarsal coalition
   - MRI: to diagnose stress fractures, osteonecrosis, soft tissue abnormalities (tendon, ligament), neoplasm, and occult osteochondritis dissecans (OCD)
   - Bone scan: to diagnose stress fractures, but MRI is superior (can concomitantly evaluate soft tissue structures)
   - Indium-tagged white blood cell (WBC) scans: to diagnose osteomyelitis (both sensitive and specific)

V. Adult Acquired Flatfoot Deformity (AAFD)

1. Critical to differentiate whether deformity is flexible or fixed
2. PTTI: most common cause of AAFD
   - Posterior tibial tendon (PTT) is primary dynamic support of arch
   - Etiology of PTTI is multifactorial:
     a. Zone of hypovascularity: 2–6 cm from tendon insertion on the navicular
     b. Arch overload from obesity or activity
     c. Inflammatory conditions [e.g., rheumatoid arthritis (RA)]
   - Spring ligament: primary static stabilizer of the TN joint
     a. Spring ligament incompetence can occur as deformity progresses.
        - Superomedial component most commonly attenuated in AAFD
        - Deltoid ligament (merges with spring ligament) may be involved
3. Presentation: medial ankle/foot pain early, progressive loss of arch, lateral ankle pain from subfibular impingement (late finding)
4. Physical examination: hindfoot valgus, loss of arch, forefoot abduction ("too many toes" on posterior view), inability to perform single-leg heel-rise, equinus contracture
   - Due to hindfoot valgus, the Achilles tendon is lateral to the axis of rotation of the subtalar joint and acts as an evertor of the calcaneus.
5. Radiographic examination
   - Negative lateral talo–first MT (Meary) angle
   - Forefoot abduction measured based on talonavicular uncoverage **(Table 10.2)**
6. Treatment: based on stage **(Table 10.5)**
   - **Caution: Flatfoot with normal TN coverage and functioning PTT is likely due to midfoot collapse from a missed Lisfranc injury. Treat with midfoot arthrodesis.**
   - Stage I
     a. Conservative: immobilization, orthotics (e.g., medial heel wedge)
     b. Surgical: synovectomy
   - Stage II
     a. Conservative: ankle–foot orthosis (AFO) or Arizona brace

Table 10.5 Stages of Adult Acquired Flatfoot Deformity

Stage	Deformity	Physical Examination	Radiographs
I	None Tenosynovitis	Able to perform single-leg heel-rise	Normal
IIA	Flatfoot deformity Flexible hindfoot Normal forefoot	Unable to perform single-leg heel-rise Mild sinus tarsi pain	Arch collapse deformity
IIB	Flatfoot deformity Flexible hindfoot Forefoot abduction ("too many toes") (> 30–40% talonavicular uncoverage)		
III	Flatfoot deformity Rigid forefoot abduction Rigid hindfoot valgus	Unable to perform single-leg heel-rise Severe sinus tarsi pain	Arch collapse deformity Subtalar arthritis
IV	Flatfoot deformity Rigid forefoot abduction Rigid hindfoot valgus Deltoid ligament compromise	Unable to perform single-leg heel-rise Severe sinus tarsi pain Ankle pain	Arch collapse deformity Subtalar arthritis Talar tilt in ankle mortise

b. Surgical:
  - FDL transfer (in phase muscle with similar dynamic function)
  - Gastrocnemius recession (if contracture present)
    - ♦ Stage IIA: medializing calcaneal osteotomy (MCO)
    - ♦ Stage IIB: lateral column lengthening (LCL) ± MCO
    - ♦ Stage IIC (fixed forefoot supination/varus): dorsal opening wedge (Cotton) medial cuneiform osteotomy
  - **Cotton osteotomy is used to correct residual forefoot varus after flatfoot reconstruction.**

- Stage III: conservative: AFO or Arizona brace; surgical: triple arthrodesis
- Stage IV:
  a. If ankle valgus is flexible: reconstruction of deltoid ligament and hindfoot
  b. If ankle deformity is rigid: tibiotalocalcaneal arthrodesis

VI. Cavovarus Foot Deformity

1. Definition: high-arched foot, often associated with hindfoot varus (cavovarus)
2. Etiology
   - Neuromuscular (NM)
     a. Unilateral: must rule out spinal cord lesion
     b. Bilateral: most commonly CMT disease
   - Idiopathic: usually bilateral, subtle
   - Traumatic: due to missed compartment syndrome or malunited talus fracture
3. Due to plantarflexed first ray and varus hindfoot
4. Positive "peek-a-boo" sign: visualization of medial side of heel from frontal view **(Fig. 10.45)**
5. Associated with lateral ankle instability, peroneal tendon injury, fifth MT stress fracture
6. Subtle cavus foot conservatively treated with physical therapy and orthotic (lateral hindfoot posting and recession of first MT head)
7. Coleman block test **(Fig. 10.46)** is used to assess hindfoot flexibility.
   - If hindfoot passively corrects when the patient stands on a wooden block placed lateral to the first ray, the varus hindfoot deformity is forefoot-driven.
     a. Treatment: first MT DF osteotomy
   - If the hindfoot does not correct, the deformity is hindfoot-contributing.
     a. Treatment: lateral calcaneal closing-wedge (Dwyer) osteotomy, lateralizing calcaneal osteotomy (LCO), and first MT DF osteotomy (ST arthrodesis for arthritic disease)
8. Charcot-Marie-Tooth (CMT) disease
   - Most common presentation: type I HMSN
   - Inheritance: autosomal dominant, chromosome 17 duplication (peripheral myelin protein)
   - TA and PB weakness overpowered by antagonist PL and PT, respectively
   - **TA is antagonist to PL; PT is antagonist to PB.**
   - PF of the first ray occurs due to the PL overpowering the TA
   - Intrinsic wasting: attempted compensation by the extrinsics (EHL, EDL, FHL, FDL) leads to claw-toe deformity.

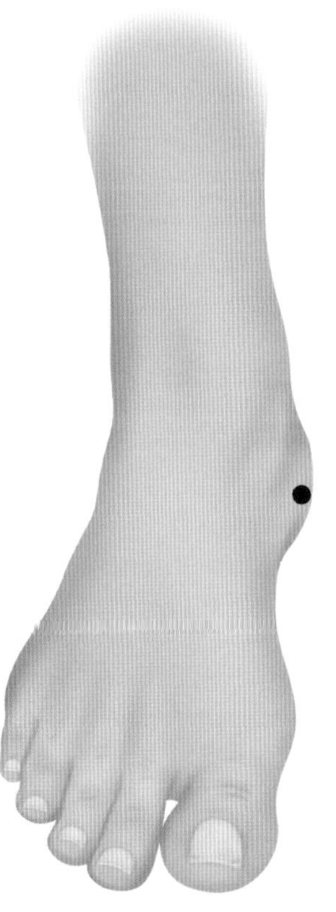

Fig. 10.45 "Peek-a-boo" heel in cavovarus foot deformity.

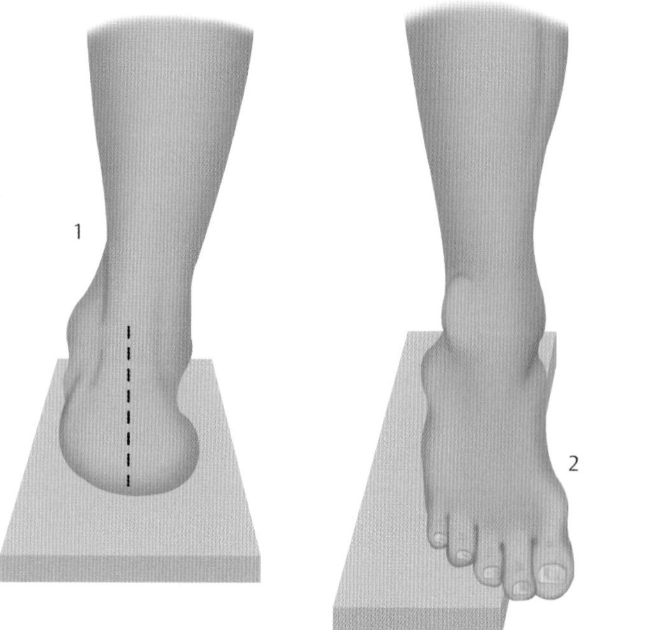

Fig. 10.46 Correction of hindfoot varus with Coleman block test (indicating forefoot-driven deformity). Hindfoot axis *(dashed line)* demonstrates correction from varus to physiologic valgus.

- Weakness of the TA leads to extensor (EDL and EHL) recruitment during the swing phase of gait, exacerbating claw-toe deformity
- Treatment of a flexible deformity (forefoot-driven hindfoot varus) involves dorsiflexion osteotomy of the first MT, transfer of PL into the PB at the level of the distal fibula, and plantar fascia release.
  a. In adolescents with flexible deformity and closed physes, surgical treatment is recommended due to the progressive nature of this disease.
- Fixed deformity (does not correct with Coleman block test)
  a. Conservative treatment can be attempted (AFO, rocker sole)
  b. Surgical treatment: LCO
    - Triple arthrodesis usually required for hindfoot correction

9. Poliomyelitis (see Chapters 4 and 11)
   - Postpolio syndrome may occur; affects about half of those with poliomyelitis

VII. Diabetic Foot Disorders

1. Pathophysiology/etiology
   - Diabetic neuropathy
     a. Sensory neuropathy
       - Polyneuropathic loss of sensation begins in a stocking-glove distribution and progresses proximally.
       - If unable to perceive a Semmes-Weinstein 5.07 monofilament, 90% of patients have lost protective sensation of their feet.
       - Medicare's Therapeutic Shoe Bill: covers extra-depth shoes and total contact inserts (three per year) for ulcer prevention in neuropathic patients
     b. Motor neuropathy
       - Most often involves the common peroneal nerve: foot drop
       - Foot intrinsics also frequently involved: claw toes
     c. Autonomic neuropathy → abnormal sweating mechanism → dry foot susceptible to fissuring cracks → portals for infection

- Peripheral vascular disease
  a. Both large and small vessels in 60–70% of patients with diabetes mellitus (DM) > 10 years
  b. Noninvasive vascular studies (essential when pulses absent):
    - Waveforms (normal: triphasic)
    - ABI: minimum value for healing: 0.5
      - Calcified vessels falsely increase ABI (> 1.3 nonphysiological)
    - Absolute toe pressures: minimum for healing: 40 mm Hg; normal: 100 mm Hg
    - Transcutaneous oxygen pressure: > 40 mm Hg
  c. Absence of hair on the toes is predictive of poor healing.
- Immune system impairment
- Metabolic deficiency
  a. Poor healing potential is indicated by total protein < 6.0 g/dL, total lymphocyte count < 1,500/mm^3, or albumin < 3.0 g/dL.

2. Clinical problems
- Ulcers
  a. Etiology: due to neuropathy and excess pressure on the plantar foot
  b. Primary risk factor for development of diabetic foot ulcer: loss of protective sensation as tested with a Semmes-Weinstein 5.07 monofilament.
  c. The rocker sole best reduces forefoot plantar pressure.
  d. Wagner-Meggitt classification (based on depth and ischemia)
    - Depth
      - Grade 0: skin intact with bony deformity, redness
        - Treatment: shoe modification (extra-depth shoe)
      - Grade 1: superficial ulcer, no exposed tendon or bone
        - Treatment: bedside incision and drainage (I&D), total-contact cast
      - Grade 2: deep ulcer with exposed tendon/joint capsule
        - Treatment: operative I&D, followed by dressing changes and total-contact casting once wound bed is healthy
        - **Grade 2 ulcer under first MT head that fails conservative management should be treated with gastrocnemius recession and PL to PB transfer.**
      - Grade 3: extensive ulcer with exposed bone (osteomyelitis by definition) or abscess
        - Treatment: same as that for grade 2
        - Partial calcanectomy is indicated for a patient with a grade 3 heel ulcer, calcaneal osteomyelitis, loss of protective sensation, and palpable pulses, who has failed conservative management.
        - No MRI needed (exposed bone: osteomyelitis)
    - Ischemia
      - Grade A: normal vascularity
      - Grade B: ischemia without gangrene
        - Noninvasive vascular studies; revascularization if indicated
      - Grade C: partial (forefoot) gangrene
        - Noninvasive vascular studies; revascularization if indicated
        - Measure albumin and total protein
          - If levels abnormal, improve nutritional status of patient preoperatively
        - Surgical treatment: partial foot amputation

- Grade D: complete foot gangrene
  - Treatment: below-knee amputation (BKA)

e. Associated equinus contracture is very common.
  - Achilles lengthening should be performed for:
    - Recurrent forefoot/midfoot ulceration
    - Ulceration with equinus deformity
    - **Patients with gastrocnemius contracture on Silfverskiöld testing and plantar forefoot ulcer should have a gastrocnemius recession.**

f. Goal: ulcer-free, functional, plantigrade foot that can fit in a brace/shoe
  - Treatment of chronic neuropathic ulcers without evidence of infection: total contact casting

- Charcot arthropathy

a. Presentation: chronic, progressive, destructive process altering bony architecture and joint alignment in patients lacking protective sensation

b. The process from bony resorption/fragmentation to bone formation/consolidation takes 6–18 months

c. Swelling/erythema/warmth typically resolve in the morning and after a short period of elevation, as opposed to osteomyelitis or abscess

d. Charlot: swelling/erythema/warmth improves with elevation (this is explained in part C).

e. Classification
  - Eichenholtz **(Table 10.6)**
  - Location:
    - Type 1: midfoot (most common)
    - Type 2: hindfoot
    - Type 3: tibiotalar joint

f. Treatment goal: achieve stage 3 (see **Table 10.6**) while maintaining alignment (prevent further collapse), ambulatory status, and soft tissue integrity
  - Initial treatment: immobilization/non–weight bearing (NWB)
    - Total-contact cast is best initially; transition to custom Charcot restraint orthotic walker (CROW) later when edema has subsided
  - Surgical management reserved for recurrent ulceration/deep infection or gross malalignment:
    - Stable deformity: ostectomy of plantar bony (usually cuboid) prominence
    - Unstable/unbraceable deformity: realignment arthrodesis; tendo-Achilles lengthening (TAL) almost always required
    - Amputation if all other measures fail

Table 10.6 Eichenholtz Classification of Charcot Arthropathy

Stage	Signs/Symptoms	Radiographs
0 (prefragmentation)	Acute inflammation (confused with infection)	Regional bone demineralization
1 (fragmentation)		Regional bone demineralization, periarticular fragmentation, joint dislocation
2 (coalescence)	Less inflammation	Absorption of bony debris, early bone healing, periosteal new bone formation
3 (resolution)	Resolved inflammation	Smoothed bone edges, bony/fibrous ankylosis

- Diabetic foot infections
  a. MRI has a high false-positive rate in the diagnosis of osteomyelitis, especially in the presence of concurrent Charcot arthropathy **(Table 10.6)**.
  b. WBC-labeled scan or dual-image technetium/indium scan is more sensitive and specific for osteomyelitis than a conventional bone scan.
  c. Deep surgical cultures (or bone biopsy) needed to identify organism
  d. Treatment
     - Broad-spectrum antibiotics after obtaining surgical cultures, then narrow antibiotic coverage based on culture results
     - Abscesses: surgical drainage and antibiotics
     - Osteomyelitis: culture-specific IV antibiotics based on bone biopsy; surgical resection of infected bone if antibiotics fail
  e. Amputation level (also see Chapter 11)
     - Transmetatarsal: no tendon transfer required; lowest energy expenditure
     - Lisfranc: must transfer peroneals to the cuboid to prevent varus, and lengthen the Achilles to prevent equinus
     - Chopart: must transfer TA to the talus and lengthen the Achilles to prevent equinus
     - Syme:
       - ♦ Lower energy expenditure than Lisfranc/Chopart amputations
       - ♦ Requires viable, uninvolved plantar heel fat pad (blood supply: branches of posterior tibial artery)
  f. Total-contact casting transfers plantar weight-bearing forces to the calf/leg
     - Maintain alignment; reduce edema and pressure on bony prominences
     - Indicated for ulcer with a healthy wound bed

VIII. Hallux Valgus

1. Adult hallux valgus
   - Definition: lateral deviation of great toe with medial deviation of first MT
   - Etiology: multifactorial
     a. Intrinsic factors: genetic predisposition (94% with a family history have maternal transmission), ligamentous laxity, anatomy (convex MT head)
     b. Extrinsic factors: shoe wear (narrow toe box, high heels)
   - Pathoanatomy **(Figs. 10.47** and **10.48)**
     a. Medial capsular attenuation
     b. Plantar-lateral migration of AbH leads to plantarflexion/pronation of phalanx.
        - Lateral translation of the plantar flexors causes them to exert valgus force on the MTP joint.
     c. Lateral deviation of the EHL and FHL causes valgus progression and pronation of the great toe.
     d. First MT head moves medially off the sesamoids, increasing the intermetatarsal angle (IMA).
     e. Secondary contracture of the lateral capsule, adductor hallucis (AdH), lateral MT-sesamoid ligament and intermetatarsal ligament
   - Radiographs **(Figs. 10.49** and **10.50)**
     a. Hallux valgus angle (HVA): angle formed by line along first MT shaft and line along shaft of proximal phalanx
        - Normal: < 15 degrees

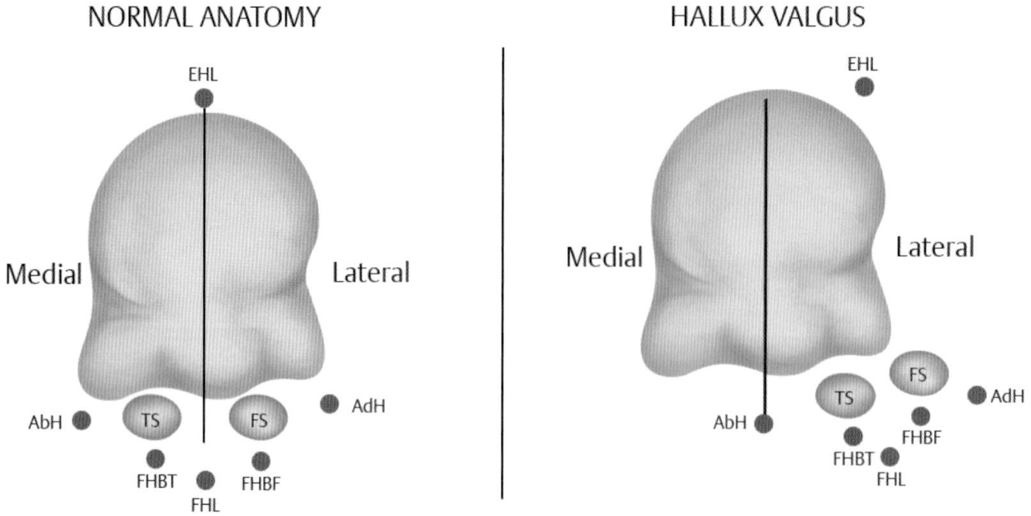

NORMAL ANATOMY
EHL
Medial
Lateral
AbH
TS
FS
AdH
FHBT
FHL
FHBF

HALLUX VALGUS
EHL
Medial
Lateral
FS
TS
AdH
AbH
FHBF
FHBT
FHL

Fig. 10.47 Flexor hallucis brevis to tibial sesamoid. AbH, abductor hallucis; AdH, adductor hallucis; EHL, extensor hallucis longus; FHBF, hallucis brevis to fibular seasmoid; FHBT, flexor hallucis brevis to tibial sesamoid; FHL, flexor hallucis longus; FS, fibular sasamoid.TS, tibial sesamoid.

b. First-second IMA: angle formed by line along first MT shaft and line along second MT shaft
   - Normal: < 9 degrees

c. Hallux valgus interphalangeus (HVI) angle: angle formed by line along shaft of proximal phalanx and line along shaft of distal phalanx
   - Normal: < 10 degrees
   - Associated with a congruent deformity

d. Distal metatarsal articular angle (DMAA): angle between line along the first MT articular surface and line perpendicular to axis of the first MT
   - Normal: < 10 degrees
   - Associated with a congruent deformity

e. First MTP joint congruity is determined by comparing the line connecting the medial and lateral edge of the first MT head articular surface with the corresponding line for the proximal phalanx **(Fig. 10.51)**
   - When these lines are parallel, the joint is congruent.
   - When these lines are divergent, the joint is incongruent.

f. In chronic or severe deformities, sesamoids are often displaced laterally.

g. If the first MTP joint is arthritic/ankylosed, a first MTP arthrodesis is warranted.

- Surgical procedures

a. The appropriate surgical treatment is based on the nature and severity of the underlying deformity.

b. Osteotomies should not be performed in isolation, to decrease recurrence rate. Other procedures include:
   - Distal soft tissue release (modified McBride)
   - Medial eminence resection and capsular imbrication

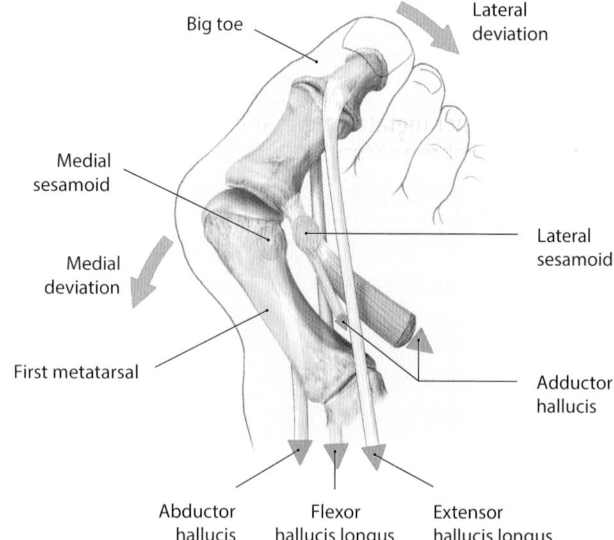

Fig. 10.48 Pathogenic mechanism of hallux valgus. (From Schuenke M, Schulte E. General Anatomy and the Musculoskeletal System: Thieme Atlas of Anatomy. New York: Thieme; 2005. Illustration by Karl Wesker.)

c. Treatment
   - IMA < 13 degrees and HVA < 40 degrees: distal MT (e.g., chevron) osteotomy, distal soft tissue release, medial eminence resection, and capsular imbrication
   - IMA > 13 degrees or HVA > 40 degrees: proximal MT osteotomy (e.g., scarf) distal soft tissue release, medial eminence resection, and capsular imbrication
   - Instability or degenerative joint disease (DJD) of the first TMT joint: Lapidus procedure (first TMT realignment arthrodesis)
     - ♦ Anatomic PF of first MT with a Lapidus procedure is needed to prevent excessive loading of the lesser MTs.
   - Arthritic first MTP or spasticity: first MTP arthrodesis
   - Increased DMAA: distal MT redirectional osteotomy and MT translational osteotomy (biplanar)
   - HVI: proximal phalanx medial closing wedge (Akin) osteotomy

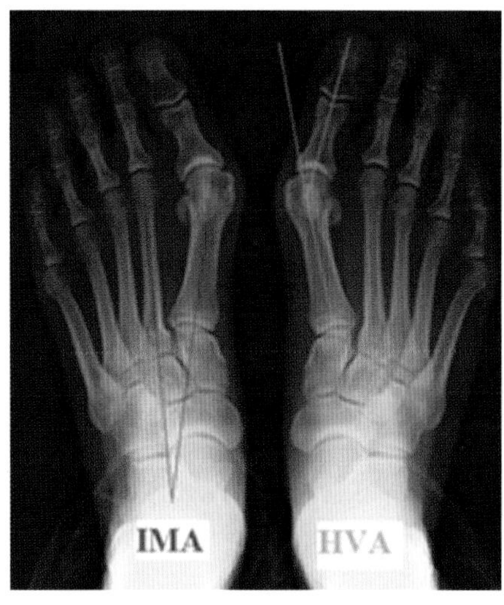

Fig. 10.49 Intermetatarsal angle (IMA) and hallux valgus angle (HVA).

- Surgical complications
  a. Avascular necrosis (AVN)
     - Distal MT osteotomy and lateral soft tissue release may be performed simultaneously without increased risk of AVN.
     - Avoid disruption of blood supply to MT head.
     - AVN: treat with first MTP fusion (bone block to restore length).
  b. Recurrence is associated with undercorrection of the IMA, high preoperative IMA and HVA, isolated soft tissue procedures or medial eminence resection, rounded first MT head, and lateral displacement of tibial sesamoid.
  c. Dorsal malunion
     - Produces transfer metatarsalgia
     - Associated with Lapidus and proximal crescentic osteotomy
     - Treatment: plantarflexion osteotomy
  d. Hallux varus can occur with:
     - Resection of fibular sesamoid (original McBride)
     - Over-resection of the medial eminence
     - Excessive lateral release
     - Overcorrection of the IMA
  e. Nonunion (highest risk associated with a Lapidus procedure)
  f. Transfer metatarsalgia: shortening (e.g., Weil, Maceira) osteotomy of the second MT should be performed if there is abnormal pressure over the longer second MT.

2. Juvenile and adolescent hallux valgus
   - Presentation: different from adult hallux valgus; varus of the first MT with a large IMA is commonly present
   - Frequently positive family history
   - Treatment
     a. If IMA ≤ 13 degrees, biplanar distal chevron osteotomy is sufficient
     b. If IMA > 13 degrees, must also do open-wedge medial cuneiform osteotomy
     c. Proximal medial cuneiform osteotomy in patients with open first MT physis
        - If arthrodesis of the first TMT is required for laxity, intervention is delayed until first MT physeal closure.
   - Complication: recurrence is most common

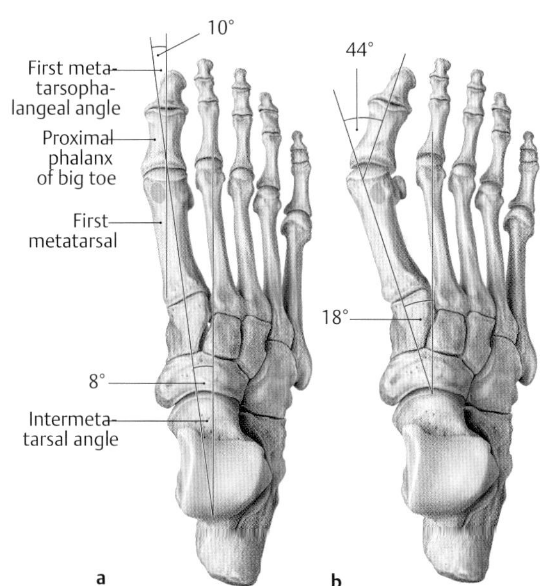

Fig. 10.50 Change in the first intermetatarsal angel and the first metatarsophalangeal angle in hallux valgus. Right foot, superior view. **(a)** Skelton of a normal right foot. **(b)** Lateral deviation of the first ray with subluxation of the metatarsophalangeal joint in hallux valgus. (From Schuenke M, Schulte E. General Anatomy and the Musculoskeletal System: Thieme Atlas of Anatomy. New York: Thieme; 2005. Illustration by Karl Wesker.)

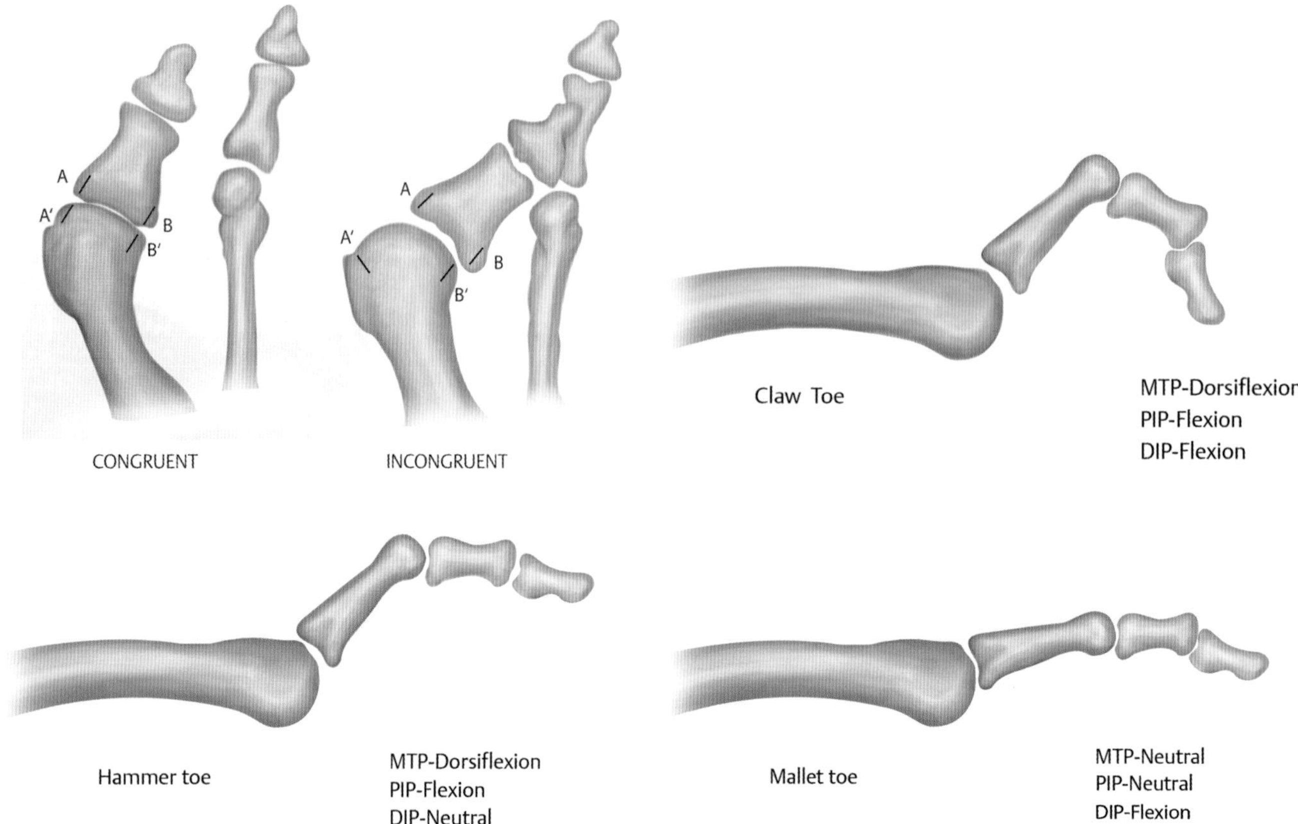

Fig. 10.51 Determination of congruency in hallux valgus deformity. If A and B on metatarsal head articular cartilage line up with A and B on proximal phalanx, then the deformity is congruent.

IX. Other First Metatarsophalangeal Disorders

1. Hallux (first MTP osteoarthritis)
   - Presentation: tenderness, limited DF due to large dorsal osteophyte, pain with grind test

   a. Classification
      - Grade 0: normal X-ray, decreased range of motion (ROM)
      - Grade I: mild osteophyte, joint space preserved, pain at extremes of ROM
      - Grade II: moderate osteophyte, joint space narrowing (< 50%)
      - Grade III: severe osteophyte formation, joint space narrowing (> 50%), significant pain but not at midrange
      - Grade IV: same as grade III with pain throughout ROM

   b. Conservative management
      - Orthotic treatment: stiff foot plate with Morton's extension

   c. Surgical management
      - Grades I and II: dorsal cheilectomy with joint debridement; consider Moberg osteotomy to increase dorsiflexion
      - Grades III and IV: gold standard—first MTP arthrodesis
      - **Young active patient with grade IV hallux rigidus are treated with a first MTP arthrodesis.**
        - ♦ Some authorities also argue that grade III with > 50% of MT head cartilage remaining can be treated with cheilectomy.

- ♦ Optimal position: neutral rotation, 10–15 degrees DF, slight valgus
  - ▪ Fuse too straight: difficulty with running
  - ▪ Fuse in valgus: excessive pressure on second toe
- ◦ Resection (Keller) of first MTP arthroplasty is only indicated for minimally ambulatory elderly patients with grade IV disease.
  - ♦ Risks: cock-up toe deformity, transfer metatarsalgia, and inability to bear weight
- ◦ Implant arthroplasty is not recommended due to poor results (e.g., aseptic loosening, mechanical failure)
  - ♦ Silastic arthroplasty: synovitis with joint destruction
    - ▪ Treatment: implant removal and synovectomy

2. Hallux varus
   - Etiology: often iatrogenic; secondary to overcorrection of hallux valgus, excessive lateral release, resection of fibular sesamoid
   - Conservative management: taping of great toe to lateral forefoot to prevent varus deviation
   - Surgical management
     a. Flexible deformity
        - ◦ Release of AbH, medial capsule, and fascia
        - ◦ Transfer of portion of EHL or EHB under transverse intermetatarsal ligament to the distal MT neck (lateral to medial)
        - ◦ Consider MT osteotomy
     b. Rigid deformity: treat with first MTP arthrodesis
3. Sesamoid problems
   - Anatomy
     a. Hallucal sesamoids lie within the two heads of the FHB tendon, separated by the crista (intersesamoid ridge)
     b. Other sesamoid attachments: plantar plate, MTP collateral ligaments, metatarsosesamoid ligaments, intersesamoid ligament, AbH and AdH
     c. Sesamoids increase the mechanical advantage of the intrinsics (FHB)
     d. Sesamoids dissipate the forces beneath the first MT head
   - Turf toe
     a. Pathogenesis: injury occurs due to forced DF, causing avulsion of the plantar plate from the base of the phalanx, leading to proximal sesamoid migration
     b. Treatment
        - ◦ Grade 1: capsular strain—stiff insole, taping, return to play
        - ◦ Grade 2: partial capsular tear—stiff insole, no athletics for 2 weeks, return to play when able to painlessly dorsiflex 60 degrees
        - ◦ Grade 3: complete tear—surgical repair
     c. Sesamoid fracture: treat with fracture boot initially, transition to sesamoid relief pad (dancer's pad), gradual return to activity
        - ◦ Symptomatic nonunions can be treated with bone grafting or partial or complete sesamoidectomy.
          - ♦ Complication of tibial sesamoid excision: hallux valgus
          - ♦ Complication of fibular sesamoid excision: hallux varus
          - ♦ Complication of excision of both sesamoids: cock-up deformity
        - ◦ Excision of the distal pole produces best results
     d. Medial sesamoid fragmentation: best treated with surgical excision
     e. Sesamoiditis: treat with anti-inflammatories
     f. Tibial sesamoid is more likely to be involved in trauma, also more likely to be bi- or multipartite

X. Lesser Toe Disorders

1. Anatomy and function
   - Stability of the lesser toes is provided by:
     a. Congruency of the MTP and interphalangeal (IP) joints
     b. Plantar plate: prevents MTP hyperextension and MT head depression
     c. Dynamic stability: tendons inserting on lesser toes [extrinsics: EDL, flexors; intrinsics: EDB, lumbricals, interossei (four dorsal, three plantar)]
        - EDL is primary extensor of the MTP joint
        - EDB extends the proximal interphalangeal (PIP) joint
        - FDL is primary plantar flexor of distal interphalangeal (DIP) joint
        - FDB is primary plantar flexor of PIP joint
        - Intrinsics flex the MTP joint and extend the IP joints
          - Pull of intrinsics is plantar to MTP joint's rotational axis
            - Plantar translation of MT head after distal MT osteotomy leads to intrinsics dorsal to axis of rotation of MTP joint, which results in "floating toe" deformity
   - Lesser toe deformities occur much more commonly in women (5:1) due to wearing high heels that are too narrow for the forefoot and that place the MTP joints in hyperextension, leading to attenuation of plantar structures, depression of the MT head, and distal fat pad migration, resulting in plantar callosities.
2. Hammer toe deformity: MTP extension, PIP flexion, DIP extension **(Fig. 10.52)**
   - Develops when the smaller intrinsics are overpowered by the extrinsics
   - Most common in second toe (longest of lesser toes), caused by short toe box
   - MTP joint appears dorsiflexed with weight bearing
     a. "Simple": corrects with elevation of the foot off the ground
     b. "Complex": does not correct (analogous to claw toe)
   - Conservative management: protective padding, tall toe box, corrective splints (flexible deformity only)
   - Surgical management: dictated by flexibility of deformity
     a. Flexible: Girdlestone-Taylor FDL flexor-to-extensor tendon transfer
     b. Fixed: PIP arthroplasty or arthrodesis
3. Claw toe deformity: PIP and DIP joint flexion with fixed MTP hyperextension
   - Etiology: cavus deformity, NM disease causing muscle imbalance, inflammatory arthropathies causing soft tissue attenuation, trauma, sequelae of compartment syndrome
   - Conservative management: orthotics to offload plantarly subluxed MT head
   - Surgical management
     a. Flexible: FDL flexor-to-extensor tendon transfer with EDB tenotomy and EDL lengthening
     b. Fixed: PIP arthrodesis or resection arthroplasty with MTP capsulotomy and extensor lengthening
        - Shortening (Weil, Maceira) osteotomy when MTP is dislocated
4. Mallet toe deformity: isolated flexion deformity at the DIP joint
   - Treatment
     a. Flexible: FDL tenotomy
     b. Fixed: DIP arthrodesis or excisional arthroplasty

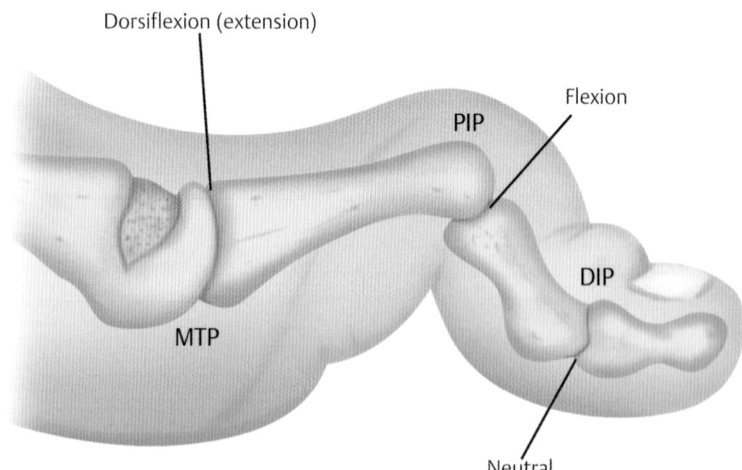

Fig. 10.52 Hammer toe deformity: metatarsophalangeal (MTP) extension, proximal interphalangeal (PIP) flexion, and distal interphalangeal (DIP) extension.

5. Crossover toe deformity
   - Crossover second toe deformity develops as a result of:
     a. Disruption of the plantar plate
     b. Attenuation of the lateral collateral ligament
   - Treatment: EDB tendon transfer to the intermetatarsal ligament with medial capsular release, flexor-to-extensor tendon transfer
     a. Distal MT osteotomy required for severe MTP subluxation/dislocation
     b. Overlapping fifth toe: release of dorsal capsule, Z-plasty of dorsal skin, EDL lengthening
     c. Underlapping ("curly") fifth toe: tenotomy of FDL equivalent to flexor to extensor transfer
     d. Weil osteotomies have been associated with floating toe (dorsiflexion) deformity at the MTP joint.
        - To avoid this complication, the osteotomy should be made parallel to the plantar surface of the foot, or a wafer of bone should be resected to avoid plantar depression of the MT head.
        - Weil osteotomies have been shown to be superior to Helal osteotomies in all respects—patient satisfaction, recurrence rate, transfer lesions, maintenance of reduction, and union rate.
     e. For severe second MTP joint deformity with subluxation or dislocation, soft tissue release alone is insufficient.
6. Metatarsophalangeal instability
   - Presentation: subluxation presenting with pain/swelling, pain with push off; drawer test (applying dorsal force to proximal phalanx while stabilizing metatarsal) reproduces pain
   - Conservative management: toe taping and lesser toe orthotics
     a. Steroid injection is contraindicated (can cause plantar plate attenuation)
   - Surgical management
     a. Isolated synovitis (stable MTP joint): MTP synovectomy, MTP joint capsule reconstruction
     b. Severe instability or deformity: add flexor-to-extensor tendon transfer for additional stability (can cause stiffness); alternatively, can do EHB rerouting deep to transverse metatarsal ligament
7. Freiberg disease
   - Lesser ray osteochondrosis most commonly involving the second MT head
   - Radiographic findings: resorption of bone adjacent to the articular surface with resultant flattening of the MT head, loose bodies, joint space narrowing
   - Surgical management
     a. For early-stage disease, debridement of all synovitis, osteophytes, and loose bodies via a dorsal incision
     b. Dorsal closing-wedge metaphyseal osteotomy (rotates preserved plantar aspect of the articular surface)
8. Bunionette deformity (tailor's bunion): prominence over fifth MT head
   - Bunionette and ipsilateral hallux valgus: "splayfoot"
   - Surgical management is based on the anatomic location of deformity:
     a. Type I (enlarged fifth MT head): lateral condylectomy
     b. Type II (lateral bowing of fifth MT diaphysis): distal chevron fifth MT osteotomy
     c. Type III (increased fourth–fifth IMA > 8 degrees): oblique diaphyseal fifth MT osteotomy
   - Proximal osteotomy should be avoided due to the tenuous blood supply at the proximal metadiaphyseal junction

XI. Degenerative Joint Disease (Osteoarthritis)

1. General
   - Often posttraumatic in the hindfoot and ankle
   - Idiopathic osteoarthritis commonly occurs in the first MTP and midfoot.
   - Lateral ankle instability, PTTI, and NM deformities contribute to DJD.
2. Midfoot (TMT) arthritis
   - Conservative management: orthotic treatment—stiff-soled shoe or steel shank–modified shoe with a rocker bottom and cushioned heel
   - Surgical management: for flatfoot deformity, realignment arthrodesis can be performed (medial column arthrodesis: fusion of first TMT and NC joints) to restore the lateral talo–first metatarsal (Meary) angle
3. Hindfoot arthritis
   - Includes subtalar (ST), talonavicular (TN) and calcaneocuboid (CC) joints
   - Conservative management: orthotic treatment—AFO or rigid lace-up leather (Arizona-type) brace
   - Surgical management: arthrodesis of single joints leads to significant limitation in hindfoot inversion/eversion (TN > ST > CC).
     a. Isolated TN fusion has a high nonunion rate.
     b. When deformity is present, surgical treatment involves triple arthrodesis
        - Ideal position: 0–5 degrees valgus, neutral abduction/adduction, plantigrade foot
        - Malunited triple arthrodesis necessitates calcaneal osteotomy (correct varus/valgus) and transverse tarsal osteotomy (restore plantigrade position).
   - ST arthritis
     a. Presentation: pain when walking on uneven surfaces
     b. Physical examination: tenderness over the sinus tarsi, pain with passive hindfoot eversion/inversion
     c. Subtalar arthrodesis has higher nonunion rate in smokers and those with a history of ankle arthrodesis.
     d. Prior calcaneal fracture with loss of height: anterior ankle impingement/pain, subfibular impingement
        - Treated with subtalar bone-block distraction arthrodesis or plantar displacing calcaneal osteotomy and subtalar arthrodesis
4. Tibiotalar arthritis
   - May be associated with rigid flatfoot deformity (stage IV), cavovarus foot deformity or lateral ankle instability; also may be associated with varus or valgus ankle deformity either at the ankle or more proximal (e.g., tibia vara)
   - Conservative management: orthotic treatment—AFO with a single rocker bottom modification or rigid lace-up leather (Arizona-type) brace
   - Surgical management
     a. Arthrodesis provides excellent pain relief
        - Optimal position of tibiotalar arthrodesis: 0–5 degrees of hindfoot valgus, 5–10 degrees of external rotation, neutral dorsiflexion
        - Add orthotic with rocker bottom sole
        - Causes arthritis in ipsilateral midfoot and hindfoot joints (ST most common)
        - Failed fusion with normal subtalar joint should be revised with compression plating and bone grafting
     b. Compared with other preoperative diagnoses, total ankle arthroplasty (TAA) has the most predictable outcomes in treatment of osteoarthritis.
        - Lower rates of failure for Agility ankle replacement when concomitant syndesmotic fusion is performed

- ♦ Persistent pain > 6 month after TAA with Agility implant is most likely due to syndesmotic nonunion
- ∘ Absolute contraindications to TAA:
  - ♦ Active infection
  - ♦ Neuropathic (Charcot) arthropathy
  - ♦ No motor function below ankle
  - ♦ Significant talar AVN
- ∘ Other contraindications include peripheral vascular disease, severe joint laxity with nonreconstructible ankle ligaments, severe osteopenia or osteoporosis
- ∘ Distraction arthroplasty has a limited role in younger patients with severe arthritis (limited data to support its use)
- ∘ No current role for soft tissue interpositional arthroplasty

XII. Rheumatoid Arthritis and Inflammatory Disorders

1. Rheumatoid arthritis
   - Forefoot more commonly involved than the midfoot or hindfoot
     a. Toes sublux or dislocate dorsally, deviate laterally into valgus, develop hammer toe deformities
        - ∘ As lesser toes deviate laterally, hallux valgus develops and worsens transfer metatarsalgia
        - ∘ Chronic synovitis: incompetence of the joint capsules and collateral ligaments

     b. Rheumatoid forefoot reconstruction: first MTP arthrodesis, lesser MT head resection with pinning of the lesser MTP joints, closed osteoclasis of the interphalangeal joints versus PIP arthroplasty
        - ∘ **For severe rheumatoid forefoot, consider first MTP arthrodesis and lesser toe MT head resections.**
        - ∘ Achieved through three well-placed longitudinal dorsal incisions
        - ∘ Most common complication of forefoot arthroplasty: intractable plantar keratosis (IPK)
   - Midfoot involvement most commonly occurs in the TN joint
   - **Isolated symmetric TN arthritis: think RA**
   - When flatfoot develops, midfoot-driven deformity must be differentiated from hindfoot-driven deformity
     a. Treat midfoot-driven deformity with a realignment midfoot arthrodesis.
     b. Treat hindfoot-driven deformity with a triple arthrodesis.
   - Tibiotalar joint involvement is best treated with ankle arthrodesis (high risk for wound complications with total ankle arthroplasty).
   - Rheumatoid patient with type 1 bunionette: treat with exostectomy
2. Seronegative spondyloarthropathy [rheumatoid factor (RF)-negative inflammatory arthropathy]
   - Presentation: in the foot as plantar fasciitis, Achilles tendinitis, or PTTI
   - Conservative management: nonsteroidal anti-inflammatory drugs (NSAIDs), salicylates, or cytotoxic drugs (directed by rheumatologist)
   - Surgical management: indicated for small joint erosions (e.g., psoriatic pencil-in-cup bony erosions), recalcitrant Achilles tendinopathy, or plantar fasciitis
3. Gout (see Chapter 1)
   - The hallux MTP joint is most often involved (50–75% of initial attacks)
     a. 90% of patients with chronic gouty attacks will have one or more episodes involving the hallux MTP joint

XIII. Nerve Disorders

1. Morton's neuroma: compressive neuropathy of the interdigital nerve, most commonly between the third and fourth MT or the second and third MT (intermetatarsal space)
   - Conservative management: wide toe box shoes, metatarsal pads to offload webspace, cortisone injections (14% get relief from first injection, 30% with multiple injections)
   - Surgical management
     a. Dorsal incision, incision of the transverse intermetatarsal (IM) ligament, and resection of the nerve 2 to 3 cm proximal to the IM ligament
     b. Most common cause of recurrent pain is inadequate resection
   - Recurrent neuroma: most common complication
     a. Bulbous enlargement of the neural stump due to inadequate proximal resection or lack of nerve retraction (nerve stump adheres to adjacent bone/soft tissue, leading to traction neuritis)
        - Surgical management: plantar incision (allows more proximal exposure), transpose new stump into muscle tissue
   - Success rate of initial excision: 80–85%; 65–75% for revision excision
2. Tarsal tunnel syndrome
   - Definition: compressive neuropathy of the tibial nerve within the fibro-osseous tarsal tunnel
   - Presentation: posteromedial ankle/heel pain with paresthesias radiating into the plantar aspect of the foot
   - Anatomy
     a. Boundaries of the tarsal tunnel: flexor retinaculum (superficially), medial talus/calcaneus/sustentaculum tali (deep), AbH (inferiorly)
     b. Contents of the tarsal tunnel: PT, FHL, FDL, posterior tibial artery, venae comitantes, tibial nerve
     c. Lateral plantar nerve may be injured during tibiotalocalcaneal (TTC) arthrodesis via a plantar approach using an intramedullary nail
   - Etiology: synovial or ganglion cysts, pigmented villonodular synovitis (PVNS), nerve sheath tumors, lipomas, fracture, varicosities, accessory muscles, tenosynovitis, pes planus, correction of cavovarus foot, or systemic diseases causing inflammatory edema (diabetes mellitus, rheumatoid arthritis, ankylosing spondylitis)
   - Physical examination
     a. Positive Tinel's sign over the nerve is often seen
     b. Sensory examination is often unreliable
     c. Assess hindfoot alignment
     d. Chronic manifestations: atrophy of the AbH (MPN) or abductor digiti quinti (ADQ; LPN)
   - Imaging/diagnostic tests
     a. Electrodiagnostic tests used to determine the level of nerve compression
        - Sensory nerve conduction study (NCS) is more commonly abnormal than motor NCS
        - Electromyogram (EMG) is less sensitive
     b. MRI can help to identify space-occupying lesions
   - Treatment
     a. Most often conservative
     b. Surgical indications:
        - Space-occupying lesions in the tarsal tunnel
        - Failure of 3–6 months of conservative treatment

c. Surgical treatment: open tarsal tunnel release (avoid endoscopic)
   - Release deep and superficial fascia of the abductor hallucis

3. Anterior tarsal tunnel syndrome
   - Etiology: compressive neuropathy of the deep peroneal nerve in the fibro-osseous tunnel beneath the inferior extensor retinaculum secondary to tightly laced shoes, anterior tibiotalar, talonavicular, or TMT osteophytes, ganglion cysts, tendinitis, or EHB compression
   - Treatment
     a. Conservative: shoe-wear modifications, alternative lacing techniques
     b. Surgical management: if conservative measures fail, incision of the inferior extensor retinaculum, osteophyte excision, capsule repair
4. Sequelae of upper motor neuron disorders
   - Most common causes: cerebrovascular accident (CVA), traumatic brain injury, spinal cord injury
   - Paralysis, spasticity, muscle imbalance, contractures, and joint subluxation
   - Most common deformity: equinovarus
     a. Equinus occurs due to overactivity of the gastrocnemius-soleus complex
        - Treat with Achilles lengthening procedure
        - Release of toe flexors is often necessary due to a tenodesis effect when the ankle is brought out of equinus
     b. Varus results from overactivity of the TA (and FHL, FDL and PT)
        - Treat with split TA tendon transfer (SPLATT) to the lateral cuneiform or cuboid or total TA transfer to lateral cuneiform
   - Surgical treatment should be delayed at least 6 months after onset to allow maximum possible recovery
   - Conservative management: PT, stretching, maintenance of joint ROM, splinting, serial casting, muscle relaxants, phenol blocks (less expensive), and botulinum injections (more expensive)
5. Peripheral nerve injury and tendon transfers
   - Conservative management: AFOs can be used initially but surgery is required to become brace-free.
   - Principles of tendon transfer:
     a. Deformity must be flexible (rigid deformity requires arthrodesis)
     b. Must have grade 4 or 5 strength to transfer (one grade is lost with transfer)
     c. Redirect a deforming force to create a restoring force
   - Peroneal nerve palsy leads to loss of active DF and eversion and equinovarus
     a. Treatment: PTT transfer through the interosseous membrane to the dorsal midfoot with Achilles lengthening; consider LCO
   - Missed compartment syndrome can lead to loss of anterior and deep posterior compartments
     a. Deformity: cavovarus (PL) and equinus (Achilles)
     b. Treatment: similar to that for peroneal nerve palsy

XIV. Heel Pain

1. Plantar heel pain
   - Plantar fasciitis
     a. Presentation: pain with the first step in the morning and after prolonged sitting
     b. Plantar fascia is the primary site of force transfer between the hindfoot and forefoot during the stance phase of gait (windlass mechanism).

c. Physical examination
   - Tenderness over the plantar medial tuberosity of the calcaneus at the plantar fascial origin
   - Associated with gastrocnemius contracture
   - **Reduced ankle dorsiflexion is the strongest independent risk factor for the development of plantar fasciitis.**

d. Conservative management (effective in > 90% of patients):
   - Stretching programs: plantar fascia–specific stretching (more effective) and Achilles tendon stretching
   - Night splints, physical therapy, anti-inflammatory medications
   - Corticosteroid injections have fallen out of favor because of risk of plantar fascial rupture

e. Surgical management (for refractory cases):
   - Limited (medial one-half) plantar fascial release
     - ♦ Complete release can jeopardize the integrity of the longitudinal arch and overload the lateral column
   - Other options include gastrocnemius recession and extracorporeal shock wave therapy (ESWT)

- Compression of the first branch of the lateral plantar (LP) (Baxter's) nerve
  a. Presents as plantar medial heel pain that can be difficult to distinguish from plantar fasciitis
     - Pain more medial over the abductor hallucis origin
  b. Compression over the nerve reproduces the pain and causes radiation into the plantar lateral foot (positive Tinel's sign)
  c. Imaging/diagnostic tests
     - MRI: may demonstrate fatty infiltration of ADQ (late finding)
     - EMG/NCS: increased motor latency within the ADQ
  d. Conservative management: activity modification, ice, NSAIDs
  e. Surgical management: if conservative measures fail, open release of the deep fascia of the abductor hallucis

- Calcaneal stress fracture
  a. Can occur after a recent increase in activity level (e.g., military recruits)
  b. If increased activity leads to pain on heel squeeze, consider calcaneal stress fracture
  c. MRI (higher specificity) preferred to bone scan since it can also evaluate surrounding soft tissues for other causes of pain
  d. Conservative management: rest, protected weight bearing

- Heel pad syndrome
  a. Presentation: pain and tenderness in the central portion of the plantar heel
     - Associated with heel pad atrophy
  b. Conservative management: cushioned shoe inserts or well-padded cast
  c. Surgical management: should be avoided; no technique can restore fat pad architecture; wound complications in this location can be devastating

2. Posterior heel pain
   - Retrocalcaneal bursitis/Haglund deformity/insertion Achilles tendinopathy
     a. Retrocalcaneal bursa lies between the anterior surface of the Achilles tendon and the posterosuperior calcaneal tuberosity
     b. Haglund deformity: enlarged prominence of the posterosuperior calcaneal tuberosity (visible on lateral foot X-ray)
     c. Retrocalcaneal bursitis may occur independently of or due to the presence of a Haglund deformity

d. Retrocalcaneal bursitis often occurs in conjunction with insertional Achilles tendinopathy

e. Insertional Achilles tendinopathy:
   - Tenderness over tendon insertion on the posterior calcaneus
   - Lateral foot X-ray: bone spur or intratendinous calcification
   - MRI may be useful to assess the degree of tendon degeneration.
   - Conservative treatment: shoe-wear modification, NSAIDs, ice
     - Heel lifts, stretching, PT (eccentric training)

f. Corticosteroid injections should be avoided (can cause Achilles rupture)

g. Surgical management
   - Retrocalcaneal bursitis: bursal debridement
   - Haglund deformity: excision of the Haglund deformity (calcaneal exostectomy)
   - Insertional Achilles tendinopathy: debridement of degenerative tendon including calcification
     - If tendon detachment (> 50%) is required for adequate debridement, reattach with suture anchors.
     - FHL tendon transfer for augmentation is indicated if > 50% of the Achilles tendon requires excision.
       - Only objective finding of FHL transfer is decreased hallucal phalangeal pressure

- Chronic Achilles tendon rupture

a. Conservative treatment: AFO; surgical treatment: FHL transfer

XV. Tendon Problems

Note: see Adult Acquired Flatfoot Deformity, above, for PT tendon issues, and Chapter 8 for Achilles tendon issues.

1. Peroneal tendons

- PL (posterolateral in fibular groove) more commonly subluxates/dislocates
- PB (anteromedial in fibular groove) more commonly tears
- Peroneal tendon pathology associated with cavovarus foot deformity

a. Increased risk of peroneal pathology with posterior fibular plating

- Pathophysiology of peroneal subluxation/dislocation: rapid dorsiflexion of an inverted foot with rapid contraction of the peroneal tendons leads to disruption of superior peroneal retinaculum
- Acute rupture of the PL can occur at or through a fracture of the os perineum.
- Imaging

a. X-rays: demonstrate retraction or fracture of the os perineum

b. Ultrasound: a dynamic tool to evaluate subluxation/dislocation

c. MRI: commonly shows false-positive longitudinal tears

- Conservative management: rest, NSAIDS, brace, physical therapy
- Surgical management:

a. Tenosynovectomy; debridement and repair for < 50% tendon degeneration

b. Fibular groove deepening is indicated if the groove is shallow.

c. Excision and tenodesis are indicated in cases of complete rupture or severely degenerative tendon (> 50%) (when repair is not possible)

d. If hindfoot varus is contributory, a lateral closing-wedge calcaneal osteotomy is necessary to correct alignment.

e. For peroneal subluxation/dislocation, the superior peroneal retinaculum must be repaired (± fibular groove deepening if necessary for stability).

f. If > 50% degeneration of both PL and PB tendons renders them both unreconstructable, FHL transfer to the fifth MT can be performed.

2. Tibialis anterior tendon
   - Complete ruptures (rare, older adults) can be repaired primarily when acute but require reconstruction with interpositional tendon grafts when chronic.
     a. Acute repair leads to improved patient outcomes, but decreased inversion and dorsiflexion strength remains a problem.
3. Stenosing FHL tenosynovitis
   - Usually seen in en-pointe dancers
   - Stenosis occurs along the course of the FHL between the posteromedial and posterolateral tubercles of the talus.
   - Physical examination: tenderness in posteromedial ankle, triggering of the hallux IP joint, painful crepitus with resisted hallux plantarflexion
   - Imaging: MRI—fluid surrounding the FHL at the level of the ankle
   - Conservative management: activity modification
     f. Surgical management: FHL tenosynovectomy and release of overlying fascia

XVI. Calcaneus Fractures

1. Extra-articular fractures
   - Tuberosity avulsion fractures **(Fig. 10.53)**
     a. May threaten posterior skin if displaced significantly; urgent operative reduction is indicated if threatened skin
   - **Beak fractures: orthopaedic emergency; requires immediate reduction and fixation due to risk of skin necrosis**
     - Treat with percutaneous lag screw technique
   - Anterior process fractures
     a. Mechanism: avulsion bifurcate ligament caused by forced inversion/PF
     b. Treatment: most often conservative
        - If > 25% displacement at the CC joint, open reduction and internal fixation (ORIF)
   - Sustentaculum fractures
     a. Rare to occur in isolation without posterior facet involvement
     b. Displaced fractures should be treated via medial approach
     c. May lead to FHL stenosis and pain with great toe flexion
2. Intraarticular fractures
   - 75% involve the posterior facet; most have some degree of displacement
   - Lateral wall "blowout": subfibular impingement/peroneal pathology
   - Heel pad crush can occur with high-energy axial loading injury.
   - Calcaneus becomes shortened, widened, and flattened, and heel falls into varus
   - 17% are open injuries: more common for wound to occur medially
   - Must evaluate for concomitant spine fractures
   - Imaging
     a. In addition to standard radiographic views, the following can be obtained: Harris (axial) view, Broden views, CT scan
     b. Bohler's angle (normal 20–40 degrees) is decreased in joint depression fractures
     c. Angle of Gissane (normal 130–145 degrees) is increased in joint depression fractures

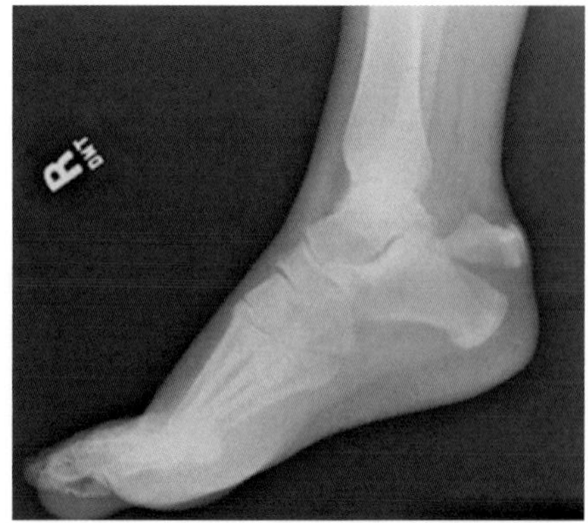

Fig. 10.53 Displaced calcaneal tuberosity avulsion (beak) fracture: surgical emergency.

- Sanders classification (based on the fracture pattern through the posterior facet on coronal oblique CT scan) **(Fig. 10.54)**
  a. Type I (nondisplaced): treatment: early motion, NWB × 6 weeks
  b. Types II and III: two- and three-part fractures
     - Treatment: ORIF indicated when posterior facet displacement > 2–3 mm, flattening of Bohler's angle, varus heel malalignment
  c. Type IV: highly comminuted, with four or more fragments
     - Treatment: ORIF with primary subtalar arthrodesis
- Prognosis:
  a. Worse outcomes in higher fracture types
  b. Surgery has better outcomes than conservative treatment for significant intra-articular displacement, flattened Bohler's angle, younger patients (age < 29 years), women, those not involved in workers compensation cases
  c. Indications for ST bone block distraction arthrodesis: significant loss of calcaneal height, decreased talocalcaneal angle, loss of talar declination, anterior ankle pain, decreased DF from tibiotalar impingement
- Complications
  a. Posttraumatic subtalar arthritis is common and may require arthrodesis (pain over sinus tarsi, decreased inversion/eversion).

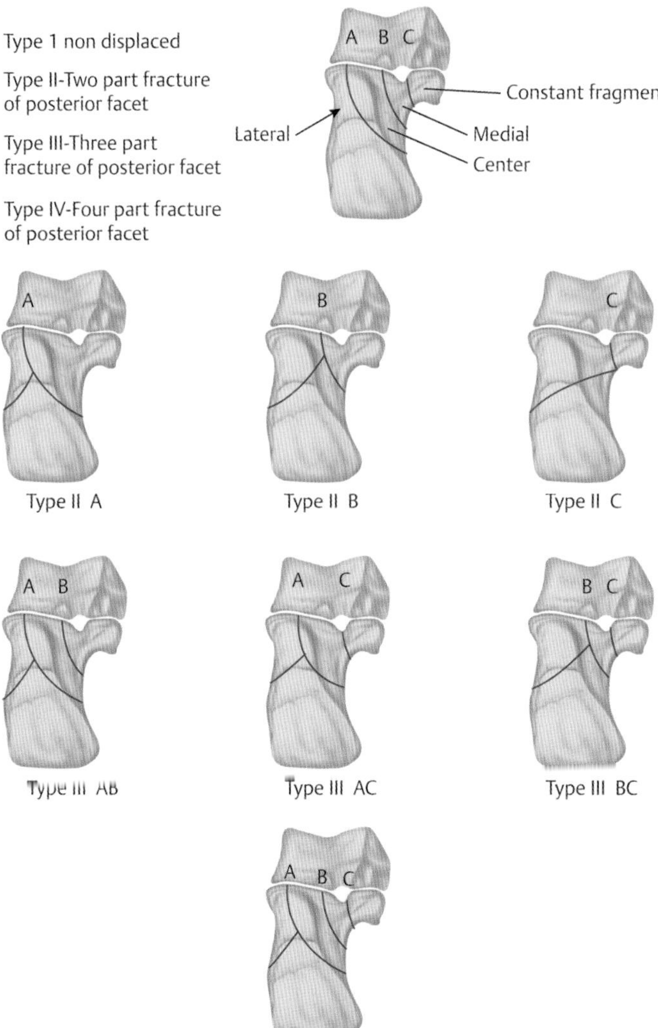

Fig. 10.54 Sanders classification, based on coronal computed tomography (CT) image through the posterior facet.

- Of displaced intra-articular calcaneal fractures treated nonoperatively, 16% require late subtalar arthrodesis.
- Male workers' compensation patients involved in heavy labor professions with an initial Bohler's angle < 0 degrees are most likely to go on to subtalar arthrodesis.

b. Delayed wound healing rate of 25% with extensile lateral approach

c. Lateral calcaneal artery (from peroneal a.) supplies flap of extensile approach to calcaneus fractures

d. Wound complications increase in open injuries, smokers, and DM

e. FHL is at risk when screws are placed from lateral to medial at the level of the sustentaculum tali (constant fragment)

f. Sural neuroma following extensile incision
- Treat with neuroma excision and burying of nerve

g. Calcaneal malunion leads to lateral wall impingement, anterior ankle impingement, and difficult shoe wear.
- Treatment: distraction osteotomy and lateral wall exostectomy

XVII. Talus Fractures

1. Second most common tarsal bone injury
2. Blood supply is provided by PT, DP, and perforating peroneal arteries.
   - Main blood supply: artery of the tarsal canal (branch of PT artery)
3. Classification
   - Talar neck fractures (Hawkins) **(Fig. 10.55)**
     a. Type I: nondisplaced
     b. Type II: displaced fracture with ST dislocation
        - Deltoid branch of PT artery (supplies half of medial talar body) is only remaining blood supply (must preserve deltoid ligament)
     c. Type III: displaced fracture with ST and tibial tendon (TT) dislocation
     d. Type IV: displaced fracture with ST, TT, and TN dislocations
   - Talar body fractures
     a. Lateral process acts as the dividing line
        - Fractures exiting posterior to this are considered body fractures
     b. Medial malleolar osteotomy often required for adequate exposure
4. Diagnosis
   - Canale oblique radiograph should be obtained to evaluate the talar neck.
   - CT scan is beneficial for preoperative planning.
5. Treatment: talar neck/body fractures with any displacement are operative.
   - Urgent closed reduction of dislocation is necessary to avoid skin compromise or neurovascular injury.
     a. Reduction is performed with plantarflexion and heel manipulation.
   - Medial neck comminution is common, leading to varus deformity if not stabilized.
   - Dual anteromedial and anterolateral incisions recommended for exposure
6. Complications
   - Posttraumatic arthritis (subtalar > tibiotalar): most common complication

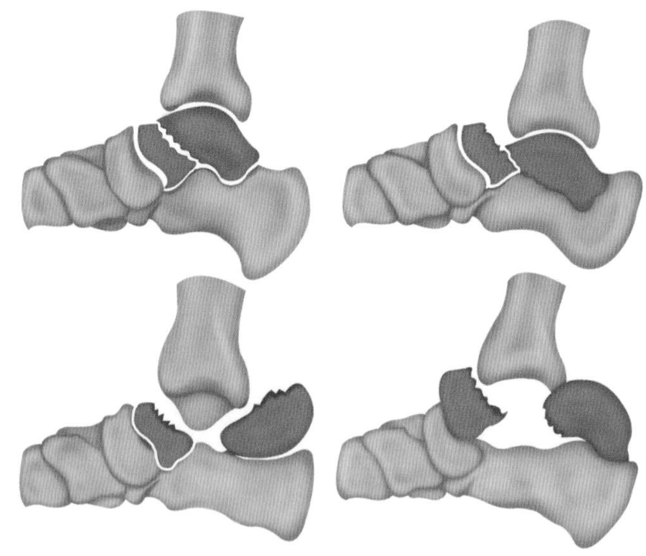

Fig. 10.55 Talar neck fractures (Hawkins).

- Varus malunion: cavovarus foot deformity limiting hindfoot eversion and causing pain on the lateral border of the foot
  a. Treat with medial opening wedge talar neck osteotomy
- Dorsal malunion: symptomatic ankle impingement limiting DF
- Avascular necrosis (second most common complication)
  a. Increases with severity of injury (approaches 100% for type IV injury)
  b. Hawkins sign: subchondral linear lucency of talar dome indicates revascularization; unlikely to develop AVN; best seen on ankle views
- Nonunion occurs in ~ 10%

7. Lateral process talus (snowboarder's) fracture
- Should be considered in cases of persistent pain after ankle sprain
- Imaging
  a. Best seen on AP ankle radiograph
  b. CT (imaging study of choice) should be performed to evaluate comminution.
- Treatment: displaced fractures should be treated with ORIF (if amenable to screw fixation) versus excision if small or highly comminuted.
  a. Resection of a 1-cm lateral process fracture leads to complete incompetence of the lateral talocalcaneal ligament.

8. Peritalar (subtalar) dislocations
- Medial dislocation (more common)
  a. Reduction obstacles: EDB, extensor retinaculum, peroneals, TN capsule
- Lateral dislocation
  a. Obstacles to closed reduction: PT, FDL, and FHL tendons
  b. Most common tarsal bone fractured with this injury pattern: cuboid
- Imaging: CT is necessary to detect presence of small intra-articular fragments
- Treatment
  a. Immobilize for 6–12 weeks (if stable); temporary fixation (if unstable)
  b. Intra-articular fracture fragments should be surgically removed.
- Complications: most common is subtalar arthritis

XVIII. Navicular and Midfoot Injuries

1. Navicular fractures
- Blood supply: dorsalis pedis supplies the dorsum; PT artery (medial plantar branch) supplies the plantar surface; both form a plexus that supplies tuberosity
  a. Central portion of the bone is relatively less vascular, so it is at increased risk for stress fracture and nonunion.
- Classification
  a. Avulsion fractures: due to dorsal TN ligaments, treat conservatively
  b. Tuberosity fractures
     - Treatment: surgical fixation required for > 5 mm displacement
       - Excise small avulsions or symptomatic nonunions
  c. Body fractures
     - Sangeorzan classification:
       - Type I: transverse coronal plane fracture, dorsal fragment < 50% of body
       - Type II: dorsal-lateral to plantar-medial fracture with medialization of the fragment and forefoot
       - Type III: central or lateral comminution

- Treatment: ORIF even for minimally displaced fractures
  - Arthrodesis when highly comminuted

d. Stress fractures
- Presentation: midfoot pain in running and jumping athletes
- Commonly occur in the central third of the navicular
- Imaging
  - MRI and bone scan can be helpful when X-rays negative
  - CT scan is the gold standard: defines complete versus incomplete, displaced versus nondisplaced
- Treatment
  - Nondisplaced fractures: NWB in cast for 6–8 weeks
    - Percutaneous screw fixation is indicated after failure of 6–8 weeks of NWB.
  - Displaced fractures or nonunion: transverse screw placement from dorsolateral to plantar medial
- Two most common complications: arthritis and AVN
  - Treatment of AVN: talonaviculocuneiform fusion with bone grating

2. TMT fracture-dislocations (Lisfranc injuries)

- Anatomy

a. Bony stability: second MT base fits into "keystone" and trapezoidal shape of the cuneiforms in the coronal plane (wider dorsally, narrower plantarly); creates a "Roman arch" configuration

b. No direct ligamentous attachment exists between the first and second MTs

c. Lisfranc ligament connects the medial cuneiform and base of second MT
- Interosseous ligament is stiffest and strongest
- Plantar ligament inserts on base of second and third MT
- **For transverse instability of the Lisfranc joint to occur, there must be an injury to both the interosseous and plantar ligament.**

d. Diagnosis
- Mechanism of action
  - Indirect: axial loading of a plantarflexed foot
  - Direct: MVA, crush injury (compartment syndrome)

e. Presentation: significant swelling, unable to bear weight, plantar ecchymosis

f. Imaging
- Weight-bearing views of both the injured and contralateral side should be obtained if possible
- Abduction stress views are another option
- "Fleck sign": avulsion from second MT base is diagnostic

g. Treatment
- Anatomic reduction is most predictive of good clinical results
  - ORIF necessary (percutaneous fixation not sufficient)
- Medial and middle columns are stabilized with screw (± plate) fixation; lateral column is temporarily fixed with Kirschner wires (K-wires) (removed at 6 weeks to maintain mobility of segment)
- **Fusion of the lateral column is never the correct approach; lateral column mobility is required for accommodation on uneven ground.**
- ORIF versus arthrodesis remains controversial.
- Primary TMT arthrodesis of medial and middle columns is indicated for purely ligamentous injuries, severe intra-articular comminution, or chronic injuries with posttraumatic arthritis.

- Midfoot realignment arthrodesis is a salvage procedure for missed chronic injuries or failed ORIF

3. Cuneiform fractures (occur in conjunction with Lisfranc injuries)
   - Medial cuneiform most common
   - Treatment: requires ORIF when displaced/unstable
4. Cuboid fractures (rarely occur in isolation)
   - "Nutcracker" fracture can occur with Lisfranc injury (abduction force)
   - Treatment:
     a. ORIF is necessary when comminution or displacement disrupts the length and alignment of the lateral column.
   - Cuboid syndrome: painful subluxation in athletes (ballet dancers)
     a. Palpable "click" as foot is brought from PF/inversion to DF/eversion

XIX. Forefoot Injuries

1. General
   - Significant displacement of an isolated MT shaft fracture is uncommon.
     a. Isolated fractures are stable (intermetatarsal ligaments at base and neck).
   - Lisfranc injury must be ruled out when there are multiple MT fractures.
   - First MT bears a third of the body weight; displaced fractures require surgery.
   - Surgical fixation of MT fractures is indicated for:
     a. > 10 degrees sagittal plane deformity
     b. Displaced fractures of three central MT shafts (inherently unstable)
   - MT base fractures: heal rapidly, high index of suspicion for Lisfranc injury
2. MT stress fractures
   - Cavovarus foot deformity leads to fifth MT stress fracture.
     a. Treatment must address foot malalignment.
   - Second MT stress fracture is most common, seen in amenorrheic dancers.
   - Most treated with weight bearing as tolerated (WBAT) in boot or hard-soled shoe
3. Fifth MT fracture
   - Zone 1 avulsion of the proximal fifth MT tuberosity secondary to inversion mechanism and pull of lateral band of plantar fascia and/or peroneus brevis **(Fig. 10.56)**

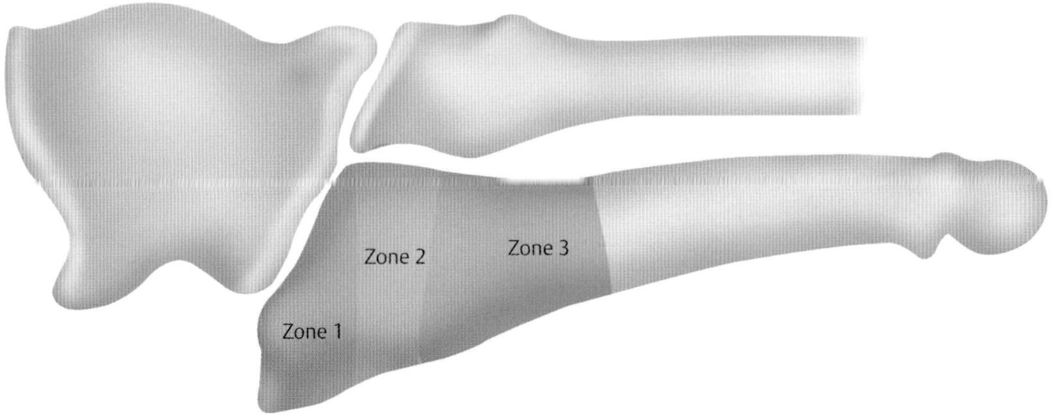

Fig. 10.56 Avulsion of the proximal fifth metatarsal (MT) tuberosity secondary to inversion mechanism and pull of the lateral band of the plantar fascia or peroneus brevis.

a. Treatment: protected weight bearing in shoe or boot

- Zone 2 (Jones fracture): involving metaphyseal-diaphyseal junction extending into the fourth–fifth intermetatarsal articulation
  a. Treatment:
    - NWB immobilization for 6 to 8 weeks
    - IM screw fixation: elite athletes, those failing conservative management
    - **Return to athletic participation prior to radiographic union leads to an increased failure rate.**
- Zone 3: fractures of proximal diaphysis (stress fractures)
  a. Slow healing time and greatest risk of nonunion
  b. Refracture rate 33% with nonoperative treatment
  c. Surgical management: treatment of choice is intramedullary screw fixation (usually in high-functioning patient)

4. Metatarsophalangeal joint injuries
   - Hallux MTP dislocation: usually dorsal due to hyperextension causing volar plate rupture at its insertion on the MT neck
   - Treatment: closed reduction should be attempted first, percutaneous pinning if joint unstable after reduction, open reduction if irreducible
5. Phalangeal fractures
   - Be aware of nail bed injury with distal phalangeal fractures (open fracture)
   - Usually nonoperative; surgery for some hallux intra-articular fractures
6. Puncture wounds
   - Most common infective organisms are *Staphylococcus* and *Streptococcus*
   - Most characteristic is *Pseudomonas*
     a. Seen if penetration goes through shoe/sneaker
     b. Most common cause of osteomyelitis
     c. Treat with local debridement and antibiotics
   - Chronic persistent pain requires surgical exploration (retained foreign body)

XX. Compartment Syndrome of the Foot

1. Anatomy **(Fig. 10.57)**
   - Medial compartment: abductor hallucis, flexor hallucis brevis
   - Central compartment: FDB, lumbricals, QP, AdH
   - Lateral compartment: flexors, abductors, and opponens of fifth toe
   - Interosseous compartment: seven interossei muscles
2. Treatment
   - Fasciotomies through three incisions: one over the second MT, one over the fourth MT, and a medial approach along the inferior border of the first MT
3. Complications
   - Claw toes can occur from an undiagnosed and untreated compartment syndrome involving the deep compartments of the foot.

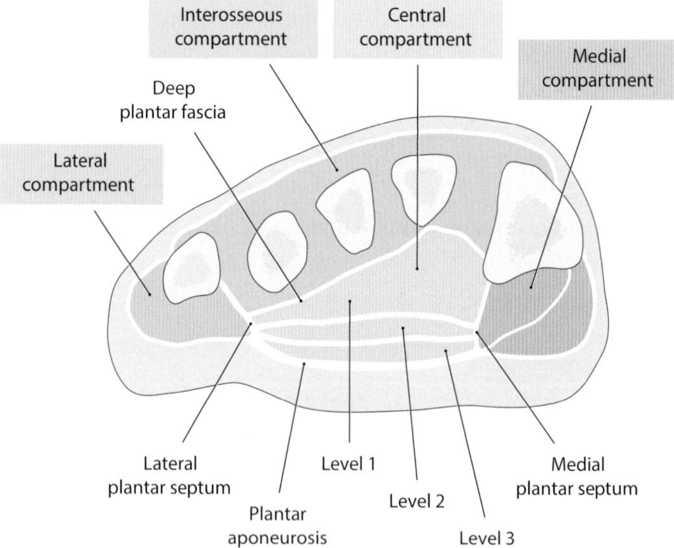

Fig. 10.57 Location of the compartments of the foot. Schematic cross section through a right foot, distal view. The different muscle compartments are indicated by color shading. (From Schuenke M, Schulte E. General Anatomy and the Musculoskeletal System: Thieme Atlas of Anatomy. New York: Thieme; 2005. Illustration by Karl Wesker.)

11

Amputations and Rehabilitation

Todd Borenstein, Gregory R. Waryasz, and Roman Hayda

I. Gait and Amputation

1. Gait **(Fig. 11.1)**
   - Walking
     a. Definitions
       - Cycle: initial heel contact to initial contact (same foot)
       - Cadence: steps per minute
       - Single-limb support: phase of gait in which body weight is supported by one leg
       - Double-limb support: period when both feet are in contact with the ground (not present in running)
       - Step: the distance from initial contact of one foot to initial contact of contralateral foot
       - Stride: the distance from initial contact to initial contact of the same foot
         - One stride = two steps **(Fig. 11.1)**
         - Running
           - Free-float phase: period when neither limb is in contact with the ground (not present in walking)
         - Gait phases
           - Stance phase: 60% of gait cycle
             - ***I*nitial contact, *L*oading response, *M*idstance, *T*erminal stance, *P*re-*S*wing; mnemonic: "I Like My Tea Pre-Sweetened"**
             - Initial contact: heel touches ground, hip is flexed, knee is extended, ankle is dorsiflexed
             - Load response: foot contacts floor, knee flexes slightly, and ankle plantar flexes to absorb energy while dorsiflexors eccentrically fire; quadriceps fire to stabilize flexed knee as limb accepts all body weight (contralateral leg comes off the ground)
             - Midstance: single limb support; hip extended and quadriceps concentrically fire to straighten the leg and progress body forward; calf muscles begin to fire as weight transitions anterior to leg and ankle begins to plantarflex
             - Terminal stance: heel rises (opposite foot is in heel strike); toes dorsiflex and toe flexors are active
             - Pre-swing: second time both limbs are on the ground; body weight transferred to other side (contralateral side in loading response), hip flexors fire to advance the limb forward; knee flexed and ankle plantar flexed

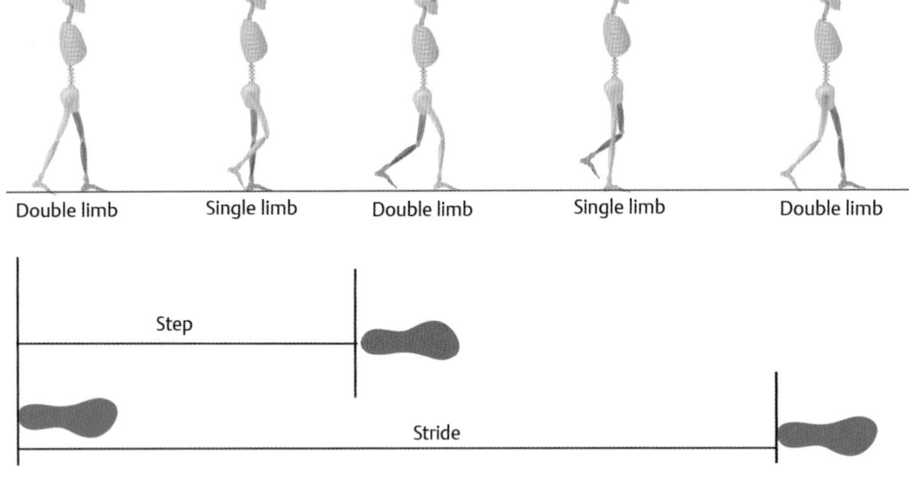

Fig. 11.1 The gait cycle.

- Just prior to heel rise in terminal stance, the posterior tibial tendon fires, which inverts the hindfoot and locks the transverse tarsal joint.
- **Hindfoot inversion in terminal stance locks the transverse tarsal joint, making the foot rigid and increasing the length of the lever arm of the Achilles tendon. This inversion optimizes heel rise/push off. Posterior tibial tendon insufficiency prevents this from happening efficiently.**
- Windlass mechanism
  - ◊ After heel rise, the plantar fascia is tightened as the metatarsophalangeal (MTP) joints extend and the longitudinal arch is accentuated, helping to further lock the transverse tarsal joint into a rigid platform.

▪ Swing phase: 40% of gait cycle
  - ***I*nitial swing (toe off), limb acceleration to *M*id-swing, limb deceleration to *T*erminal swing; mnemonic: "In My Teapot"**
  - Initial swing: hip flexed, knee flexed, ankle dorsiflexed (single-limb support)
  - Mid-swing: knee extends, hip and ankle stay flexed
  - Terminal swing: hamstrings decelerate the leg, and hip and ankle stay flexed as walker transitions to heel strike

▪ Normal gait prerequisites
  - Stance phase stability
  - Swing phase ground clearance
  - Foot position before initial contact
  - Energy-efficient step length and speed

♦ Gait dynamics
  ▪ Energy-efficient gait lessens the excursion of the center of gravity.
  ▪ Center of gravity **(Fig. 11.2)**
    - Located anterior to T10, average of 33 cm above the hip
    - Vertical displacement: 5 cm; follows sinusoidal curve
    - Lateral displacement, transfer of body weight to limb: 6 cm; also follows sinusoidal curve
  ▪ Line of gravity **(Fig. 11.2)**
    - Passes anterior to S2

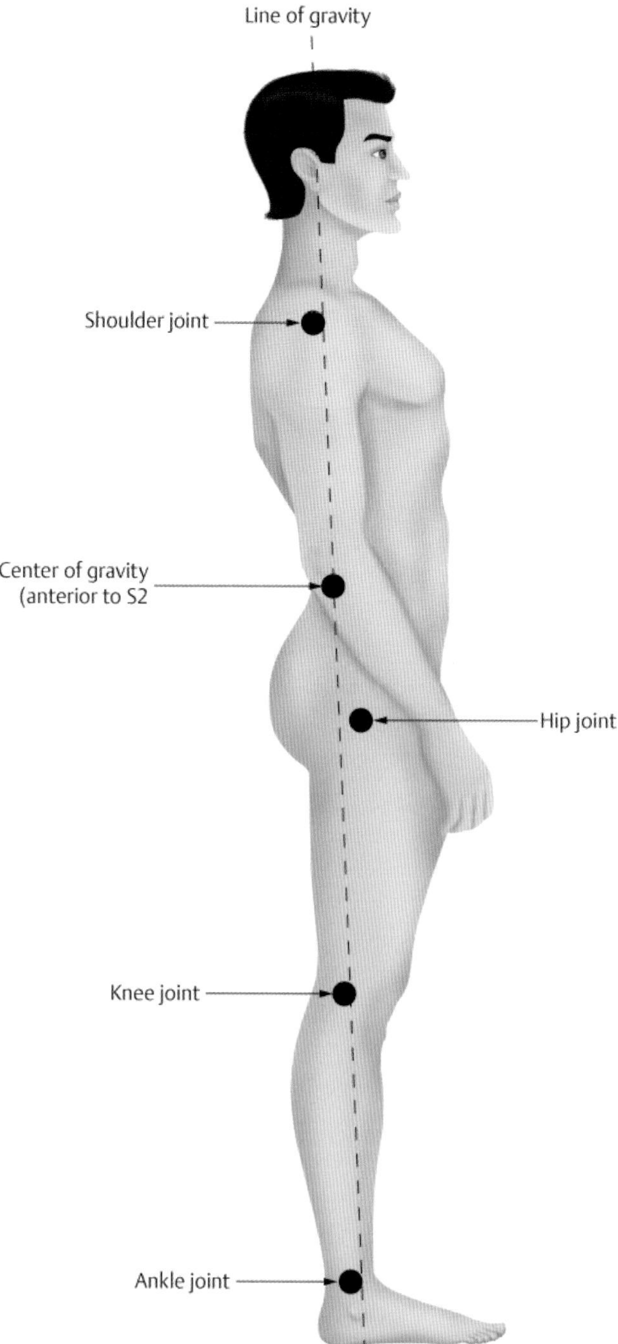

Fig. 11.2 The center of gravity of the body relative to the knee and hip joints.

- Reference for moment arm to the center of the joint under consideration, can be used to calculate joint forces
  - ◊ Line of gravity passes anterior to hip joint and posterior to the knee joint, the weight of the body hyperextends these joints, which are resisted by the iliofemoral ligament at the hip and the ligamentous apparatus of the knee

♦ Determinants of gait: six factors that help minimize excursion of the body's center of gravity

- ▪ Pelvic rotation: occurs horizontally about a vertical axis
  - Lessens the center of mass deviation
  - Reduces impact on floor contact

- Pelvic tilt: the non–weight-bearing side drops 5 degrees to reduce superior deviation
- Knee flexion in stance: stance phase limb is flexed to 15 degrees at loading
  - Dampen impact at loading
  - Lowers the center of gravity to decrease energy expenditure
- Foot and ankle motion: impact of loading is dampened through ankle plantarflexion
  - Increased stability at midstance
  - Increased efficiency during push-off
- Knee motion: knee extends while ankle plantarflexes after mid-stance to restore limb length
  - Diminishes fall of pelvis at contralateral heel strike
- Lateral pelvic displacement: displacement of the center of gravity over the stance limb
  - Increases stance-phase stability

♦ Muscle action
- Agonists and antagonists work together during the gait cycle.
- Eccentric contraction of an antagonist muscle dampens the activity of an agonist causing deceleration, and lengthening the muscle during active resistance of an opposing force.
  - Eccentric contraction is associated with highest tensile forces on muscle tendon unit and is associated with tears of major tendons.
  - **Achilles, patellar, and quadriceps tendon tears are often associated with eccentric muscle contractions, such as occur during deceleration from a jump or preventing a fall.**
- Concentric muscle contraction shortens the muscle to move a joint through space.
- During swing phase the limb is advanced forward by concentric contraction of the hip flexors and decelerated during terminal swing by eccentric contraction of the hip extensors.
- Muscle contraction forces at the ankle during stance **(Fig. 11.3)**:
  - During initial contact dorsiflexors (tibialis anterior) eccentrically contract to slow ankle plantarflexion and prevent the foot from slapping the floor.
    - ◊ Maximum electrical activity of tibialis anterior during initial contact
  - Then plantar flexors eccentrically contract during stance to slow ankle dorsiflexion.
  - Concentric contraction by plantar flexors for heel; off at end of stance phase

♦ Pathological gait **(Table 11.1)**
- Muscle weakness decreases the ability to move a joint normally through space.
- Grading of motor weakness **(Table 11.2)**
  - Walking patterns develop based on the specific muscle weakness and the ability of the individual to acquire a substitution pattern.
  - Example: abductor lurch (Trendelenburg) gait (weak hip abductors)
    - ◊ Superior gluteal nerve (L4,5) or muscle injury
    - ◊ Contralateral pelvis drops; as a result the trunk lurches to the weakened side to maintain balance **(Fig. 11.4)**.

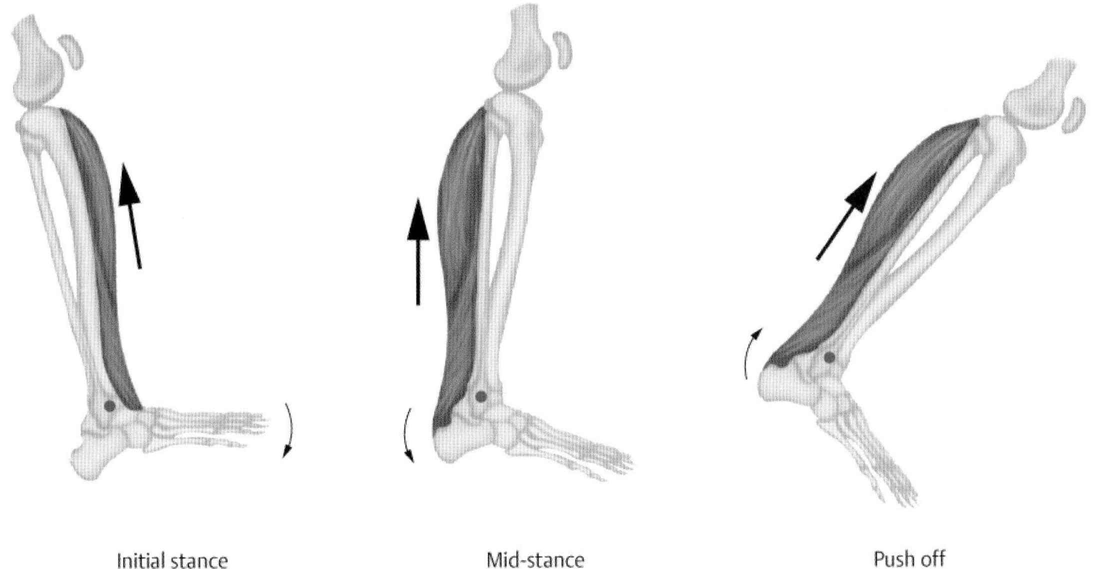

Fig. 11.3 Leg muscle action during gait. The *large arrows* indicate the direction of muscle contraction. The *small arrows* indicate the direction of joint motion. When the arrows are in different directions, this indicates eccentric contraction. The *dot* indicates the axis of movement. The tibialis anterior eccentrically contracts during initial stance to control foot contact to ground. Plantar flexors eccentrically control ankle dorsiflexion at midstance followed by concentric contraction of plantar flexors during push-off.

- Neurologic conditions may affect gait by producing muscle weakness, loss of balance, and reduced coordination between agonists and antagonists with or without joint contracture.
  - Steppage gait: foot drop
    - ◊ Equinus and varus foot and back-set knees; result of the loss of tibialis anterior and peroneal muscles (peroneal nerve)
  - Knee hyperextension: spasticity of ankle plantar flexor or knee extensors during stance phase; may also be the result of quadriceps weakness to prevent knee buckling with weight bearing
  - Hip scissoring: overactive hip adductors
  - Knee flexion contracture: hamstring spasticity
  - Flatfoot gait: weak gastrocnemius from posterior tibial nerve injury or muscle tear
  - Stroke: equinovarus, spastic gastrocnemius/soleus ± tibialis anterior and tibialis posterior
    - ◊ Split anterior tibial tendon transfer and gastrocnemius recession to correct
- Antalgic gait: shortened stance phase on a painful limb; contralateral swing phase is more rapid

Table 11.1 Gait Alteration Patterns from Muscle Weakness

Abnormal Gait	Muscle Weakness
Abductor lurch (Trendelenburg)	Gluteus medius
Hip hyperextension/lurch	Gluteus maximus
Back knee gait	Quadriceps
Flatfoot	Gastrocnemius/soleus
Steppage gait/foot drop	Tibialis anterior

Table 11.2 Grading of Muscle Weakness

Grade	Description
0/5	No contraction
1/5	Muscle flicker, no movement
2/5	Movement with gravity eliminated
3/5	Movement against gravity
4/5	Movement against some resistance
5/5	Movement against full resistance/normal strength

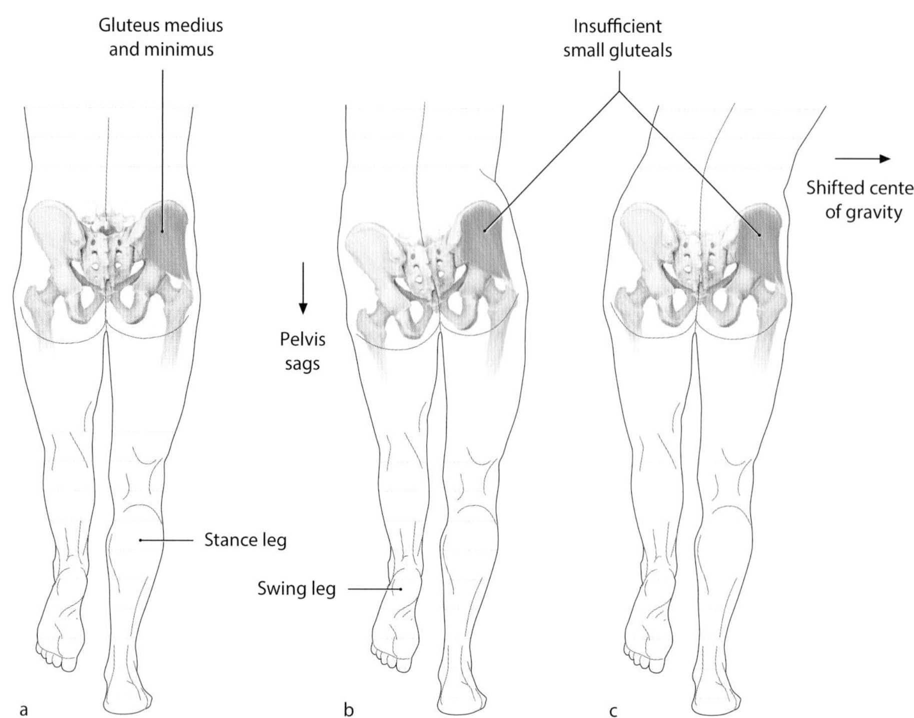

Fig. 11.4 Trendelenburg gait and stance. **(a)** Normal function of gluteals (abductors) keeping pelvis level. **(b,c)** Weak or nonfunctioning gluteals fail to control the relationship of the iliac wing and greater trochanter resulting in either **(b)** dropping of the opposite pelvis or **(c)** compensation by shifting the center of gravity over the affected hip. (From Schuenke M, Schulte E. General Anatomy and the Musculoskeletal System: Thieme Atlas of Anatomy. New York: Thieme; 2005. Illustration by Karl Wesker.)

- Hemiplegia: prolonged stance and double-limb support
  - Gait impairments as a result of excessive plantarflexion, weakness, and balance problems
    - ◊ Associated with ankle equinus, limitation of knee flexion, increased hip flexion
- Leg length discrepancy
  - Increased mechanical work by long leg
  - Increased stance time and step length on longer leg
  - Overall walking velocity is slower
  - Increased ground reaction forces on long leg
- Crutches and canes ameliorate instability and pain.
  - Crutches increase stability.
    - ◊ To be touchdown weight bearing, a patient must use double axillary crutches.
  - A cane shifts the center of gravity to the affected side when used in the contralateral hand.
    - ◊ Decreases the joint reactive force by decreasing the moment arm between the center of gravity and the femoral head
- Arthritis: forces across the knee may be four to seven times body weight
  - 70% through the medial compartment
- Water walking: decreases joint contact forces as result of the effect of buoyancy

2. Amputations
   - Treatment of peripheral vascular disease, trauma, tumor, infection or a congenital anomaly
   - Metabolic cost of amputee gait
     a. Metabolic cost of walking is increased with proximal-level amputations.
        - Inversely proportional to length of the residual limb and number of preserved joints

Table 11.3 Energy Expenditure for Ambulation

Amputation Level	Energy Above Baseline (%)	Speed (m/min)
Long transtibial	10	70
Average transtibial	25	60
Short transtibial	40	50
Bilateral transtibial	41	50
Transfemoral	65	40
Wheelchair	0–8	70

b. Energy expenditure compared with normal limb (**Table 11.3**):
  - Transfemoral, 65% more
  - Transfemoral in vascular patient, 100% more
  - Bilateral transtibial, 40% more
  - Short transtibial, 25% more
  - Long transtibial, 10% more
  - **Note: a unilateral transfemoral amputation entails a higher energy expenditure than a bilateral transtibial amputation.**

- Load transfer
  a. The soft tissue envelope acts as an interface between the bone of the residual limb and the prosthetic socket.
    - Ideally composed of a secure muscle mass covering the bone end and full-thickness skin that can tolerate direct pressure
    - A mobile nonadherent soft tissue envelope decreases shear forces.
  b. Load transfer occurs either directly or indirectly
    - Direct load transfer: occurs in knee or ankle disarticulations
      - ♦ Load transferred directly through terminal weight-bearing surface
      - ♦ Intimacy of prosthetic device is necessary only for suspension
    - Indirect load transfer: occurs when the amputation is through a long bone, i.e., transfemoral or transtibial
      - ♦ Load is transferred indirectly by total contact method
      - ♦ Must have intimate fit of the prosthetic socket
- Amputations in the dysvascular patient
  a. Patients with diabetes and peripheral vascular disease
    - Special wound healing and soft tissue considerations
      - ♦ Peripheral neuropathy most important risk factor
      - ♦ Total contact casts can reduce pressure and shear stress on wounds
      - ♦ May perform myoplasty instead of myodesis
        - ▪ Avoid further compromise of blood supply to muscle
        - ▪ **Myoplasty: suturing muscle directly to muscle to cover bone end**
        - ▪ **Myodesis: suturing muscle or tendon directly to bone end**
          - Amputations commonly for nonhealing wounds and infections

II. Wound Healing Considerations

1. Vascular supply
   - Transcutaneous oxygen tension > 40 mm Hg (gold standard)

   a. Measure of oxygenation and vascular supply
   b. Most predictive factor for successful wound healing
   c. > 40 mm Hg good wound healing, < 20 mm Hg poor wound healing
   d. Ideally > 45 mm Hg
- Hemoglobin > 10 g/dL
- Doppler pressure > 70 mm Hg
   a. Minimum inflow pressure to support wound healing
- Toe pressure > 40 mm Hg
- Ischemic index > 0.5
   a. Ratio of Doppler pressure at the level compared with the brachial systolic pressure
   b. An index of > 1 can be falsely elevated due to vascular calcifications.

2. Nutritional and immune status
- Serum albumin > 3.0 g/dL
   a. < 3.0 g/dL indicates a patient is malnourished
- Total lymphocyte > 1,500/mm^3
   a. Total lymphocyte < 1,500/mm^3 indicates immune deficiency
- High rate of wound failure in patients with malnutrition or immune deficiency
- Should delay amputation until nutritional parameters can be improved by nutritional support
- Pediatric amputations
   a. Usually performed for congenital limb deficiencies, trauma, or tumors
   b. Congenital amputations are the result of failure of formation.
      ◦ Amputations are rarely indicated for upper extremity congenital limb deficiencies; even rudimentary appendages can be useful.
      ◦ In the lower extremity, amputation of an unstable segment may allow for direct load transfer and improved walking.
         ♦ Absent fibula: Syme amputation
         ♦ Absent tibia: knee disarticulation
   c. Overgrowth is the most common complication in transosseous pediatric amputations, most commonly at the humerus
      ◦ Also seen in diaphyseal amputations of fibula, tibia, and femur
      ◦ Best method to predictably resolve this is surgical revision with adequate resection of bone
      ◦ Osteochondral stump capping has unpredictable results.
      ◦ Disarticulation is the only reliable measure to prevent overgrowth and subsequent revision surgeries.
         ♦ Maintain maximum residual limb length by preserving growth plates
   d. Prosthetic fitting
      ◦ Upper limb: at 4–6 months of age (sitting), 2–3 years for active device
      ◦ Lower limb: at 8–12 months of age
- Amputations in the trauma patient
   a. There are grading scales for evaluating mangled extremities that act as guidelines to determine if a limb is salvageable
      ◦ LEAP (Lower Extremity Assessment Project): severe soft tissue injury most important factor in decision making
      ◦ MESS (Mangled Extremity Severity Score): takes into consideration age, shock, limb ischemia, and energy of skeletal soft tissue injury
         ♦ Helpful as guide, but not proven to be sufficiently sensitive

b. Patient factors always a consideration:
   - Physiological, psychological, social, economic resources (self-efficacy); substance abuse history
   - May sway decision in "gray area" scenarios

c. Indications for immediate amputation
   - Grade IIIB and IIIC tibial injuries with uncontrollable hemorrhage
     - Typically from multiple levels of arterial/venous injury
     - Life versus limb: patients in extremis or very critically ill
   - Crush injury with warm ischemia time > 6 hours
   - Incomplete traumatic amputations with significantly injured distal segment

d. "Gray area" indications with high risk for prolonged reconstruction with complications and resulting in poor function
   - Significant segmental bone or muscle loss
   - Open tibia fractures associated with open foot injuries
   - Significant nerve injury
     - Lack of plantar sensation on exam is not a reliable clinical indicator of significant nerve injury; may be neurapraxia
       - Exploration of tibial nerve required

e. Amputation level
   - Amputate at most distal, viable level followed by open wound management
     - Closure or coverage when patient condition is stable and soft tissue stabilized
   - Amputation through the zone of injury caused by a blast mechanism predictive for the development of heterotopic ossification
     - Role of limb salvage in the trauma patient
       - Used in "gray area" scenarios when patient factors sway decision to limb salvage
       - SIP (Sickness Impact Profile) and return to work *not* significantly different at 2 and 7 years between limb salvage and amputation in severe limb threatening injuries
         - A salvaged lower limb that is insensate on the weight-bearing surface with associated functional muscle and bone loss is unlikely to provide a durable weight-bearing surface.
       - Lifetime costs incurred are thought to be higher with amputation than with limb salvage.
         - Western society: costs associated with prosthetics
       - Complication rates
         - Severe open tibia fractures managed by limb salvage have high rates of complications, including increased hospitalizations, infection, multiple surgeries

- Musculoskeletal tumors

  a. The goal of surgery is to remove the tumor with negative margins.

  b. Limb salvage versus amputation
     - Based on expected functional outcome if acceptable margins can be obtained with limb salvage
     - There is controversy regarding the outcomes of limb salvage versus amputation.
     - Limb salvage patients tend to be more sedentary.
     - Amputees tend to be more active.

- Technical considerations
  a. Skin flaps should be full thickness.
  b. Periosteal stripping helps minimize regenerative bone overgrowth.
  c. Wounds should not be closed under tension.
  d. Muscle should be secured to bone (myodesis) at resting tension as opposed to secured to antagonist muscle (myoplasty).
     - Especially adductor in transfemoral amputation
  e. Stable residual limb mass reduces atrophy and provides a stable soft tissue envelope over bone.
  f. All transected nerves form neuromas.
     - The nerve end should be far away from potential pressure areas.
  g. Compressive dressings postoperatively help with swelling and pain.
  h. Early prosthetic fitting is done at 5–21 days.
- Complications
  a. Pain
     - Phantom limb sensation occurs in most adults
     - Phantom dysesthesia in the absent limb
     - Complex regional pain syndrome is a common cause of residual pain.
       - May be treated with α-blocking agents
  b. Edema
     - Postoperative edema may prevent wound healing.
     - Rigid dressings and compression help reduce edema.
     - Chronic swelling can cause verrucous hyperplasia.
       - Should be treated with total contact casting
  c. Joint contractures
     - Hip and knee flexion contractures occur if the respective muscles are anchored with the joints in a flexed position during surgery.
     - Avoided with correct positioning during recovery (keeping knee fully extended and prone lying for the hip)
  d. Wound failure to heal
     - Most often in diabetics
     - If not amenable to local care, excision of a wedge of soft tissue and bone with tension-free soft tissue closure is preferred.
- Upper limb amputations
  a. Benefits of limb salvage
     - Sensation is crucial for function in the upper limb.
     - A partially sensate, partially functional salvaged limb is often more functional than an insensate prosthesis.
  b. Wrist disarticulation
     - Advantages
       - Preserves more forearm rotation because preserves distal radioulnar joint (DRUJ) compared with transradial
       - Flare of distal radius helps suspend prosthesis
     - Disadvantages
       - Cosmetic issues
         - Prosthesis is longer than contralateral limb
         - Motor and battery of myoelectric components cannot be hidden
         - Transradial amputation and elbow disarticulation
           - A nonfunctioning hand and forearm is best treated with a transradial amputation or elbow disarticulation.

- Optimum length of transradial amputation is at junction of middle and distal thirds.
  - ◊ Myoelectric components can be hidden.
- Length and shape of elbow disarticulation provides improved lever arm; epicondyles can enhance suspension.

▪ Transhumeral amputation
- Often limited prosthetic use due to discomfort and difficulty using prosthesis—elbow (flexion/extension) and hand functions (hand open/close) performed sequentially. Patients adapt using single upper extremity.

- Lower limb amputations

a. Toe and ray amputations
- ∘ Patients with ischemia do well after toe amputations because they ambulate with a propulsive gait pattern.
- ∘ Great toe should be amputated distal to the flexor hallucis brevis (FHB) insertion
- ∘ Isolated second-toe amputations are performed distal to the proximal phalanx metaphyseal flare to prevent late hallux valgus.
- ∘ Single outer ray amputations function well in shoes.
- ∘ Resection of more than one ray creates a narrow forefoot, leading to difficulty in shoe fitting.
- ∘ Central ray amputations have wound healing issues:
  - ♦ Rarely gets better results than midfoot amputations

b. Transmetatarsal and midfoot amputations (Lisfranc and Chopart)
- ∘ Long plantar flap is myocutaneous and the preferred flap
- ∘ Transmetatarsal amputations should be through proximal metaphyses to help prevent ulcer formation.
  - ♦ May bevel metatarsals on plantar surface and medial and lateral border
- ∘ Achilles tendon lengthening should be performed to help prevent equinus or equinovarus.
  - ♦ Result of overpull from gastrocnemius and posterior tibialis and short lever arm of absent forefoot
- ∘ Equinovarus can be corrected with tibialis anterior transfer to the neck of the talus.
  - ♦ Insertion site of the peroneus brevis and tertius at the base of the fifth metatarsal should be preserved.
  - ♦ Act as antagonists to posterior tibial tendon to prevent supination/inversion of the foot
- ∘ Avoid hindfoot amputations in patients with diabetes and vascular disease.

c. Ankle disarticulation (Syme)
- ∘ Allows direct load transfer, rarely has issues with ulcers and tissue breakdown
- ∘ Provides stable gait pattern
- ∘ Despite being more proximal, is more energy efficient than midfoot amputations such as Lisfranc or Chopart amputations
- ∘ Less energy efficient than a transmetatarsal amputation
- ∘ Posterior tibial artery supplies the heel pad and must be patent
  - ♦ Patients with an ankle-brachial index (ABI) < 0.5 in the posterior tibial artery have decreased healing rates.
- ∘ Remove malleoli and metaphyseal flares.

- The heel pad should be secured to the tibia either anteriorly with drill holes or posteriorly using the Achilles tendon.
  - Avoid hypermobile heel pad to ensure good results.

d. Transtibial amputation (below knee)
- The soft tissue envelope is created using a long posterior myocutaneous flap.
  - "Dog ears" at the edge of a long posterior flap are left intact because of the risk of injury to the saphenous and sural arteries. Flap necrosis is also a risk.
- Optimum bone length is at least 12 cm below the joint line but longer is better; provides soft tissue cover and room for prosthetic components
- Posterior muscle secured to beveled anterior tibia by myodesis
- Cylindrical shape preferred
- Rigid dressings are used in the early postoperative period.
- Early prosthesis fitting in 5–21 days depending on wound healing and if the residual limb is able to transfer load.
- Ertl modification, in which a bone bridge between the fibula and the tibia is created, was proposed to create a more stable platform for load transfer by enlarging the stable surface area.

e. Knee disarticulation
- Use long posterior flap with gastrocnemius as end padding
- The patella is sutured to the cruciate ligaments, leaving the patella on the anterior femur.
- Findings from the LEAP study suggest this to be the level of slowest walking speed and least self-reported satisfaction.
  - May be due to amputation through zone of injury in LEAP study and shorter follow-up (24 month)
- Patients report less pain compared with transtibial and transfemoral amputations.
- Usually used in nonambulatory patients
- Entails a muscle balanced amputation with a stable weight-bearing platform; allows direct load transfer
- Can use polycentric knee; maintains the knee center close to the anatomic joint line

f. Transfemoral amputation (above knee)
- Increases energy cost of walking
- Patients with transfemoral amputations and peripheral vascular disease usually do not ambulate well.
- **Transfemoral amputees may use close to maximum energy expenditure and may not regain the capacity to walk, especially the elderly and dysvascular patient.**
- A bone cut 12 cm above the knee center maintains symmetric joint lines and helps accommodate the prosthesis.
  - More proximal amputations have less adductor control and less surface area for prosthetic fitting.
  - To incorporate a rotator that allows for patient controlled rotation of the prosthesis to help with positional changes, the bone cut should be 3 cm more proximal.
- Greater femoral length gives a greater level arm, better for optimum limb advancement, better sitting balance, better adduction, more surface area for socket.
- Adductor myodesis is important to maintain femoral adduction: most important surgical consideration to successful patient function

- Restore tension on adductor magnus: anchored to lateral femur with femur held in adduction
- Mechanical axis near normal after amputation: limb should be in slight adduction
- Major deforming force is flexion and abduction
  - Adductor myodesis helps prevent this.
  - Distal third amputation results in 70% loss of adduction moment.

g. Hip disarticulation
   - High energy expenditure of walking; few patients ambulate
   - Patient sits in the prosthesis and uses torso to advance the limb forward

3. Prostheses
   - Upper limb

a. Upper limb biomechanics
   - The shoulder is the center of rotation.
   - The elbow acts as a caliper to position the hand in space.
   - Normally multiple joint actions occur simultaneously; with a prosthesis, they must occur sequentially.

b. Timing of prosthetic fitting
   - Should be done as soon as possible, even before complete wound healing
   - In unilateral amputations, patients can learn adaptive strategies leading to low prosthetic use.
   - < 30% use when fitted later than 30 days of transradial amputation

c. Two types of prostheses
   - Myoelectric prosthesis
     - Utilizes external battery and surface electrodes to control movement
     - Indications: transradial amputations, sedentary work, overhead activities
     - Advantages: better cosmesis, no straps or harnessing
     - Disadvantages: heavy, costly, less sensory feedback, requires frequent maintenance
   - Body powered prosthesis
     - Utilizes cables and harnesses to mechanically maneuver prosthesis through shoulder and arm movement
       - Harness ring of figure-of-8 brace should be at spinous process of C7
     - Indications: worker performing heavy labor
     - Advantages: durable, moderate cost, high sensory feedback
     - Disadvantages: poor cosmesis, requires upper body movement to power prosthesis

d. Below-elbow amputation
   - Body-powered prostheses
     - One-cable system
     - Terminal device activated by shoulder flexion and abduction
     - Appropriate for worker performing heavy labor
   - Myoelectric prostheses for sedentary work

e. Above-elbow amputation
   - Body-powered prosthesis
     - Two-cable system: control elbow flexion and terminal device
     - Two motions make for less functional outcomes and heavier prostheses
     - Elbow flexion and extension are controlled by shoulder extension and depression.

- Hybrid prosthetic system uses both myoelectric and body-powered components: provides best function

f. Proximal transhumeral and shoulder disarticulation amputations
   - Limited function is achieved with a manual shoulder joint positioned with contralateral hand, with prosthetic components

- Lower limb

a. Most important factor when prescribing components for a lower limb prosthesis in adults is their current and potential functional levels.
   - K1: household ambulator
   - K2: limited community ambulator
   - K3: unlimited community ambulator
   - K4: child, active adult or athlete

b. Prosthetic feet
   - Single-axis foot: ankle hinge provides plantar and dorsiflexion
   - Solid ankle, cushioned heel (SACH) foot; use discontinued
     - Was the standard; useful for patients with low activity levels
     - Led to overload of contralateral foot; use discontinued
   - o Dynamic response foot
     - Flexible keel deforms under load and absorbs energy
       - Soft heel can lead to knee extension
       - Hard heel can lead to knee flexion
     - Allow many normal activities, including running on uneven ground
     - Articulated and nonarticulated
       - Articulated dynamic response foot
         - Inversion/eversion, rotation of foot
         - Useful for activities on uneven surfaces
           - Young active patients
       - Nonarticulated dynamic response foot
         - Short or long keels
         - Short keels are not as responsive, indicated for moderate activity and ambulation
         - Long keels are more responsive, indicated for high-demand activities

c. Prosthetic knees
   - Used in patients with transfemoral amputations and knee disarticulations
   - Alignment stability: position of the prosthetic knee in relation to the patient's line of weight bearing **(Fig. 11.2)**
     - Center of rotation of prosthesis posterior to line of weight bearing allows control in stance but makes flexion difficult.
     - Center of rotation of prosthesis anterior to line of weight bearing makes flexion easier but allows less control.
   - Six basic types of knee prostheses:
     - Polycentric knee: moving center of rotation provides different stability characteristics during the gait cycle.
       - In stance, center of rotation kept posterior to line of gravity to aid in knee extension
       - Recommended for patients with transfemoral amputations, knee disarticulations, bilateral amputations
     - Constant friction knee: a hinge that dampens the knee swing by friction

        - Most common knee prosthesis in children
        - Only single-speed walking, not good for older patients
        - Stability in stance relies only on alignment
    - Stance phase control (weight activated) knee: functions like constant friction knee during swing phase but freezes via high friction brake when weight is applied to the limb
        - For older patients (safety knee)
        - Not for bilateral use
    - Fluid control (hydraulic and pneumatic) knee: allows variable cadence, can change speed of walking
        - Decrease knee flexion allows earlier swing through
        - Best for young, active patients
    - Variable friction (cadence control) knee: allows walking at different speeds but is not durable
    - Manual locking knee: consists of constant friction knee that has a lock in extension, can be unlocked
        - Used in weak and unstable patients
- Newer knee prostheses
    - Computerized power knee
        - Heavier, allows for normal gait and stair climbing
        - Also good choice for an active young patient
    - Rheo knee
        - Magnetorheological fluid
            - Intensity of magnetic field changes fluid viscosity
            - Load application impacts resistance

d. Suspension systems

- Suspension is provided in lower extremity prostheses through socket design and suspension sleeves
- Sockets
    - Provide comfortable control and even pressure distribution
    - Suction sockets provide airtight seal and are the primary socket modality
    - Transfemoral sockets
        - Quadrilateral sockets have a posterior brim that provides a shelf for the ischial tuberosity **(Fig. 11.5)**.
            - Narrow anteroposterior (AP) diameter
            - Difficult to keep femur in adduction
        - Narrow mediolateral transfemoral sockets distribute forces more evenly.
            - More anatomic, contain ischial tuberosity
            - Enhance rotational control
    - Transtibial sockets: weight bearing by patellar tendon loads all areas of residual limb that tolerate weight
        - Patella tendon bearing supracondylar/suprapatellar socket
            - Has proximal extensions over distal femoral condyles and patella
            - Recommended when the residual limb is short to increase surface area for pressure distribution
        - Pressure from the brim of the prosthesis can lead to peroneal nerve palsy
- Prosthetic sleeves
    - Friction and negative pressure are used for suspension.

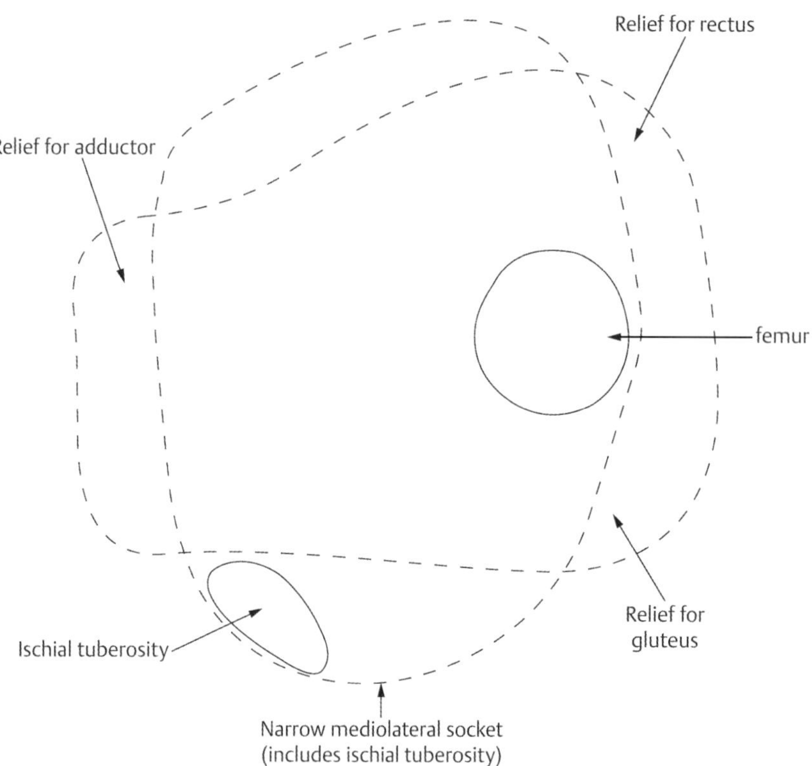

Fig. 11.5 Transfemoral amputation sockets: the quadrilateral versus the mediolateral socket. The dashed line is the quadrilateral socket.

- ♦ Transtibial suspension
  - ▪ Gel liner with a locking pin is preferred method
  - ▪ Sleeve rolls over stump and locking pin locks into socket
  - ▪ Allows unrestricted knee flexion, minimal piston action
  - ▪ Best used in young patients without stump volume fluctuation
- ♦ Transfemoral suspension
  - ▪ Negative pressure (vacuum) suspension frequently used
  - ▪ Stable body weight required for intimate fit

e. Common prosthetic problems
- ○ Skin problems
  - ♦ Contact dermatitis, cysts, scars
  - ♦ Painful residual limb caused by heterotrophic ossification, bony prominences, poor fitting prosthesis, neuromas, etc.
  - ♦ Residual limb ulcers are first treated with local wound care and adjustment of the residual limb–prosthesis interface
- ○ Prosthetic feet problems
  - ♦ Plantarflexed prosthetic foot or heel that is too soft can lead to excessive knee extension.
  - ♦ Dorsiflexed prosthetic foot or heel that is too hard can lead to excessive knee flexion.
- ○ Transtibial prosthetic problems
  - ♦ Swing-phase pistoning: ineffective suspension
  - ♦ Stance-phase pistoning: poor socket fit
  - ♦ Alignment problems
    - ▪ Medialized prosthesis
      - • Leads to varus strain on knee
      - • Pressure points distal/lateral and proximal/medial

- Lateralized prosthesis
  - Leads to valgus strain on knee
  - Pressure points distal/medial and proximal/lateral; usually fibula head
- Anterior prosthesis leads to knee extension.
- Posterior prosthesis leads to knee flexion.

♦ Problems related to the foot
- Same as prosthetic feet problems cited above

◦ Transfemoral prosthetic problems

♦ Lateral trunk bending: short prosthesis, weak hip abductors

♦ Abducted gait: poor socket fit medially

♦ Circumducted gait: long prosthesis, excessive knee friction

♦ Increased lumbar lordosis: hip flexion contractures, weak hip extensors, and insufficient anterior socket support

♦ Terminal snap: inadequate knee flexion

♦ Medial whip: caused by varus knee, excessive external rotation of knee, or muscle weakness

♦ Lateral whip: caused by valgus knee, internal rotation of knee, or muscle weakness

◦ Stair climbing

♦ Amputees tend to ascend stairs leading with the normal limb

♦ Descend stairs leading with the prosthetic limb

4. Orthoses
- Description
  a. An orthosis is a device used to control the motion of body segments and to manage painful joints, muscle weakness, and joint instability or contracture.
  b. Can be static, dynamic, or a combination
     - Static orthoses are rigid devices used to support the body part in a particular position.
     - Dynamic orthoses are devices that control body motion for optimum function.
  c. Generally not indicated for correction of fixed or spastic deformities that are not easily controlled manually
- Shoes
  a. Cushioned (SACH) or negative heels are used with a rigid ankle to reduce knee flexion moment
  b. Extra depth shoes with a high toe box are used to limit pressure over bony prominences, especially in diabetics.
  c. Plantar surface of an insensate foot is protected using pressure dissipating material
  d. Steel shanks can be used to extend the foot lever and prevent deformity at the toe break seen after a partial first ray amputation
     - Also used to treat metatarsalgia and hallux rigidus (Morton's extension)
  e. Rocker soles help transfer the body weight forward while walking and can lessen the bending force on an arthritic or stiff midfoot or ankle.
     - Used to nonsurgically relieve push-off pain from a Lisfranc nonunion; unloads the tarsometatarsal (TMT) junction
     - Used to treat metatarsalgia, hallux rigidus, with steel shanks
- Foot orthoses
  a. Three types: rigid, semi-rigid, soft
     - Rigid: limit joint motion, stabilize flexible deformities

- Semi-rigid: allow dorsiflexion and/or plantarflexion
- Soft: best shock absorbing capacity; accommodate fixed-foot deformities, especially with neuropathy

b. A heel cup is a rigid plastic insert.

- Covers the plantar surface of the heel and extends posteriorly, medially, and laterally
- Used to prevent lateral calcaneal shift in flexible flatfoot

c. University of California Biomechanics Lab (UCBL) orthosis

- Encompasses the heel and midfoot with rigid medial, lateral, and posterior walls
- Recommended as initial nonsurgical management for adult acquired flatfoot deformity
  - ♦ Elderly patients with a sedentary lifestyle have the highest patient satisfaction with this management.

d. Arizona ankle foot orthosis

- Combines the UCBL orthosis with a laced ankle support
- Provides more rigid hindfoot support

• Ankle–foot orthosis (AFO)

a. Consists of a footplate with stirrups, uprights, and calf band

b. Used to control the ankle joint

c. May be rigid to prevent ankle motion or can allow free or spring-assisted motion

d. Ankle position indirectly affects knee stability; ankle plantarflexion provides the knee with an extension force, and ankle dorsiflexion provides the knee with a flexion force.

e. After a hindfoot fusion, the primary goals are absorption of the ground reactive force, protection of the fusion sites, and protection of the midfoot.

f. Can be useful nonsurgical method of treating adult acquired flatfoot deformity

g. Nonarticulating AFO

- Used for equinus deformity
- Place flexion force on the knee during weight acceptance
- Described by the amount of rigidity of the brace

h. Articulating AFO

- Allows more natural gait pattern
- Used for drop foot
- Can be used if subtalar motion is present
- Adjustable ankle joints can set the desired range of ankle dorsiflexion and plantarflexion.

• Knee–ankle–foot orthosis (KAFO)

a. Extends from upper thigh to foot

b. Used to control an unstable or paralyzed knee joint

- Weak or paralyzed quadriceps
- Provides medial and lateral joint stability

c. Includes knee orthoses

- Elastic knee orthoses for treatment of patellar disease
- Metal and plastic used for an unstable anterior cruciate ligament

d. Knee joints

- Multiple types of knee joints, including single axis, posterior offset, polycentric, and dynamic (active extension with spring or coil)

- Hip–knee–ankle orthosis
  a. AFO plus a mechanical knee joint, thigh uprights, hip joint, and waist band
  b. Provides hip and pelvic stability
  c. Rarely used by paraplegic adults because it is cumbersome and requires large energy expenditures
  d. Children with lumbar myelomeningocele use reciprocating gait orthoses
    - Modified hip–knee–ankle–foot orthosis (HKAFO) for standing and simulated walk
- Elbow orthosis
  a. Hinged elbow brace provides limited stability for unstable elbows
  b. Dynamic spring-loaded orthoses have been used to treat elbow flexion and extension contractures.
- Wrist–hand orthosis
  a. Most commonly used for postoperative care after injury or reconstructive surgery
  b. Opponens splint pre-positions thumb but impairs tactile sensation
  c. Wrist-driven hand orthoses are used in lower cervical quadriplegics
    - Can be body powered by tenodesis or motor driven
    - Patients with injury at C5 can use ratchet orthosis.
    - Patients with injury at C6 can use wrist-driven, extensor-activated orthosis to provide pinch.
- Fracture braces
  a. Valuable treatment for isolated fractures of humerus, tibia and fibula
  b. Can be used in simple foot and ankle fractures, ankle sprains, simple hand injuries
- Pediatric orthoses
  a. Dynamic orthoses are used by children to control motion but limit immobilization.
  b. Pavlik harness is used for developmental dysplasia of the hip.
- Spine orthoses
  a. Cervical spine
    - Various collars, halo vests
  b. Thoracolumbar spine
    - Mechanically stabilize the back, reduces pain
    - Three-point orthoses achieve control through length of lever arm and limitation of motion.

5. Stroke and closed head injury rehabilitation
  - Description
    a. Adult acquired spasticity secondary to stroke or closed head injury
      - Balance is best predictor of function
      - Nonsurgical treatment
        - ♦ Orthotics, serial casting, motor point nerve blocks
        - ♦ Splinting a joint in neutral does not prevent contractures.
        - ♦ Intervention is necessary when functional ranging is insufficient.
        - ♦ Local anesthetic injections before casting can relieve pain and allow for maximum correction.
        - ♦ Open nerve blocks may be warranted to prevent injecting nerves with large sensory contributions.
      - Surgical treatment
        - ♦ Should be delayed until patient develops maximal spontaneous motor recovery: 6 months for stroke, 12–18 for traumatic brain injury (TBI)

- ♦ Patients should be screened for cognitive deficits, motivation, and body image awareness.
- ♦ Patients must have adequate short-term memory for learning.
- ♦ **Increased risk of heterotopic ossification in patients with traumatic brain injury**

- Lower limb
  - a. Balance is the best predictor of a patient's ability to ambulate after acquired brain injury.
  - b. Treatment goals for dynamic ankle equinus
    - ◦ Ankle stability in neutral position during initial floor contact
    - ◦ Ankle clearance during swing phase
  - c. Nonsurgical treatment
    - ◦ Adjustable AFO with ankle dorsiflexion and plantarflexion stop at neutral for use during the recovery period.
  - d. Surgical treatment
    - ◦ Motor balancing surgery: required when the dynamic equinus overcomes the orthosis and the brace will not stay in place
    - ◦ Split or complete lateral transfer of tibialis anterior: used for out-of-phase tibialis anterior muscle activity during gait, producing a dynamic varus deformity
- Upper limb
  - a. Nonfunctional goals
    - ◦ Surgical release of static contracture performed for nursing care and hygiene when contractures are causing skin maceration or breakdown
  - b. Functional goals
    - ◦ Improve upper extremity tracking (arm swing) during walking
    - ◦ Increase prehensile hand function
    - ◦ May allow one-handed patient to become two-handed by increasing hand function
      - ♦ When the goal is functional improvement, patients need to be screened for cognitive capacity, motivation, and body image awareness.
      - ♦ Muscle unit lengthening of the agonist deforming muscle along with motor balancing tendon transfers of the antagonists are used to achieve muscle balance.

6. Spinal cord injury rehabilitation
   - Mobility
     - a. Level of the spinal cord injury determines mobility
     - b. Injury at C4 and higher: requires high back and head support
     - c. Injury at C5: allows for mouth-driven wheelchair
     - d. Injury at C6: patients can use manual wheelchairs and flexor hinge wrist–hand orthoses
     - e. Transfers are dependent with C4 injury, assisted with C5 injury, and independent with C6 injury.
   - Activities of daily living
     - a. Patients with injury at C6 can groom and dress themselves.
     - b. Patients with injury at C7 can cut meat and can control bowel and bladder via rectal stimulation and intermittent catheterization.
   - Autonomic dysreflexia
     - a. Potentially catastrophic hypertensive event can occur with injuries above T6.
     - b. Acute sympathetic hyperactivity
     - c. Usually caused by obstructed urinary catheter or fecal impaction

d. Treatment: catheterize patient, control blood pressure with antihypertensives

- Surgery

a. Spinal fusion used to prevent late development of pain and deformity
   - Anterior or posterior fusion or both with internal fixation should be performed soon after injury.

b. Spasticity and contracture may cause hygiene issues or pressure ulcers.
   - Urosepsis is most common cause of death.
   - Pressure sores are preventable with proper bedding, frequent turns.
   - Percutaneous motor nerve blocks can be used to treat deformities.
   - When deformity is a static contracture, muscle release or disarticulation may improve sitting or transfer ability.

7. Postpolio syndrome

- Polio is a viral disease affecting the anterior horn cells of the spinal cord.

a. Sensation is intact; motor weakness

b. Postpolio syndrome is not reactivation of the virus but further inactivation of nerve cells as a result of aging.

c. Occurs after middle age

- Affected patients use a large amount of their capacity for activities of daily living.
- Treatment

a. Limited exercise combined with periods of rest: best method to optimize function of muscles

b. Contracture release, arthrodesis, tendon transfers when the deformity overcomes functional capacity

c. Lightweight orthoses help patients remain functionally independent

8. Physical therapy and rehabilitation

- Strongest negative predictor for successful outcome from rehabilitation for chronic disorders is high pre-rehabilitation pain intensity.
- Exercise types

a. Isotonic: constant muscle tension as muscle changes length

b. Isoinertial: application of a muscle contraction throughout the range of motion (ROM) against a constant resistance/load where the measurement system considers acceleration and velocity to keep the same inertia even if the direction of the ROM changes

c. Isometric: muscle contraction without joint motion (length same)

d. Isokinetic: fixed muscle contraction speed with varying resistance throughout ROM
   - Biking at constant speed with varied resistance

- Muscle contraction

a. Concentric: muscle shortening during a contraction

b. Eccentric: muscle lengthening during a contraction
   - Eccentric contractions are useful in treating late-stage tendinopathies
   - Proven to be as successful as surgery for patellar tendinopathy (jumper's knee)
   - Also commonly used in Achilles tendinopathy

c. Most efficient way to strengthen skeletal muscle

- Exercise definitions

a. Periodization: conditioning program in which changes in training specificity, intensity, and volume are organized into cycles to help make strength/endurance gains

b. Plyometrics: utilizes the stretch-shortening cycle (eccentric–amortization/pause–concentric) to train muscles, connective tissue, and the nervous system; starts with eccentric loading of a muscle, a brief pause/transition phase, and then a rapid contraction to generate a forceful movement

- Range of motion
  a. Exercise programs for musculoskeletal rehab should primarily focus on nonpainful ROM
  b. Active: motion of a joint that a patient can actively do without assistance
  c. Active assist: motion of a joint that a patient does with assistance from a therapist to increase the motion
  d. Passive: the motion of a joint that a therapist can put a patient through
- Stretching types
  a. Static: slow and constant stretch
  b. Ballistic: active muscular effort through a bouncing movement
  c. Dynamic: increasing flexibility through sport-specific movements; often part of a warm-up
  d. Proprioceptive neuromuscular facilitation (PNF): utilizes passive and isometric stretching. The muscle is passively stretched, then isometrically contracted against resistance in the stretched position. Next, it is passively stretched again by post-isometric relaxation through the resulting increased ROM.
  e. Active-isolated stretching (AIS): method in which the athlete actively contracts the agonist muscle to isolate a stretch to the targeted muscle, then holds the maximal stretch position for 1 to 2 seconds. The stretch is then released and repeated six to 10 times.
- Open versus closed kinetic chain exercises
  a. Open kinetic chain exercises
     - Movements against resistance with the foot or hand not in contact with a fixed surface
     - **Open chain exercises are avoided in early anterior cruciate ligament (ACL) rehab to prevent creating greater shear stresses on the graft.**
     - Examples: knee extensions, biceps curls
  b. Closed kinetic chain exercises
     - Movements against resistance with the foot or hand in contact with the ground, wall, or other fixed surface and is therefore making the limb weight bearing
     - Examples: squats, push-ups, leg press
     - Preferred in earlier rehabilitation stages
     - Safer and protective due to the compressive nature of the applied loads
       - ♦ Less shear, translation, and distraction of the joints within the chain

9. Physical therapy modalities and techniques
   - Functional capacity evaluation: systematic measurement of a patient's ability to perform meaningful tasks
     a. Helps to assess recovery, determine goals, assist in returning patient to work
   - Work hardening/simulation: replication of work activities in controlled environment to help return an injured worker to the premorbid level of function
   - Ultrasound: applies deep thermal energy at 0.8 to 3 MHz to deep tissues.
   - Pulsed ultrasound: used for localized deep-tissue massage for reduction of edema in acute injuries

- Phonophoresis: utilizes ultrasound to deliver medications to tissues locally
- Neuromuscular electrical stimulation (NMES): modality using electrical stimulators including burst-modulated alternating current. Useful to maintain muscle mass and strength during prolonged immobilization
- Transcutaneous electrical nerve stimulation (TENS): form of electrical stimulation for acute and chronic pain
- High-voltage stimulation (HVS): uses a monophasic pulse to act on negatively charged plasma proteins in the acute setting of injury to create an electrical potential to result in less edema at the injury site
- Cryotherapy/ice: cools tissue to 0 to 23°C to decrease local tissue metabolism, promote vasoconstriction, decrease edema or hemorrhage, decrease muscle efficiency, and improve pain relief by blunting neuromuscular transmission
- Heat: warming tissue to 37 to 43°C; typically helpful for spasms, abdominal muscle cramping, menstrual cramps, and superficial thrombophlebitis
- Iontophoresis: delivery of a charged medication through the skin via direct electrical stimulation. Medications delivered through this modality include dexamethasone, lidocaine, and acetate.

12

Biomechanics and Biostatistics

Gregory R. Waryasz and Michael J. Rainbow

I. Newtonian Mechanics

1. Vectors and scalars
   - Vector **(Fig. 12.1)**
     a. Magnitude and direction (orientation)
     b. Direction specified by
        - Angle
        - **Useful values: sine (30 degrees) = cosine (60 degrees) = 0.5, sine (45 degrees) = cosine (45 degrees) ≈ 0.7, sine (60 degrees) = cosine (30 degrees) ≈ 0.9**
        - Resolved into components along x, y, and z axes
     c. Examples: velocity, acceleration, force, moment
   - Scalar
     a. Magnitude only
     b. Examples: mass, time, temperature, speed
2. Mass properties
   - Mass: property of a physical body that determines its resistance to changes in velocity (acceleration) and the strength of the gravitational attraction to other bodies
     a. Units: kilograms (kg)
   - Density: amount of mass per unit area, or per unit volume
     a. Units: kg/m^2 (per unit area) or kg/m^3 (per unit volume)
     a. Symbol: Greek letter rho, ρ
   - Center of mass (COM): unique, imaginary point at which all the mass of an object can be considered to be concentrated.
     a. The COM of the human body is located within the pelvis/lower abdomen (anterior to S2) during standing and gait **(Fig. 12.2a, b)**
     b. COM location depends on the distribution of mass (e.g., relative position of body segments) **(Fig. 12.2c)**
     c. **Since there are equal amounts of mass on each side of the COM in a given plane, the COM is the point of balance.**
   - Mass moment of inertia: distribution of the mass of an object about a given axis
     a. Mass multiplied by length squared ($I_0 = r^2 * m$), where I_0 is the mass moment of inertia, r^2 is the distance of the mass from the axis, and m is the mass.
     b. Resistance to rotation about an axis
     c. **Moment of inertia is the rotational analog to mass**

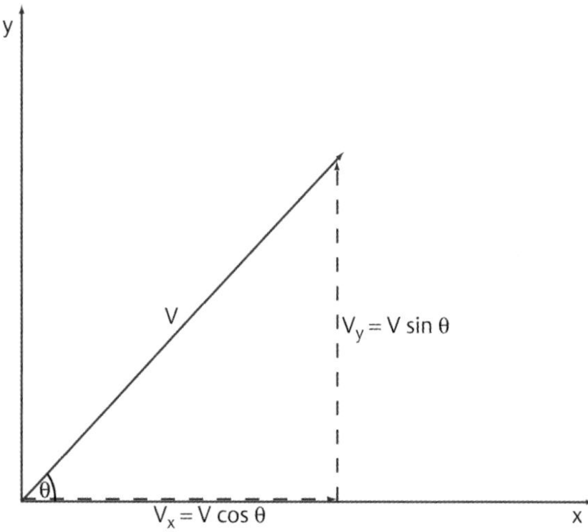

Fig. 12.1 Vector: basic definition. Vector **V** has magnitude V and direction θ. **V** can be broken into two vectors directed along the x and y axes with magnitudes $V_x = V * \cos(\theta)$ and $V_y = V * \sin(\theta)$, respectively.

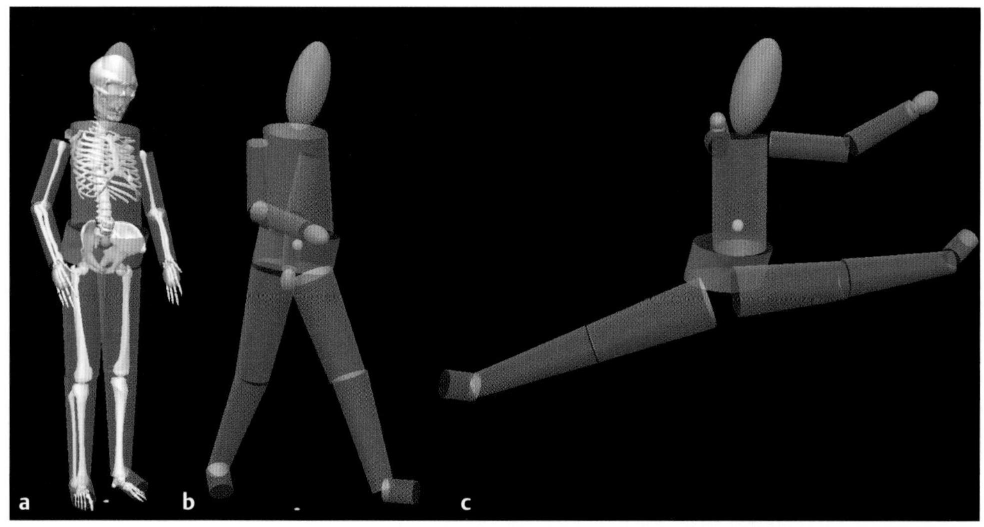

Fig. 12.2 (a,b) The center of mass (COM) of the human body is located within the pelvis/lower abdomen (anterior to S2) during standing and gait. **(c)** COM location depends on the distribution of mass (e.g., relative position of body segments).

- Polar moment of inertia: measure of the difficulty to turn a cross section about an axis perpendicular to it (J = r^4)
  a. Greater polar moment of inertia increases a beam's resistance to torsion
- Area moment of inertia: property of a cross section that characterizes its deflection under loading or I_A = r^4
  a. Greater area moment of inertia requires more stress to deflect a beam

3. Velocity and speed
   - Velocity is a vector quantity equal to distance/time along a direction.
   - Speed is a scalar quantity equal to distance/time.
   - Units: meters/second (meters per second)
4. Acceleration
   - Acceleration is a vector quantity.
   - Magnitude is equal to speed/time or distance/ time^2.
   - Units: meters/second^2
   - Example: acceleration due to gravity, *g*, is 9.81 m/s^2
5. Angular velocity (ω)
   - $\omega = v/r$, where *v* is the tangential velocity of an object and *r* is the distance to the axis of rotation
   - Units: radians/second (360 degrees/s = 2*PI radians/s)
   - **Some joints are capable of very high angular velocities; for example, the shoulder can internally rotate at ~9,000 deg/s or 1500 rpm during a baseball pitch**
6. Angular acceleration (α)
   - $\alpha = \omega$/time
   - Units: radians/s^2 or degrees/s^2
7. Force = mass * acceleration (Newton's second law)
   - **Layman's description: a push or a pull**
   - Force is a vector (magnitude and direction).
   - Units: newtons (N) = kg * m/s^2
8. Moment (torque): force * perpendicular distance **(Fig. 12.3)**
   - **Layman's description: rotational force**
   - Perpendicular distance is called moment arm or lever arm.
   - Units: newton-meters

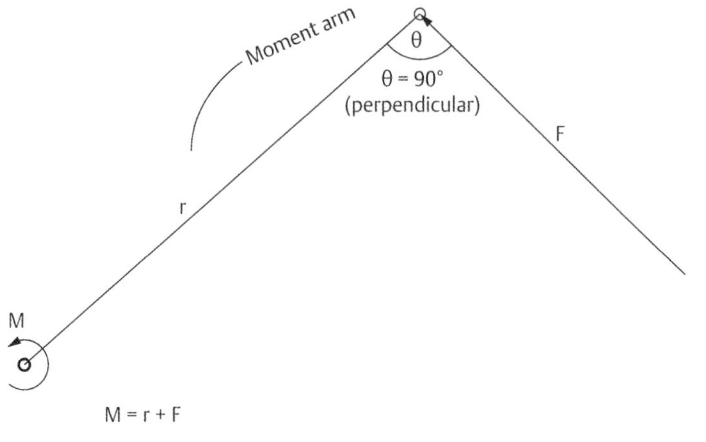

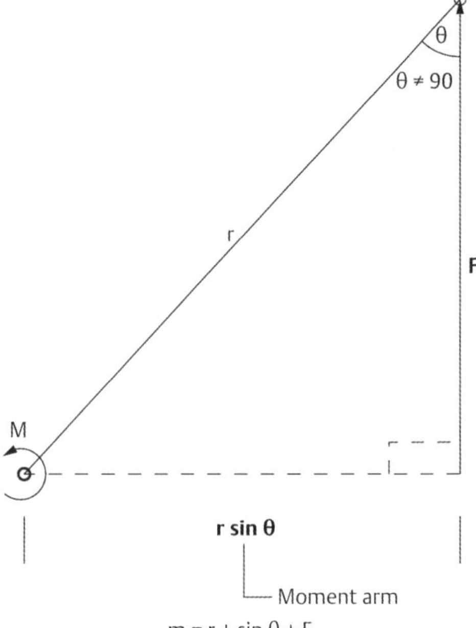

Fig. 12.3 Moment or torque is equal to the moment arm (lever arm) * force. Moment arm is perpendicular distance from the point of force application to the applied moment. **(a)** Case 1: force is perpendicular to *r*. **(b)** Case 2: force is not perpendicular to *r*. Moment arm is the perpendicular distance *r* * sin Θ. M, moment arm; f, force.

- Moment is a vector (magnitude and direction).
- **In biomechanics, moment is often computed about a joint's center of rotation.**

9. Work (*W*): force and the displacement it causes (work = force * distance)
   - Energy: ability to perform work
   - Units: joules
10. Power (*P*): energy per unit time
    - *P* = force * velocity
    - *P* = moment * angular velocity
    - Units: joules/second or watts
    - **During jogging, the power burst of the ankle joint at push-off is ~800 watts. For comparison, the power consumption of a smart phone during a phone call is ~3 watts.**
11. Newton's laws
    - First law (inertia): If net force is zero, body will not move or will move with constant velocity
    - Second law: Force is equal to mass multiplied by acceleration ($F = m * A$)
    - **The rotational analog of newton's second law is $M = I * \alpha$, where *M* is the moment, *I* is the mass moment of inertia, and α is angular acceleration.**
      a. Example: weight = mass * acceleration due to gravity ($w = m * g$)
    - Third law (action-reaction): For every action there is an equal and opposite reaction
      a. Example: ground reaction force and weight **(Fig. 12.4)**

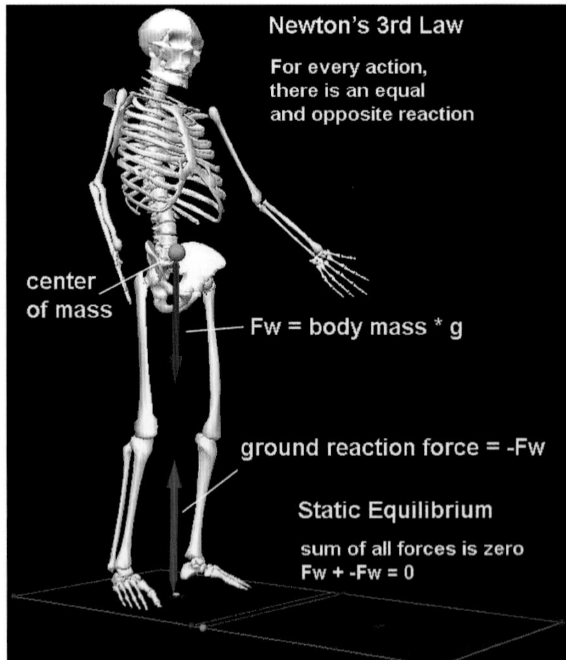

Fig. 12.4 Statics: actions of forces and moments on rigid objects in a system in static equilibrium. Example: during quiet standing, ground reaction force is equal and opposite to weight. FW, ground reaction force; g, acceleration due to gravity.

II. Application of Newtonian Mechanics

1. Statics: actions of forces and moments on rigid objects in a system in static equilibrium **(Fig. 12.4)**

- Sum of all forces = 0
- Sum of all moments = 0

2. Dynamics: bodies accelerating and related forces and moments
   - Sum of all forces = mass * acceleration
   - Sum of all moments = moment of inertia * angular acceleration
3. Analysis
   - Definitions of forces **(Fig. 12.5)**
     a. Normal force is perpendicular to surface it acts on.

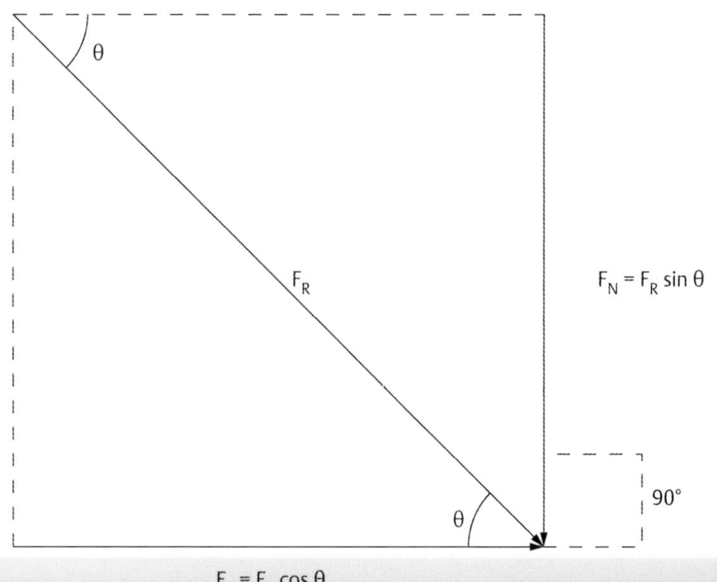

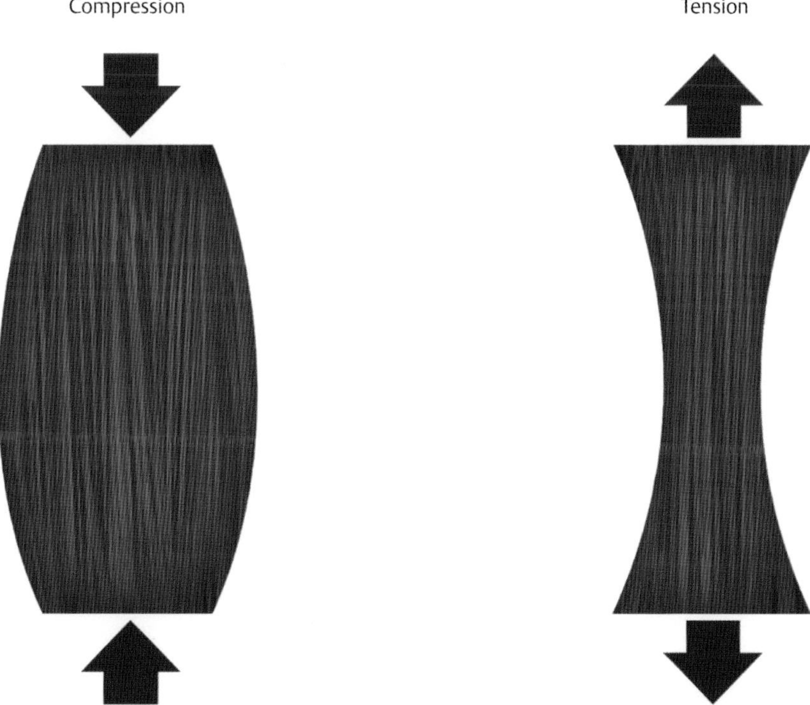

Fig. 12.5 Definitions of forces. **(a)** The force F_R acting at an angle to the surface is broken into a normal force F_N perpendicular to the surface and a tangential force F_T that is parallel to the surface. **(b)** Example of forces acting in compression and tension.

b. Tangential force is parallel to surface it acts on.
c. Compressive force shortens a body in the direction of the force.
d. Tensile force lengthens a body in the direction of the force.

- Free-body diagram: used to solve statics and dynamics problems
  a. Draw only one body that contains unknowns being solved.
  b. Draw all known forces and moments at their points of application.
  c. Draw unknown forces and moments including those due to bodies that are in contact.
  d. Do not include internal forces that originate and terminate within the free body.
- Example statics problem: determine muscle-tendon force of the biceps when holding a ball **(Fig. 12.6)**.

III. Biomechanics

1. Definitions
   - Biomechanics: study of structure and function of living organisms using principles of mechanics
   - Kinematics: study of motion without consideration of causes of motion
   - Kinetics: study of motion and its causes (forces, moments)
   - Kinesiology: study of human motions/movements
2. Overview of joints and their characteristics
   - Degrees of freedom
     a. Number of translational and rotational motions a joint possesses out of a total possible of six (three x, y, and z rotations and three x, y, and z translations)
        - **Examples: The hip joint has three rotational degrees of freedom, the wrist has two rotational degrees of freedom (flexion-extension, and radial-ulnar deviation), and the patella has six degrees of freedom.**

     b. Rolling and sliding: joints roll and slide to maintain congruence (e.g., knee joint and knee total joint)
     c. Mechanical approximations of human joints: joints are modeled as mechanical joints with varying degrees of freedom **(Fig. 12.7)**
   - Friction: force that acts in the opposite direction to movement
     a. Coefficient of friction is the ratio of the force of friction and the normal force. Examples: 0.002 to 0.04 for human joints, metal on ultrahigh molecular weight polyethylene (UHMWPE) is 0.05 to 0.15

IV. Biomechanics of Individual Joints

1. Shoulder
   - Combination of glenohumeral and scapulothoracic motion
     a. Abduction: 120 degrees of glenohumeral motion and 60 degrees of scapulothoracic motion at a 2:1 ratio; total abduction is 165 degrees
   - Arthrodesis: 15 to 20 degrees abduction, 20 to 25 degrees forward flexion, 40 to 50 degrees internal rotation
2. Elbow
   - Range of motion (ROM): 150 degrees of flexion, 0 degrees of extension, 90 degrees of pronation, 90 degrees of supination
     a. Functional ROM is 30 to 130 degrees (extension/flexion), 50 degrees (pronation/supination)

1.

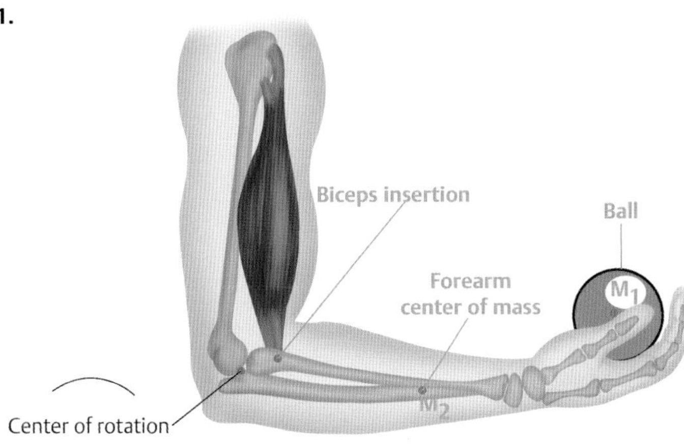

2.

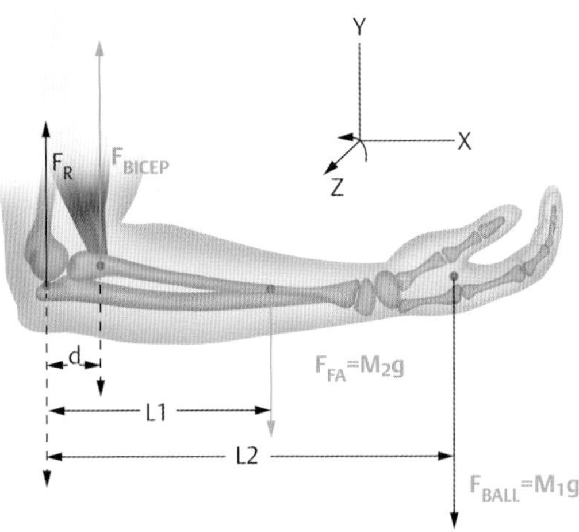

3.

(A) (B)

$\sum F = 0. \sum M = 0$ (Compute moment about center of rotation)

(A) $F_R + F_{BICEP} - F_{FA} - F_{BALL} = 0 = \sum F$

(B) $(F_R * 0^0) + (F_{BICEP} * d) - (F_{FA} * L_1) - (F_{BALL} * L_2) = 0 \sum M$

$$F_{BICEP} = \frac{F_{FA} L_1 + F_{BALL} L_2}{d}$$

Could plug in to (A) and solve for joint reaction force

Fig. 12.6 Example statics problem: determine muscle-tendon force of the biceps when holding a ball. F_R is the joint reaction force, F_{BICEP} is the force exerted by the bicep, F_{FA} is the weight of the forearm, and F_{BALL} is the weight of the ball. 1, physical scenario; 2, translated to force vectors; 3, static equation.

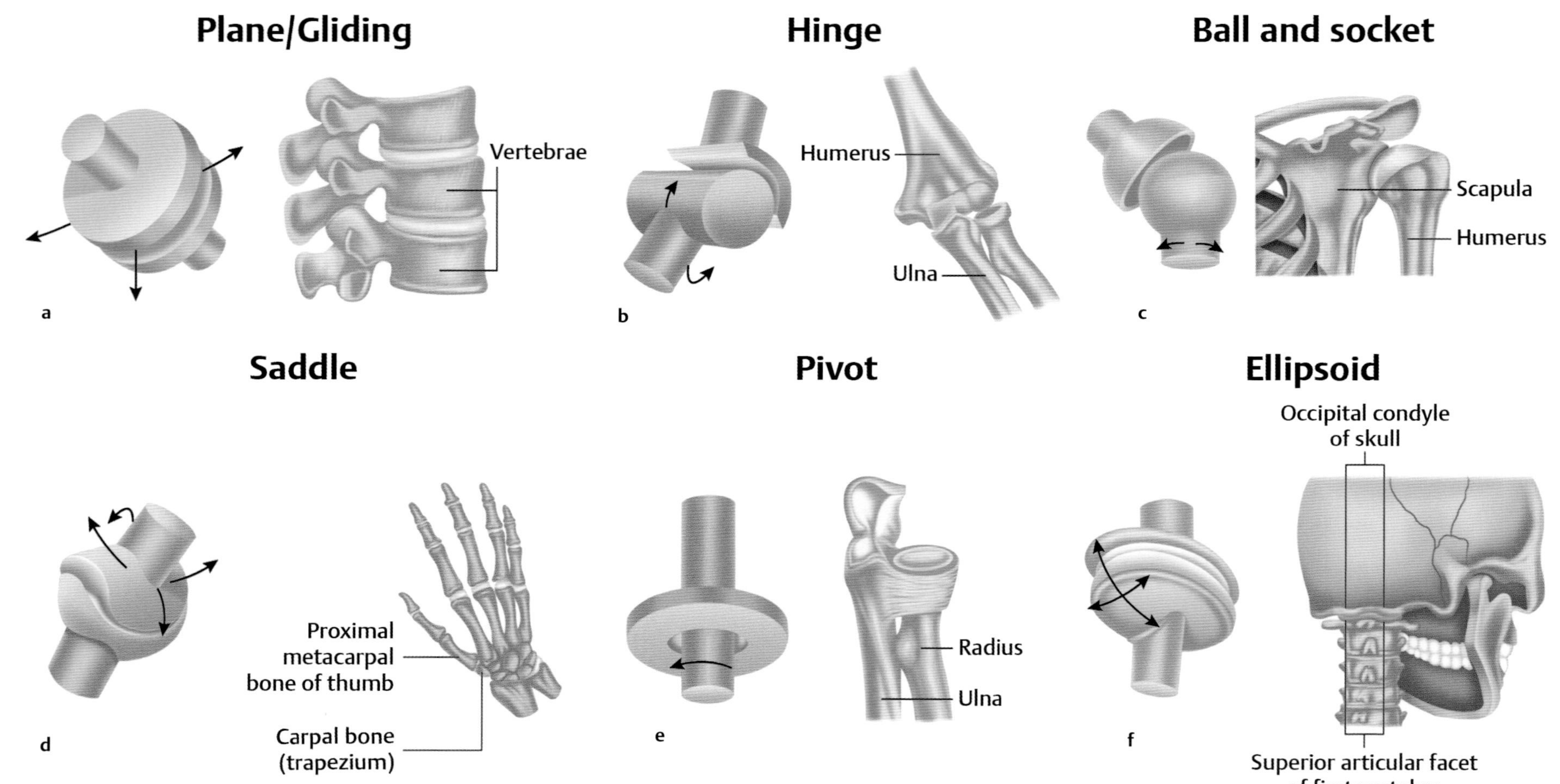

Fig. 12.7 The classification of joints by shape. The *arrows* indicate the direction in which the skeletal elements can move around the axis or axes of the joint. Amphiarthroses (not shown here) are "stiff" because their mobility is greatly restricted by the shape of their articular surfaces and by tight ligaments (examples are the proximal tibiofibular joint and sacroiliac joint). **(a)** Plane/gliding joint. The only movement allowed is a translation (sliding) of one member on the other (example: vertebral facet joint). **(b)** Hinge joint. This joint has one axis of motion, resulting in two primary movements (example: parts of the elbow joint). **(c)** Ball-and-socket joint. This type of joint has three mutually perpendicular axes of motion, resulting in six primary movements (example: hip joint). **(d)** Saddle joint. This is a biaxial joint with four primary movements (example: the carpometacarpal joint of the thumb). **(e)** Pivot joint. This is a uniaxial joint with two primary movements (example: the proximal radioulnar joint). **(f)** Ellipsoid joint. The only movement allowed is a translation (sliding) of one member on the other (example: vertebral facet joint).

- Arthrodesis
    a. Unilateral: 90 degrees of flexion
    b. Bilateral: 110 degrees of flexion for hand to reach mouth, 65 degrees of flexion for perineal hygiene

3. Hand/wrist
    - Wrist ROM: 65 degrees of flexion, 70–90 degrees of extension, 20 degrees of radial deviation, 35 degrees of ulnar deviation
        a. Functional ROM: 10 degrees of flexion, 35 degrees of extension, 0 degrees of radial deviation, 15 degrees of ulnar deviation
    - Wrist arthrodesis: 10 to 20 degrees of extension; if bilateral, then fuse contralateral wrist at 0 to 10 degrees of palmar flexion or do a total wrist arthroplasty
    - Hand ROM: metacarpophalangeal (MCP) joint is 100 degrees of flexion and 60 degrees of abduction/adduction; proximal interphalangeal (PIP) joint is 110 degrees; distal interphalangeal (DIP) joint is 80 degrees of flexion.
    - Hand joint arthrodesis: finger MCP 20–40 degrees of flexion, PIP 40–50 degrees of flexion, DIP 0–5 degrees of flexion; thumb MCP 25 degrees of flexion, interphalangeal (IP) 20 degrees of flexion.
4. Hip
    - Ball-and-socket joint
    - ROM: 115 degrees of flexion, 30 degrees of extension, 50 degrees of abduction, 30 degrees of adduction, 45 degrees of internal rotation, 45 degrees of external rotation
    - Joint reaction force can be three to six times body weight
    - Trendelenburg gait is essentially a reduction in joint reaction force and abductor moment by shifting weight over the affected hip. This gait pattern compensates for weak hip abductors.
        a. A cane in the opposite hand can produce an additional moment to reduce the hip abduction moment.
    - Arthrodesis position is 25–30 degrees of flexion, 0 degrees of abduction/rotation.
5. Knee
    - Flexion and extension involve rolling and sliding. Posterior rollback maximizes flexion.
    - "Screw home mechanism": tibia externally rotates during last 15 degrees of extension
    - ROM: 0 degrees of extension, 130 degrees of flexion
        a. At full extension there is minimal rotation; at 90 degrees of flexion can achieve 45 degrees of external rotation and 30 degrees of internal rotation
        b. Require 110 degrees of flexion to rise from a chair after total knee arthroplasty (TKA)
    - Patella slides 7 cm caudally during full flexion
    - Stabilizers: anterior cruciate ligament (ACL)/posterior cruciate ligament (PCL) for anterior and posterior
    - Arthrodesis: 0 to 7 degrees of valgus, 10 to 15 degrees of flexion
    - Mechanical axis **(Fig. 12.8)**
        a. Anatomic axis of the femur is along the shaft.
        b. Mechanical axis of the femur is the femoral head center to the knee center.
        c. Anatomic axis of the tibia is along the shaft.
        d. Mechanical axis of the tibia is the center of the plateau to the center of the ankle.
    - Patella: increases lever arm to increase extension, loss of 30% extension power after patellectomy

6. Foot and ankle
   - Ankle joint (tibiotalar) (also known as talocrural joint)
     a. ROM: 25 degrees of dorsiflexion, 35 degrees of plantarflexion, 5 degrees of rotation
     b. Arthrodesis: neutral dorsiflexion, 5–10 degrees of external rotation, 0–5 degrees of hindfoot valgus
   - Subtalar joint (talus-calcaneus)
     a. ROM: 5 degrees of pronation, 20 degrees of supination; functional ROM is 6 degrees
   - Transverse tarsal joint (talus–navicular, calcaneal–cuboid)
     a. Inversion/eversion
   - Foot
     b. Three arches
        - Medial longitudinal
        - Lateral longitudinal
        - Transverse
7. Spine
   - ROM
     a. Occiput-C1: 13 degrees of flexion/extension, 8 degrees of lateral bending, 0 degrees of rotation
     b. C1–C2: 10 degrees of flexion/extension, 0 degrees of lateral bending, 45 degrees of rotation
     c. C2–C7: 10–15 degrees of flexion/extension, 8–10 degrees of lateral bending, 10 degrees of rotation
     d. T-spine: 5 degrees of flexion/extension, 6 degrees of lateral bending, 8 degrees of rotation
     e. L-spine: 15–20 degrees of flexion/extension, 2–5 degrees of lateral bending, 3–6 degrees of rotation
   - Alignment
     a. Normal is 55 to 60 degrees of lumbar; most lordosis at L4-S1

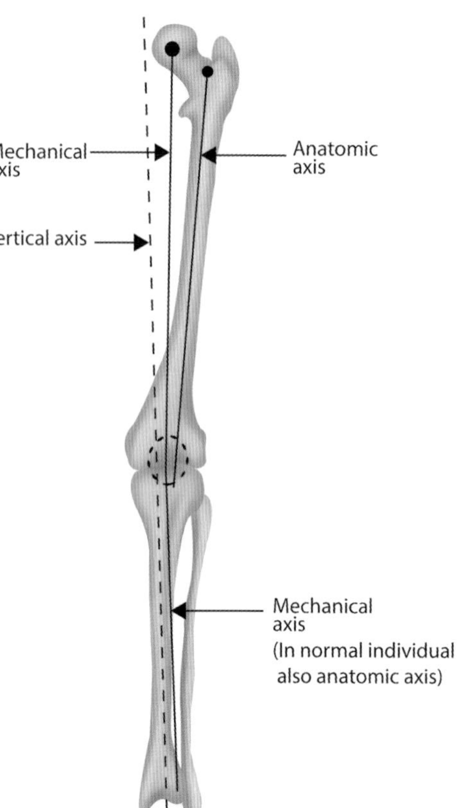

Fig. 12.8 Mechanical axis. Lower extremities axes.

V. Biomaterials

1. The basics
   - Structural properties: depends on shape
     a. Bending stiffness, torsional stiffness, axial stiffness
   - Material properties: independent of shape
     a. Elasticity, yield point, brittle-ductile, toughness
2. Definitions
   - Loads: forces acting on an object (e.g., compression, tension, shear, torsion)
   - Load relaxation: decreased peak loads over time with the same amount of elongation
   - Deformation: elastic is temporary, plastic is permanent
   - Elasticity: ability for a structure to return to its original shape once load is removed
   - Stress: force divided by area (N/m^2) **(Fig. 12.9)**
     a. Normal stresses are perpendicular to the acting surface.
     b. Shear stresses are parallel to the acting surface.
     c. Stress relaxation: decrease in stress under constant strain
     d. ACL graft in reconstruction undergoes stress relaxation

- Strain: measure of deformation due to loading **(Fig. 12.10)**
  a. In one-dimension: change in length/original length
  b. Can result from either normal or shear stresses
  c. Strain rate is the strain divided by the time that the load is applied
- Hooke's law: stress is proportional to strain to a limit (the elastic zone)
- Young's modulus of elasticity (*E*) **(Fig. 12.11)**
  a. *E* = stress/strain where *E* is the slope in the elastic range of the stress strain curve.
  b. A material with a higher *E* is resistant to greater forces than those with a lower *E*.
  c. Defined as stress at failure divided by strain at failure

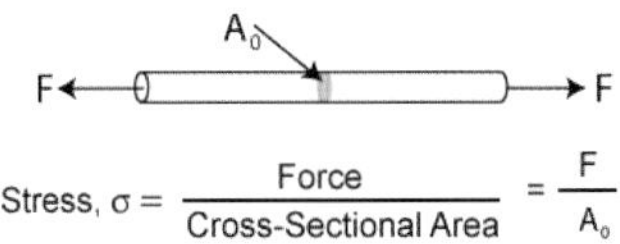

Fig. 12.9 Stress: force divided by cross-sectional area (N/m^2).

3. Stress-strain curve **(Fig. 12.12)**
   - **Relative elastic modulus of common orthopaedic materials (in descending order)**
     a. Ceramics
     b. Cobalt-chrome alloy
     c. Stainless steel
     d. Titanium
     e. Cortical bone
     f. Polymethylmethacrylate (PMMA) (cement)
     g. Polyethylene
     h. Cancellous bone
     i. Tendon/ligament
     j. Cartilage
   - Elastic deformation: when the stress/strain curve is linear and the applied force to the material is linear to the displacement; the material returns to its resting shape after the force is removed; stiffer materials have a steeper slope.
   - **The steeper the slope, the stiffer the material. Brittle materials have a steep slope and essentially no plastic deformation before failing.**
   - Yield point (elastic limit): transition point on the stress/strain curve where the force applied creates a nonlinear change in displacement; after this point, the material undergoes plastic deformation.
   - Plastic deformation: when the stress/strain curve is nonlinear, and the applied force leads to displacement that does not return to its resting shape after the force is removed (permanently deformed)
   - Energy (measured in joules): Energy absorbed by the material is equal to the area under the curve (elastic and plastic zones).
   - Ultimate strength and failure point: maximum strength of a material until failure where the material breaks
     a. Material with little plastic deformation is brittle (ceramic for example)
     b. Material with large range of plastic deformation is ductile (copper for example)
   - Toughness (strain energy, joules/m^2): material that can absorb large amount of energy before failure; has a large area under the curve from plastic deformation
   - **Materials that are both strong and ductile are tough because they can absorb high amounts of energy prior to failure, as seen by the large area under the curve.**
   - Strong: amount of force required for a material to reach its failure point

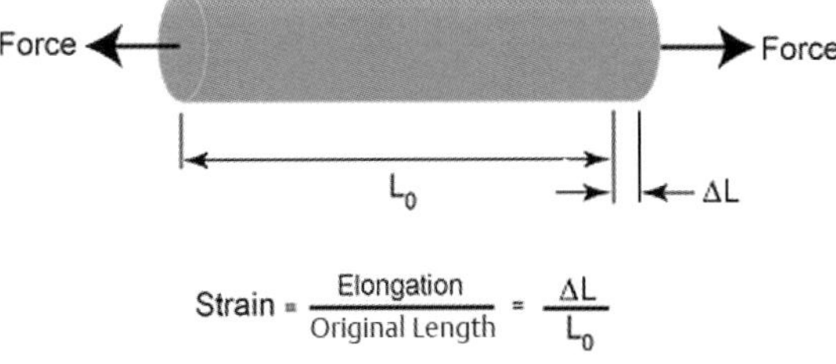

Fig. 12.10 Strain: measure of deformation due to loading.

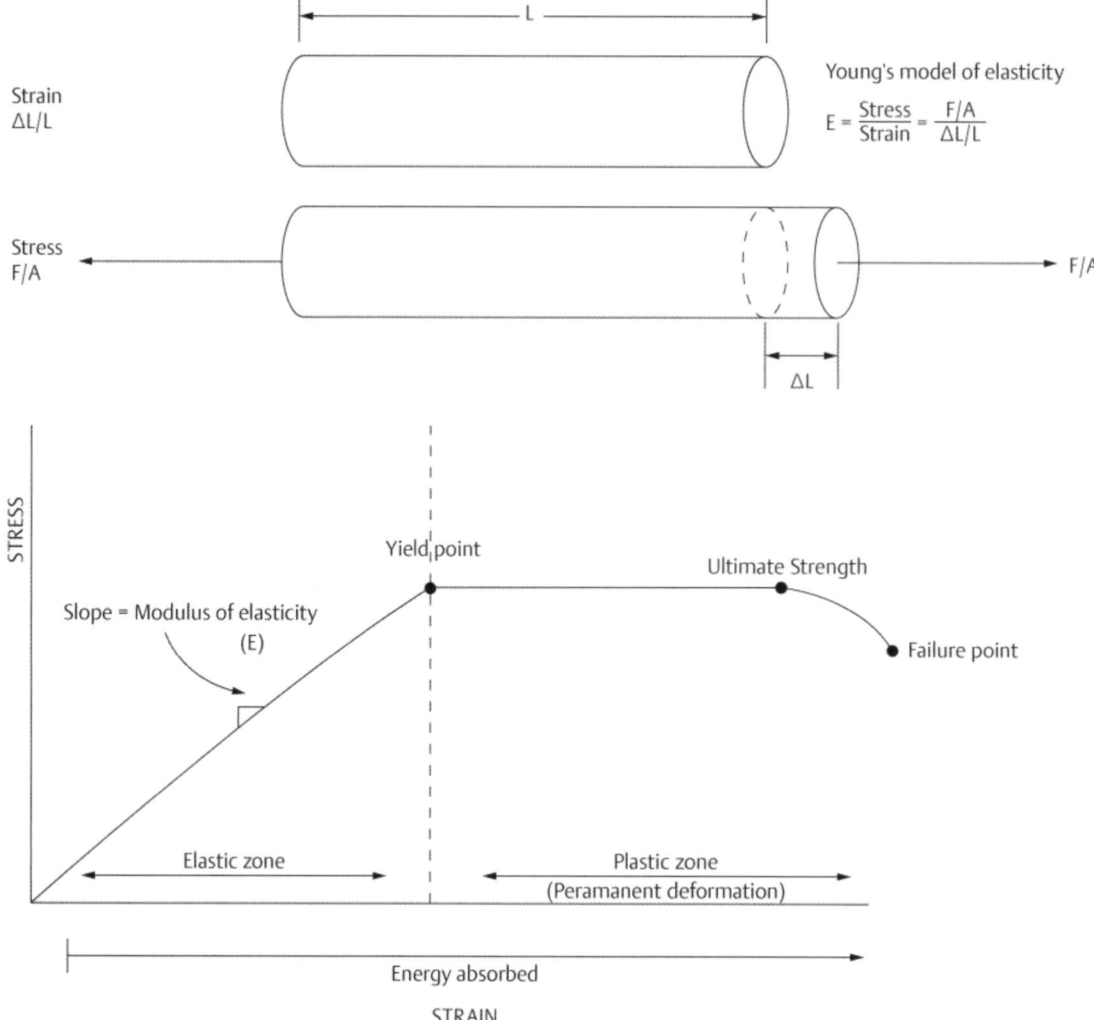

Fig. 12.11 Characteristics of the stress-strain curve. A, cross-sectional area; F, force; L, length.

4. Materials **(Table 12.1)**
   - Brittle: small amount of deformation between elastic limit and breaking point; therefore, these materials display little to no plastic deformation prior to failure.
     a. Examples: PMMA, concrete, glass, cast iron
        - **Brittle = Hard; small plastic curve**
   - Ductile: large amount of deformation between elastic limit and breaking point; therefore, these materials undergo a large amount of plastic deformation prior to failure.
     a. Examples: steel, aluminum, nylon, Teflon
        - **Ductile = Tough; large plastic curve**
   - Viscoelastics: time-rate dependent stress-strain behavior; load magnitude and rate determine characteristics; display hysteresis (characteristics depend on current and past environment); tensile strength is affected by the rate of applied strain.

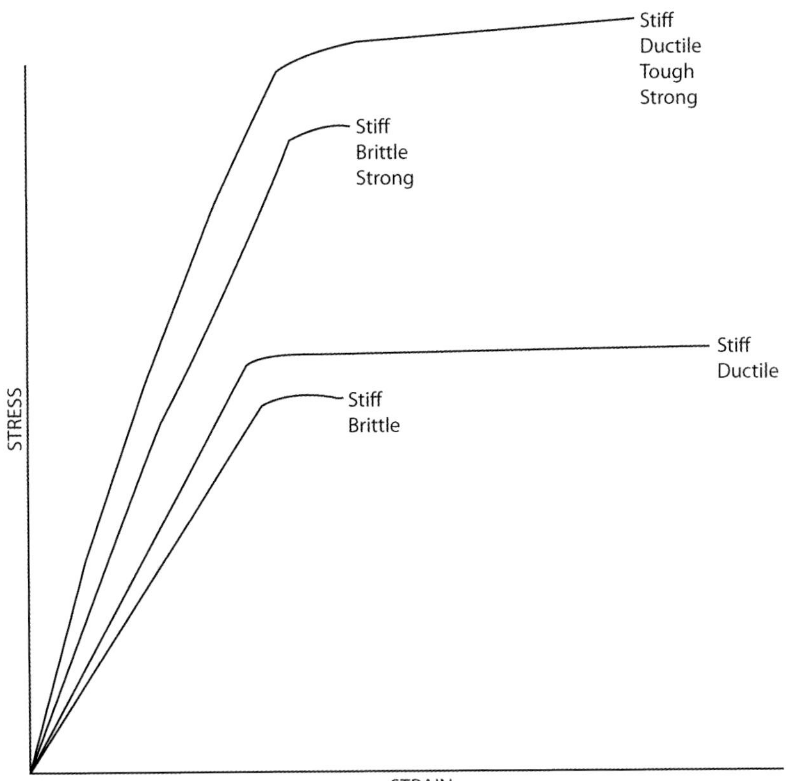

Fig. 12.12 Stress-strain curve for brittle versus ductile materials.

   a. Examples: bone and ligaments
- Isotropics: mechanical properties remain the same independent of direction of load
   a. Example: golf ball
- Anisotropics: mechanical properties change based on direction of load
- **Bone is an anisotropic material, allowing for fractures to occur with varying directions of force applied.**
   a. Example: bone can withstand greater axial loading than radial loads.
- Homogeneous: uniform structure or composition

5. Metals
   - Definitions
      a. Fatigue failure: function of cyclic loading with stresses below ultimate tensile strength; steps are initiation of a crack, crack propagation, and catastrophic failure; most common cause of failure in orthopaedics
         - Endurance limit: maximum stress allowable to keep a material from failing independent of total number of loading cycles
      b. Creep (cold flow): continual/progressive deformation due to constant force over an extended period of time
      c. Toughness: ability of a material to absorb energy and plastically deform without fracturing
   - Corrosion: chemical dissolving of metals
      a. Galvanic: between different metals and results in electrochemical destruction; examples: between cobalt-chrome and stainless steel, between plate and screws if different metals are used

Table 12.1 Young's Modulus Order

Tantalum	Stiffness
Alumina ceramica	Highest
Zirconia-reinforced alumina ceramica	
Zirconia ceramic	
Cobalt-chrome alloy	
Stainless steel	
Titanium alloy	
Cortical bone	
Cement (PMMA)	
Polyethylene (UHMWPE)	
Cancellous bone	
Tendon/ligament	
Cartilage	Lowest

Abbreviations: PMMA, polymethylmethacrylate; UHMWPE, ultrahigh molecular weight polyethylene.

- Electrochemical potential created between two metals in physical contact when immersed in a medium that is conductive
- 316L stainless steel and cobalt-chromium are highly susceptible to galvanic corrosion
- Titanium undergoes self-passivation forming a protective surface oxide leading to immunity to galvanic corrosion

b. Crevice: fatigue crack with low oxygen tension; example: holes in plates or uncemented acetabular cup
   - 316L stainless steel is most likely metal to experience crevice corrosion

c. Stress: areas with high stress gradients

d. Fretting: due to abrasion from small movements under load or micromotion; example: modular arthroplasty with tapered junctions

e. Pitting: localized but symmetric corrosion that forms "pits" on metal surfaces

f. Oxidative corrosion: chemical reaction involving a change in the oxidation state of polyethylene or metal

g. Degradation corrosion: degradation from exposure to a harsh environment

- Metal types used in orthopaedics

  a. Steel (316L)
     - Iron-carbon, chromium, nickel, molybdenum, manganese
     - Modulus of elasticity is more stiff than with titanium

  b. Titanium
     - Poor resistance to wear, can lead to histocytic response
     - Most closely emulates axial and torsional stiffness of bone; has similar Young modulus of elasticity to bone
     - Forms titanium oxide (TiO_2) when exposed to oxygen. This process of self-passivation covers the surface of titanium and titanium alloys with a nonreactive ceramic coating to make the material very biocompatible.

  c. Cobalt (cobalt-chrome alloys)
     - Chromium, molybdenum, cobalt are in cobalt alloy.
     - Less metal debris in total hip than with titanium

  d. Tantalum
     - Very resistant to corrosion
     - Often used in implants where bony ingrowth is desired

- Nonmetal materials

  a. Polyethylene: UHMWPE
     - Viscoelastic and highly susceptible to abrasion
     - Wear to UHMWPE is most likely caused by third-body inclusions.
     - Thermoplastic: altered by temperature and high-dose radiation
       - ♦ Gamma-irradiation: increases polymer chain cross-linking to improve wear characteristics (reduce fatigue and fracture)
       - ♦ Annealing: to decrease free radicals
     - Particles 0.1 to 1.0 μm are most reactive
     - Catastrophic wear in total joints is due to varus knee alignment, thin inserts < 6 mm, flat/nonconforming surfaces, and heat treatments to the insert
     - Polyethylene fretting wear is from the back side of the insert in total knee arthroplasty, leading to osteolysis.

  b. PMMA (bone cement): acts as a grout to mechanically interlock with bone
     - Ultimate strength achieved at 24 hours
     - Reduction of porosity increases strength and decreases cracking (vacuum mixing, centrifugation)

- Cementing can lead to a precipitous drop in blood pressure.
- Wear leads to macrophage response (prosthesis loosening).

c. Silicone: used in non–weight-bearing joints; displays poor strength and wear; a complication is synovitis

d. Ceramics: metallic and nonmetallic elements (alumina or zirconium dioxide)
   - Characteristics: brittle, high modulus, high compressive strength, low tensile strength, low yield strain, poor crack resistance
   - Less friction and diminished wear
   - Can be coated in calcium phosphate (hydroxyapatite) to increase attachment and promote bone healing
   - Undergoes mainly elastic deformation prior to failure, has very little capacity for any plastic deformation prior to fracture

e. Polyactic acid: coated carbon and new polymer reinforced by carbon fibers

- Implants

a. Screws
   - Pitch: distance between adjacent threads
   - Lead: distance traveled in one revolution or turn
   - Root/core diameter: refers to minimal/inner diameter
   - Outer diameter: functions to improve pullout strength
   - Working distance: the distance of bone traversed by a screw
   - Maximize pullout strength with larger outer diameter, small root diameter, and fine pitch
     - ♦ Increase resistance to pullout of screw in osteoporosis by screw placement parallel to the trabecular pattern, good cortical bone purchase, using a locking screw or fixed angle construct, and augmentation with PMMA.

b. Plates
   - Locking: absorb axial forces from screws
     - ♦ Does not compress to bone
     - ♦ Reduce interfragmentary strain more than conventional plating
   - Nonlocking: assist in reduction; if possible, should be placed on tension side of long bones to minimize bending stresses in the plate
     - ♦ Compression plating with concave bend (ends bowed toward bone) helps to create compression of the far and near cortices of a fracture; useful for transverse fractures
     - ♦ Limited contact dynamic compression (LCDC) plates have less implant-bone-contact–induced osteopenia than standard compression plating.
     - ♦ Dynamic compression plating achieves compression by eccentric placement of a cortical screw into a hole in the plate.
   - Hybrid: nonlocked aide in reduction; locked screws create a fixed device
   - Working distance of plate/screw: the length between the two screws closest to the fracture; a shorter distance increases stiffness.
     - ♦ **Bending rigidity is t^3 where t is plate thickness**

c. Intramedullary nails
   - High polar moment of inertia allows for rigidity and strength to torsional forces
   - Torsional (polar moment of inertia) and bending (area moment of inertia) rigidity
   - Larger nails lead to increased rigidity and strength
   - Bending rigidity is r^4 where r is the radius

- Titanium nails can bend more easily than stainless steel and therefore require less axial force to drive the nail down the canal, reducing risk of iatrogenic comminution.
- Interlocking screws most likely to fracture in the region inside the nail due to four-point bending of the screw from the nail

d. External fixation

- Allows fracture ends to come into contact
- Conventional fixator
  - Enhance stability techniques
  - Increasing the number of pins
    - **Larger diameter pins**
    - **Decrease bone–rod distance**
    - **Pins/rods in different planes**
    - **Increased space between pins**
    - **Central pins close to fracture**
    - **Peripheral pins far from fracture**
    - **Increased mass of rods or double stack the rods**
    - **Fracture end contact**
- Circular (Ilizarov)
  - Enhance stability techniques
    - Larger diameter wires/additional wires
    - Decreased ring diameter
    - Using olive wires
    - Wires/pins crossing at 90-degree angles
    - Increased wire tension (130 kg)
    - Central rings close to fracture site
    - Decrease spacing between rings
    - Increased number of rings

e. Biological fit/bone implant unit

- Interference fit: mechanical or press fit relies on fibrous tissue interface
- Interlocking fit: PMMA microinterlocking to cancellous bone
- Biological fit: tissue ingrowth
- Bone resorption if the material has increased modulus (*E*)
- Implant failure in materials with decreased modulus (*E*)
- Optimal pore size for bone ingrowth is 50 to 150 μm

6. Bone

- Mechanical properties: collagen has low elastic modulus, good tensile strength, and poor compressive strength. Calcium hydroxyapatite is stiff, brittle, and has good compressive strength.
- Bone is viscoelastic
  a. Its force-deformation characteristics are dependent on the rate of loading.
- Bone is anisotropic
  a. Its modulus is dependent on the direction of loading.
  b. it is weakest in shear, then tension, then compression.
- Mineral content determines elastic modulus.
- Cortical bone is best for torque resistance.
- Cancellous bone is best for resisting compressive and shear forces.
  a. 25% as dense, 10% as stiff, and 500% more ductile than cortical bone

- Aging bone adaptation increases inner and outer diameter to offset changes in mechanical properties.
- There is a 15 to 30% fracture rate of cortical structural allografts used in oncological and arthroplasty surgery due to failure of remodeling and remaining devascularized.
- Fracture callus helps to minimize stress at a healing fracture site by increasing the diameter of the bone.
- **Moment of inertia is proportional to r^4; fracture callus increases the radius at the fracture site, therefore increasing the moment of inertia and stiffness.**
- Stress shielding: decrease in physiological stress in bone due to a stiffer structure load sharing
  a. When it occurs from implants, it leads to osteoporosis in adjacent bone, as there are decreased normal bone stresses.
  b. Cartilage exhibits stress shielding of the solid matrix components due to its high water content.
- Fracture forces
  a. Tension: muscle pulling leads to transverse fractures.
  b. Compression: axial loading of cancellous bone leads to crush or compression fractures. Bone is strongest in compression.
  c. Shear: fracture is parallel to the applied load. Bone is weakest in response to shear stresses.
  d. Bending: can produce a transverse, oblique, or butterfly fragment. Segmental fractures are due to four-point bending. The greatest tensile stresses are at the periosteal surface.
  e. Torsion: results in spiral fracture
  f. Comminution: results from the amount of energy transferred to the bone

7. Ligaments
   - Fibers oriented parallel if they resist major joint stresses, but can be in any direction
   - Prolonged immobilization lowers yield point and tensile strength.
8. Tendons
   - Fibers arranged parallel
   - Strong in tension only; demonstrate creep and stress relaxation
9. Articular cartilage
   - Biphasic: solid phase depends on structural matrix; fluid phase is due to deformation and shift of water in the solid matrix
   - Solid component is subject to stress shielding.

VI. Biostatistics

1. Research principles
   - Study types
     a. Prospective: assesses outcomes in future
     b. Retrospective: assesses outcomes in the past
     c. Longitudinal: assesses outcomes at different points in time
     d. Observational
        - Case report: single patient
        - Case series: a few patients with a particular injury
        - Case-control: a few patients with a particular disease compared with control

- ◦ Cohort: patients with similar characteristics or exposure studied over time; either prospective or retrospective
- ◦ Cross-sectional study design: population is studied at a specific time and all measurements are made with no follow-up. These studies help describe prevalence of a disease at one specific instance in time.

- Types of studies
  a. Level 1: randomized controlled studies; systematic review of level 1 randomized controlled trials; testing a gold-standard diagnostic criterion
  b. Level 2: prospective cohort study; poor-quality randomized controlled study; systematic review of level 2 studies; developing a diagnostic criteria
  c. Level 3: case-control study; retrospective cohort study; systematic review of level 3 studies
  d. Level 4: case series; case-control studies with poor reference standard
  e. Level 5: expert opinion
- Problems encountered in research
  a. Confounding variables: factors outside the scope of the study that can possibly influence the outcome
  b. Internal validity: deals with the research design quality and how well the study is controlled and can be reproduced
  c. External validity: ability to extrapolate the study to a whole population of interest
  d. Bias: unintentional systematic error that poses a threat to the internal validity of a study; examples include subject selection, loss to follow-up, observer bias, and recall bias
     - ◦ Computer random number generators help prevent selection bias.
     - ◦ Washout period bias: time between therapies so the effect of the first therapy is allowed to wear off

2. Epidemiology
   - Definitions
     a. Prevalence: all diagnoses of an existing disease in a population
     b. Incidence: number of new diagnoses of a disease in a specific time interval
     c. Relative risk: ratio between two incidences in a cohort. The treated/exposed cohort is the numerator and the untreated/unexposed cohort is the denominator. Estimates probability.
        - ◦ If > 1, the incidence of the outcome is greater in the treated/exposed cohort.
        - ◦ If = 1, the incidence of an outcome is the same between cohorts.
        - ◦ If < 1, the incidence of an outcome is higher in the untreated/unexposed cohort.
     a. Odds ratio: the probabilities of outcome in two cohorts in a case-control study.
   - Contingency table **(Tables 12.2** and **12.3)**
     a. Sensitivity: positive test in patients who actually have the disease (True positives/Total patients with the disease)
     b. Specificity: negative test in patient who actually does not have the disease (True negative/Total patients without the disease)

Table 12.2 Contingency Table

	Disease Present	**Disease Absent**
Diagnostic Test Positive	True positives (A)	False positives (B)
Diagnostic Test Negative	False negatives (C)	True negatives (D)

Table 12.3 Contingency Table Equations

Sensitivity	= A/A+C
Specificity	= D/B+D
Positive predictive value	= A/A+B
Negative predictive value	= D/D+C
Positive likelihood ratio	= Sensitivity/ (1 – Specificity)
Negative likelihood ratio	= (1 – Sensitivity)/Specificity

c. Positive predictive value: how well a positive test correlates with an actual disease present (True positives/Total patients with positive test result)

d. Negative predictive value: how well a negative test correlates with an actual disease not present (True negatives/Total patients with negative test result)

e. Likelihood ratios: probability of a disease in a test result
   - A value of 1: no increase or decrease in probability of disease
   - Positive likelihood ratio: > 1.0, indicates high probability of a disease as long as the test result is positive
   - Negative likelihood ratio: < 1.0, indicates high probability of no disease as long as the test result is negative
   - **Tests with higher sensitivities tend to be better screening tests.**

- Hypothesis testing

  a. Definitions
   - Descriptive statistics
     - Mean: sum of all scores divided by the total number of samples
     - Median: the middle value in the sample score set
     - Mode: most frequent score seen in a sample
     - Standard deviation: a value calculated to describe the variability of the data collected; 68.27% of the values lie within 1 standard deviation of the mean.
     - Variance: quantity equal to the standard deviation squared
     - Confidence interval: a calculated value to quantitatively describe the precision of the mean, odds ratio, or relative risk
       - 95% confidence interval means that it is 95% accepted that the value will fall within the data points
   - Effect size: estimated magnitude of the difference in the means between two groups

- Statistical test types (short definitions)

  a. Student *t*-test: compares two groups
   - Dependent (paired) samples *t*-test: compares continuous and normally distributed data from subjects at two different points in time
   - Independent samples *t*-test: compares continuous and normally distributed data from two separate subject groups

  b. ANOVA (analysis of variance): appropriate for three or more groups of continuous and normally distributed data

  c. MANOVA (multivariate analysis of variance): a variation of ANOVA, reserved for three or more groups with multiple independent variables

  d. ANCOVA (analysis of covariance): used when a statistical analysis has confounding factors

  e. Post hoc testing: to be completed after ANOVA to determine differences between all combinations of each pair within three or more groups

f. Correlation and regression
   - Correlation coefficient: describes how well two variables are related

g. Tests for categorical data
   - Chi square: used for two or more categorical data groups
   - Fisher exact test: similar to Chi square, but better for smaller groups or when the number of a specific outcome is very low

- Error

a. Type 1 (α error): false-positive error; probability that the test result is wrong when the null hypothesis is rejected (usually *p* = 0.05)

b. Type 2 (β error): false-negative error; probability that a test result is wrong when the study does not reject the null hypothesis (accepting the null hypothesis when it is in fact not true; accepted at 20%)

   - Statistical power of a study is one minus type 2 error. Power is the probability of finding a significant association in a research study when one truly exists.

c. Accuracy: ability of a study to identify true positives and true negatives
   - **Power is a function of the frequency of the disease and the number of individuals tested.**

Index

Note: Page references followed by *f* and *t* indicate figures and tables, respectively.

D

M

N

Q

R

S

T

U